AF518230

Spectral Domain Optical Coherence Tomography in Macular Diseases

Carsten H. Meyer • Sandeep Saxena
SriniVas R. Sadda
Editors

Spectral Domain Optical Coherence Tomography in Macular Diseases

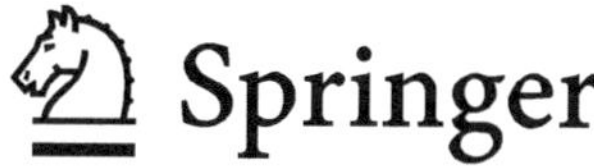

Springer

Editors
Carsten H. Meyer
Pallas Klinik
Aarau
Switzerland

SriniVas R. Sadda
Doheny Eye Institute
Los Angeles
USA

Sandeep Saxena
Department of Ophthalmology
King George's Medical University
Lucknow
India

ISBN 978-81-322-3608-5 ISBN 978-81-322-3610-8 (eBook)
DOI 10.1007/978-81-322-3610-8

Library of Congress Control Number: 2016953002

Printed on acid-free paper

This Springer imprint is published by Springer Nature
The registered company is Springer (India) Pvt. Ltd.
The registered company address is 7th Floor, Vijaya Building, 17 Barakhamba Road, New Delhi 110 001, India

Foreword

Undoubtedly, optical coherence tomography has changed the approach of clinicians in their daily practice. The evolution of technology from time domain to spectral domain and swept source OCT increased the possibilities of imaging the retinal and choroidal details. Newer evaluations are now available to better understand the diseases and to find new biomarkers for retinal and choroidal pathologies. From measurement to morphology could be the right description of changes occurring from time domain to spectral domain. The possibility to visualize retinal and choroidal morphology in real life and not only post-mortem allowed a better understanding not only of the tissue damage but in particular of its recovery: the dynamic healing process of idiopathic macular holes after surgical repair, of optic pit-related retinoschisis and neurosensory retinal detachment, or of color and visual impairment and its recovery after systemic or intravitreal pharmacological treatments are just few examples of the advantages of the OCTs. Thanks to the OCT images, we learned about the new pathologic characteristics of retinal diseases like in age-related macular degeneration, the outer retinal tubulations or the differences between drusen and reticular pseudodrusen, in myopia the macular retinoschisis, and in juxtafoveal macular telangiectasia the degenerative cysts of Muller cells. Optical coherence tomography images have played an important role in the study of vitreomacular interface. The classification of vitreomacular adhesion, traction, and macular hole introduced a new approach not only based on the slit lamp fundus evaluation but also on the changes visible with OCT. There is no doubt that imaging the choroid before the advent of OCT was almost impossible. In ocular oncology, the differences between choroidal melanoma, metastasis, osteoma, hamartoma, hemangioma, lymphoma, and granuloma are better delineated with OCT than with ultrasounds. In uveitis, the possibility to visualize and measure changes in choroidal thickness provided a better diagnosis and a more accurate control of the treatment effect. In central serous choroidopathy, the visualization of an increased thickness of the choroid supported the enrollment of the choroid in this disease. However, the real changes occurred in everyday clinical practice, changing the approach for diagnosis and treatment. Undoubtedly, for many ophthalmologists, not only for retinal specialists, OCT is the leading tool for their practice. The number of fluorescein angiography examinations has been reduced in the last 10 years with an important increase of OCT procedures. The future will be even more interesting with the full introduction of OCT angiography, wide-field OCT, and adaptive OCT.

In this text, Professors Meyer, Saxena, and Sadda have assembled a very well-known group of imaging specialists. The topics described go from technology to clinical use through a series of published paper reviews. Reading this book is a perfect way to update our knowledge on OCT.

I wish you a good reading.

Giovanni Staurenghi
Professor, Department of Ophthalmology
University Eye Clinic
Toronto, ON, Canada

University Eye Clinic
Department of Biomedical
and Clinical Science "Luigi Sacco"
"Luigi Sacco" Hospital
Milan, Italy

Preface

Optical coherence tomography (OCT) is an imaging technology based on the principle of low-coherence interferometry. Optical coherence tomography provides a noninvasive, noncontact, transpupillary technique for real time in vivo imaging of the retina.

Optical coherence tomography is an ever evolving technology that has revolutionized ophthalmic imaging. This technology has played essential roles in ophthalmology as well as other branches of medicine. The technology has been adapted to produce noninvasive, high-resolution images of both the anterior segment (cornea and structures at the angles) and posterior pole (retina, choroid, sclera, and optic disk). With rapid evolution in technology and improved cellular level resolution, clinical use of OCT has been extended to retinal diseases with more complex morphological features.

Three-dimensional imaging with its increased potential in interpreting retinal morphology provides a global perspective to various retinal diseases. This allows effortless localization of images for monitoring disease progression and response to therapy. Preservation of retinal topography enables visualization of subtle changes associated with the disease. Enface OCT provides a new dimension in our understanding of the vitreoretinal interface.

Optical coherence tomography angiography is based on the same technology as conventional OCT imaging but selectively detects signals associated with motion corresponding to blood flow in the fundus. Thus, OCT angiography noninvasively visualizes three-dimensional retinal and choroidal vascular networks and enables visualization of these networks in en face sections, as in fluorescein and indocyanine green angiography. Increasing attention is being paid to potential clinical applications of this technology in retinal ischemic diseases and macular diseases.

Swept source OCT devices allow wider regions of the eye to be scanned and visualize more precise details of deeper structures such as the choroid and sclera. Swept source OCT provides simultaneous high-quality visualization of the vitreous, retina, and choroid.

The emergence of intraoperative OCT is linked to the concept of an image-guided intervention that facilitates high precision in clinical diagnosis. This technology aims to create image overlays during the surgical intervention in order to assist the surgeon to better visualize and manage living tissues.

Spectral domain optical coherence tomography has proved useful in identifying various biomarkers for imaging in several ocular diseases. Spectral domain OCT-based imaging parameters have also been documented as prognostic biomarkers in various neurological diseases.

Hyperspectral imaging is an emerging technology which identifies materials or detects biochemical and metabolic processes within the retina. It also provides a feasible method for measurement and analysis of vascular oxygen content in healthy and diseased retina.

This text is an effort to provide an in-depth current knowledge of optical coherence tomography in macular diseases by experts in their respective fields from across the globe.

Aarau, Switzerland Carsten H. Meyer
Lucknow, India Sandeep Saxena
Los Angeles, USA SriniVas R. Sadda

Contents

Contributors

Levent Akduman, MD Department of Ophthalmology, Saint Louis University, Saint Louis, MO, USA

Pooja Bansal, MD Senior Research Associates, R.P. Centre AIIMS, New Delhi, India

Susanne Binder, MD Department of Ophthalmology, Rudolf Foundation Clinic, Karl Landsteiner Institute for Retinal Research and Imaging, Vienna, Austria

Zachary M. Bodnar, MD Department of Ophthalmology, Saint Louis University, Saint Louis, MO, USA

WengOnn Chan, MB, ChB, MPhil South Australian Institute of Ophthalmology, Royal Adelaide Hospital, Adelaide, Australia

Peter Charbel Issa, MD Department of Ophthalmology, University of Bonn, Bonn, Germany

Gemmy Cheung, MBBS, FRCOphth Singapore Eye Research Institute, Singapore National Eye Center, Singapore, Singapore

Victor Chong, MD, FRCS, FRCOphth Oxford Eye Hospital, Oxford, UK

Manor Hospital, Oxford, UK

London Medical, London, UK

Aude Couturier, MD Department of Ophthalmology, Hôpital Lariboisière, Universitè Paris, Paris, France

Ankit Desai, MD Department of Ophthalmology, Henry Ford Hospital, Detroit, MI, USA

Ali Dirani, MD Department of Ophthalmology, University of Lausanne, HôpitalOphtalmique Jules Gonin, Lausanne, Switzerland

Jay S. Duker, MD, PhD New England Eye Center, Tufts Medical Center and Tufts Unviersity School of Medicine, Boston, MA, USA

Xavier Fagan, MBBS, FRANZCO Ringwood Eye Specialists, Melbourne, Australia

Michel E. Farah, MD Department of Ophthalmology, Federal University of São Paulo, Sao Paulo, Brazil

Samia Fatum, MD Oxford Eye Hospital, Oxford, Oxfordshire, UK

Daniela Ferrara, MD, PhD Tufts University School of Medicine, Boston, MA, USA

Monika Fleckenstein, MD Department of Ophthalmology, University of Bonn, Bonn, Germany

Angie H.C. Fong, FRCS Department of Ophthalmology and Visual Sciences, The Chinese University of Hong Kong, Hong Kong, China

Ana C. Garcia, MD Department of Ophthalmology, Federal University of São Paulo, Sao Paulo, Brazil

Alain Gaudric, MD Department of Ophthalmology, Hôpital Lariboisière, Université Paris, Paris, France

Jagjit S. Gilhotra, MBBS, FRANZCO South Australian Institute of Ophthalmology, Royal Adelaide Hospital, Adelaide, Australia

Carl Glittenberg, MD Department of Ophthalmology, Rudolf Foundation Clinic, Karl Landsteiner Institute for Retinal Research and Imaging, Vienna, Austria

Varun Gogia, MD Senior Research Associates, R.P. Centre AIIMS, New Delhi, India

Masanori Hangai, MD, PhD Department of Ophthalmology and Visual Sciences, Graduate School of Medicine Kyoto University, Kyoto, Japan

Department of Ophthalmology, Doheny Eye Institute, University of Southern California, Los Angeles, CA, USA

Tjebo F.C. Heeren, MD Department of Ophthalmology, University of Bonn, Bonn, Germany

Frank G. Holz, MD Department of Ophthalmology, University of Bonn, Bonn, Germany

Tomohiro Iida, MD Department of Ophthalmology, Tokyo Women's Medical University School of Medicine, Tokyo, Japan

Yasushi Ikuno, MD Department of Ophthalmology, Osaka University Medical School, Osaka, Japan

Ghazal Ismail, MS Department of Ophthalmology, King George's Medical University, Lucknow, UP, India

Peter Kroll, MD Department of Ophthalmology, Philipps University, Marburg, Germany

Timothy Y.Y. Lai, FRCS, FRCOphth Department of Ophthalmology & Visual Sciences, The Chinese University of Hong Kong, Hong Kong, China

Jessica Lee, MD New York Eye & Ear Infirmary of Mount Sinai, New York, NY, USA

Lyndell Lim, MBBS, FRANZCO Department of Ophthalmologist, Centre for Eye Research Australia, Royal Victorian Eye, Ear Hospital and Royal Melbourne Hospital, Melbourne, Australia

Moritz Lindner, MD Department of Ophthalmology, University of Bonn, Bonn, Germany

Vicky H.J. Lu Singapore National Eye Center, Singapore, Singapore

Lyubomyr Lytvynchuk, MD, PhD Department of Ophthalmology, Rudolf Foundation Clinic, Karl Landsteiner Institute for Retinal Research and Imaging, Vienna, Austria

Ichiro Maruko, MD Department of Ophthalmology, Tokyo Women's Medical University School of Medicine, Tokyo, Japan

Carsten H. Meyer, MD, FEBO, FMH Department of Ophthalmology, Pallas Klinik, Aarau, Switzerland

Simone Müller, MD Department of Ophthalmology, University of Bonn, Bonn, Germany

Elizabeth Pearce, MD Department of Optometry, Moorfields Eye Hospital, London, UK

Fernando M. Penha, MD, PhD Bascom Palmer Eye Institute, University of Miami, Miami, FL, USA

Prateep Phadikar, MBBS Department of Ophthalmology, King George's Medical University, Lucknow, UP, India

Eduardo B. Rodrigues, MD Department of Ophthalmology, Federal University of São Paulo, Sao Paulo, Brazil

Andre Romano, MD Department of Ophthalmology, Federal University Sao Paulo, Sao Paulo, Brazil

University of Miami, Miller School of Medicine, Miami, FL, USA

Neovista Eye Center, Americana, Brazil

Richard B. Rosen, MD, DSc(Hon), FACS, FASRS, CRA Retinal Services, New York Eye and Ear Infirmary of Mount Sinai, New York, NY, USA

Department of Ophthalmology, Ican School of Medicine at Mount Sinai, New York, NY, USA

Philip J. Rosenfeld, MD, PhD Bascom Palmer Eye Institute, Miami, FL, USA

Surabhi Ruia, MS Department of Ophthalmology, King George's Medical University, Lucknow, UP, India

SriniVas R. Sadda, MD Doheny Eye Institute, David Geffen School of Medicine, University of California – Los Angeles, Los Angeles, CA, USA

Sandeep Saxena, MS FRCSEd FRCS FRCOphth FAICO Department of Ophthalmology, King George's Medical University, Lucknow, UP, India

Karen B. Schaal, MD Bascom Palmer Eye Institute, Miami, FL, USA

Ursula Schmidt-Erfurth, MD Department of Ophthalmology and Optometry, Medical University of Vienna, Vienna, Austria

Steffen Schmitz-Valckenberg, MD Department of Ophthalmology, University of Bonn, Bonn, Germany

Shivani Sinha, MS Department of Ophthalmology, King George's Medical University, Lucknow, UP, India

Khushboo Srivastav, MS Department of Ophthalmology, King Georges Medical University, Lucknow, India

Julia Steinberg, MD Department of Ophthalmology, University of Bonn, Bonn, Germany

Colin S. Tan, MBBS, MMed, FRCSEd National Healthcare Group Eye Institute, Tan TockSeng Hospital, Singapore, Singapore

National Healthcare Group Eye Institute, Fundus Image Reading Center, Singapore, Singapore

Anna C.S. Tan, MMed Singapore Eye Research Institute, Singapore National Eye Center, Singapore, Singapore

Michael D. Tibbetts, MD New England Eye Center, Tufts Medical Center and Tufts Unviersity School of Medicine, Boston, MA, USA

Reinhard Told, MD, PhD Department of Ophthalmology, Medical University of Vienna, Vienna, Austria

Pradeep Venkatesh, MD R.P. Centre AIIMS, New Delhi, India

Sebastian M. Waldstein, MD Department of Ophthalmology and Optometry, Medical University of Vienna, Vienna, Austria

Thomas J. Wolfensberger, MD, MBA Department of Ophthalmology, University of Lausanne, HôpitalOphtalmique Jules Gonin, Lausanne, Switzerland

Ute E.K. Wolf-Schnurrbusch, MD Department of Ophthalmology, University Hospital Bern, Inselspital, University Bern, Bern, Switzerland

Edmund Y.M. Wong, MMed, FRCSED Singapore National Eye Center, Singapore, Singapore

About the Editors

Dr. Dr. Carsten H. Meyer, M.D., FEBO, FMH, is Professor of Ophthalmology and Head of the Department at Pallas Klinik, Aarau, Switzerland. He completed his medical educationQ1 in Freiburg (Germany), Innsbruck (Austria), and Oxford (England), and a Vitreoretinal Research Fellowship at Duke University, Durham, USA. He is a specialist in vitreoretinal diseases and has published extensively on the subject. He has several book chapters and a textbook on vitreoretinal surgery to his credit. He is an editorial board member of 8 ophthalmic journals and serves as a reviewer in more than 50 peer-reviewed journals.

Dr. Sandeep Saxena, M.S., FRCSEd, FRCS, FRCOphth, FAMS, FAICO, is a Professor of Ophthalmology and Chief of Retina Service in the Department of Ophthalmology in King George's Medical University at Lucknow, India. He has over 115 publications in indexed, peer-reviewed journals. He has published 14 textbooks and has written 31 book chapters with leading international publishers. Dr. Saxena serves as member editorial board of *International Journal of Retina and Vitreous*. He has designed an instrument called "Saxena Retinal Grid-520 and 428" (two models), Ocular Instruments, USA, for adult and pediatric use.

Dr. SriniVas R. Sadda, M.D., is the President and Chief Scientific Officer of the Doheny Eye Institute, the Stephen J. Ryan–Arnold and Mabel Beckman Endowed Chair, and Professor of Ophthalmology, at the University of California, Los Angeles (UCLA), USA. He has more than 280 peer-reviewed publications and 13 book chapters. Dr. Sadda also serves as an editorial board member of *Ophthalmic Surgery, Lasers & Imaging*, *Retina*, and *Ophthalmology*. He is also an editor of the fifth edition of the Ryan's Retina textbook.

Part I
Essentials of Optical Coherence Tomography

1 Optical Coherence Tomography: A Primer

Shivani Sinha, Prateep Phadikar, and Sandeep Saxena

Contents

1.1 Introduction

Optical coherence tomography (OCT) is a noninvasive, non-contact transpupillary interferometric technique for real time *in vivo* imaging of retinal microstructures. It is equivalent to ultrasound B-mode imaging with the use of light instead of sound. Long-wavelength light (near infrared 840 nm) with wide-spectrum range allows penetration into the scattering medium.

S. Sinha, M.S. • P. Phadikar, MBBS
S. Saxena, MS,FRCSEd,FRCS,FRCOphth, FAICO (✉)
Department of Ophthalmology, King George's Medical University, Lucknow, UP, India
e-mail: sandeepsaxena2020@gmail.com

C.H. Meyer et al. (eds.), *Spectral Domain Optical Coherence Tomography in Macular Diseases*,
DOI 10.1007/978-81-322-3610-8_1

This allows achievement of image with micrometer resolution ranging from 1 to 10 μm.

The latest commercial instruments have an axial resolution of approximately 5 μm, while a resolution of approximately 2 μm is achieved with research instruments. The lateral resolution is usually about 20 μm due to diffraction caused by the pupil. The image acquisition time is less than 2 s and is limited by the patient's ability to avoid eye movements. The scanning speed of the instrument is a crucial parameter in determining the amount of data available for a single OCT dataset (Ryan 2013).

1.2 Basic Principle

The principle of OCT is based upon low-coherence interferometry, where the backscatter from outer retinal tissues can be differentiated from that of inner tissues, due to the difference in time taken by the reflected light to reach the sensor. As the differences between the most superficial and the deepest layers in the retina are around 300–400 μm, the difference in time of arrival is very small and requires interferometry for measurement. The low coherent light creates an interference pattern allowing a better depth resolution. The low coherent light is optically split into two arms, the reference arm and the sample arm, before entering the eye. The reference arm is aimed at a mirror at known distance and is thereby reflected. The sample arm enters the eye and reflects back from the tissues at different depth. Changing the position of the mirror changes the amount of interference at different tissue depths. A higher interference pattern is achieved as long as the two reflected light waves resemble each other. This is attained by maintaining similar distance between the reflected light from the reference and sample arm. As the optical properties of the eye add noise and slightly change the reflected reference arm light wave, the interference is never perfect. The sensor measures the energy of the interferogram and displays it as the OCT signal intensity (Podoleanu 2012).

There are two main OCT methods: time domain OCT (TD-OCT) and Fourier domain OCT. Fourier domain methods can be implemented in two formats:

(i) Spectrometer based (SB)
(ii) Swept source (SS)

Each method, SB-OCT or SS-OCT, has its own merits and demerits. The depth resolution achieved is dependent on the bandwidth of the optical source in the TD-OCT and SB-OCT and on the tuning bandwidth in the SS-OCT.

1.2.1 Time Domain Optical Coherence Tomography

TD-OCT setup has a broadband optical source and a processing unit that employs a single photodetector. The sample arm light wave as reflected from tissue at different depth of the retina creates an interference pattern with the reflected reference arm light wave. Mirror is used for reflection of the reference arm light wave. By moving this mirror to match the optical path of the sample arm reflected by different depth of tissue, an axial A-scan is constructed. This setup limits the scanning speed to a few thousand A-scans per second. By collecting adjacent A-scans along a transversal coordinate, a cross-sectional image, known as B-scan, is obtained.

1.2.2 Spectral Domain Optical Coherence Tomography

Spectral domain OCT (SD-OCT) also utilizes a broadband optical source, a processing unit, and a spectrometer. Fourier domain transformation utilizes an array of detectors in place of a moving mirror to acquire an A-scan concurrently. This increases the scanning speed to about 200 times faster than TD-OCT. The high sampling density achieved with the scanning speed of SD-OCT produces high-quality individual B-scan images. The large, dense raster scans make it possible to acquire detailed topographical images of individual retina layers, known as segmentation maps. This enables visualization and quantitative evaluation of the corresponding retinal structures. Commercially available SD-OCT devices have scanning rates of 18,000–70,000 A-scans/s. Some of the commercially available SD-OCT devices include: Cirrus OCT (Carl Zeiss Meditec, Dublin, CA, USA), Spectralis OCT (Heidelberg Engineering, Heidelberg, Germany), 3D-OCT 2000 (Topcon, Tokyo, Japan), Bioptigen SD-OCT (Bioptigen, Research Triangle Park, NC, USA), and RTVue (Optovue, Fremont, CA, USA).

1.2.3 Swept-Source Optical Coherence Tomography

Swept source utilizes a tunable laser that sweeps across a narrow band of wavelength with each scan. The processing unit comprises of a complementary metal oxide semiconductor camera and two fast parallel photodiode detectors. The spectral interference patterns obtained undergoes reverse Fourier transform to generate an A-scan image. The scan speed of swept-source instruments, 100,000 A-scans/s, is twice that of SD-OCT devices. This facilitates faster acquisition of B-scans, as well as wider field B-scans (12 mm vs 6–9 mm with conventional SD-OCT). A wider scan images the optic nerve and macula on the same scan. Simultaneous high-quality visualization of the vitreous, retina, and choroid is realized. At present, SS-OCT is not widely available commercially, with the DRI-OCT 1 (Topcon) being the only commercially available device. A different OCT has been compared in Table 1.1.

1.3 Scanning Protocol

The three scanning protocols are:

(i) Macular cube scan
(ii) Line scan
(iii) C-scan

1.3.1 Macular Cube Scans

They are volume scans similar to computed tomography or magnetic resonance scans that acquire volumetric cubes of data. Rapid series B-scans are acquired, generally in a 6 mm × 6 mm square area centered on the fovea. Manual centering of the cube scans other areas of interest besides the fovea. Similarly, optic nerve topographic scans are cube scans centered on the optic nerve. The Cirrus HD-OCT (Carl Zeiss Meditec Inc., CA, USA) provides two macular cube scan protocols. The 512 × 128 protocol analyzes 128 horizontal scans at high resolution (512 A-scans per B-scan). The 200 × 200 protocol achieves faster imaging at the cost of resolution. It takes 1.6 s to acquire 200 horizontal scans (200 A-scans per B-scan). As the average foveal thickness is 160–180 microns, the resolution of A-scan is less than 4 microns theoretically. In Heidelberg Spectralis volume scan uses a scanning protocol with fast 25 B-scans, each of which consists of 512 A-scans or a dense 1024 × 49 default scanning protocol. The Topcon 3D OCT has a 512 × 128 and a 256 × 256 scanning protocol. In RTVue 3D macular scans have a 4 mm × 4 mm macular cube scan with 101 B-scans each consisting of 512 A-scans and a MM5 protocol. Raster and radial scans are also available to scan the macula.

1.3.2 Line Scans, Cross Lines, and Raster Scans

SD-OCT line scans are a single B-scan composed of a higher number of A-scans than the macular cube scans enabling higher resolution scans of the retinal tissue. In Cirrus 5-line raster, five horizontal 6 mm lines are scanned four times and averaged. Oversampling increases the signal-noise ratio, thereby increasing the resolution of the image. The five lines in the raster can be integrated to obtain a single line scan consisting of 20 averaged B-scans. The RTVue uses cross line scans consisting of horizontal and vertical lines scans. In Heidelberg 7-line raster scans are used.

Table 1.1 Some of the commercially available SD-OCT devices

Device (manufacturer)	Axial resolution	Scanning rate	Special characteristics	Scans available
3D-OCT 2000 (Topcon, Tokyo, Japan)	5 μm	27 kHz	Fundus camera	Fast map, box scan 5- and 9-line raster, line scan 12-line radial scans
Bioptigen SD-OCT (Bioptigen, Research Triangle Park, NC, USA)	4 μm	20 kHz	Designed for research	Rectangular volume, mixed volume Linear scan Radial volume
Cirrus HD-OCT (Carl Zeiss Meditec, Dublin, CA, USA)	5 μm	27 kHz		Macular cube 5-line raster scan, 1-line raster scan
RTVue-100 (Optovue, Fremont, CA, USA)	5 μm	27 kHz		3D macular scan, MM5 Line scan, HD scan, cross line, HD cross line Radial slicer, MM6 MM5 mesh scan
Spectral OCT SLO (Opko, Miami, FL, USA)	6 μm	27 kHz	Microperimetry	3D macular scan Line scan
Spectralis OCT (Heidelberg Engineering, Heidelberg, Germany)	8 μm	40 kHz	Eye-tracking fluorescein ICG angiography, autofluorescence	Volume scans 7-line raster scan

1.3.3 C-Scans

The C-scans are also known as en face image or OCT fundus image. The literal meaning of the term en face is "on the face." En face image is obtained by summating data from all B-scans and has the same appearance as a red-free image of fundus. These provide with a global overview of the morphology of the retinal surface.

1.4 Three-Dimensional Spectral Domain Optical Coherence Tomography

The high scanning speed of the SD-OCT allows multiple B-scans to be obtained and thus acquires a large dataset for the macular cube. The inbuilt software, 3D-volume rendering, in Cirrus HD-OCT (Carl Zeiss Meditec Inc., CA, USA) reconstructs a three-dimensional image of the whole retinal cube. The three planes of 3D SD-OCT are the X, Y, and Z planes. The X plane corresponds to the horizontal B-scan or cross section. The Y plane is the vertically reconstructed B-scan. The Z plane or the coronal plane (C-scan) corresponds to the reconstructed en face image of the retina.

1.5 Topographical Maps

A topographical map of the individual retinal layers, internal limiting membrane (ILM) and retinal pigment epithelium (RPE) are generated by 3D segmentation analysis. The ILM segmentation map is color-coded pale blue; the RPE/choriocapillaris complex is brown or cream. These maps provide an effortless pictorial representation of the morphological alterations as well as localization of the pathology. The topographical map of the retina represents the thickness of the retina, between ILM and RPE, with a cold/warm color scale. The color coding provides a global representation of the difference in thickness of the retina in comparison to a normative database.

1.6 Masking

Masking is another feature of the SD-OCT, useful when visualizing the three-dimensional retinal cube. Masking of the tissue below a desired layer from cutting enables peeling back of the tissues above the desired layer. By applying the internal limiting membrane (ILM) mask, the tissue below the ILM is preserved from being cut, and the ILM and the tissues above this layer can be peeled back. "Niche" allows for masking in two dimensions, the X and Y planes simultaneously. These facilitate imaging of the retinal pathology at various depths.

1.7 Retinal Pigment Epithelium Fit

The RPE fit feature of the Cirrus HD-OCT (Carl Zeiss Meditec Inc., CA, USA) is an important advancement to understand various retinal pathology (Lumbroso et al. 2009). It provides C-scan images adapted to retinal curvature. En face images that follow the curvature of posterior pole can be obtained. RPE fit software identifies RPE/choriocapillaris complex to display it as a curved 3D section plane. The software adapts to concavity of RPE/choriocapillaris (Wei et al. 2012). Sections with thickness varying from 2 to 20 μm can be obtained with thinner sections known as slices and thicker sections known as slabs. Blood vessels of the choroid can be seen by changing the thickness of sections. A slab of selective thickness, the slab thickness of interest, can be studied by selecting and adjusting the anterior and posterior boundaries represented by two separable same-color dashed lines. The slab image represents an average signal intensity value for each A-scan location through the selected depth of the slab.

1.8 Optical Coherence Tomography Interpretation

1.8.1 Qualitative Data Analysis

Qualitative interpretation reviews individual line scans of the imaged retina and assess the pathology on the basis of knowledge of normal anatomy. Comparison with the previous scans allows assessment of course of the underlying disease and response to treatment. There are three things to be taken care of: registration, sampling error, and subjective evaluation. Registration implies that future line scans must be registered to past scans so that precisely same anatomic areas are scanned. Sampling error is important as to rule out any pathology, so multiple line scans through the macula is examined. Line scans in quantitative assessment tends to be individualized as qualitative numbers are lacking.

1.8.2 Quantitative Data Analysis

The inbuilt software in commercially available OCT devices are capable of analyzing the thickness of the total retina, individual layers like retinal nerve fiber layer, and the macular volume. This is facilitated by the software's ability to distinguish inner and outer boundaries of the retina. Unlike time domain OCT mapping, which measures the total retinal thickness as distance from the photoreceptor inner and outer segments (IS/OS) junction to the ILM, the SD-OCT thickness mapping strictly corresponds to anatomical retinal thickness, that is, the distance from the RPE to the ILM.

1.8.3 Mapping Retinal Thickness

In the context of a thickness map the early treatment of diabetic retinopathy study (ETDRS) grid is superimposed on the fovea. The grid has an innermost circle of 1 mm diameter centered at the fovea, an inner circle of 3 mm, and an outer circle of 6 mm diameter. The outer two circles are divided into superior, nasal, inferior, and temporal quadrants. Average thickness values for each sector are indicated numerically and also by a color scale. A color-coded representation demonstrates the difference in the retinal thickness with age-matched normative database.

1.9 Recent International Nomenclature for Optical Coherence Tomography

Recently, an international panel with expertise in retinal imaging reached a consensus for OCT imaging terminology (Staurenghi et al. 2014). They suggested the terms band, layer, and zone for the layers of the retina. The term band refers to the three-dimensional structure of the retinal layers anatomically. The term zone describes those regions on OCT whose anatomical correlation is not clearly delineated. The RPE/Bruch's complex is one of the layers ascribed as zone as they are inseparable owing to interdigitation of cellular structure or tissue.

1.10 Interpretation of Normal Retinal Layers

Histologically, the retina consists of ten layers, four of them are cellular and two are neuronal junctions. The axonal layers, nerve fiber layer, and plexiform layers are capable of potent light scatter and hence are hyperreflective. The light scattering potential of nuclear layers is lower. The first layer visible on OCT images is the hyperreflective ILM line at the vitreoretinal interface. The hyperreflective retinal nerve fiber layer lies next to this layer. Outer to this is a hyporeflective ganglion cell layer. Subsequently, hyperreflective plexiform layers are imaged with an inner nuclear layer situated between them. The relatively thick hyporeflective outer nuclear layer is visible next. A thin hyperreflective line underneath the outer nuclear layer corresponds to the location of the external limiting membrane (ELM). The

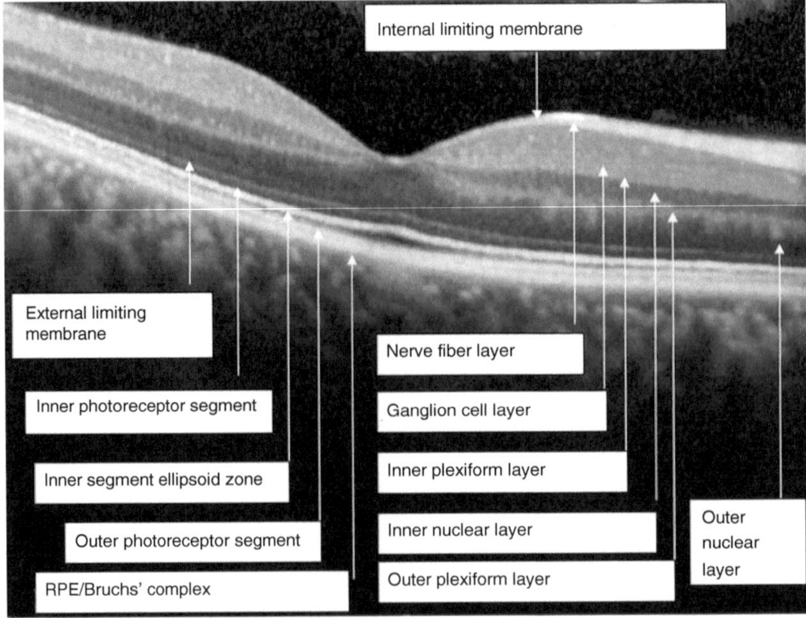

Fig. 1.1 Reflectivity of different layers on optical coherence tomography (Heidelberg Engineering)

hyperreflective layer of photoreceptor junction of inner and outer segments, currently termed as the photoreceptor inner segment ellipsoid zone, lies beneath this layer. Due to the increased length of outer cone segments in the central fovea, this line is slightly elevated in the foveal region. The outermost layer imaged is the hyperreflective RPE-Bruch's complex. The choriocapillaris and the choroid are visible outer to the RPE-Bruch's zone. The fovea is recognized on a cross-sectional image by its characteristic depression, due to the thinning of the retina with the absence of the inner layers at the macula (Fig. 1.1) (Table 1.2).

Table 1.2 Reflectivity of different layers on optical coherence tomography.

Layer	OCT finding	Nomenclature
1	Hyperreflective	Posterior cortical vitreous
2	Hyporeflective	Pre-retinal space
3	Hyperreflective	Nerve fiber layer
4	Hyporeflective	Ganglion cell layer
5	Hyperreflective	Inner plexiform layer
6	Hyporeflective	Inner nuclear layer
7	Hyperreflective	Outer plexiform layer
8	Hyporeflective band	Inner half, Henle's nerve fiber layer; outer half, outer nuclear layer
9	Hyperreflective	External limiting membrane
10	Hyporeflective	Myoid zone of the photoreceptors
11	Hyperreflective	Ellipsoid zone of the photoreceptors
12	Hyporeflective	Outer segments of the photoreceptors
12	Hyporeflective	Cone interdigitation with RPE
13	Hyperreflective band	RPE-Bruch's membrane complex. On occasion this can be separated into more than 1 band
14	Thin layer of moderate reflectivity in inner choroid	Choriocapillaris

Adapted from: Staurenghi et al. (2014). The IN.OCT Consensus

1.11 Imaging of the Outer Retina

A high-resolution SD-OCT provides an in vivo cellular level resolution imaging of the outer retina. Four bands have been distinguished in the outer retina. The first band, the innermost and faintest band, is attributed to the ELM and represents the junction of the Muller cells with photoreceptors (Drexler et al. 2003). Anatomical correlation of the second band has been controversial. In the past, the second highly reflective band was considered to be junction of the photoreceptor inner and outer segments (IS/OS) (Ko et al. 2004; Srinivasan et al. 2006). The third band is commonly referred to as the cone outer segment tips (COST) line, or Verhoeff's membrane, representing ensheathment of cone outer segments by RPE cell apical processes (Oishi et al. 2010; Puche et al. 2010; Srinivasan et al. 2008; Zawadzki et al. 2005). The outermost highly reflective fourth band is believed to represent the RPE with contribution from the Bruch's membrane and the choriocapillaris (Spaide and Curcio 2011).

Various studies demonstrated that the length of the photoreceptor inner and outer segments is roughly the same (Anger et al. 2004; Drexler et al. 2003; Hogan et al. 1971; Krebs and Krebs 1991; Spaide 2012). They suggested that the IS/OS band should form a plane midway between the ELM and RPE. On the contrary, the second reflective band was observed to lie significantly closer to the ELM than to the RPE. Using ultrahigh-resolution SD-OCT, Fernandez et al. were able to demonstrate the anatomy of human foveal cone photoreceptors, including visualization and identification of the myoid and ellipsoid zones of the inner segment of the photoreceptors (Fernandez et al. 2008). Based on published histology, a model of the outer retina was drawn to scale by Spaide and Curcio (2011). They compared the layers reflected on OCT to its anatomical correlate. They observed that the second band on OCT correlated with the photoreceptor inner segment ellipsoid zone (EZ). Lu et al., by comparative alignment of OCT bands with an anatomically correct model of the outer retina (using freshly isolated living retinas from the leopard frog), also suggested EZ to be responsible for contributing to the second reflective band (Lu et al. 2012).

Yamuchi et al. observed that the origin of the EZ was due to the biological activities of the photoreceptor cells. The EZ and ELM visualized on SD-OCT image of the retina of a live rat was observed to fade or be entirely absent after euthanasia (Yamuchi et al. 2013).

1.12 Basic Optical Coherence Tomography Interpretation of Macular Pathology

The OCT reflects the optical properties of the imaged tissue in terms of signal intensity. The reflectivity of retinal layers is determined by the arrangement of their structures, their biological densities, and degree of pigmentation. The areas can be hyperreflective or hyporeflective depending upon the amount of light being reflected compared to surrounding areas. Shadowing and reverse shadowing depends upon the amount of light being absorbed by surrounding tissue. Structures which absorb more light compared to the surrounding tissue cause optical shadowing and decreased visualization of outer layers. Reverse shadowing occurs when there is loss/atrophy of pigmented tissue that allows excessive light to be transmitted through to the outer layers. Other than the gray scale image, false color coding system is also attributed by the image processing algorithm for distinguishing the different layers of the retina. Structures with high biological reflectivity are represented by red, medium reflectivity with yellow/green, and those with low reflectivity by blue.

Pathological features that can be hyperreflective are epiretinal membranes and hard exudates. Areas with higher fluid content, e.g., intraretinal cysts and intraretinal and subretinal fluid accumulation, are usually hyporeflective. Vitreous debris, larger retinal vessels, hard exudates, and highly pigmented areas cause shadowing. The RPE is a major source of light absorption on OCT scanning, so atrophy of the RPE causes reverse shadowing with increased reflectivity from the choroid.

1.13 Spectral Domain Optical Coherence Tomography-Based Classification Systems

Several authors established the correlation of visual acuity with the integrity of EZ in diabetic retinopathy. Maheshwary et al. (2010) evaluated the ellipsoid zone, 500 microns in either direction of the fovea on horizontal and vertical SD-OCT images in patients with diabetic macular edema. The length of disruption was graded, and grades from each patient's horizontal and vertical scan were added to yield a global disruption scale. The percentage disruption of photoreceptor EZ was found to be an important predictor of visual acuity in diabetic macular edema. Sharma et al. put forth a simplified, comprehensive, and physician-friendly grading for EZ disruption (Sharma et al. 2014). The terms focal disruption, disruption localized to the subfoveal area, and global EZ disruption, generalized disruption throughout the macular cube, were defined. EZ disruption was found to be significantly associated with the severity of retinopathy. The length of the grade of disruption was observed to significantly correlate with impairment in visual acuity.

Subsequent studies established the role of the external limiting membrane (ELM) in maintaining the structure of the retina. On ultrastructural analyses of the junction proteins at the ELM, it was found that these junction proteins occludin, junction adhesion molecule, and zonula occludens-1 are tight junction proteins, similar to those found between RPE cells. The ELM is considered the third blood retinal barrier. Decrease in the occludin content at the level of ELM, along with swelling of the glial Muller cells in diabetes, leads to fluid accumulation in the macula (Omri et al. 2010). Mehalow et al. observed that the shortening of the photoreceptor inner segment might be a secondary consequence of the

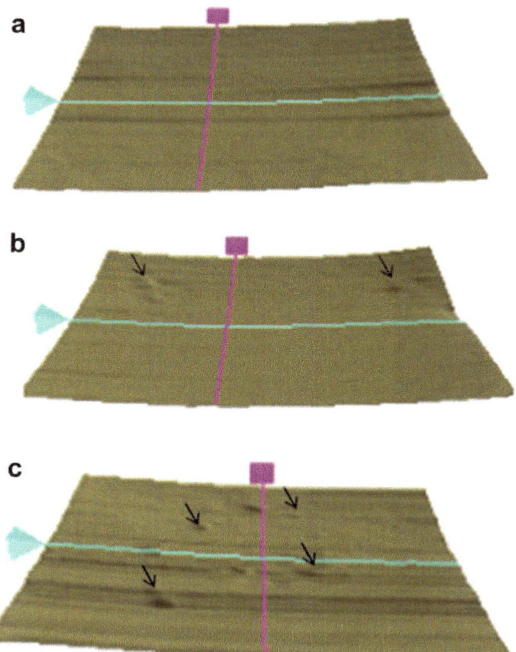

Fig. 1.2 Retinal pigment epithelium segmentation maps showing topographic alterations in diabetic retinopathy. (**a**) Grade 0: No RPE alteration. (**b**) Grade 1: Focal – alteration in up to two quadrants of the map (*black arrow*). (**c**) Grade 2: Global – alteration in more than two quadrants (*black arrows*)

fragmented ELM. Jain et al. published a novel grading system of photoreceptor ELM and EZ disruption, establishing that the disruption of ELM occurred before disruption of the EZ (Jain et al. 2013). The grades of ELM and EZ disruption predict the severity of the disease and visual outcome in patients with diabetic retinopathy. Another classification system was proposed on the basis of variability in the reflectivity level of EZ on SD-OCT (Murakami et al. 2012). Relatively homogeneous and continuous ELM band was described as intact, whereas absent or discontinuous ELM band was described as disrupted. In a classification by Sharma et al based on alteration of RPE was graded into three categories – grade 0: no RPE alteration; grade 1: focal (alteration predominantly in up to two quadrants of the map) and grade 2: global (alteration in more than two quadrants of the map) (Fig. 1.2) (Sharma et al. 2015)

1.14 Optical Coherence Tomography Angiography

OCT angiography identifies retinal circulation using the intrinsic motion of the blood cells in the vessel. It is based on comparison of repeated OCT scans of the eye acquired at the same position in the retina (Spaide et al. 2014). With the structures of the retina remaining static, blood flow in the vasculature or movement of the eye itself causes changes in the scans. After software processing for correction for eye movements, the difference between OCT images due to blood flow remains. Imaging data is acquired with a high speed OCT system (70,000 A-scans per second or more), and high-quality en face maps of vasculature are obtained noninvasively without the use of any exogenous dye. The angiographic image is generated by comparison with corresponding OCT B-scans of a volumetric scan, allowing for registration and correlation of vasculature with the structural B-scan. The vasculature at different depths of the retina can also be individually visualized. This feature is useful in retinal pathologies like diabetic retinopathy, retinal vein occlusion, age-related macular degeneration, and macular telangiectasias (Paulerkhoff et al. 2015).

1.15 Enhanced Depth Imaging

Imaging full-thickness choroid is technically challenging because of the attenuation of signal by pigment cells in RPE. OCT using 800 nm wavelength is unsuitable for posterior ocular tissue imaging.

Two systems are available:

(i) High-penetration OCT
(ii) Enhanced depth imaging (EDI)

Fourier transform decodes interferometric signals into two conjugate images; one of these two images is shown with the retina facing toward the top of the screen. To visualize deeper structures like the choroid and sclera, peak sensitivity is placed posteriorly. The upside-down conjugate image of these structures is visualized. This feature is available in commonly used OCT, and the need to invert the image has been eliminated in these OCT (Mrejen and Spaide 2013, Spaide et al 2008). Deep choroidal images are enhanced by taking an inverted image and multiple B-scan averaging (50–100 images) to improve signal to noise ratio.

1.16 Artifacts on Optical Coherence Tomography

Artifacts are a common occurrence resulting during OCT image acquisition, image processing, and analysis by the software or movement of the eye (Duker et al. 2013). Artifacts are important to identify as they may affect the qualitative or quantitative interpretation of images. Mirror artifact is only seen in SD-OCT devices as the Fourier domain devices generate two OCT mirror images around a zero-delay line. The ghost mirror image (image with lesser resolution) is not visualized by the operator unless it is moved close to the zero-delay line. This happens when the OCT machine is pushed very close to the eye, or with eyes with large axial length. Vignetting results when a part of the OCT beam is blocked by the iris characterized by a loss of signal over one side of the image. Misalignment artifact occurs in patients with poor fixation or eccentric fixation. The normal foveal depression is not aligned with the center of the ETDRS map. Software breakdown results due to misidentification of the inner or outer retinal boundaries due to underlying pathologies like epiretinal membrane, RPE atrophy, etc. These result in inaccurate quantitative measurements and topographical mapping. Momentary blockage of image acquisition during blink results in partial loss of data. These blink artifacts are recognized as black horizontal bars across the OCT image. Motion artifacts occur due to distortion or repeat scanning of the same area due to movement of the eye during OCT scanning. Out of range error is an operator-induced error. It occurs when the patient's head is not aligned properly on the machine. In this B-scan is shifted out of the scanning range. These artifacts should be identified before clinical decision-making by visualizing the color-coded maps and correlating the OCT images with the fundus image.

References

Anger EM, Unterhuber A, Hermann B, Sattmann H, Schubert C et al (2004) Ultrahigh-resolution optical coherence tomography of the monkey fovea: identification of retinal sublayers by correlation with semithin histology sections. Exp Eye Res 78:1117–1125

Drexler W, Sattmann H, Hermann B, Ko TH, Stur M et al (2003) Enhanced visualization of macular pathology with the use of ultrahigh-resolution optical coherence tomography. Arch Ophthalmol 121:695–706

Duker JS, Waheed NK, Goldman D (2013) Handbook of retinal OCT: optical coherence tomography. Elsevier Health Sciences, London

Fernandez EJ, Hermann B, Povazay B, Unterhuber A, Sattmann H et al (2008) Ultrahigh- resolution optical coherence tomography and pancorrection for cellular imaging of the living human retina. Opt Express 16:11083–11094

Hogan JA, Alvarado MJ, Weddell JE (1971) Histology of the human eye. An atlas and textbook. WB Saunders, Philadelphia

Jain A, Saxena S, Khanna VK et al (2013) Status of serum VEGF and ICAM-1 and its association with external limiting membrane and inner segment-outer segment junction disruption in type 2 diabetes mellitus. Mol Vis 19:1760–1768

Ko TH, Fujimoto JG, Duker JS, Paunescu LA, Drexler W et al (2004) Comparison of ultrahigh- and standard-resolution optical coherence tomography for imaging macular hole pathology and repair. Ophthalmology 111:2033–2043

Krebs W, Krebs I (1991) Primate retina and choroid. In: Atlas of fine structure in man and monkey. Springer, New York

Lu RW, Curcio CA, Zhang Y, Zhang QX, Pittler SJ et al (2012) Investigation of the hyper-reflective inner/outer segment band in optical coherence tomography of living frog retina. J Biomed Opt 17:060504

Lumbroso B, Rispoli M (2009) Guide to interpreting spectral domain optical coherence tomography, 2nd edn. chapter 4. Jaypee highlights. pp 33–34

Maheshwary AS, Oster SF et al (2010) The association between percent disruption of the photoreceptor inner segment-outer segment junction and visual acuity in diabetic macular edema. Am J Ophthalmol 150: 63–67

Mehalow AK, Kameya S, Smith RS et al (2003) CRB1 is essential for external limiting membrane integrity and photoreceptor morphogenesis in the mammalian retina. Hum Mol Genet 12:2179–2189

Mrejen S, Spaide RF (2013) OCT: Imaging of choroid and beyond. Surv Ophthalmol 58:387–429

Murakami T, Nishijima K, Akagi T, Uji A, Horii T et al (2012) Optical coherence tomographic reflectivity of photoreceptors beneath cystoid spaces in diabetic macular edema. Invest Ophthalmol Vis Sci 53: 1506–1511

Oishi A, Hata M, Shimozono M, Mandai M, Nishida A, Kurimoto Y (2010) The significance of external limiting membrane status for visual acuity in age-related macular degeneration. Am J Ophthalmol 150:27–32

Omri S, Omri B et al (2010) The outer limiting membrane (OLM) revisited: clinical implications. Clin Ophthalmol 4:183–195

Paulerkhoff D, Heimes D, Spital G (2015) OCT ANGIOGRAPHY is this future of macular diagnosis? Klin Monbl Augenheilkd 232:1069–1076

Podoleanu GA (2012) Optical coherence tomography. J Microsc 10:1365–2818

Puche N, Querques G, Benhamou N, Tick S, Mimoun G et al (2010) High-resolution spectral domain optical coherence tomography features in adult onset foveomacular vitelliform dystrophy. Br J Ophthalmol 94:1190–1196

Ryan SJ (2013) Retina, 5th edn. Elsevier, Health Sciences, London

Sharma SR, Saxena S et al (2014) The association of grades of photoreceptor inner segment- ellipsoid band disruption with severity of retinopathy in type 2 diabetes mellitus. J Case Rep Stud 2:205

Sharma SR, Saxena S, Srivastav K, Shukla RK, Mishra N et al (2015) Nitric oxide and oxidative stress is associated with severity of diabetic retinopathy and retinal structural alterations. Clinical and Experimental Ophthalmology, 43:429–436

Spaide RF (2012) Questioning optical coherence tomography. Ophthalmology 119:2203–2204

Spaide RF, Curcio CA (2011b) Anatomical correlates to the bands seen in the outer retina by optical coherence tomography: literature review and model. Retina 31:1609–1619

Spaide RF, Koizumi H, Poconni ML (2008) Enhanced depth imaging spectral domain optical coherence tomography. Am J Ophthalmol 146:496–500

Spaide RF, Klancnik JM, Cooney MJ (2014) Retinal vascular layers imaged by fluorescein angiography and optical coherence tomography angiography. JAMA Ophthalmol 133:E1–E6

Srinivasan VJ, Ko TH, Wojtkowski M, Carvalho M, Clermont A et al (2006) Noninvasive volumetric imaging and morphometry of the rodent retina with high-speed, ultrahigh-resolution optical coherence tomography. Invest Ophthalmol Vis Sci 47: 5522–5528

Srinivasan VJ, Monson BK, Wojtkowski M, Bilonick RA, Gorczynska I et al (2008) Characterization of outer retinal morphology with high-speed, ultrahigh-resolution optical coherence tomography. Invest Ophthalmol Vis Sci 49:1571–1579

Staurenghi G, Sadda S et al (2014) Proposed lexicon for anatomic landmarks in normal posterior segment spectral-domain optical coherence tomography. The IN.OCT consensus. Ophthalmology 121:1572–1578

Wei J, Lumbroso B, Jang B, Davis J, inventors; Optovue, Inc., assignee (2012) Computer-aided diagnosis of retinal pathologies using frontal en-face views of optical coherence tomography. United States patent application US 13/360,503

Yamauchi Y, Yagi H, Usui Y et al (2011) Biological activity is the likely origin of the intersection between the photoreceptor inner and outer segments of the rat retina as determined by optical coherence tomography. Clin Ophthalmol 5:1649–1653

Zawadzki RJ, Jones SM, Olivier SS, Zhao M, Bower BA et al (2005) Adaptive-optics optical coherence tomography for high- resolution and high- speed 3D retinal in vivo imaging. Opt Express 13:8532–8546

2 Three-Dimensional Spectral Domain Optical Coherence Tomography

Surabhi Ruia and Sandeep Saxena

Contents

Electronic supplementary material The online version of this chapter (doi:10.1007/978-81-322-3610-8_2) contains supplementary material, which is available to authorized users.

S. Ruia, MS • S. Saxena, MS,FRCSEd,FRCS, FRCOphth,FAICO (✉)
Department of Ophthalmology, King George's Medical University, Lucknow, UP, India
e-mail: sandeepsaxena2020@gmail.com

2.1 Introduction

Optical coherence tomography (OCT) is an ever evolving technology that has revolutionized ophthalmic imaging. With the advent of spectral domain technology, an unparalleled micrometer axial resolution of 5–10 μm is achieved. With more data acquisition per scanning session, volumetric analysis and three-dimensional imaging are realized (Puliafito et al. 1995; Regatieri et al. 2012; Yannuzzi et al. 2004). Three-dimensional OCT generates OCT fundus images that enable precise registration of OCT images with the image of fundus on standard ophthalmoscopic examination techniques (Podoleanu and Jackson 1998; Podoleanu et al. 1998). This allows effortless localization of images for monitoring disease progression and response to therapy. Preservation of retinal topography enables visualization of subtle changes associated with the disease. With rapid evolution in technology, clinical usage of OCT has extended to diseases with more complex morphological features. Improved cellular level resolution has extended the application of spectral domain OCT to retinal degenerations and dystrophies. Three-dimensional imaging, with its increased potential in elucidating retinal morphology, provides a global perspective to various retinal diseases (Saxena and Meredith 2006).

C.H. Meyer et al. (eds.), *Spectral Domain Optical Coherence Tomography in Macular Diseases*,
DOI 10.1007/978-81-322-3610-8_2

2.1.1 Scanning Protocol

In the Cirrus HD-OCT (Carl Zeiss Meditec Inc., CA, USA), two macular cube scans are available through a square grid of 6×6 mm. The 512×128 protocol analyzes 128 horizontal scans at high resolution (512 A-scans per B-scan). The 200×200 protocol achieves faster imaging with good resolution. Cube scan analysis incorporates an algorithm for identification of two layers: internal limiting membrane (ILM) and retinal pigment epithelium (RPE). The ILM and RPE are presented in their entirety as three-dimensional surface maps (Fig. 2.1). The ILM-RPE thickness map gives a complete image of changes in retinal thickness with false color coding. These can be rotated for view from various perspectives.

The three-dimensional reconstructed macular cube gives a comprehensive image of all the retinal layers. Three orthogonal planes are outlined for imaging of the cube (Fig. 2.2):

The X plane parallel to the front of the cube corresponds to the horizontal B-scan or cross section.

The Y plane parallel to the side of the cube corresponds to the vertically reconstructed B-scan.

The Z plane or the coronal plane parallel to the top of the cube corresponds to the reconstructed *en face* image of the retina or the *OCT fundus image*.

2.1.2 Three-Dimensional Scan

Three-dimensional reconstruction displays the entire retinal cube data. Image can be studied along either of the three orthogonal planes. An image can be cropped to study a section of interest in either of the plane. The entire 3D cube can be rotated for viewing from any perspective. False color-coding images can be obtained. Other than cropping of the image along the X, Y, or Z plane, niche editing, i.e., cropping of a quadrant of tissue image simultaneously along two planes, is also possible. Masking pertains to the additional option of preserving the tissues below a specific layer of interest. RPE mask, masks from cutting the tissue below the RPE, and thereby

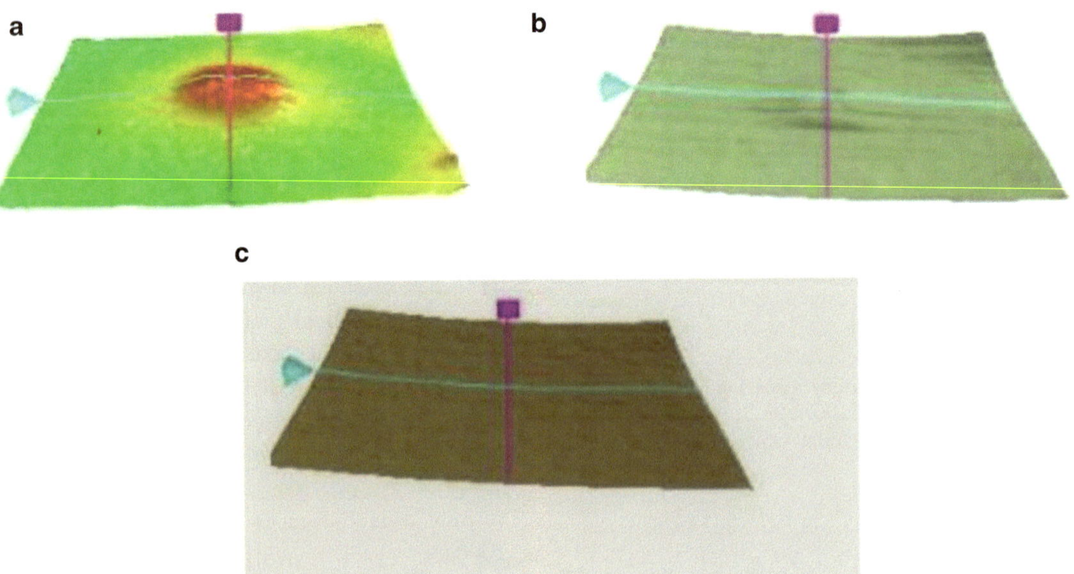

Fig. 2.1 Three-dimensional segmentation maps. (**a**) Internal limiting membrane-retinal pigment epithelium (ILM-RPE) thickness map. (**b**) ILM surface contour segmentation map.(**c**) RPE surface topography map

enables peeling back the tissue above the RPE. This feature allows for localizing and studying in detail the pathologies at deeper layers of the retinal cube.

2.2 Macular Diseases

2.2.1 Dry Age-Related Macular Degeneration

Geographic atrophy (GA) and drusens are known to be distinguishing features of nonexudative (dry) age-related macular degeneration (AMD). The volume and number of drusen are known to be biomarkers for severity of the disease (Yi et al. 2009). Segmented RPE surface topography maps on macular thickness analyses show contour alteration due to underlying drusens. SD-OCT made possible the ultrastructural characterization of drusen (Khanifar et al. 2008). They are characterized by smooth or jagged elevations of the RPE layer, with varied reflectivity in relation to reflectivity of the photoreceptor layer and RPE (Hee et al. 1996; Srinivasan et al. 2006a). The *summed-voxel projection*, a representative two-dimensional en face image created by B-scans along the anterior-posterior axis of a three-dimensional OCT stack, orients the drusen seen tomographically, with respect to retinal vasculature seen on fundus photographs. Geographic atrophy results from the loss of the photoreceptor layer, RPE, and choriocapillaris. In most cases, GA first appears in the parafoveal location and progresses around the fovea with concomitant loss of central visual acuity. These are identified on sequential imaging of three-dimensional retinal cube along the orthogonal planes. The RPE contour map gives the complete image of the lateral extent of the atrophy surrounded by a transitional area. In transitional areas the photoreceptor dysfunction precedes the appearance and progression of GA (Curcio et al. 1996). Advanced macular visualization helps identify disruption of inner segment ellipsoid segment (EZ) of photoreceptors along areas of the spread of GA.

2.2.2 Exudative Age-Related Macular Degeneration

In classic neovascularization (CNV), SD-OCT illustrates a hyperreflective mass that extends above the RPE, raising the neuroretina (Fig. 2.3). Intraretinal edema and neovascular mass surrounded by areas of neurosensory or pigment epithelium detachment (PED) indicate active CNV. Occult neovascular membranes are located between the RPE and Bruch's membrane. Hemorrhagic subretinal fluid and serous elevation of RPE are differentiated on the basis of reflectivity profile. The high resolution of SD-OCT allows precise imaging of minute areas of intraretinal or

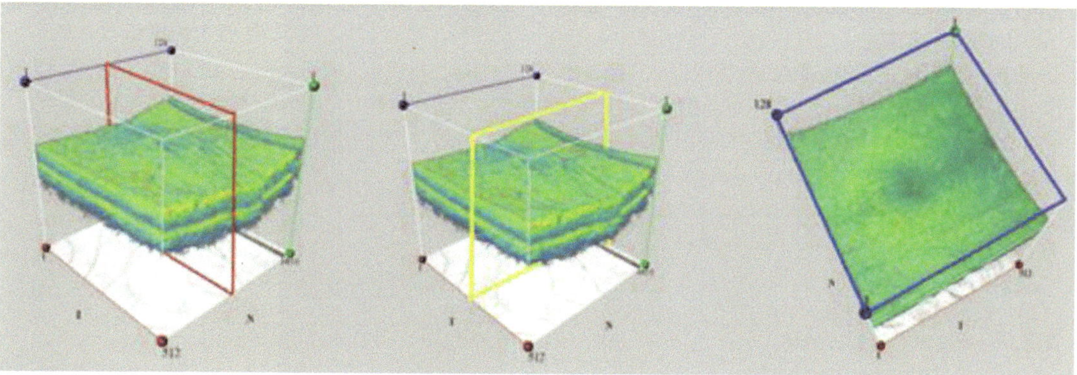

Fig. 2.2 Three-dimensional spectral domain optical coherence tomography showing orthogonal planes X (*red*), Y (*yellow*), and Z (*blue*) planes

subretinal fluid and their localization to specific layers. Alterations in ILM-RPE thickness maps with changes in foveal contour and surface alteration of RPE topography map are useful indicators for early identification of occult cases as well as for monitoring progression of CNV. Sequential imaging of the three-dimensional cube in the Z plane provides with en face imaging of the retina at a defined depth especially at the level of RPE. Three-dimensional SD-OCT has superseded fluorescein angiography in subclinical identification of the retinochoroidal anastomosis (Querques et al. 2011). Changes in height of PED, obliteration of subretinal space, and progression of CNV are visual guides on follow-up of cases (Ahlers et al. 2008). RPE tears are known to complicate PED (Chang and Sarraf 2007; Leitritz et al. 2008). Tangential stress on RPE due to the increasing height of RPE detachment, rapid contraction of regressing CNV, and treatment with anti-vascular endothelial growth factor (anti-VEGF) therapy are probable causes of RPE tear (Chan et al. 2007; Chan et al. 2010; Chiang et al. 2008; Gass 1984; Lafaut et al. 2001; Shiraki et al. 2001). Three-dimensional SD-OCT with its unparallel topographical view of retinal layers identifies and localizes RPE tear particularly subclinically (Saxena et al. 2012d). The RPE tear is visualized as absence of RPE underneath the neurosensory retina with focal interruption of the RPE signal and a hyperreflective retracted RPE edge (Fig. 2.4). Associated CNV is responsible for hyperreflection in sub-RPE space. The RPE tear creates an area where photoreceptors have no RPE support affecting the visual acuity, especially in cases where fovea is involved (Albert et al. 2011). With time, fibroproliferative changes obliterate the subretinal space. This has been correlated with histological studies that revealed rolled up margins of the RPE tear along with the fibrovascular membrane over remains of outer segments (Leitritz et al. 2008).

2.2.3 Central Serous Chorioretinopathy

Central serous chorioretinopathy (CSC) is a disorder of RPE-choriocapillaris complex (Spaide 2005). It is characterized by serous detachments of the neurosensory retina (Fig. 2.5). Disruption of the choroidal circulation, followed by decompensation of RPE, allows exudation from the choroidal vasculature to pass into the subretinal space (Guyer et al. 1994; Piccolino et al. 2005; Scheider

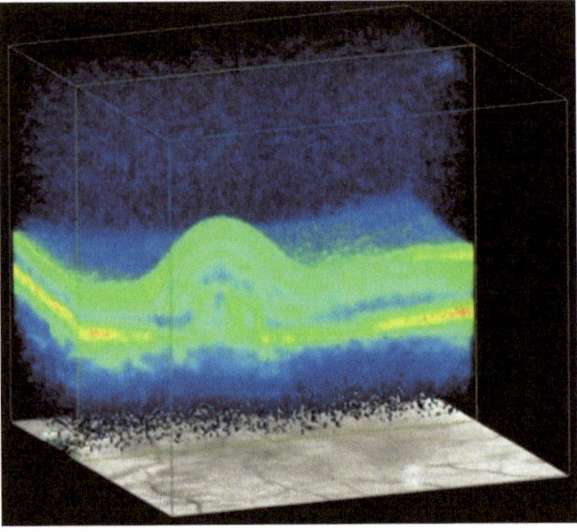

Fig. 2.3 Three-dimensional imaging of exudative age-related macular degeneration. Classic neovascular membrane forms a hyperreflective nonhomogeneous fusiform mass located in front of the retinal pigment epithelium. Cystic cavities present above the lesion. Bruch's membrane and RPE are also interrupted at the area of the neovascularization

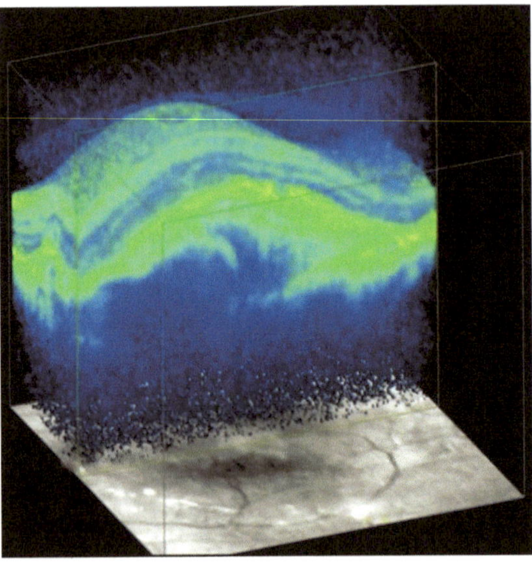

Fig. 2.4 Three-dimensional imaging of retinal pigment epithelium tear with hyperreflective edges

et al. 1993). Pigment epithelium detachment is not an uncommon finding in these cases and is usually located within or at the edge of the sensory retinal detachment (Figs. 2.5, 2.6). Diffuse RPE atrophy or alterations characterize chronic CSC. Subretinal fluid may be cloudy due to the presence of fibrin in chronic or recurrent cases (Mitarai et al. 2006; Ojima et al. 2007). A better understanding of the pathogenesis has been gained with advent of OCT (Kamppeter and Jonas 2003; Lida et al. 2000; Mitarai et al. 2006; Piccolino and Borgia 1994). SD-OCT succeeded fluorescein angiography by identifying defects in the RPE layer in the areas of PED corresponding to sites of leakage (Fujimoto et al. 2008; Hussain et al. 2006; Montero and Ruiz-Moreno 2005). Three-dimensional OCT localizes these leakage sites precisely (Wang et al. 2011). Three-dimensional surface RPE maps confirm both PEDs and RPE alterations. Surface topography map of ILM reveals the presence and location of subclinical CSC with changes in surface contour. False color-coded ILM-RPE maps provide with progressive analysis of thickness (Fig. 2.6). Subretinal fibrin deposition in chronic CSC has been demonstrated on 3D SD-OCT (Saxena et al. 2011). Hyperreflectivity in the subretinal space with fibrin deposition corresponds to clinically observed yellowish white subretinal exudate (Fig. 2.7).

Alteration in the photoreceptor outer segment (OS) and EZ is visualized inner to the detached neurosensory retina (Ojima et al. 2007). The increased thickness of the OS in acute phase gradually decreases with reattachment. Punctuate or granular appearance of the OS occurs more frequently in cases of chronic or recurrent

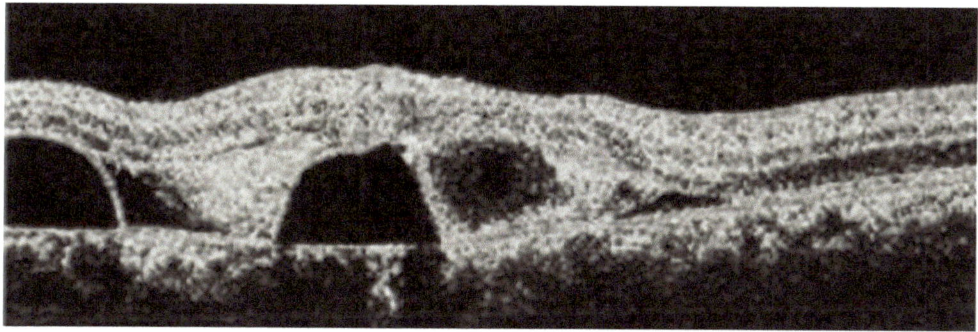

Fig. 2.5 Central serous chorioretinopathy. Spectral domain optical coherence tomography cross section showing pigment epithelium detachment associated with neurosensory detachment

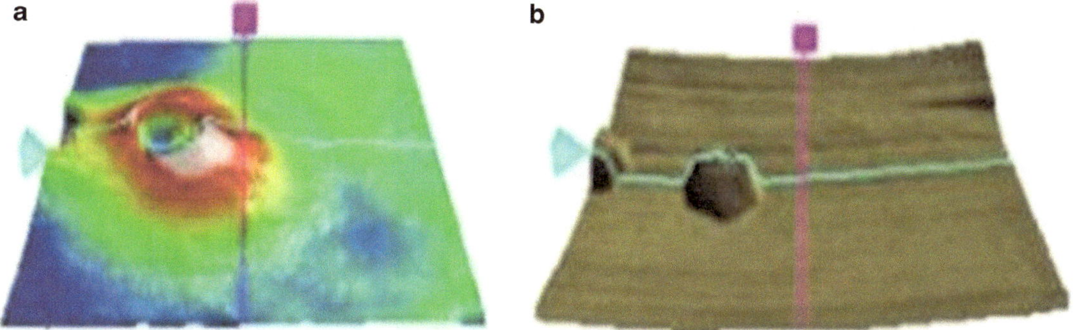

Fig. 2.6 Central serous chorioretinopathy. (**a**) Surface topography maps with false color-coded internal limiting membrane-retinal pigment epithelium (ILM-RPE) thickness depicting increased retinal thickness. (**b**) Surface map of RPE showing pigment epithelium detachment

CSC. The latter appearance is probably due to the accumulation of the shed OS. After retinal reattachment, the EZ gradually becomes clear, implying normalization of the assembly of the OS due to regular phagocytosis resumed by the RPE. Thus a detailed morphological assessment of the disease is obtained.

2.2.4 Nonproliferative Diabetic Retinopathy and Diabetic Macular Edema

OCT has been an indispensable ancillary investigation for characterization of intraretinal cystoid spaces in diabetic macular edema. The thickness of the subretinal space is greatest at the central fovea and declines peripherally. Serous retinal detachment is seen as a subretinal fluid accumulation with elevation of neurosensory retina from RPE (Figs. 2.8, 2.9). 3D SD-OCT is a supportive investigative tool for evaluation and follow-up of patients with diabetic retinopathy. Involvement of the outer plexiform layer, inner plexiform, and ganglion cell layer with global extent of edema is well defined with sequential imaging in the three orthogonal planes. Cotton wool spots, due to retinal ischemia, appear as regions of increased reflectivity of the retinal nerve fiber layer and inner neurosensory retina. Hard exudates are identifiable as hyperreflective foci in the outer retinal layers with posterior shadowing. Color-coded retinal thickness maps pick up the earlier stages of diabetic retinopathy with ILM surface topography depicting the absence of foveal depression. RPE changes may also reflect previous laser photocoagulation, which are visualized on RPE segmentation map. High-resolution imaging enables better evaluation of the integrity of the photoreceptor layer, both at baseline and after resolution of diabetic macular edema.

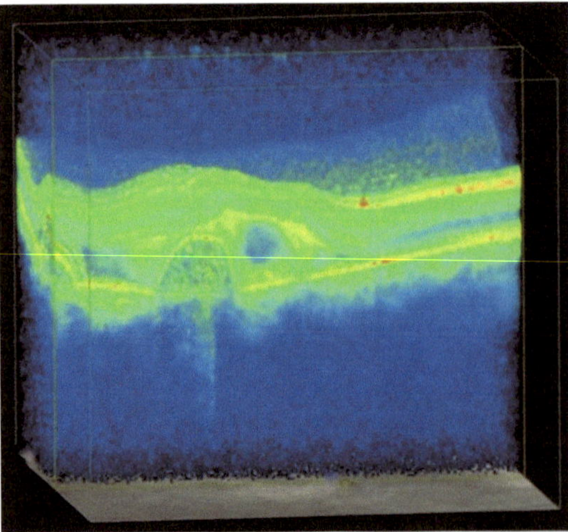

Fig. 2.7 Three-dimensional imaging of central serous chorioretinopathy. Neurosensory detachment from retinal pigment epithelium. The photoreceptors follow the neurosensory retina along the anterior boundary of detachment. In cases of prolonged detachment, these segments of the photoreceptors become altered and granular. Hyperreflective subretinal depicts fibrin deposition in the subretinal space. Pigment epithelium detachment is associated with detachment of the neuroepithelium

2.2.5 Proliferative Diabetic Retinopathy

Three-dimensional SD-OCT is an auxiliary investigative tool for portraying neovascularization, hemorrhage, and preretinal fibrosis in proliferative diabetic retinopathy. With imaging of vitreoretinal interface, visualization of subhyaloid hemorrhage relative to the ILM and posterior hyaloid face, extent of the lesion, and structural alteration of layers of the retina below the hemorrhage are well defined (Kroll et al. 1999; Punjabi et al. 2008). Structural changes in the retina below the hemorrhage predict the visual outcome post therapy. Distinction of preretinal membranes, visible as thin reflective bands anterior to the retina, from detached posterior vitreous is made easy. The posterior hyaloid typically has a lower reflectivity than a preretinal membrane due to the optical transparency of the vitreous. Presence, localization, and extent of retinal traction are well visualized (Srinivasan et al. 2006a). Retinal thinning corresponding to retinal atrophy occurs in the region of previous photocoagulation treatment. The vitreous gel plays a key role in causing effects at vitreoretinal interface with fibrovascular proliferation or epiretinal mem-

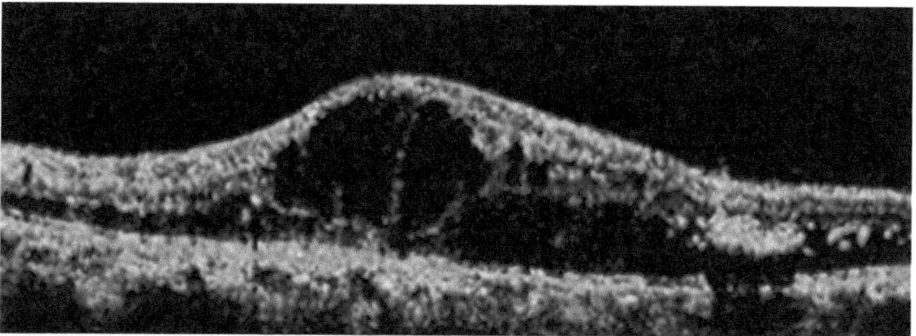

Fig. 2.8 Spectral domain optical coherence imaging of nonproliferative diabetic retinopathy showing cystoid macular edema

brane (ERM) formation at later stages of diabetic retinopathy. Presence and severity of macular traction and distortion of retinal contour due to ERM are well studied. Uniform attachment or multiple surface adhesions with retinal striae or focal tenting of the inner retina are better visualized on 3D SD-OCT. Evaluation of vitreoretinal interface has helped better understand the pathophysiology of the disease and planning for surgery (Gallemore et al. 2000).

2.2.6 Retinal Vein Occlusion

Occlusion of the retinal venous system is the second most common retinal vascular disease after diabetic retinopathy (Spaide et al. 2003). OCT findings in retinal vein occlusion include cystoid macular edema, ERM, pseudoholes, lamellar holes, and subhyaloid or preretinal hemorrhages (Arevalo et al. 2013; Spaide et al. 2003). The extent of involvement of edema depends on the territory of the occluded vessel. Hemorrhages are localized to the nerve fiber layer and outer plexiform layer. Edematous changes in the inner nuclear and ganglion cell layer appear as diffuse thickening with hyporeflective spaces. Cystic changes localize to the inner and outer nuclear layer, and serous retinal detachments may occur with neurosensory retina detachment from RPE. Alteration in external limiting membrane (ELM) as well as EZ is also observed. With 3D SD-OCT, improved monitoring of macular edema, with changes in retinal contour in response to treatment and correlation with post-resolution visual acuity, has been realized. Spatial extent of macular edema is better discerned with scans along the three orthogonal planes (Yamaike et al. 2008). OCT plays a pivotal role in quantitatively monitoring the changes in retinal thickness after treatment, such as intravitreal triamcinolone or anti-VEGF therapy (Greenberg et al. 2002).

2.2.7 Retinal Artery Occlusion

Central retinal artery occlusion is an unfavorable ocular condition that results in profound and permanent loss of vision. On OCT, the affected area demonstrates increased thickness and reflectivity in the inner retina corresponding to edema of the retinal layers. The ganglion cell layer and inner nuclear layer are affected in proportion to the duration of ischemia, whereas outer nuclear and plexiform layers and photoreceptors show no damage (Wojtkowski et al. 2005). Three-dimensional OCT will enhance the irregular macular contour due to ischemia-induced edema of the inner retinal layers. These findings correlate with the histopathology where ischemic necrosis of the inner layers is observed. Hyperreflectivity of the inner retinal layers causes shadowing of the optical signal of the outer layers and RPE/choriocapillaris complex, mimicking retinal edema. The marked difference from retinal edema due to other retinal vascular diseases is lack of cystic spaces of low reflectivity. No correlation has been found with extent of initial macular edema and visual improvement (Schmidt et al. 2006). Branch retinal artery occlusion and cilioretinal artery occlusion shows similar hyperreflectivity localized to the distribution of the artery involved. After the resolution of retinal edema, the inner retina becomes atrophic in a few days due to reperfusion injury (Saxena et al. 2013b). Later on with washout of oxidative stress biomarkers, recovery of retinal thickness termed pseudo normalization, is observed. Retinal atrophy sets in by 3 months with formation of an acellular scar of the inner retinal layers. False color-coded thickness maps are useful in monitoring these changes.

2.2.8 Macular Hole

Visualization of vitreofoveal interface with SD-OCT improved the understanding of pathophysiology of progression of a macular hole. Anteroposterior vitreous and tangential traction explain the sequel of subtle changes in the outer retinal layers of the fovea, elevation of foveal contour in the foveal pit region, followed by formation of a foveal pseudocyst that characterizes an impending macular hole. Retinal tissue remains at the base of a pseudocyst. Three-dimensional SD-OCT demonstrates vitreoretinal interface between the cone of the posterior hyaloid and the inner retinal surface of the foveal pit. Three-dimensional views of the ILM show elevation of the roof of the foveal cyst in the foveal pit. Incompletely detached posterior hyaloid exhibits an oblique pull over the retinal surface with a clinical appearance of crescent or horseshoe retinal defect. Full-thickness macular holes are characterized by disruption of retinal layers up to the RPE with involvement of photoreceptor layers (Figs. 2.10, 2.11, and 2.12). Detachment of vitreous from retinal surface at posterior pole and in later stages from the disk is observed. Full-thickness macular holes are visualized as a cone-shaped steepening of the fovea with variation in extent and base. The size of a macular hole has been documented to affect anatomical and visual success post surgery. Variable amount of intraretinal edema surrounding the hole is present with increase in retinal thickness. Disruption of the photoreceptor layer is a useful predictor of visual outcome post surgery (Hangai et al 2007; Inoue et al 2009; Srinivasan et al. 2006a, b). SD-OCT is useful in evaluating the preoperative macular hole configuration and postoperative resolution (Altaweel and Ip 2003; Tilanus et al. 1999; Ullrich et al. 2002).

SD-OCT also improved the differentiation of lamellar holes and pseudomacular holes (Witkin et al. 2006). Lamellar holes earlier defined as defects in the fovea, due to the avulsion of the roof of a cystoid macular edema, is now described on OCT as dehiscence in the inner fovea with intact outer retinal layers at the base of the hole (Haouchine et al. 2004). Macular pseudohole is described as steepening of foveal contour due to ERM contraction and a normal or slightly increased central and paracentral retinal thickness (Haouchine et al. 2004). Three-dimensional volume rendering illustrates the vertical edges of the foveal pit with a U shape of the fovea (Fig. 2.13). Outer retinal layers are intact.

2.2.9 Epiretinal Membrane

The epiretinal membrane (ERM) is a nonvascular fibrocellular proliferation that develops on the surface of the ILM and causes a spectrum of

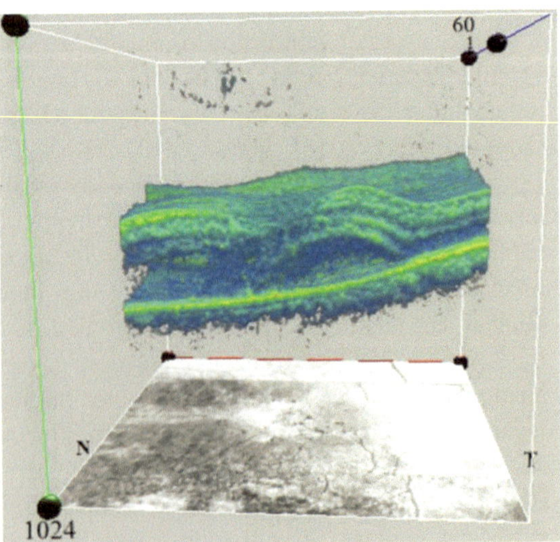

Fig. 2.9 Three-dimensional imaging of nonproliferative diabetic retinopathy showing intraretinal edema along with serous retinal detachment

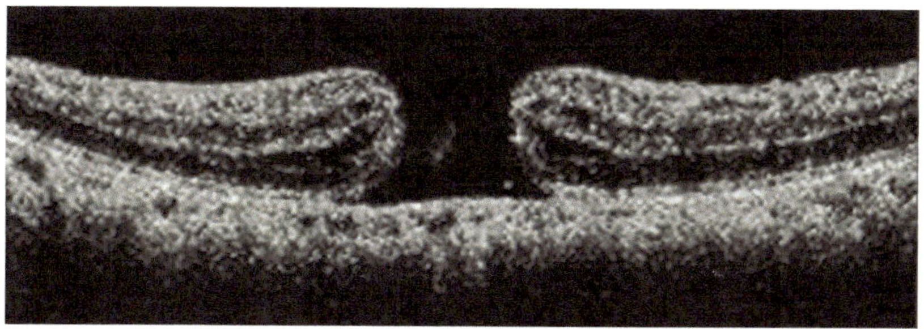

Fig. 2.10 Cross-sectional spectral domain OCT of full-thickness macular hole

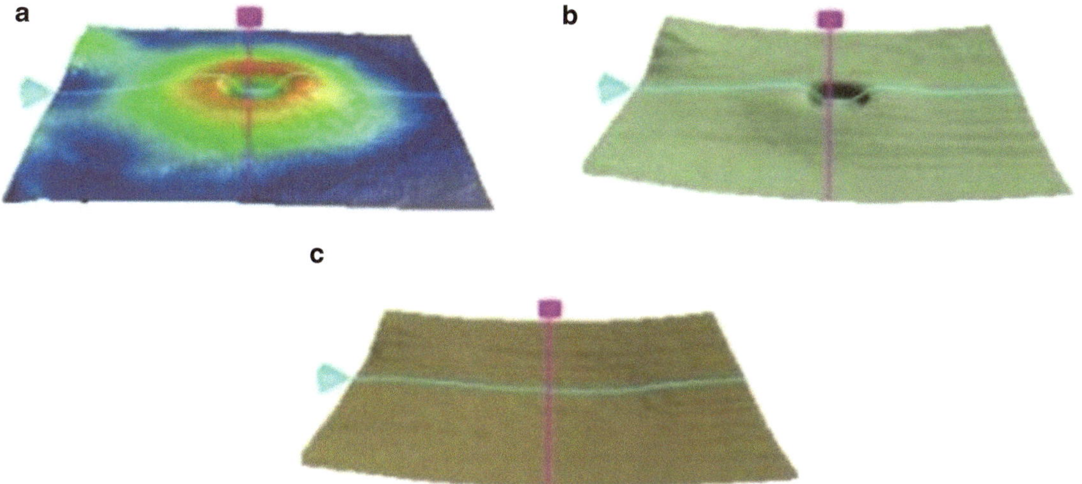

Fig. 2.11 Figure showing (**a**) false color coded internal limiting membrane-retinal pigment epithelium (ILM-RPE) thickness map demonstrating thickened retina, loss of foveal contour and surface distortion due to epiretinal membrane, (**b**) ILM surface topography map with presence of radial folds due to epiretinal membrane (**c**) and normal RPE topography map in the same eye

changes such as increase in retinal thickening, loss of foveal contour, distortion of the retinal surface, vascular tortuosity, cystic changes, intraretinal fluid accumulation, foveoschisis, and formation of macular pseudoholes. ERM in healthy eyes is localized between ILM and the vitreous body interface (Koizumi et al. 2008). From cellophane macular reflex to macular pucker, ERM has been classified on clinical as well as on OCT findings (Gass 1997; Mori et al. 2004; Wilkins et al. 1996). SD-OCT, besides detecting the focal and broad-based attachments of the ERM to the retina, enhances the resolution of intraretinal architectural morphology (Fig. 2.14). Retinal thickness and integrity of the EZ are known to be prognostic factors of visual acuity after ERM surgery (Wong et al. 2005). Thicker and opaque membranes may cause partial posterior vitreous detachment with persistent vitreomacular adhesions leading to cystoid macular edema. Posterior vitreous detachments also may cause tractional retinal detachment or retinal breaks. Absence of posterior vitreous detachment helps differentiate vitreomacular traction from idiopathic ERM, although both the entities significantly overlap (Koerner and Garweg 1999; Legarreta et al. 2008). ERM with vitreomacular and vitreopapillary adhesions has been described in diabetic retinopathy and Eales' disease (Ophir and Martinez 2011; Saxena et al. 2012a). With three-dimensional imaging in diabetic retinopathy, ERM with

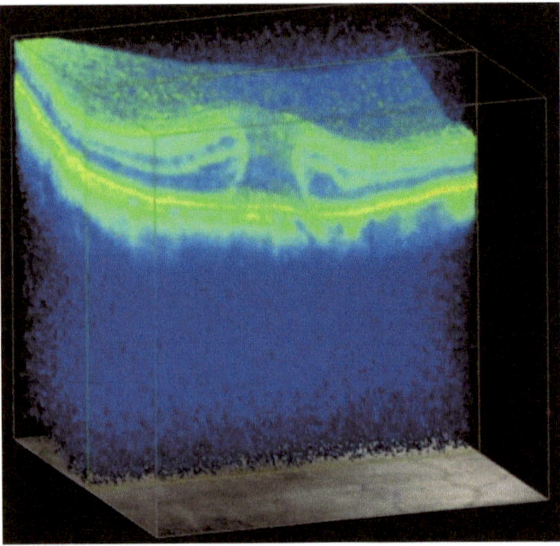

Fig. 2.12 Three-dimensional imaging showing stage IV macular hole. Cystoid macular edema forms a ring around the margins of the hole. These pseudocysts are located in the internal and external nuclear layers

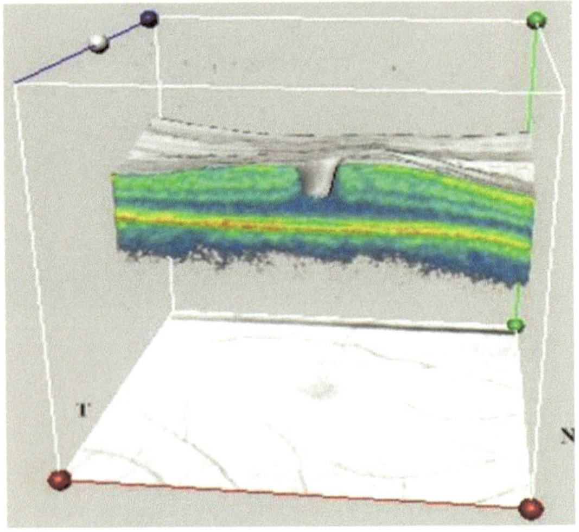

Fig. 2.13 Three-dimensional imaging showing pseudomacular hole with steep foveal contour. Preservation of the outer layers of retina

nontractional vitreoretinal interfaces were identified as fine foldings seen on ILM maps, which disappeared after ILM peeling (Abe et al. 2013). ILM segmentation maps demonstrate parallel or radiating folds due to vitreoretinal interaction at sites of adhesion of ERM. Color-coded ILM-RPE thickness maps identify intraretinal fluid accumulation causing elevation of foveal contour (Fig. 2.15). Three-dimensional imaging allows better characterization of ERM including visualization of extent of ERM, cleavage planes formed between retinal layers, evaluation of vitreoretinal surface for attachment sites and its configuration, and assessment of thickness of the ERM (Elbendary 2010). The identification of presence and localization of adhesions of ERM to inner retina help in preoperative planning in membrane peeling or delamination. Sequential imaging of the retinal cube in all the three planes gives a high-resolution representation of all the intraretinal layers identifying extent and location of alteration in functionally relevant structures including the photoreceptor layer. Restoration of the anatomy post surgery can be well demonstrated on OCT. Three-dimensional SD-OCT gives unprecedented visualization of ERM (Figs. 2.13 and 2.14).

2.2.10 Vitreomacular Traction Syndrome

Vitreomacular traction (VMT) is a distinct clinical entity which results from persistent attachment of vitreous to the macula in the presence of incomplete posterior vitreous detachment. Asymptomatic disease course of VMT occurs due to spontaneous detachment of vitreous from macula with restoration of structural retinal changes (Hikichi et al. 1995). Persistent traction leads to structural changes of retinal contour with progressive retinal edema, distortion of retinal architecture, detachment of fovea, or full-thickness macular hole formation (Gallemore et al. 2000; Yamada and Kishi 2005). Vitreopapillary adhesion may influence the vectors of force at the vitreoretinal interface causing a centrifugal tangential contraction which can result in idiopathic ERM (Wang et al. 2009). Coexisting macular diseases classifies VMT as concurrent. Vitreopapillary and vitreomacular traction have been described in diabetic retinopathy (Karatas et al. 2005; Ophir and Martinez 2011; An OCT based classification by the International Vitreomacular Traction study group subclassified VMT with attachment of 1500 μm or less as focal, whereas VMT with attachment of more than 1500 μm as broad (Duker et al. 2013). Three-dimensional imaging gives a comprehensive view of vitreoretinal interface changes and a global perspective to the structural alteration of retinal layers caused by VMT (Ito et al. 2000; Chang et al. 2008). SD-OCT discerns retinoschisis of the outer retinal layers. Structural alteration of the photoreceptor layer correlates well with visual dysfunction, metamorphopsia. Surface topography ILM map shows corresponding elevation of ILM at the points of vitreous attachments at foveal and extrafoveal locations. A cleavage plane due to infolding of the retina can be observed as a corresponding dip over the ILM map. A false color-coded ILM-RPE map highlights the changes in macular thickness. Introduction of ocriplasmin, a pharmacological means of vitreolysis, has increased the significance of evaluation of the vitreomacular interface with SD-OCT. A detailed evaluation of the attachment site reinforces the role of 3D OCT in identifying suitable cases for ocriplasmin therapy (Figs. 2.16, 2.17, and 2.18).

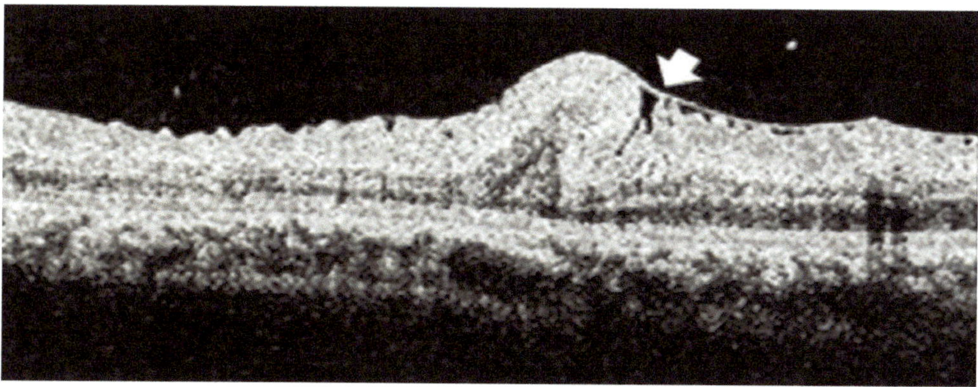

Fig. 2.14 Spectral domain OCT cross-sectional imaging showing hyperreflective, taut, and continuous epiretinal membrane (ERM) exerting traction on the retinal surface, causing folds on the internal limiting membrane and the inner retinal layers. Arrow marks the partial separation of ERM from the retinal surface

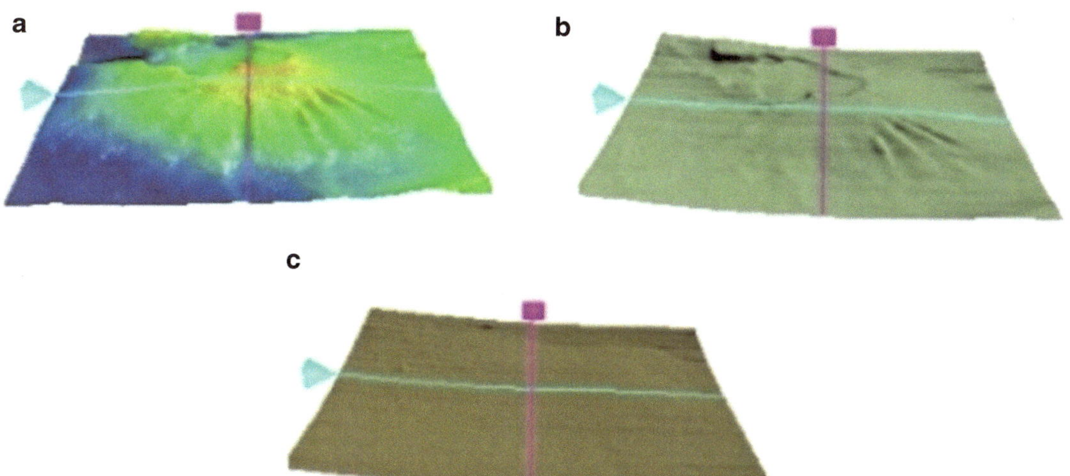

Fig. 2.15 Figure showing (**a**) false color coded internal limiting membrane-retinal pigment epithelium (ILM-RPE) thickness map demonstrating thickened retina, loss of foveal contour and surface distortion due to epiretinal membrane, (**b**) ILM surface topography map with presence of radial folds due to epiretinal membrane (**c**) and normal RPE topography map in the same eye

2.2.11 Eales' Disease

Eales' disease is an idiopathic inflammatory venous occlusive disease and primarily affects the peripheral retina of young men. It is characterized by stages of venous inflammation (periphlebitis), peripheral capillary nonperfusion, and retinal neovascularization. SD-OCT offers high-resolution imaging of the retina in cases of Eales' disease. Appreciation of ERM, retinal folds, and hyperplastic RPE are well discerned. Retinoschisis in a case of Eales' disease has also been detected with the help of SD-OCT (Saxena and Kumar 2000). Saxena and Kumar have also reported the involvement of macula in Eales' disease. Vitreopapillary and vitreomacular tractions with ERM leading to vitreomaculopathy have been documented (Saxena et al. 2012a).

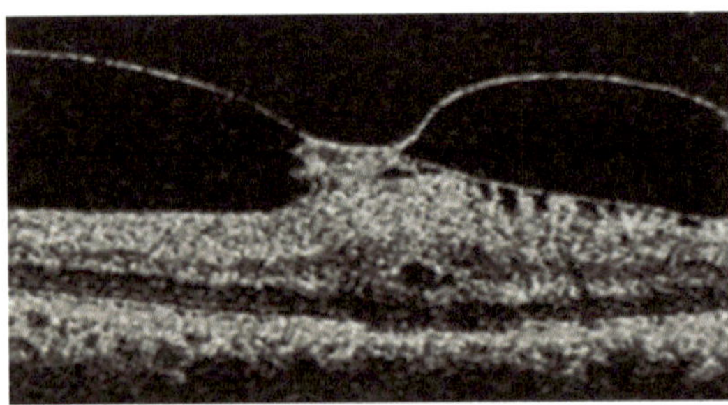

Fig. 2.16 Cross-sectional spectral domain-OCT imaging of vitreomacular traction. Partially adherent vitreous exerting traction on the retinal surface, causing the foveal depression to disappear. The inner retinal layers are pulled up into a cone at the site of traction

Anomalous posterior vitreous detachment is not the cause of vitreomacular or vitreopapillary traction in these cases. Microstructural changes in the retina due to vector forces of the fibrous traction bands are well discerned with the help of three-dimensional SD-OCT (Fig. 2.19). The ILM-RPE segmentation maps are useful in depicting the topographical changes due to traction caused by fibrous bands. These maps reveal the surface alterations on the retina, internal limiting membrane, and the changes in retinal thickness.

2.2.12 Macular Dystrophies

Stargardt disease (STGD) is an autosomal recessive macular dystrophy, linked to mutation of the ABCA4 gene, characterized by early onset, rapid progression, and poor visual outcome. Fundus flavimaculatus (FFM) is a variant dystrophy with late onset and slow progression. The ABCA4 gene codes for a transport protein that is involved in the visual cycle and located in the photoreceptor outer segments. Mutation in ABCA4 results in abnormal accumulation in RPE and consequent RPE degeneration and photoreceptor disruption. Both dystrophies are characterized by macular atrophy and fleck-like deposits in the retina of varying size and shapes (Querques et al. 2006). SD-OCT is helpful in these cases in revealing photoreceptor disruption and appropriate localization of the flecks in different layers of

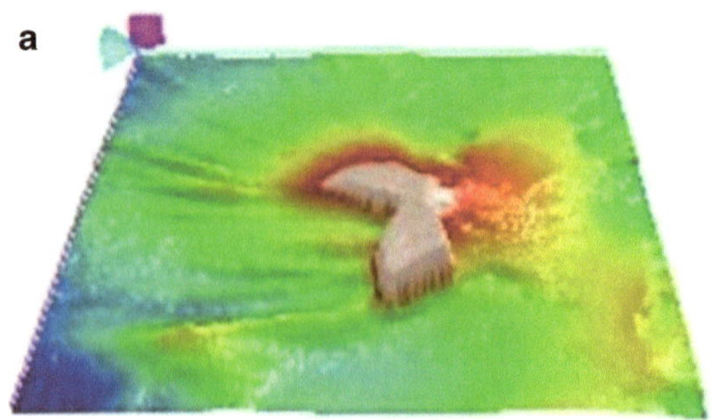

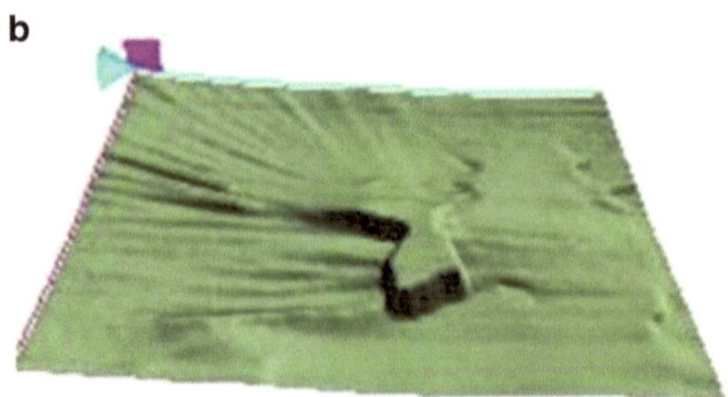

Fig. 2.17 (**a**) Internal limiting membrane-retinal pigment epithelium (ILM-RPE) thickness map with false color coding demonstrating thickened retina, presence of radial folds and elevated ILM cone at the site of adhesion to vitreous. (**b**) Surface topography internal limiting membrane (ILM) map depicting surface elevation at the site of adherence with vitreous surrounded by radiating folds

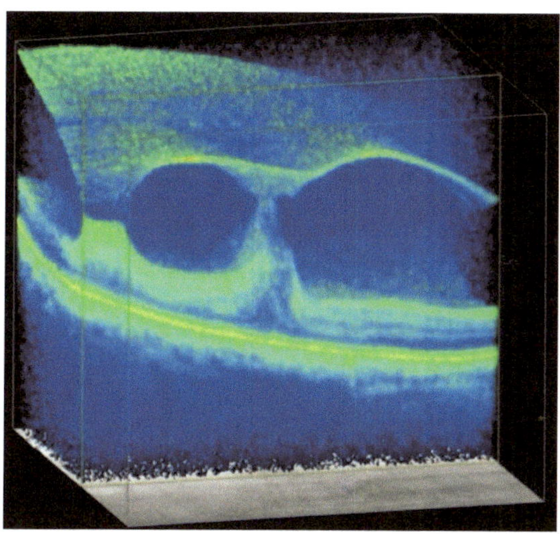

Fig. 2.18 Three-dimensional imaging along the X plane showing vitreoretinal interaction with elevation of inner retinal layers at sites of persistent attachment of vitreous

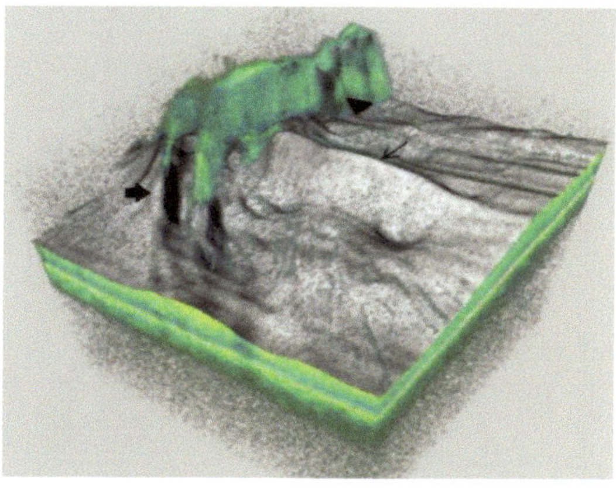

Fig. 2.19 Eales' disease. Three-dimensional spectral domain optical coherence tomography showing vitreomacular traction (*arrow*) highlighted on the internal limiting membrane (*gray tone*) due to fibrous proliferation in Eales' disease (Reprinted with permission from Saxena et al.)

the retina and their anatomic configuration with one another (Querques et al. 2009). Voigt et al. (2010) demonstrated presence of flecks at five different levels in FFM. They reported flecks at the level of outer segment of the photoreceptors, the RPE interdigitations, at and beneath the RPE/Bruch membrane complex, interface of photoreceptors and external limiting membrane, and a few flecks at the level of outer nuclear layer. Verdina et al. (2012) showed the absence of isolated flecks at ONL and reported that there was a presence of anatomical connection between all the hyperreflective flecks at the level of ONL with the one present at the level of RPE. These represent the different appearances or stages of the same lesion. On SD-OCT, flecks at the level of RPE correspond to areas with disruption of ellipsoid zone of the photoreceptor.

Three-dimensional SD-OCT imaging provides novel insight into the in vivo retinal morphology and pathogenesis of STGD and FFM (Saxena et al. 2012e). The atrophic area in fovea may be surrounded by a transition zone which is hypothesized to represent areas in the process of photoreceptor disruption. Macular visualization on SD-OCT demonstrates central macular atrophy with loss of the photoreceptor layer, marked thinning of outer nuclear layer, and residual neurosensory retina. Peripheral retinal layers are structurally normal. Segmentation maps provide ancillary findings. The ILM-RPE thickness maps reveal two concentric ring-like patterns for the two zones in both STGD and FFM. The inner zone of accentuated foveal depression, surrounded by an outer transitional zone, is visualized. Analysis of a single ILM map gives a better definition of the two zones in the case of FFM as compared to STGD. A segmentation map of RPE demonstrates the flecks as surface irregularities. The distribution of flecks on a RPE topography map further distinguish the two variants; a widespread distribution of flecks all over the posterior pole is a feature of STGD, whereas in FFM, flecks are present only along the vascular arcades. Irregular hyperreflectivity below the RPE was more prominent in the subfoveal area in the case of Stargardt (Figs. 2.20 and 2.21).

2.2.13 Foveal Retinoschisis

X-linked foveal retinoschisis is caused by mutations in the XLRS1 gene on chromosome Xp22 encoding *retinoschisin*, which is primarily expressed in the photoreceptor and bipolar cells. The disease is characterized by degeneration of

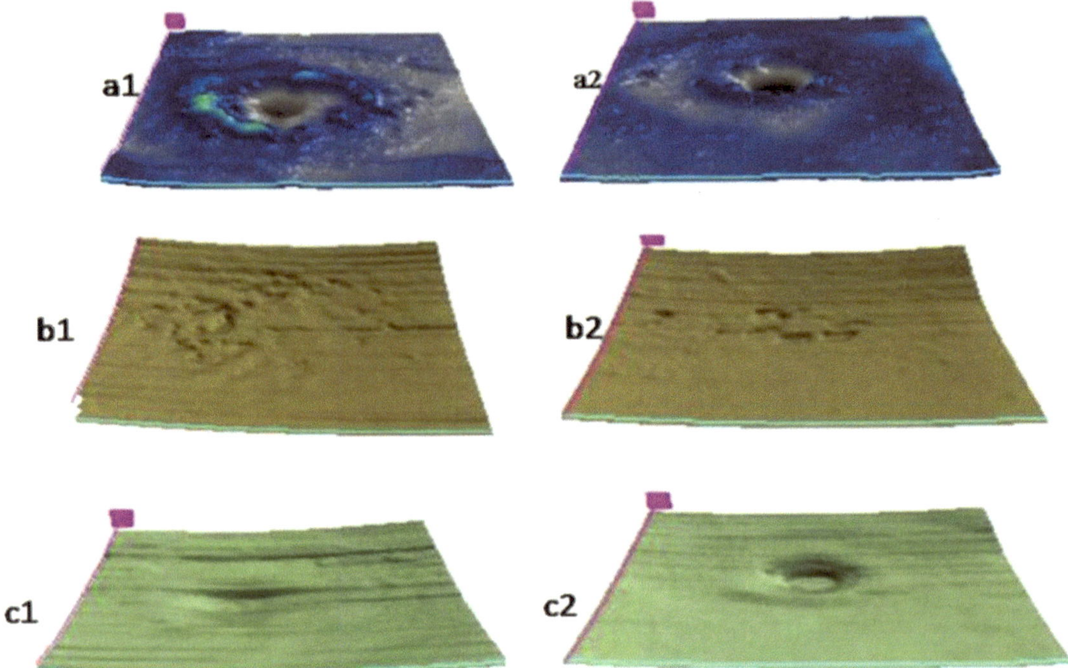

Fig. 2.20 Internal limiting membrane-retinal pigment epithelium (ILM-RPE) maps showing the two areas of central macular atrophy and the transitional zone in Stargardt disease (**a1**) and fundus flavimaculatus (**a2**), respectively. RPE maps showing irregularities corresponding to the flecks, more widespread in Stargardt disease (**b1**) as compared to FFM (**b2**). The ILM map shows the two zones of central macular atrophy and the transitional zone much more distinct in fundus flavimaculatus as two concentric rings (**c2**) as compared to Stargardt disease (**c1**)

vitreous and splitting of the retina. Bilateral asymmetric involvement occurs. Macular changes are present in almost all cases. Intraretinal cysts or schitic cavities form in the macula; however studies have documented no significant correlation between visual acuity and size of intraretinal cyst (Apushkin et al. 2005). Schisis at the level of the retinal nerve fiber layer, ganglion cell layer, outer plexiform layer, inner nuclear layer, and outer nuclear layer is observed. Bullous and atrophic morphological subtypes have been classified based on clinical and OCT findings (Eriksson et al. 2004; Greene and Shakin 2004). Bullous retinoschisis have been documented in a younger age group with involvement of all the retinal layers with increased retinal thickness. With advancement of the disease, the retina becomes atrophic with foveal contour flattening, widening, and minor RPE changes. Schisis within the inner nuclear layer of perifoveal areas is observed (Yanoff and Fine 1989). Disruption of the ELM and EZ occurs in almost all cases. These changes have been correlated with findings on histopathology (Condon et al. 1986). Three-dimensional imaging well defines the extent and configuration of splitting (Gerth et al. 2008; Prenner et al. 2006). The foveal contour changes along with elevation of the outer retinal layers due to traction are well enhanced (Saxena et al. 2013a). Vitreous veils, overlying the schisis, causing traction on inner retinal layers are observed. OCT also reveals subclinical schisis areas or extension to the optic disc area or beyond. Color-coded ILM-RPE thickness maps and ILM maps show elevation or tenting in the foveal area due to subclinical traction. SD-OCT is an important adjunct for assessment of foveal retinoschisis (Figs. 2.22 and 2.23).

2.2.14 Toxoplasma

Ocular toxoplasmosis is known to occur either in a congenital or a postnatal acquired form. Congenital toxoplasma becomes clinically apparent decades later. Acquired toxoplasmosis is the most common cause of infectious retinitis in immunocompetent individuals. Bilateral development may occur during the acute phase of the infection or more commonly many months to years later. The hallmark is a necrotizing retinochoroiditis satellite lesion adjacent to old hyperpigmented scars accompanied by vitreous inflammation and anterior uveitis along with vasculitis. Clinical course varies from benign self-limited disease to vision-threatening cases depending on involvement of critical structures.

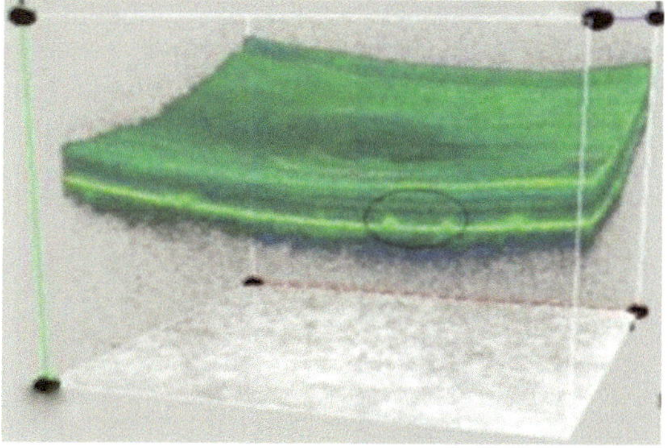

Fig. 2.21 Three-dimensional visualization shows flecks at the level of retinal pigment epithelium (enclosed in *black circle*) in an eye with Fundus flavimaculatus

Toxoplasma retinochoroiditis can be associated with severe morbidity if the disease extends to the macula and optic nerve, or if there are complications such as retinal detachment due to necrotic hole formation or tractional changes or neovascularization.

Spectral domain OCT in active toxoplasmosis enabled identification of morphological features underestimated on clinical examination (Monnet et al. 2009; Orefice et al. 2007). SD-OCT imaging revealed features like diffuse macular edema, VMT, maculoschisis, and relative hyperreflectivity of choriocapillaris/choroid in the central atrophic area and posterior vitreous detachment. Absent retinal nerve fiber layer, splitting of layers of the retina at the outer nuclear layer, and discontinuation of the photoreceptor layer are conspicuous subclinical findings well visualized on a 3D macular cube (Garg et al. 2009). Retinal thinning in the scar area correlates with a histopathological finding of severe destruction of the infected area with chorioretinal adhesion. OCT imaging has been found to be helpful in cases with better visual acuity with localization of lesion in parafoveal areas or with intact neurosensory layer. Three-dimensional SD-OCT allows comprehensive imaging of excavated lesion in healed cases (Saxena et al. 2010). The RPE segmentation maps accentuate the excavated scar/atrophy, as it illustrates increased thickness at the periphery of the lesion with loss of RPE in the center of the lesion (Figs. 2.24, 2.25 and 2.26).

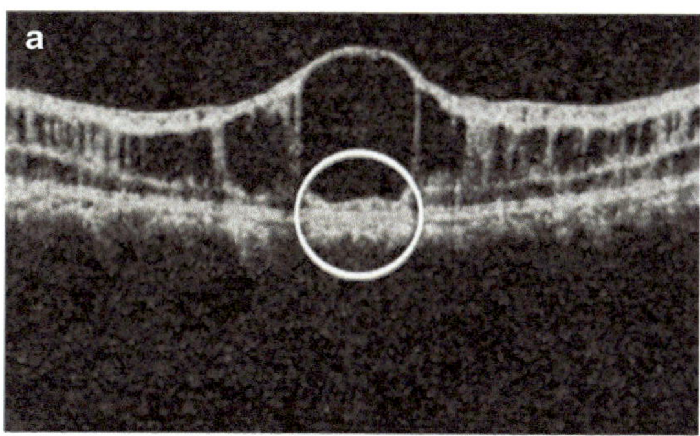

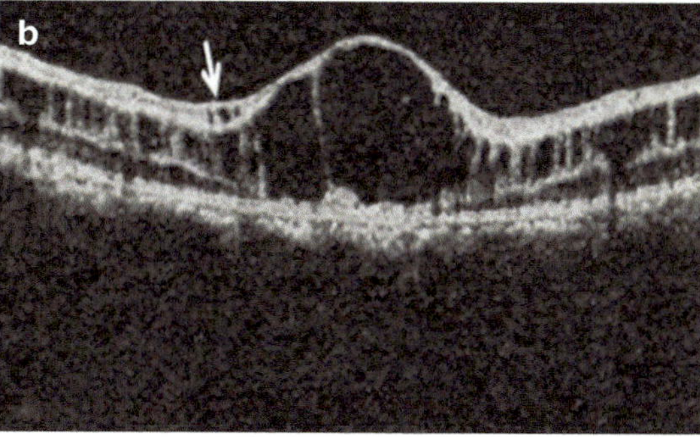

Fig. 2.22 Spectral domain OCT showing foveal retinoschisis. (**a**) Disruption of the outer nuclear layer, external limiting membrane, and inner segment ellipsoid zone (*circle*). (**b**) SD-OCT showing two large central cysts with intervening connecting palisade in outer plexiform layer in the foveal region. Three small cysts are observed in the inner nuclear layer (*arrow*)

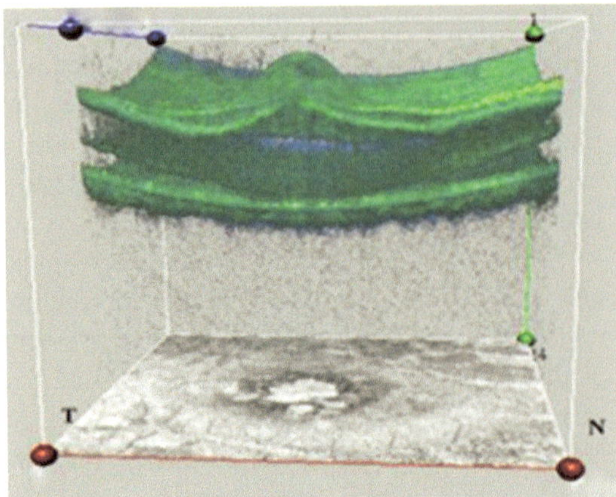

Fig. 2.23 Three-dimensional image showing tractional elevation of inner layers of the retina leading to tenting in that region and schisis in the inner nuclear layer

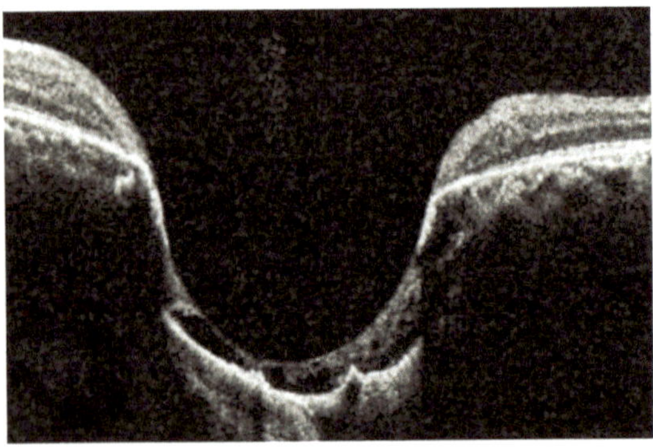

Fig. 2.24 Spectral domain OCT image scan through the center of a toxoplasma lesion showing with discontinuation of photoreceptor layer, inner segment ellipsoid zone, relative hyperreflectivity of choriocapillaris, and increased thickness of retinal pigment epithelium at periphery

2.2.15 Choroidal Tuberculoma

Intraocular involvement in tuberculosis is believed to develop via a hematogenous spread from the lung. Tuberculosis can have a variety of ocular manifestations and consequently may mimic a number of ocular inflammatory diseases. A definitive diagnosis of ocular TB requires a combination of clinical signs consistent with known patterns of ocular TB and a demonstration of the mycobacterium by means of culture, DNA amplification from ocular samples, or a positive response to a week of therapeutic trial of antitubercular therapy. The common presenting manifestation of intraocular TB is reported to be choroidal tubercles, tuberculomas, and serpiginous choroiditis (Gupta et al. 2015). Choroidal tuberculomas are known to present as solitary subretinal mass, mimicking a choroidal tumor. Exudative retinal detachment is common in the area surrounding the tuberculoma and is responsive to antitubercular treatment (Bodaghi and Le Hoang 2000; Salman et al. 2006). Enhanced depth imaging SD-OCT, improves the visibility of the choroid (Spaide et al. 2008). Three-dimensional SD-OCT imaging of choroidal tuberculoma well documents the spatial visualization of the elevated retina (Saxena et al. 2013c). Hyperplastic RPE with proliferating RPE cells and granular outer plexiform layer due to phagocytosed photoreceptor cells is observed. This results from chronicity of the underlying lesion abutting the retina. 3D SD-OCT exquisitely demonstrates the response to antitubercular therapy with decrease in retinal elevation and resolution of the subfoveal neurosensory detachment (Figs. 2.27, and 2.28).

2.2.16 Welder's Arc Maculopathy

Light emitted during the use of welding tools affects the eye in various ways. Ultraviolet emission affects the cornea and lens, while the infrared radiation damages the retina, primarily affecting the macula. Three-dimensional SD-OCT comprehends the topographical alteration in photic maculopathy (Saxena et al. 2014). Photoreceptors are the main focus of damage. Advanced macular visualization on 3D SD-OCT shows disruption of EZ in the subfoveal area. Presence of cystoid changes at the photoreceptor layer along with hyperreflective material in the area of disruption is observed (Cellini et al. 2011). These changes may not present in the acute phase requiring SD-OCT imaging at follow-up to appreciate the damage to the outer

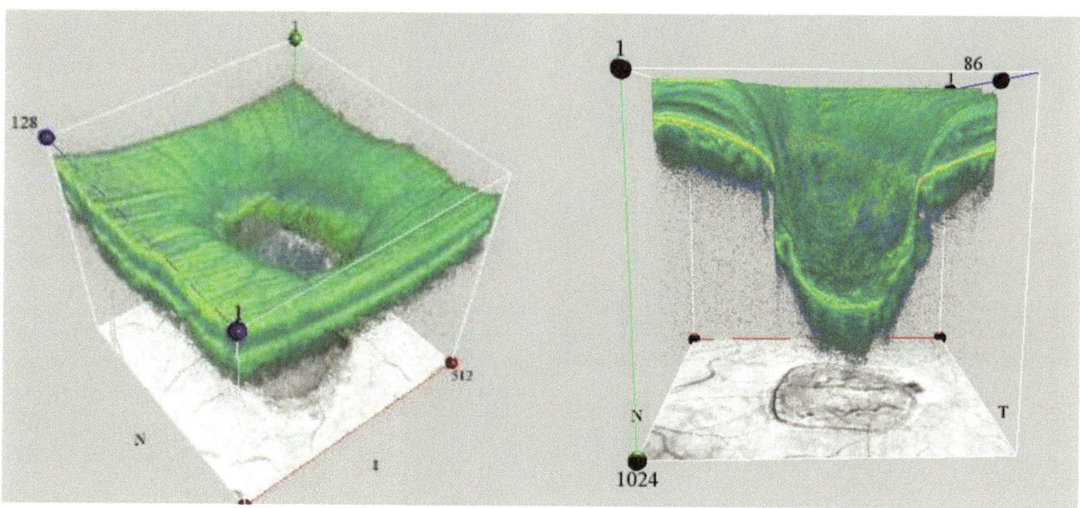

Fig. 2.25 Three-dimensional imaging showing the excavated central toxoplasma scar with central thinning of the retina and discontinuation of the photoreceptor layer

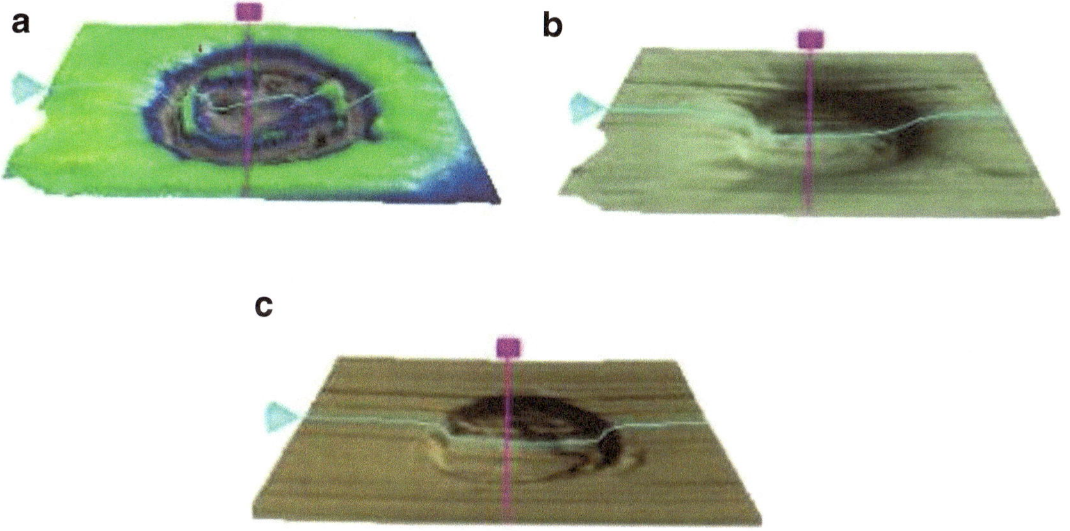

Fig. 2.26 Segmentation maps. (**a**) Internal limiting membrane-retinal pigment epithelium (ILM-RPE) thickness map showing atrophic central toxoplasma scar. (**b**) Excavated scar evident on ILM contour map. (**c**) RPE atrophy with increased thickness at periphery

retinal layers with time (Bonyadi 2013). Chronic changes observed in photic injury by welding arc, solar retinopathy, and distant lightning strike are similar (Bonyadi et al. 2011). Solar radiation is responsible for reduced phagocytosis of the OS. This results in increased accumulation of the OS in the outer retina and subretinal space. The hyperreflective material in the area of photodisruption of EZ may result from increased accumulation of the cone OS. Ingestion of pho-

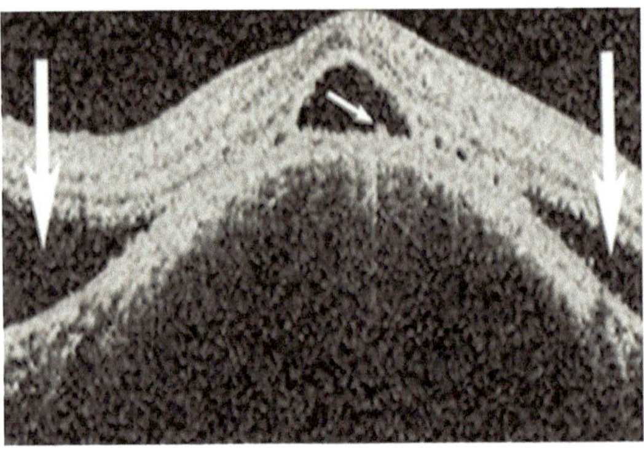

Fig. 2.27 Spectral domain optical coherence tomography of choroidal tuberculoma showing subfoveal neurosensory detachment and proliferating retinal pigment epithelial cells (*small white arrow*) with parafoveal serous retinal detachment (*large white arrows*)

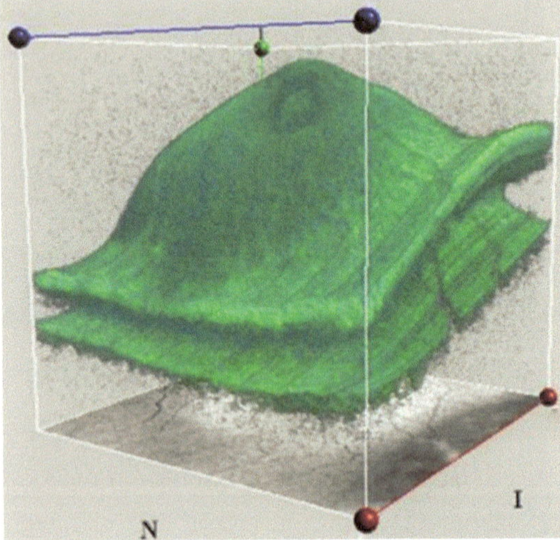

Fig. 2.28 Three-dimensional OCT of tuberculoma with exudative retinal detachment

tosensitizing drugs such as hydrochlorothiazide, furosemide, allopurinol, benzodiazepines, and fluphenazine increase the risk of photic maculopathy (Power et al. 1991) (Figs. 2.29 and 2.30).

2.2.17 Choroidal Metastasis

Intraocular metastasis is considered the most common malignancy of the eye. The frequency of choroidal metastasis is estimated to be approximately 2–7 % (Eliassi-Rad et al. 1996). Intraocular metastasis might well be the only sight of involvement of the disease with no systemic primary lesion. The most common location for choroidal metastases is the posterior pole of the globe. Up to 40 % of lesions have been reported to be in the macular region.

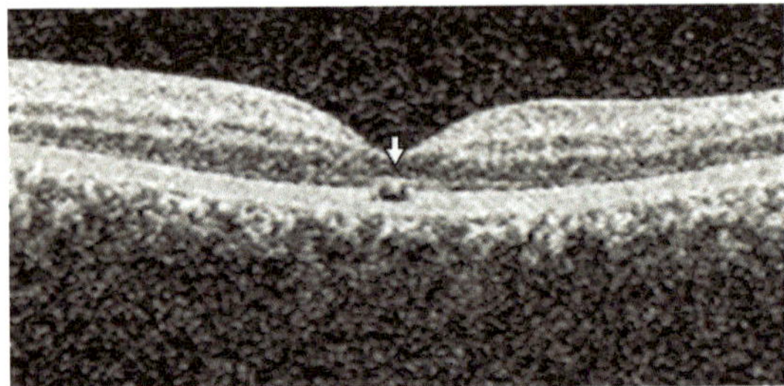

Fig. 2.29 Cross-sectional spectral domain optical coherence tomography showing disruption of the inner segment ellipsoid zone with presence of hyperreflective material in the area of defect in an eye with Welder's arc maculopathy

The distribution of tumors within the choroid is speculated to be related to its vascular characteristics (Ferry and Font 1974). Abundant supply of posterior ciliary arteries to the choroid allows a greater flow of tumor emboli to the posterior uvea as compared to fewer anterior ciliary vessels supplying the anterior uvea. The common primary sites of cancer are the breast, lung, and gastrointestinal tract with rarer presentation with metastasis due to endometrial carcinoma. Symptoms range from being asymptomatic to painless visual loss by involvement of the macular area or an associated exudative retinal detachment. Diagnosis of ocular metastases is based primarily on clinical findings supplemented by imaging studies like fluorescein angiography and ultrasonography (Arevalo et al. 2005; Perez-Alvarez et al. 2009). SD-OCT clearly outlines the changes in the retinal architecture due to the underlying choroidal mass (Fig. 2.29). 3D SD-OCT features of the retina following choroidal metastasis due to breast, lung, and uterine endometrial carcinoma have been reported (Saxena et al. 2012b, c).

Metastatic lesion shows retinal elevation with intraretinal splitting or associated neurosensory retinal detachment with subretinal fluid overlying a thickened hyperreflective RPE-choriocapillaris complex. Large cystoid spaces localized between the inner and outer retina, in the outer plexiform layer, and occasionally in the inner plexiform layer are observed. These cystoid spaces are not of uniform thickness, and multiple bridging strands traverse them. RPE segmentation map with false color-coding layer reveals hyperplastic, irregular, and disfigured RPE. The photoreceptor layer is anteriorly displaced by subretinal fluid. This outer photoreceptor layer shows the presence of granularity with low reflective particles representing phagocytosed outer photoreceptor cells. Neurosensory detachment results from effusion of fluid from the underlying choroidal lesion. However, at places where the choroidal lesion tightly abuts the retina, a shearing force of effusing fluid does not create a cleavage plane between the RPE and neurosensory retina; instead splitting of retinal layers occurs due to retinal degeneration.

SD-OCT elegantly differentiates metastatic lesions from primary choroidal pathology like melanoma, osteoma, disciform scar, and subretinal hemorrhage. Changes at the level of the photoreceptor help in prognosticating the disease. Imaging defines the number, size, depth, and location of the lesion relative to the fovea and helps in identifying the treatment modality. SD-OCT helps follow up the patient both prior to and post treatment (Figs. 2.31 and 2.32).

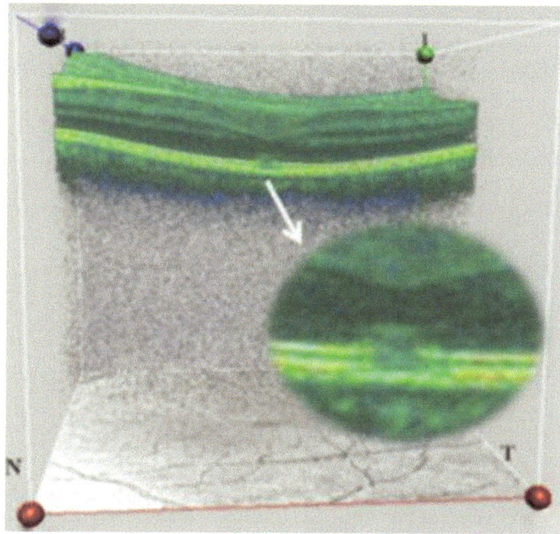

Fig. 2.30 Advanced three-dimensional analyses showing defect in the inner segment ellipsoid zone with significant hyperreflective material in the area of disruption in an eye with Welder's arc maculopathy

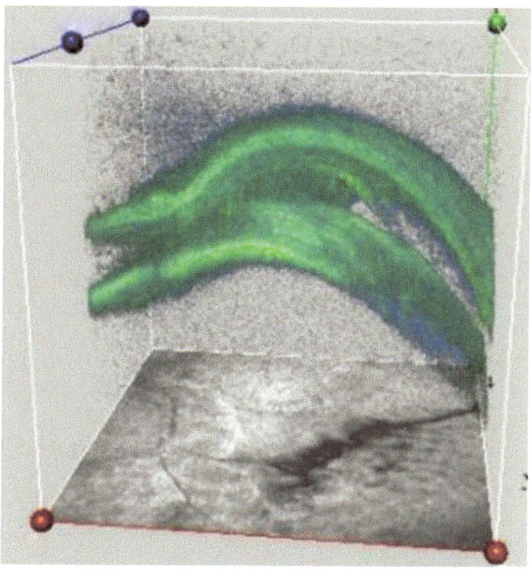

Fig. 2.31 Three-dimensional imaging of choroidal metastasis from endometrial carcinoma showing neurosensory detachment

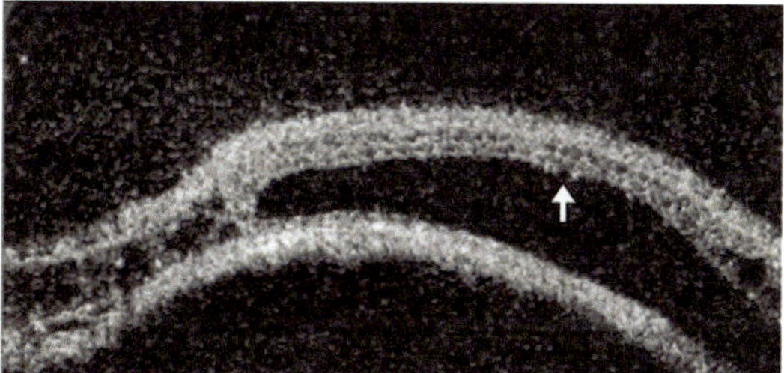

Fig. 2.32 Spectral domain optical coherence tomography of the retina over the tumor mass shows neurosensory detachment with splitting of the retinal layers at some places. Large cystoid spaces are noticed that are localized in the outer plexiform layer with multiple bridging strands crossing in the cystoid spaces. Occasional tiny pockets of cystoid changes are seen in the inner retina. In areas of neurosensory detachment, the outer photoreceptor layer shows the presence of granularity (*arrow*)

References

Abe S, Yamamoto T, Kashiwagi Y et al (2013) Three-dimensional imaging of the inner limiting membrane folding on the vitreomacular interface in diabetic macular edema. Jpn J Ophthalmol 57:553–562

Ahlers C, Geitzenauer W, Simader C et al (2008) New perspectives in diagnostics: high resolution optical coherence tomography for age related macular degeneration. Ophthalmologe 105:248–254

Albert C, Bernd K, Sascha F (2011) Retinal pigment epithelium tears secondary to age-related macular degeneration—a simultaneous confocal scanning laser ophthalmoscopy and spectral-domain optical coherence tomography study. Arch Ophthalmol 129:575–579

Altaweel M, Ip M (2003) Macular hole: improved understanding of pathogenesis, staging, and management based on optical coherence tomography. Semin Ophthalmol 18:58–66

Apushkin MA, Fishman GA, Janowicz MJ (2005) Correlation of optical coherence tomography findings with visual acuity and macular lesions in patients with X-linked retinoschisis. Ophthalmology 112:495–501

Arevalo JF, Fernandez CF, Garcia RA (2005) Optical coherence tomography characteristics of choroidal metastasis. Ophthalmology 112:1612–1619

Arevalo JF, Lasave AF, Arias JD et al (2013) Clinical applications of optical coherence tomography in the posterior pole: the 2011 José Manuel Espino Lecture – Part II. Clin Ophthalmol 7:2181–2206

Bodaghi B, Le Hoang P (2000) Ocular tuberculosis. Curr Opin Ophthalmol 11:443–448

Bonyadi MH (2013) Early and late spectral domain optical coherence tomography features of acute welding maculopathy. J Ophthalmic Vis Res 8:391–392

Bonyadi MH, Soheilian R, Soheilian M et al (2011) Spectral-domain optical coherence tomography features of mild and severe acute solar retinopathy. Ophthalmic Surg Lasers Imaging 42:e84–e86

Cellini M, Gattegna R, Toschi PG et al (2011) Multifocal electroretinogram and optical coherence tomography spectral-domain in arc welding macular injury: a case report. BMC Ophthalmol 11:40

Chang LK, Sarraf D (2007) Tears of the retinal pigment epithelium: an old problem in a new era. Retina 27:523–534

Chan CK, Meyer CH, Gross JG et al (2007) Retinal pigment epithelial tears after intravitreal bevacizumab injection for neovascular age related macular degeneration. Retina 27:541–555

Chang LK, Fine HF, Spaide RF et al (2008) Ultrastructural correlation of spectral-domain optical coherence tomographic findings in vitreomacular traction syndrome. Am J Ophthalmol 146:121–127

Chan CK, Abraham P, Meyer CH et al (2010) Optical coherence tomography-measured pigment epithelial detachment height as a predictor for retinal pigment epithelial tears associated with intravitreal bevacizumab injections. Retina 30:203–211

Chiang A, Chang LK, Sarraf D et al (2008) Predictors of anti-VEGF associated retinal pigment epithelial tear using FA and OCT analysis. Retina 28:1265–1269

Condon GP, Brownstein S, Wang NS (1986) Congenital hereditary (juvenile X-linked) retinoschisis: histopathologic and ultrastructural findings in three eyes. Arch Ophthalmol 104:576–583

Curcio CA, Medeiros NE, Millican CL (1996) Photoreceptor loss in age-related macular degeneration. Invest Ophthalmol Vis Sci 37:1236–1249

Duker JS, Kaiser PK, Binder S et al (2013) The International vitreomacular traction study group classification of vitreomacular adhesion, traction and macular hole. Ophthalmology 120:2611–2619

Elbendary AM (2010) Three dimensional characterization of epiretinal membrane using spectral domain optical coherence tomography. Saudi J Ophthalmol 24:37–43

Eliassi-Rad B, Albert DM, Green WR (1996) Frequency of ocular metastases in patients dying of cancer in eye bank populations. Br J Ophthalmol 80:125–128

Eriksson U, Larsson E, Holmstrom G (2004) Optical coherence tomography in the diagnosis of juvenile X linked retinoschisis. Acta Ophthalmol Scand 82:218–223

Ferry AP, Font RL (1974) Carcinoma metastatic to the eye and orbit: a clinicopathologic study of 227 cases. Arch Ophthalmol 92:276–286

Fujimoto H, Gomi F, Wakabayashi T et al (2008) Morphologic changes in acute central serous chorioretinopathy evaluated by Fourier-domain optical coherence tomography. Ophthalmology 115:1494–1500

Gallemore RP, Jumper JM, McCuen BW et al (2000) Diagnosis of vitreoretinal adhesions in macular disease with optical coherence tomography. Retina 20:115–120

Garg S, Mets MB, Bearelly S et al (2009) Imaging of congenital toxoplasmosis macular scars with optical coherence tomography. Retina 29:631–637

Gass JD (1984) Pathogenesis of the tears of the RPE. Br J Ophthalmol 68:513–519

Gass JD (1997) Stereoscopic atlas of macular diseases: diagnosis and treatment. Mosby, St. Louis Missouri

Gerth C, Zawadzki RJ, Werner JS et al (2008) Retinal morphological changes of patients with X-linked retinoschisis evaluated by Fourier-domain optical coherence tomography. Arch Ophthalmol 126:807–811

Greenberg PB, Martidis A, Rogers AH et al (2002) Intravitreal triamcinolone acetonide for macular oedema due to central retinal vein occlusion. Br J Ophthalmol 86:247–248

Greene JM, Shakin EP (2004) Optical coherence tomography findings in foveal schisis. Arch Ophthalmol 122:1066–1067

Gupta V, Shoughy SS, Mahajan S et al (2015) Clinics of ocular tuberculosis. Ocul Immunol Inflamm 23:14–24

Guyer DR, Yannuzzi LA, Slakter JS et al (1994) Digital indocyanine green videoangiography of central serous chorioretinopathy. Arch Ophthalmol 112:1057–1062

Hangai M, Ojima Y, Gotoh N et al (2007) Three-dimensional imaging of macular holes with high-speed optical coherence tomography. Ophthalmology 114:763–773

Haouchine B, Massin P, Tadayoni R et al (2004) Diagnosis of macular pseudoholes and lamellar macular holes by optical coherence tomography. Am J Ophthalmol 138:732–739

Hee MR, Baumal CR, Puliafito CA et al (1996) Optical coherence tomography of age-related macular degeneration and choroidal neovascularization. Ophthalmology 103:1260–1270

Hikichi T, Yoshida A, Trempe CL (1995) Course of vitreomacular traction syndrome. Am J Ophthalmol 119:55–61

Hussain N, Baskar A, Ram LM et al (2006) Optical coherence tomographic pattern of fluorescein angiographic leakage site in acute central serous chorioretinopathy. Clin Experiment Ophthalmol 34:137–140

Inoue M, Watanabe Y, Arakawa A et al (2009) Spectral-domain optical coherence tomography images of inner/outer segment junctions and macular hole surgery outcomes. Graefes Arch Clin Exp Ophthalmol 247:325–330

Ito Y, Terasaki H, Mori M et al (2000) Three-dimensional optical coherence tomography of vitreomacular traction syndrome before and after vitrectomy. Retina 20:403–405

Kamppeter B, Jonas JB (2003) Central serous chorioretinopathy imaged by optical coherence tomography. Arch Ophthalmol 121:742–743

Karatas M, Ramirez JA, Ophir A (2005) Diabetic vitreopapillary traction and macular oedema. Eye 19:676–682

Khanifar AA, Koreishi AF, Izatt JA et al (2008) Drusen ultrastructure imaging with spectral domain optical coherence tomography in age-related macular degeneration. Ophthalmology 115:1883–1890

Koerner F, Garweg J (1999) Vitrectomy for macular pucker and vitreomacular traction syndrome. Doc Ophthalmol 97:449–458

Koizumi H, Spaide RF, Fisher YL et al (2008) Three dimensional evaluation of vitreomacular traction and epiretinal membrane using spectral domain optical coherence tomography. Am J Ophthalmol 145:509–517

Kroll P, Wiegand W, Schmidt J (1999) Vitreopapillary traction in proliferative diabetic vitreoretinopathy. Br J Ophthalmol 83:261–264

Lafaut BA, Aisenbrey S, VandenBroecke C et al (2001) Clinicopathological correlation of retinal pigment epithelial tears in exudative age related macular degeneration: pretear, tear, and scarred tear. Br J Ophthalmol 85:454–460

Legarreta JE, Gregori G, Knighton RW et al (2008) Three-dimensional spectral-domain optical coherence tomography images of the retina in the presence of epiretinal membranes. Am J Ophthalmol 145:1023–1030

Leitritz M, Gelisken F, Inhoffen W et al (2008) Can the risk of retinal pigment epithelium tears after bevacizumab treatment be predicted? An optical coherence tomography study. Eye 22:1504–1507

Lida T, Hagimura N, Sato T et al (2000) Evaluation of central serous chorioretinopathy with optical coherence tomography. Am J Ophthalmol 129:16–20

Mitarai K, Gomi F, Tano Y (2006) Three-dimensional optical coherence tomographic findings in central serous chorioretinopathy. Graefes Arch Clin Exp Ophthalmol 244:1415–1420

Monnet D, Averous K, Delair E et al (2009) Optical coherence tomography in ocular toxoplasmosis. Int J Med Sci 6:137–138

Montero JA, Ruiz-Moreno JM (2005) Optical coherence tomography characterisation of idiopathic central serous chorioretinopathy. Br J Ophthalmol 89:562–564

Mori K, Gehlbach PL, Sano A et al (2004) Comparison of epiretinal membranes of differing pathogenesis using optical coherence tomography. Retina 24:57–62

Ojima Y, Hangai M, Sasahara M et al (2007) Three-dimensional imaging of the foveal photoreceptor layer in central serous chorioretinopathy using high-speed optical coherence tomography. Ophthalmology 114:2197–2207

Ophir A, Martinez MR (2011) Epiretinal membranes and incomplete posterior vitreous detachment in diabetic macular edema, detected by spectral-domain optical coherence tomography. Invest Ophthalmol Vis Sci 52:6414–6420

Orefice JL, Costa RA, Orefice F et al (2007) Vitreoretinal morphology in active ocular toxoplasmosis: a prospective study by optical coherence tomography. Br J Ophthalmol 91:773–780

Perez-Alvarez MJ, Arriola-Villalobos P, Reche-Frutos J et al (2009) Choroidal metastasis from a breast carcinoma. Diagnosis and follow-up with optical coherence tomography and fluorescein angiography and autofluorescence with HRA-II (Heidelberg Retina Angiograph). Arch Soc Esp Oftalmol 84:267–270

Piccolino FC, Borgia L (1994) Central serous chorioretinopathy and indocyanine green angiography. Retina 14:231–242

Piccolino FC, Longrais RR, Ravera G et al (2005) The foveal photoreceptor layer and visual acuity loss in central serous chorioretinopathy. Am J Ophthalmol 139:87–99

Podoleanu AG, Jackson DA (1998) Combined optical coherence tomograph and scanning laser ophthalmoscope. Electron Lett 34:1088–1090

Podoleanu AG, Seeger M, Dobre GM et al (1998) Transversal and longitudinal images from the retina of the living eye using low coherence reflectometry. J Biomed Opt 3:12–20

Power WJ, Travers SP, Mooney DJ (1991) Welding arc maculopathy and fluphenazine. Br J Ophthalmol 75:433–435

Prenner JL, Capone A Jr, Ciaccia S et al (2006) Congenital X-linked retinoschisis classification system. Retina 26:S61–S64

Puliafito CA, Hee MR, Lin CP et al (1995) Imaging of macular diseases with optical coherence tomography. Ophthalmology 102:217–229

Punjabi OS, Flynn HW Jr, Knighton RW et al (2008) Spectral domain optical coherence tomography for proliferative diabetic retinopathy with subhyaloid hemorrhage. Ophthalmic Surg Lasers Imaging 39: 494–496

Querques G, Leveziel N, Benhamou N et al (2006) Analysis of retinal flecks in fundus flavimaculatus using optical coherence tomography. Br J Ophthalmol 90:1157–1162

Querques G, Prato R, Coscas G et al (2009) In vivo visualization of photoreceptor layer and lipofuscin accumulation in Stargardt's disease and fundus flavimaculatus by high resolution spectral-domain optical coherence tomography. Clin Ophthalmol 3:693–699

Querques G, Avellis FO, Querques L et al (2011) Three dimensional spectral domain optical coherence tomography features of retinal-choroidal anastomosis. Graefes Arch Clin Exp Ophthalmol 250:165–173

Regatieri CV, Branchini L, Fujimoto JG et al (2012) Choroidal imaging using spectral-domain optical coherence tomography. Retina 32:865–876

Salman A, Parmar P, Rajamohan M et al (2006) Optical coherence tomography in choroidal tuberculosis. Am J Ophthalmol 142:170–172

Saxena S, Kumar D (2000) Macular involvement in Eales disease. Ann Ophthalmol 32:98–100

Saxena S, Meredith TA (2006) Optical coherence tomography. In: Saxnea S, Meredith TA (eds) Optical coherence tomography in retinal diseases, 1st edn. McGraw-Hill publishers, New York

Saxena S, Rastogi RAK, Vishvkarma K et al (2010) Spectral-domain optical coherence tomography in healed ocular toxoplasmosis. J Ocul Biol Dis Inform 3:109–111

Saxena S, Sinha N, Sharma S (2011) Three-dimensional imaging by spectral domain optical coherence tomography in central serous chorioretinopathy with fibrin. J Ocul Biol Dis Inform 4:149–153

Saxena S, Jain A, Akduman L (2012) Vitreopapillary and vitreomacular traction in proliferative Eales' disease. BMJ Case Rep. doi:10.1136/bcr-2012-007231

Saxena S, Jain A, Akduman L (2012b) Three-dimensional spectral domain optical coherence tomography of retina in choroidal metastasis due to breast and lung carcinoma. J Ocul Biol Dis Infor 5:9–12

Saxena S, Jain A, Sharma SR, Meyer CH (2012c) Three-dimensional spectral domain optical coherence tomography of retina in choroidal metastasis due to uterine endometrial carcinoma. BMJ Case Rep 11:2012

Saxena S, Mishra N, Meyer CH (2012d) 3D spectral domain OCT in spontaneous retinal pigment epithelial tear. J Ocul Biol Dis Infor 5:70–76

Saxena S, Mishra N, Meyer CH (2012e) Three-dimensional spectral domain optical coherence tomography in Stargardt disease and fundus flavimaculatus. J Ocul Biol Dis Infor 5:13–18

Saxena S, Manisha, Meyer CH (2013a) Three-dimensional spectral domain optical coherence tomography in X linked foveal retinoschisis. BMJ Case Rep. doi:10.1136/bcr-2012-007661

Saxena S, Mishra N, Meyer CH et al (2013b) Ischaemia-reperfusion injury in central retinal artery occlusion. BMJ Case Rep. doi:10.1136/bcr-2013-201415

Saxena S, Singhal V, Akduman L (2013c) Three-dimensional spectral domain optical coherence tomography imaging of the retina in choroidal tuberculoma. BMJ Case Rep. doi:10.1136/bcr-2012-008156

Saxena S, Mishra N, Meyer CH (2014) Three-dimensional spectral domain optical coherence tomography in chronic exposure to welding arc. BMJ Case Rep

Scheider A, Nasemann JE, Lund OE (1993) Fluorescein and indocyanine green angiographies of central serous choroidopathy by scanning laser ophthalmoscopy. Am J Ophthalmol 115:50–56

Schmidt D, Kube T, Feltgen N (2006) Central retinal artery occlusion: findings in optical coherence tomography and functional correlations. Eur J Med Res 11:250–252

Shiraki K, Kohno T, Ataka S et al (2001) Thinning and small holes at an impending tear of a retinal pigment epithelial detachment. Graefes Arch Clin Exp Ophthalmol 239:430–436

Spaide RF (2005) Central serous chorioretinopathy. In: Holz FG, Spaide RF (eds) Medical retina essentials in ophthalmology. Springer, New York

Spaide RF, Lee JK, Klancnik JK Jr et al (2003) Optical coherence tomography of branch retinal vein occlusion. Retina 23:343–347

Spaide RF, Koizumi H, Pozzoni MC (2008) Enhanced depth imaging spectral-domain optical coherence tomography. Am J Ophthalmol 146:496–500

Srinivasan VJ, Wojtkowski M, Witkin AJ et al (2006a) High-definition and 3-dimensional imaging of macular pathologies with high-speed ultrahigh-resolution optical coherence tomography. Ophthalmology 113:2054–2065

Srinivasan VJ, Ko TH, Wojtkowski M et al (2006b) Noninvasive volumetric imaging and morphometry of the rodent retina with high-speed, ultrahigh-resolution optical coherence tomography. Invest Ophthalmol Vis Sci 47:5522–5528

Tilanus MA, Cuypers MH, Bemelmans NA et al (1999) Predictive value of pattern VEP, pattern ERG and hole size in macular hole surgery. Graefes Arch Clin Exp Ophthalmol 237:629–635

Ullrich S, Haritoglou C, Gass C et al (2002) Macular hole size as a prognostic factor in macular hole surgery. Br J Ophthalmol 86:390–393

Verdina T, Tsang SH, Greenstein VC et al (2012) Functional analysis of retinal flecks in stargardt disease. J Clin Exp Ophthalmol 3:6

Voigt M, Querques G, Atmani K et al (2010) Analysis of retinal flecks in fundus flavimaculatus using high-definition spectral-domain optical coherence tomography. Am J Ophthalmol 150:330

Wang MY, Nguyen D, Hindoyan N et al (2009) Vitreopapillary adhesion in macular hole and macular pucker. Retina 29:644–650

Wang GH, Zhang J, Zhang D et al (2011) Value of three dimensional optical coherence tomography and fundus photochromy in correlating the fluorescein

leaking sites of acute central serous chorioretinopathy. Med Princ Pract 20:283–286
Wilkins JR, Puliafito CA, Hee MR et al (1996) Characterization of epiretinal membranes using optical coherence tomography. Ophthalmology 103:2142–2151
Witkin AJ, Ko TH, Fujimoto JG et al (2006) Redefining lamellar holes and the vitreomacular interface: an ultrahigh-resolution optical coherence tomography study. Ophthalmology 113:388–397
Wojtkowski M, Srinivasan V, Fujimoto JG et al (2005) Three-dimensional retinal imaging with highspeed ultrahigh-resolution optical coherence tomography. Ophthalmology 112:1734–1746
Wong JG, Sachdev N, Beaumont PE et al (2005) Visual outcomes following vitrectomy and peeling of epiretinal membrane. Clin Experiment Ophthalmol 33:373–378
Yamada N, Kishi S (2005) Tomographic features and surgical outcomes of vitreomacular traction syndrome. Am J Ophthalmol 139:112–117
Yamaike N, Tsujikawa A, Ota M et al (2008) Three dimensional imaging of cystoid macular edema in retinal vein occlusion. Ophthalmology 115:355–362
Yannuzzi LA, Ober MD, Slakter JS et al (2004) Ophthalmic fundus imaging: today and beyond. Am J Ophthalmol 137:511–524
Yanoff M, Fine BS (1989) Ocular pathology. A text and atlas. Mosby, St. Louis Missouri
Yi K, Mujat M, Park BH et al (2009) Spectral domain optical coherence tomography for quantitative evaluation of drusen and associated structural changes in non-neovascular age-related macular degeneration. Br J Ophthalmol 93:176–181

En Face Optical Coherence Tomography

3

Jessica Lee and Richard B. Rosen

Contents

J. Lee, MD
New York Eye & Ear Infirmary of Mount Sinai, New York, NY, USA

Department of Ophthalmology, Icahn School of Medicine at Mount Sinai, New York, NY, USA

R.B. Rosen, MD, DSc(Hon), FACS, FASRS, CRA (✉)
Retinal Services, New York Eye and Ear Infirmary of Mount Sinai, New York, NY, USA

Department of Ophthalmology, Icahn School of Medicine at Mount Sinai, New York, NY, USA
e-mail: rrosen@nyee.edu

3.1 Introduction

En face optical coherence tomography (OCT) (face-to-face, from French – opposite) is OCT in the standard fundus image perspective of the retina. It incorporates all of the cross-sectional information of conventional sagittal (B-scan) OCT but provides a full field view. En face is the viewpoint captured by ophthalmoscopes, fundus cameras, fluorescein and ICG angiograms, and microperimetry (Fig. 3.1)

Optical coherence tomography (OCT) was a major leap forward providing clinicians access to the cross-sectional details of the retina. Early OCT images, however, had limited resolution of the retinal layers and provided limited lesion localization. The evolution of OCT from time-domain (TD)-OCT to spectral-domain (SD)-OCT has led to better sensitivity and faster acquisition speeds of cross-sectional (B-scan) images. The improved resolution of OCT images has allowed better localization of retinal details, enabling more accurate diagnosis of pathology. OCT has revolutionized the diagnosis and treatment of retinal diseases offering a noninvasive virtual "optical biopsy" of the retina in real time (Fig. 3.2).

As OCT technology advanced, it became increasingly evident that localization of the cross-sectional information was almost as important as the features detected by the technique. In 1997, Podoleanu et al. introduced the concept of en face OCT paired with corresponding scanning laser ophthalmoscopic (SLO) imaging (Podoleanu

C.H. Meyer et al. (eds.), *Spectral Domain Optical Coherence Tomography in Macular Diseases*,
DOI 10.1007/978-81-322-3610-8_3

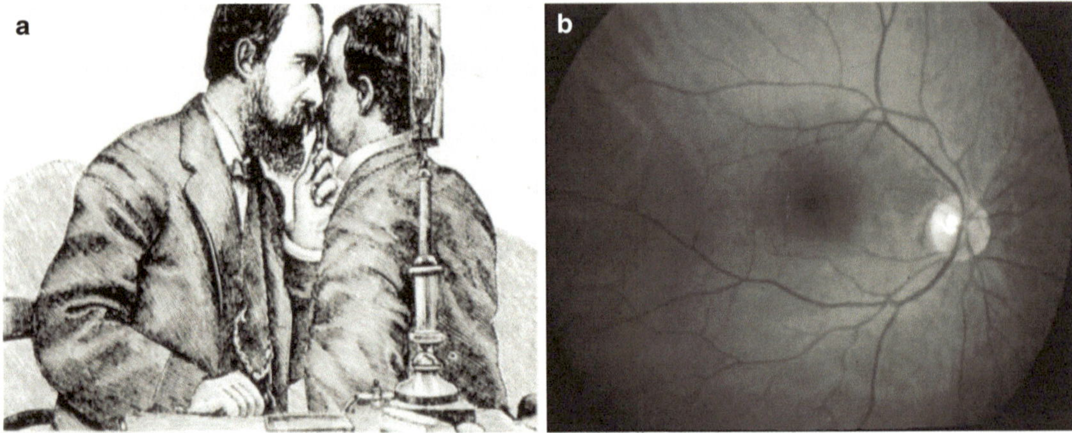

Fig. 3.1 (**a**) Direct fundus examination. (**b**) Standard fundus (en face) view right eye

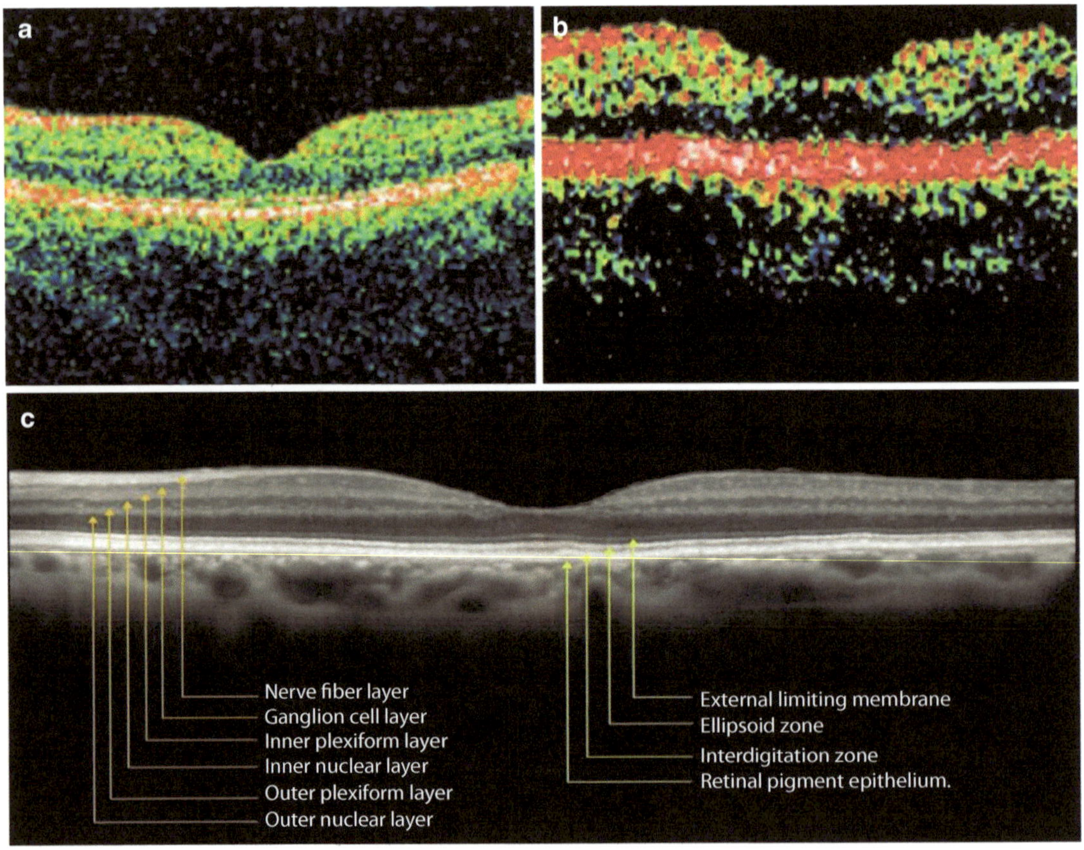

Fig. 3.2 The evolution of optical coherence tomography. (**a**) Time-domain OCT image (1997). (**b**) Time-domain OCT (2001). (**c**) Spectral-domain optical coherence tomography image from the macula of a normal eye. The following retinal layers are labeled: nerve fiber layer, ganglion cell layer, inner plexiform layer, inner nuclear layer, outer plexiform layer, outer nuclear layer, external limiting membrane, ellipsoid zone (previously referred to as the IS-OS junction), interdigitation zone, and retinal pigment epithelium

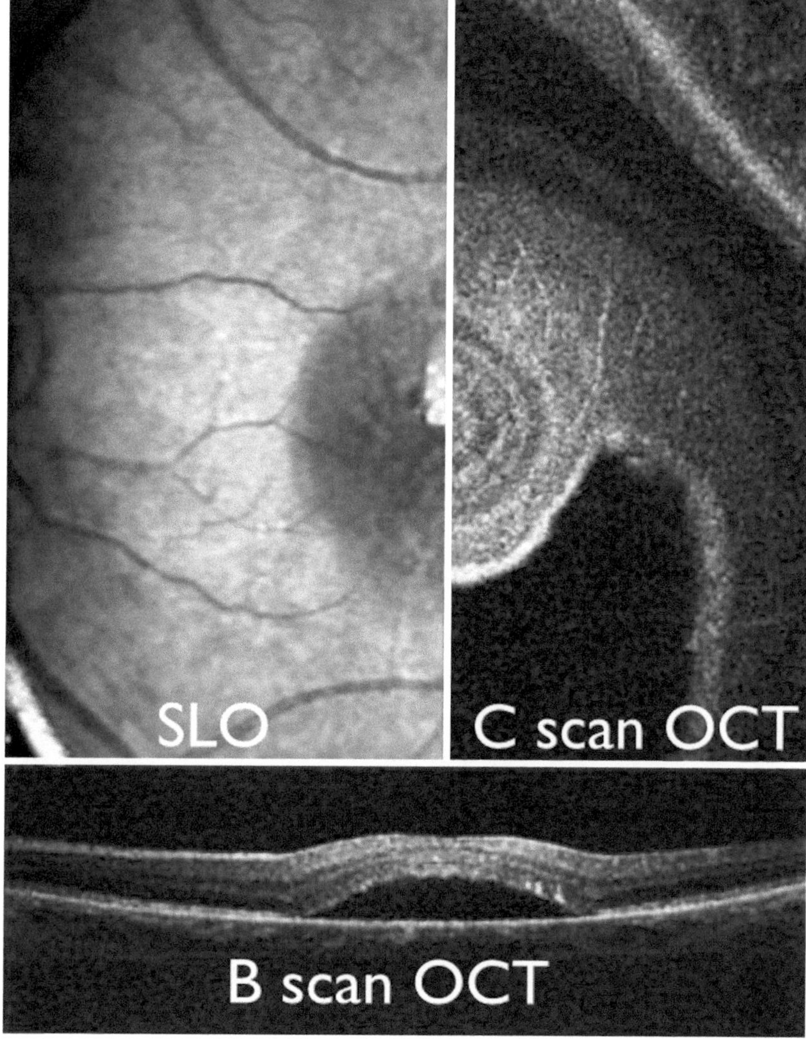

Fig. 3.3 Simultaneous time-domain scanning laser ophthalmoscopy (*SLO*)/en face (*C-scan*) OCT and *B-scan* OCT of a patient with central serous retinopathy. The split image view is used to show the relationship between the surface appearance and internal structure seen with the en face OCT

et al. 1997). Signals from transverse scans of the retina were split between a confocal optical path to produce an SLO image and a Michelson interferometer which generated a series of en face OCT images at progressive depths.

En face imaging using TD-OCT employed lateral scanners with z-axis stages to control depth generating scans in both the transverse and axial directions. The transverse linear scans (T-scans) combined to create C-scan (coronal planar) images. B-scan (sagittal planar) cross-sectional planar images could also be constructed from this optical configuration. C-scan images when generated from axial scans as in the cases of SD-OCT or swept-source (SS)-OCT are constructed by post-processing 3D OCT volumes (Podoleanu 2013) (Fig. 3.3).

The A-scan data is processed through several steps which include zero padding, fast Fourier transformation (FFT), data resampling, spectral shaping, and apodization to render en face images from the 3D volume of A-scans (Bradu and Podoleanu 2014). The time it takes to obtain the transverse scans plus the time required to analyze the scans determines how long it takes to produce an en face image (Zhang and Kang 2010).

Advancements in SD-OCT and swept-source (SS)-OCT technology combined with the use of graphic processing unit cards has helped minimize the time needed to image and process the data allowing for improved en face imaging quality and even approaching real-time en face imaging capabilities.

3.2 Unique Features of En Face Optical Coherence Tomography

There are several features of en face OCT imaging which provide unique clinical advantages. *Familiarity of perspective* is first on the list since en face OCT reveals the retinal surface and subsurface structural details in the orientation of the standard ophthalmoscope. With this perspective, the orientation of features is familiar and intuitive for the examiner to appreciate. The shapes and dimensions of pathological lesions revealed below the retinal surface are more easily interpreted than when transposed into a series of cross sections as provided by standard B-scan OCT imaging.

En face OCT enables precise registration with other imaging modalities, giving the clinician the ability to investigate features with a variety of structural and functional filters. The en face perspective, combined with vertical and horizontal B-scan OCT images, allow the clinician to survey a retinal or choroidal lesion using a convergence of orthogonal views. The ability to simultaneously study surface details provided by scanning laser ophthalmoscopy (SLO) along with en face OCT internal details is often helpful in educating the clinician as to the surface appearance of deeper retinal lesions (Fig. 3.4).

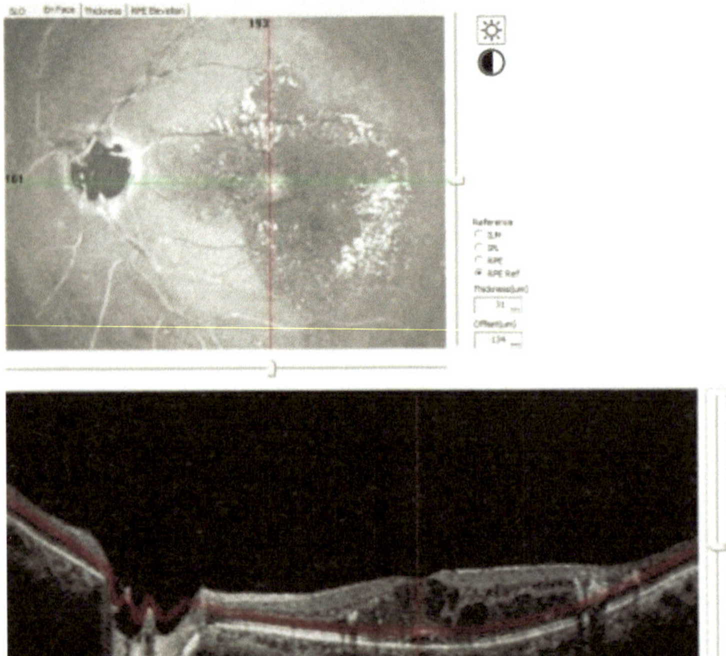

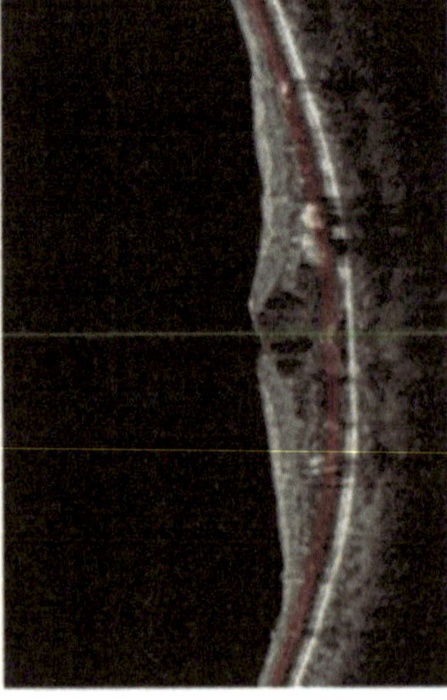

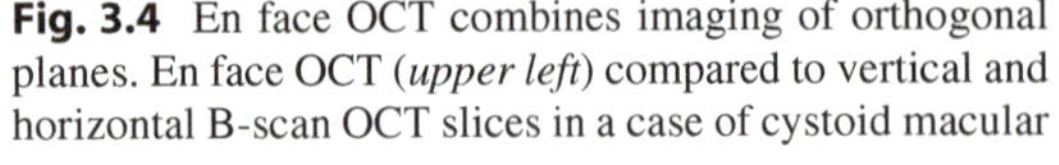

Fig. 3.4 En face OCT combines imaging of orthogonal planes. En face OCT (*upper left*) compared to vertical and horizontal B-scan OCT slices in a case of cystoid macular edema. The en face image reveals the full extent of the outer retinal disturbance

En face OCT reveals each layer of the retina as a separate surface. The contour of the slice will vary depending on which layer of the retina is used as the reference curvature. Choosing the internal limiting membrane vs the retinal pigment epithelium when segmenting the macula will have very different appearances (Figs. 3.5 and 3.6)

The en face perspective can often reveal small lesions that could be easily be missed if only single B-scan OCT slices are used. Since patients will typically fixate using the best part of their retina, small disturbances are preferentially avoided resulting in B-scan OCTs which can appear normal even in abnormal eyes. The expanse of the C-scan view can often pick up these features which can then be reexamined in a B-scan OCT cross-sectional images (Fig. 3.7).

With en face OCT, the extent and expanse of a lesion can be better appreciated. The en face perspective can show the lateral as well as the vertical extent of lesions (Figs. 3.8 and 3.9).

3.3 Vitreomacular Interface

Structural and dimensional details of vitreomacular interface disorders such as epiretinal membranes (ERM) and macular holes can be better delineated with en face OCT. Using en face OCT, certain patterns of idiopathic epiretinal membranes have been identified. Plaques were found to be the most common feature in patients with ERM. The plaques seen on en face OCT correspond generally to localized areas of tight adherence between the retina and the membrane on standard OCT sections. Retinal starfolds were not as common as plaques in patients with ERM and may possibly precede the development of these plaques. Diffuse retinal folds were least commonly seen on en face imaging in patients with an ERM. The identification of certain patterns of ERM seen on en face OCT complements the standard OCT images and can aid surgical planning of membrane peeling (Rispoli et al. 2012) (Fig. 3.10).

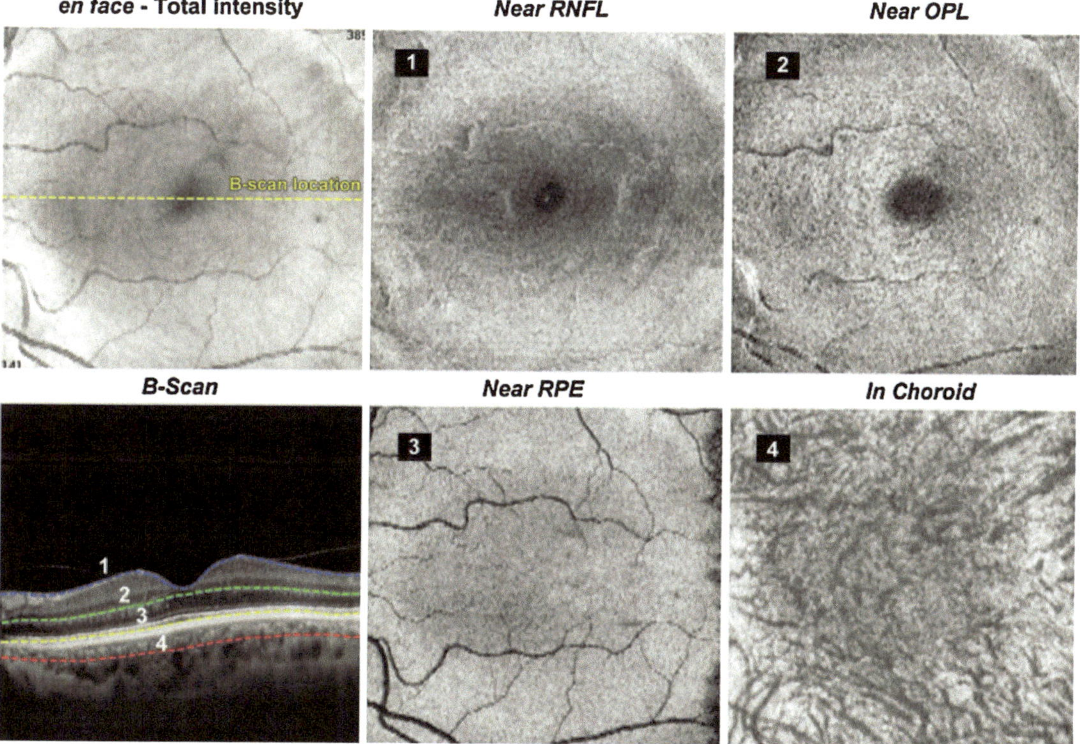

Fig. 3.5 SD-OCT (Avanti) en face of the segmented layers of the macula at progressively deeper layers

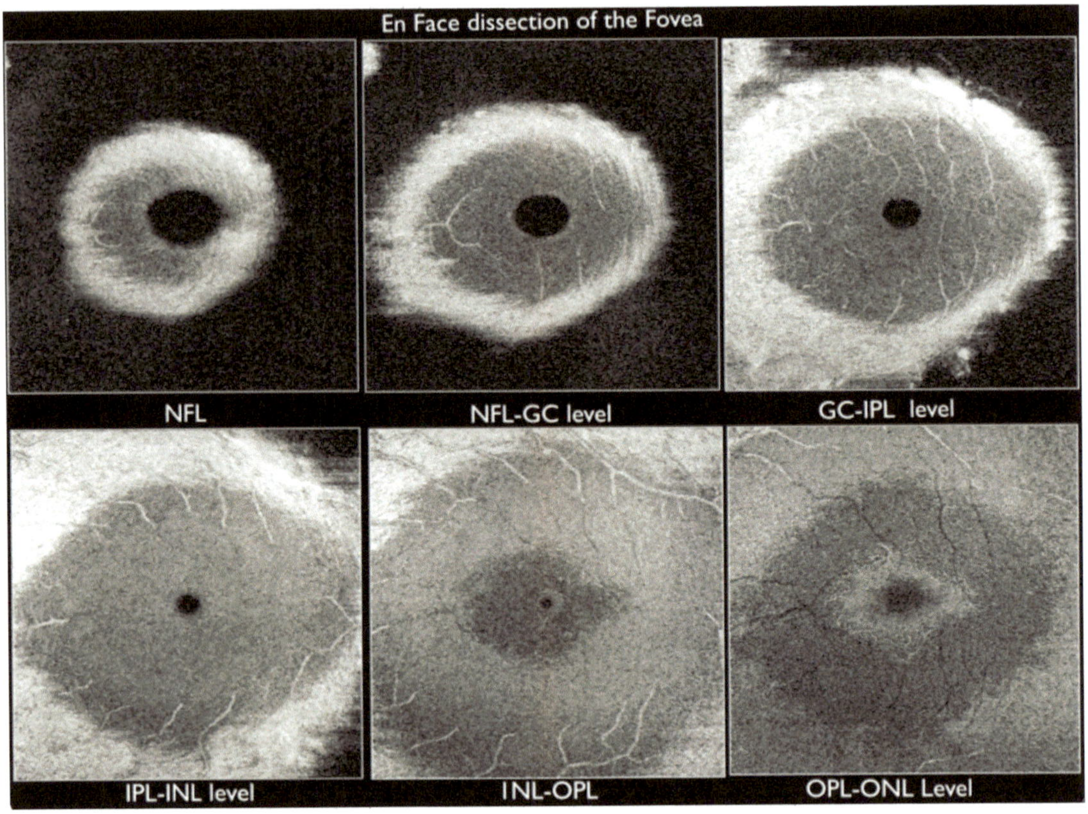

En Face dissection of the Fovea

NFL

NFL-GC level

GC-IPL level

IPL-INL level

INL-OPL

OPL-ONL Level

Fig. 3.6 High-resolution SD-OCT en face dissection of the central macula showing different retinal layers. The unique curvature of the fovea is not easily compensated for by the flattening processing resulting in multiple concentric zones of sequential layers

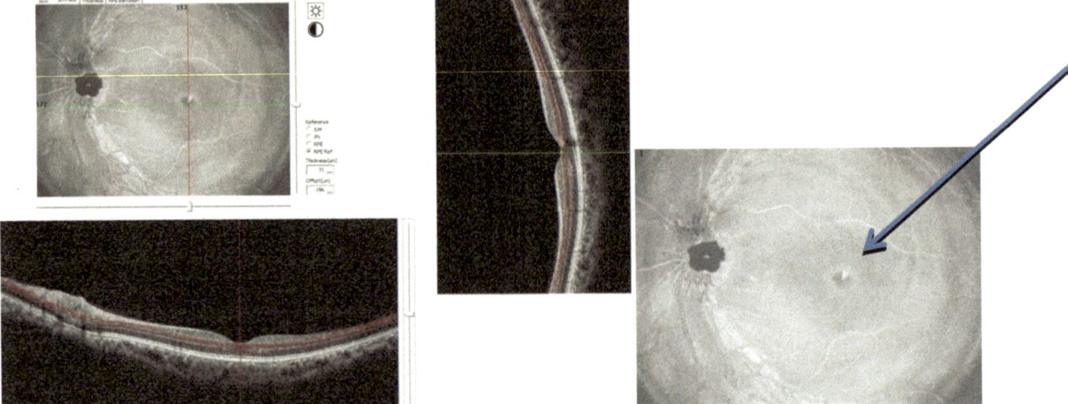

Fig. 3.7 En face OCT identification of a small occult parafoveal intraretinal lesion that was overlooked on standard B-scan OCT

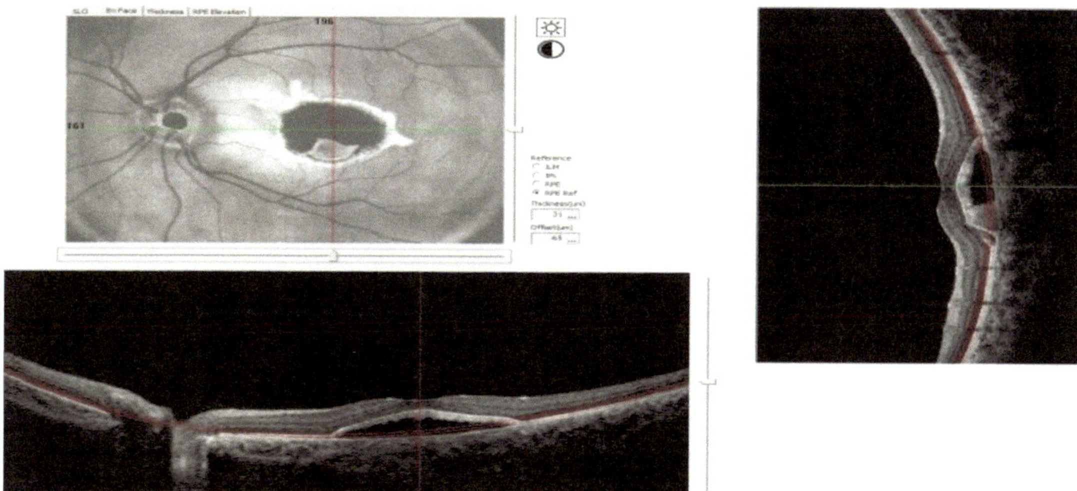

Fig. 3.8 En face OCT and B-scan OCT of pigment epithelial detachment. Note the hypo-reflective center representing the low density serous fluid surrounded by a bright hyper-reflective overlying RPE signal

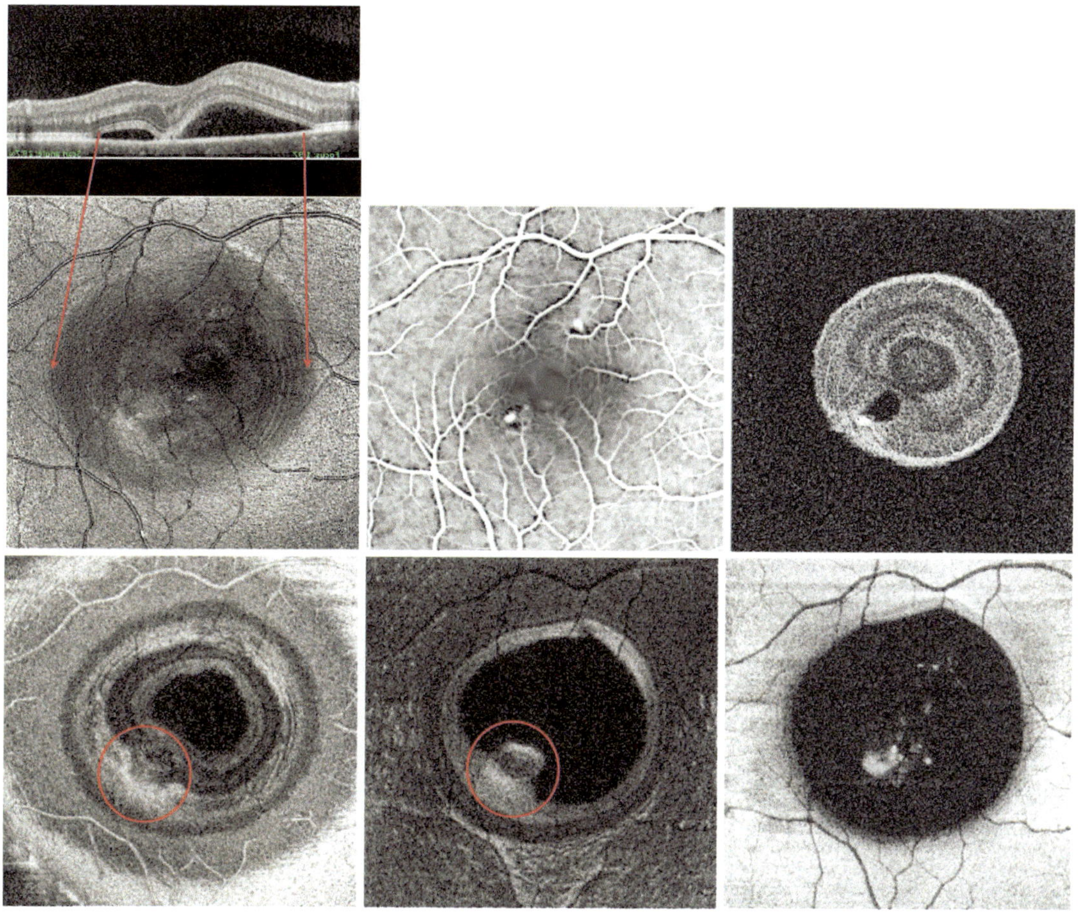

Fig. 3.9 En face images of central serous chorioretinopathy the demonstrating lateral extent of lesion and concentric rings produced by the cut through multiple retinal layers. The horizontal B-scan OCT is seen on top (*upper right*) directly above the SLO (*middle left*) of the macular surface. A corresponding fluorescein angiogram (*middle second row image*) shows a focal leak at the level of the RPE corresponding to an inferior temporal dip in the serous elevation. The lower level of images shows progressively deeper slices moving to the right through the serous elevation. At the RPE level (*lower right*), the isolated RPE disturbance is isolated and surrounded by the shadow of the overlying serous bleb

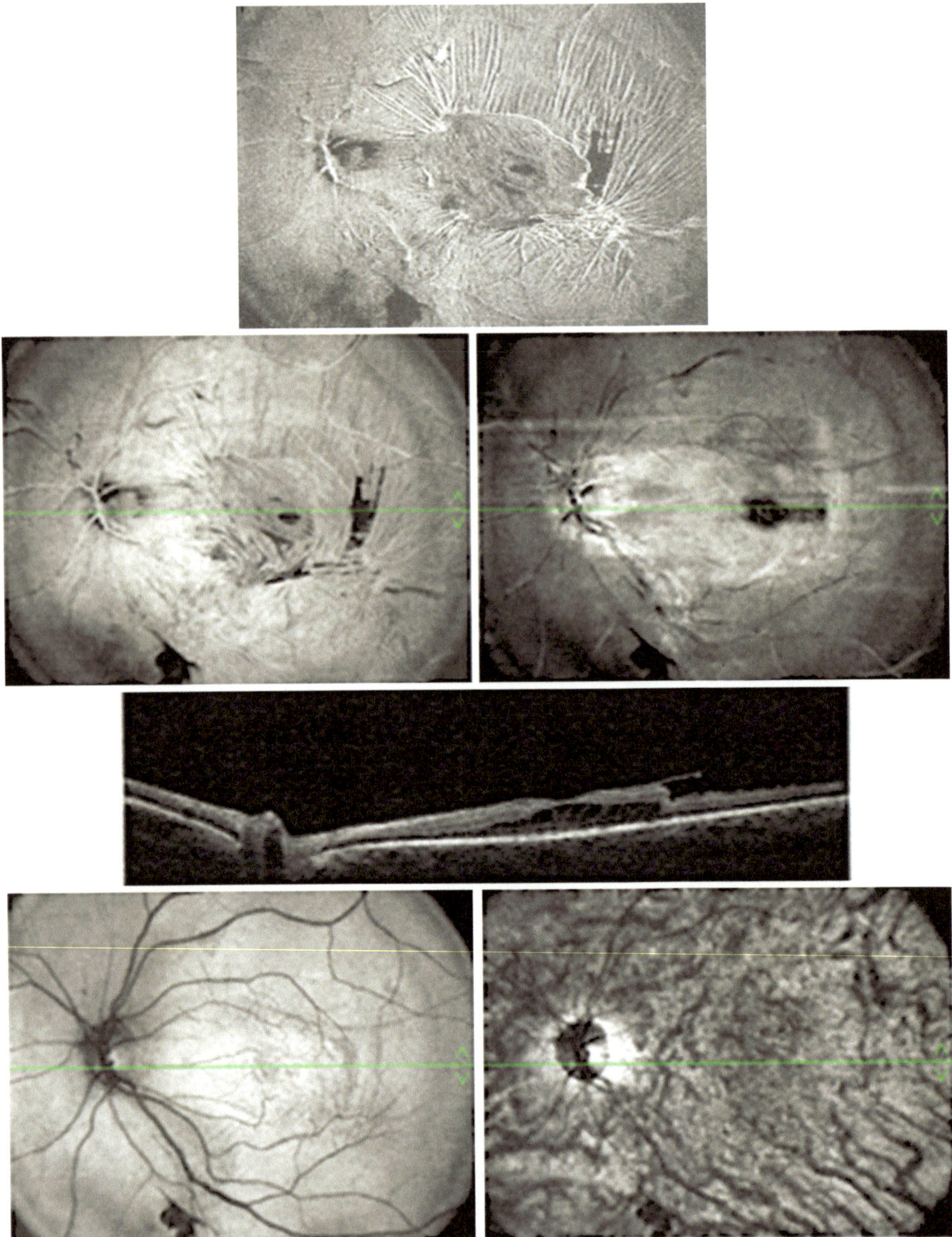

Fig. 3.10 Epiretinal membrane. En face OCT shows the disturbance to the anatomy which is most evident in the upper and lower left images, leaving the choroid untouched. The details of the plaque-like pattern of the ERM can be better appreciated with en face OCT

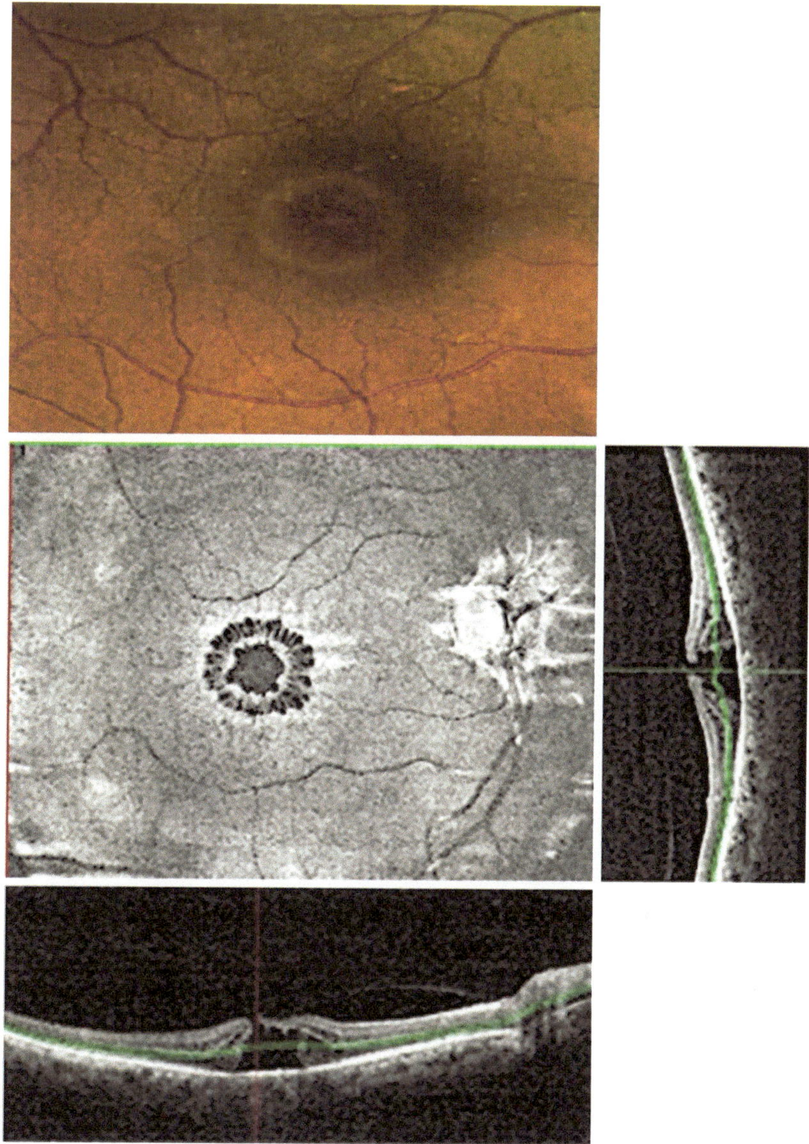

Fig. 3.11 Macular hole. The en face OCT shows a symmetric petaloid, cystoid edematous pattern with lines of centrifugal tension surrounding the macular hole

3.4 Macular Hole

En face imaging of macular holes can similarly aid in preoperative planning and postoperative follow-up. The completeness of the removal of the internal limiting membrane in macular hole surgery can be elucidated with en face imaging (Alkabes et al. 2011) (Fig. 3.11).

3.5 Branch Retinal Vein Occlusion

En face images performed at the level of the internal limiting membrane and inner plexiform layer can reveal areas of high and low reflectivity which represent intraretinal hemorrhage and exudates that are main features of retinal vein occlusions (Fig. 3.12).

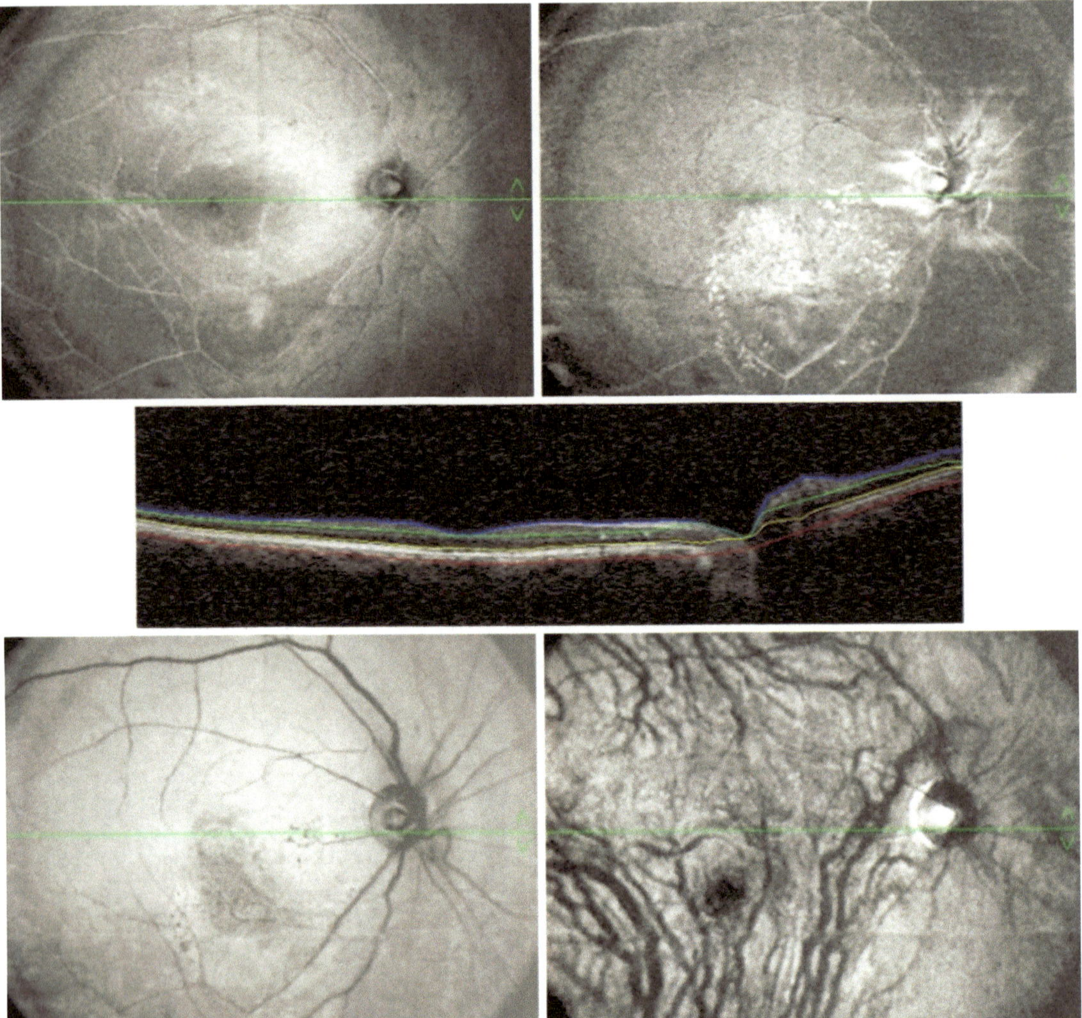

Fig. 3.12 Branch retinal vein occlusion. En face OCT shows more extensive involvement in middle and deep retinal layers than is evident from B-scan OCT image which shows the levels of segmentation

3.6 Age-Related Macular Degeneration

En face OCT imaging of pathologic features of age-related macular degeneration (AMD) such as drusen, geographic atrophy, and choroidal neovascularization can be combined with standard B-scan OCT to better monitor disease progression. Geographic atrophy is characterized by the loss of photoreceptors cells, retinal pigment epithelium (RPE), and the choriocapillaris layer. En face OCT enables the affected multiple layers to be closely examined. The OCT signals have greater signal penetration through the areas of atrophic RPE and choriocapillaris and allow for better visualization of the choriocapillaris. The areas of geographic atrophy often enlarge and coalesce over time in a slowly progressive nature. En face OCT can be used to identify the margins of geographic atrophy and quantify the amount of disease progression

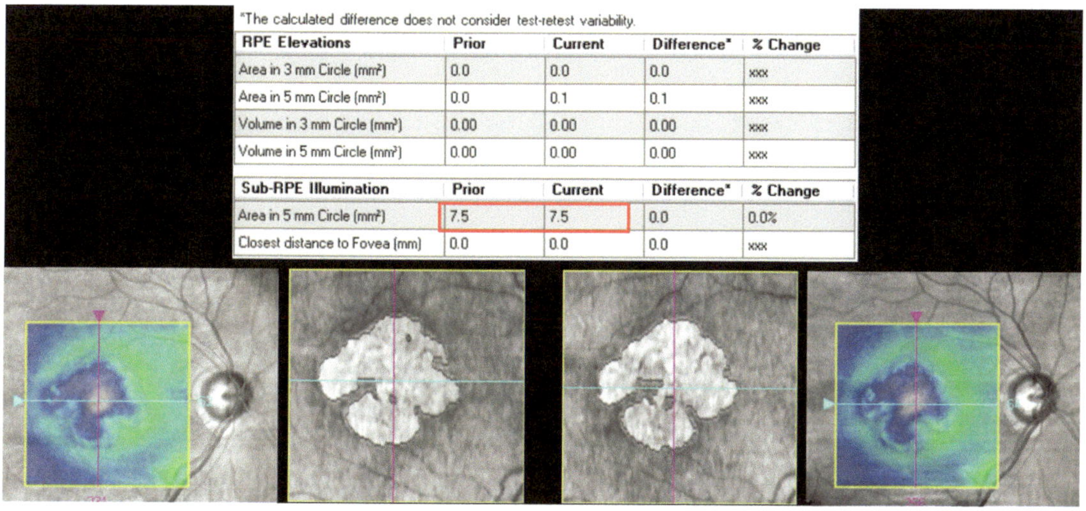

*The calculated difference does not consider test-retest variability.

RPE Elevations	Prior	Current	Difference*	% Change
Area in 3 mm Circle (mm²)	0.0	0.0	0.0	xxx
Area in 5 mm Circle (mm²)	0.0	0.1	0.1	xxx
Volume in 3 mm Circle (mm³)	0.00	0.00	0.00	xxx
Volume in 5 mm Circle (mm³)	0.00	0.00	0.00	xxx

Sub-RPE Illumination	Prior	Current	Difference*	% Change
Area in 5 mm Circle (mm²)	7.5	7.5	0.0	0.0%
Closest distance to Fovea (mm)	0.0	0.0	0.0	xxx

Fig. 3.13 En face OCT of geographic atrophy in 4/2012 compared to 5/2012. Area of sub-RPE illumination in 5 mm circle measured to have no change

and even predict the progression of geographic atrophy (Nunes et al. 2013) (Fig. 3.13).

Recently, Flores-Moreno et al. described using en face swept-source OCT with fluorescein angiography (FA) and/or ICG angiography (FA) for neovascular AMD. En face images at RPE level revealed changes in all 38 eyes that were studied. There were no differences in the horizontal and vertical diameters of the neovascular complex area, measured with en face OCT and the FA. En face OCT is a rapid, noninvasive imaging modality that can complement fluorescein angiography in evaluating and treating neovascular AMD (Flores-Moreno et al. 2015).

3.7 Retinitis Pigmentosa

Photoreceptor dystrophies such as retinitis pigmentosa can be visualized in a different perspective with en face OCT combining the frontal view of disease with the B-scan cross-sectional views. In retinitis pigmentosa, the cross-sectional OCT often shows normal retinal contour in the macula with increasing atrophic changes in the periphery. En face imaging of retinitis pigmentosa corresponds with these changes seen on cross-sectional OCT demonstrating a central island of hyper-reflective surrounded by a ring of hyporeflectivity representing areas of atrophy (Fig. 3.14).

3.8 Multiple Evanescent White Dot Syndrome

Multiple evanescent white dot syndrome (MEWDS) is characterized by numerous small discrete, white lesions deep in the outer retina or at the retinal pigment epithelium level. These inflammatory white lesions may appear subtle on standard fundus photos but can be readily identified with en face OCT. The en face OCT scans can pass through the level between the inner and outer segment of the photoreceptors with the retinal pigment epithelium serving as the reference surface retinal contour. As the en face OCT passes through the junctions of the inner and outer photoreceptors and the interdigitation zone, multiple irregular lesions are identified (de Bats et al. 2014) (Fig. 3.15).

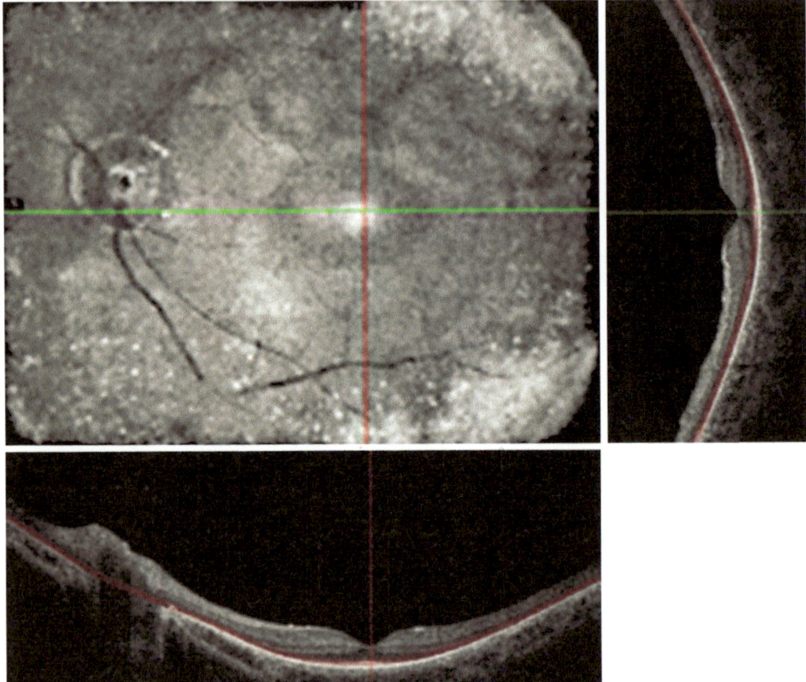

Fig. 3.14 En face and B-scan images of retinitis pigmentosa. B-scan OCT shows extreme thinning peripherally where photoreceptor layer is gone with hyper-reflective layer in subfoveal region corresponding to surviving photoreceptors with disrupted ellipsoid layers in the perifoveal area. En face OCT: hyper-reflective island of surviving outer retina centrally surrounded by hypo-reflective ring and snowflake-like peripheral hyper-reflectance of RPE

3.9 Diabetic Maculopathy

Diabetic maculopathy presents with a variety of lesion from microaneurysms, brawny edema, and cystoid edema before deteriorating into atrophy. En face OCT can help delineate the lateral extent and foveal involvement better than individual B-scan slices (Fig. 3.16).

3.10 Choroidal Disease

In vivo imaging of the choroid has been limited to the use of ICG angiography and enhanced depth imaging with SD-OCT. With the use of en face OCT imaging, detailed in vivo reconstructions of the choroidal vasculature can be studied as well as choroidal pathologies such as central serous chorioretinopathy (CSCR) and choroidal rupture.

In CSCR, en face OCT is able to localize the focal leak point seen in both FA and ICGA, the size and location of serous detachments, pigment epithelium detachments, and the presence of thickened fibrinous fluid (van Velthoven et al. 2005) (Figs. 3.17 and 3.18).

3.11 En Face Imaging Optical Coherence Tomography Enables Multimodal Imaging

Along with simultaneous confocal SLO imaging, en face OCT technology has been developed to offer the possibility of combining OCT/SLO with fluorescein imaging. By com-

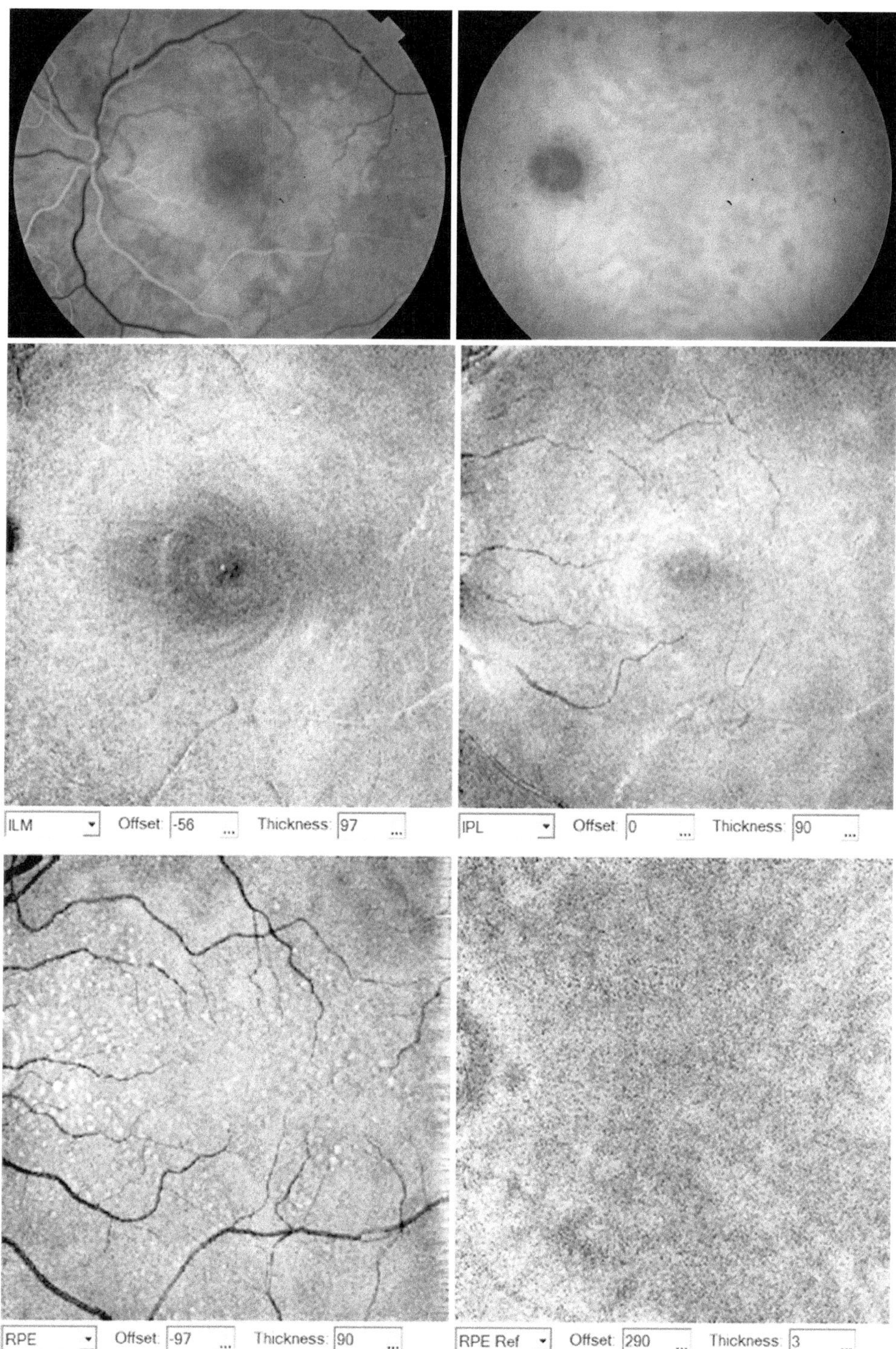

Fig. 3.15 Multiple evanescent white dot syndrome: Early FA (*upper image*) showing diffuse placoid hyperfluorescence. Late ICG (*second level*) showing focal hypofluorescent spots. En face OCT sequence (*above*): shows underlying multiple granular lesions best seen at the level of the junction between the inner and outer segments of photoreceptors. En face OCT of white dot lesions overlaid on fundus photo (*bottom*)

Fig. 3.15 (continued)

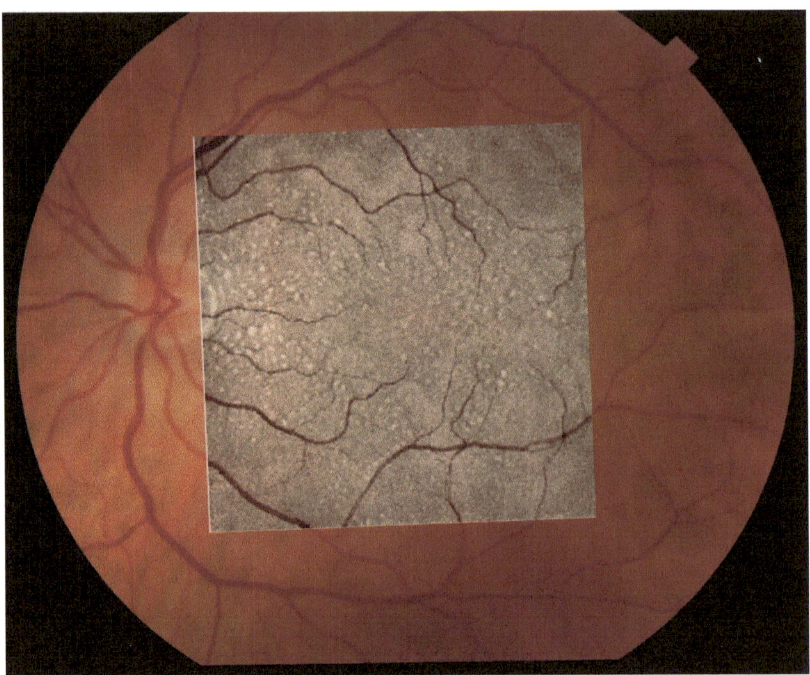

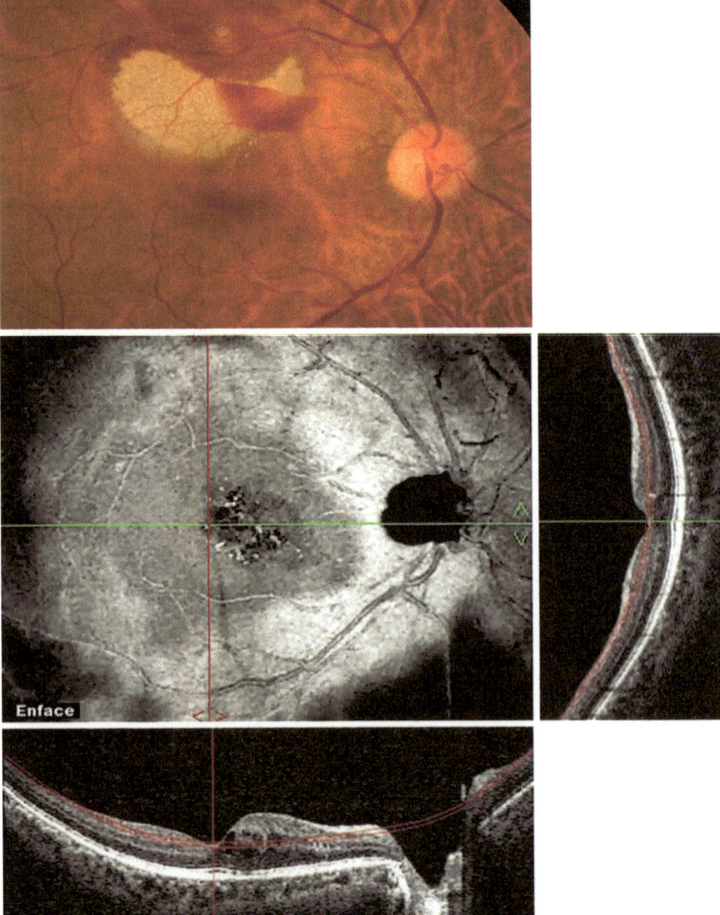

Fig. 3.16 En face OCT of non-proliferative diabetic retinopathy showing cystoid edema and exudates in the deeper layers which are barely evident on the color image. Center involving edema appears more extensive than suggested by accompanying B-scan OCT slices

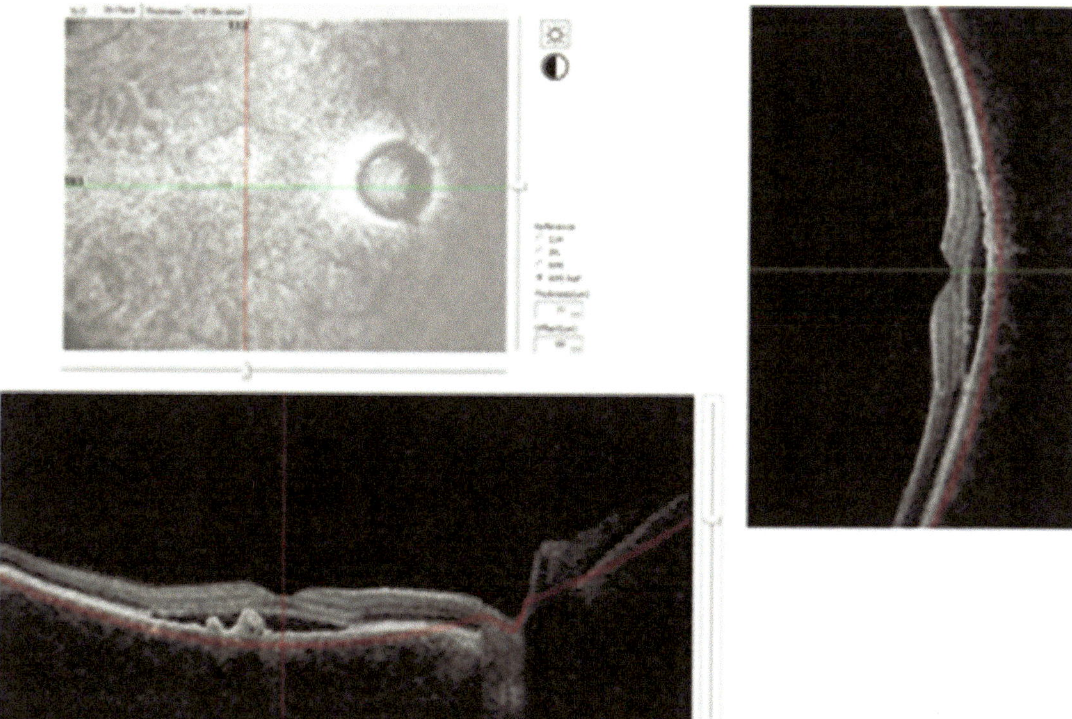

Fig. 3.17 Choroidal disruption in central serous chorioretinopathy. En face section parallel to the RPE shows a highly reflective area corresponding to the area of choroidal thickening, serous detachment, small pigment epithelium detachment, and irregularities of the outer photoreceptor segment seen on the longitudinal scan

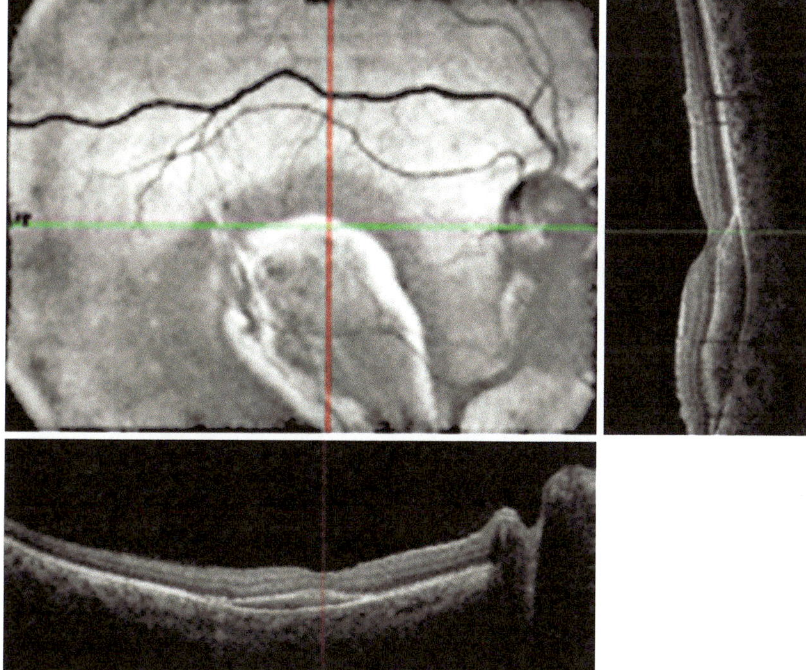

Fig. 3.18 Occult choroidal rupture with subretinal hemorrhage following head trauma. The en face OCT reveals the break and shows its relation to the overlying blood

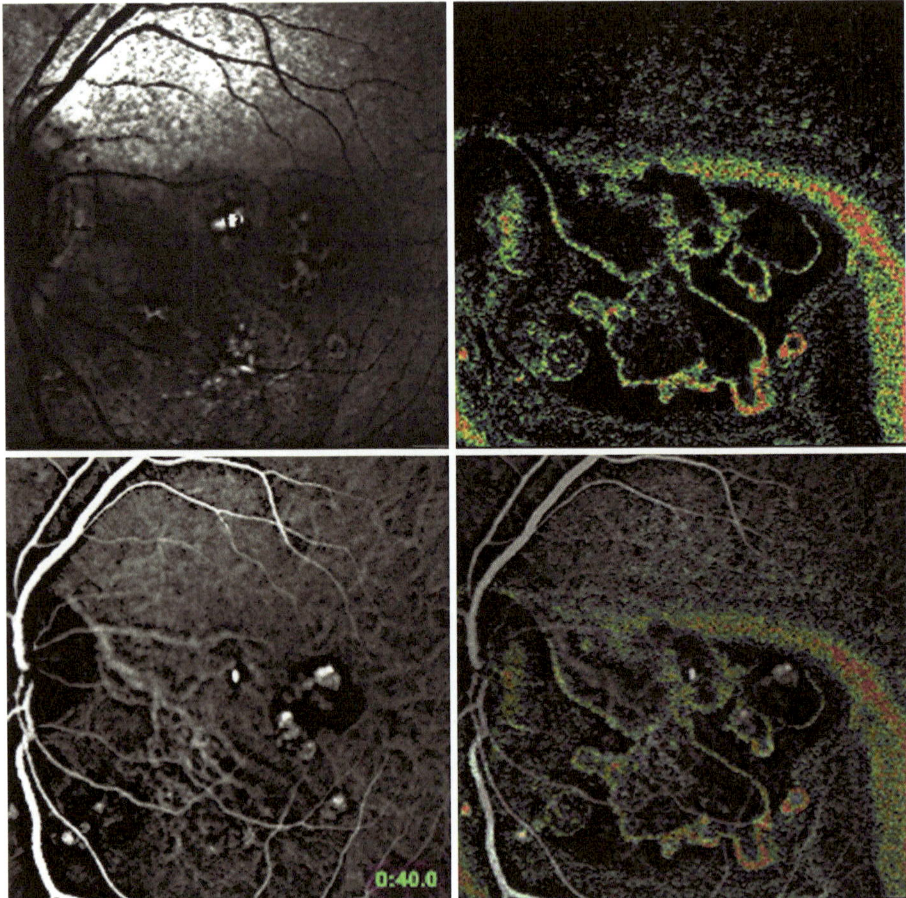

Fig. 3.19 ICG/OCT/SLO set of a patient with polypoidal choroidal vasculopathy. The SLO image (*upper left*) shows hemorrhages and pigmentary disturbances. The simultaneous en face OCT (*upper right*) shows the outline of the multi-lobular polypoidal serous detachments which distort the surface of the macula. Mid arterial-venous ICG phase (*lower left*) demonstrates a leash of deep abnormal vessels with hyperfluorescent bulbous endings. The combined OCT/ICG image (*lower right*) shows the overlying serous elevation surrounding the vessels and hot spots

bining en face OCT with ICG angiography, additional retinal and choroidal vessel details can be elucidated. Indocyanine green (ICG) angiography and OCT share similar spectral bands that facilitate the combination of these two imaging modalities. The most widely used band for retinal OCT of the retina is 820–920 nm, while ICG is usually excited at 806 nm and fluoresces in the band 810–860 nm with a peak at 830 nm. Figure 3.19 demonstrates the utility of the system in the evaluation of a retina of a patient with polypoidal choroidal vasculopathy, an unusual variant of neovascular macular degeneration (Rosen et al. 2009).

3.12 En Face Optical Coherence Tomography Correlated with Microperimetry

Retinal lesions identified on en face OCT can be functionally correlated with symptomatic scotomas and objectively characterized with overlay of microperimetry (Fig. 3.20).

En face OCT provides high-resolution cross-sectional OCT information in a clinically familiar perspective. Using en face OCT, individual retinal layers can be peeled layer by layer to examine the extent of pathology in specific regions. En face OCT serves as adjunctive imaging modality that can be combined with

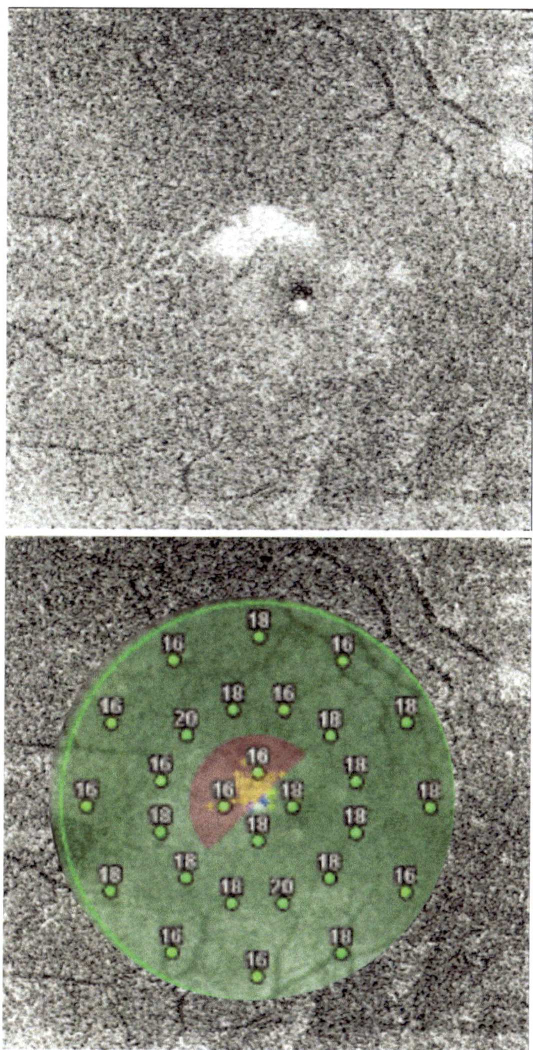

Fig. 3.20 Occult mid retinal infarct revealed by en face OCT but difficult to see with B-scan OCT imaging. Corresponding microperimetry testing with combined OCT/SLO microperimetry was able to detect and localize this lesion weeks after its onset

traditional fundus imaging, fluorescein angiography, and functional testing such as microperimetry.

OCT angiography with split-spectrum amplitude-decorrelation angiography (SSADA) algorithm allows OCT to provide noninvasive, three-dimensional mapping of the retina and choroidal microvasculature (Yali et al. 2012). OCT angiography has already been applied to identify vascular changes seen in diabetic retinopathy. Ishibazawa et al. used OCT angiography to image microaneurysms, venous beading, neovascularization, and nonperfused areas (Ishibazawa et al. 2015) (Fig. 3.21).

Using OCT angiography, the areas of nonperfusion and neovascularization were quantified. There are advantages of using OCT angiography over traditional imaging modalities for diabetic retinopathy, including the ability of OCT angiography using the SSADA analysis to separately image and measure the deep and superficial retinal and choroidal capillary layers. Novel ways of using OCT angiography have been recently introduced including using OCTA-coded perfusion density mapping to discriminate and quantitate progressive retinal perfusion changes in diabetic retinopathy (Agemy et al. 2015) (Fig. 3.22).

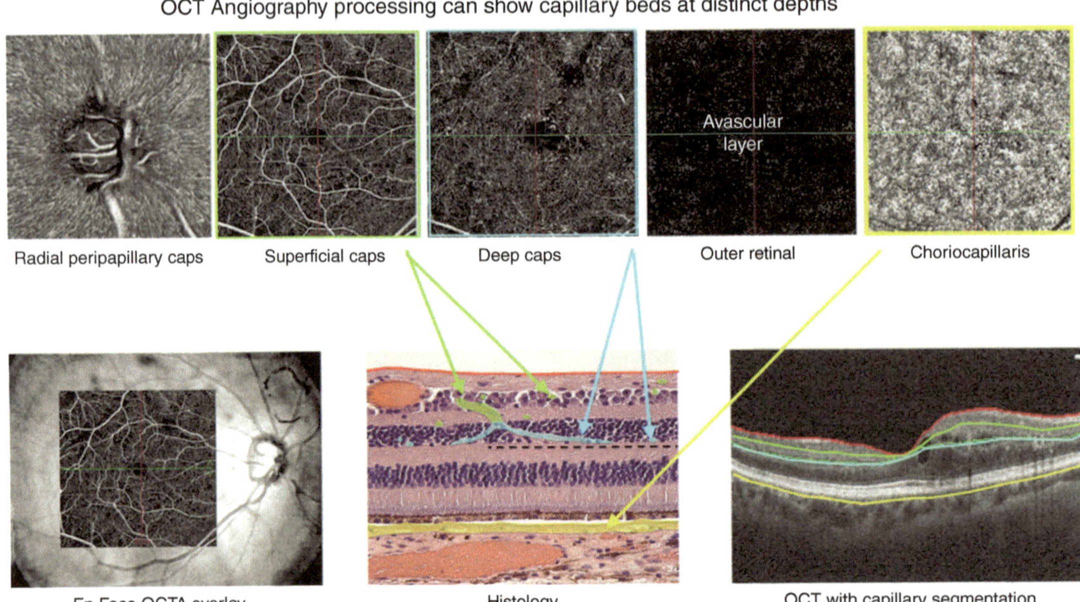

Fig. 3.21 OCT angiography (SSADA) showing radial peripapillary, superficial, deep, and choroidal capillary beds. Motion contrast processing of en face OCT is necessary to isolate blood flow and produce noninvasive angiograms

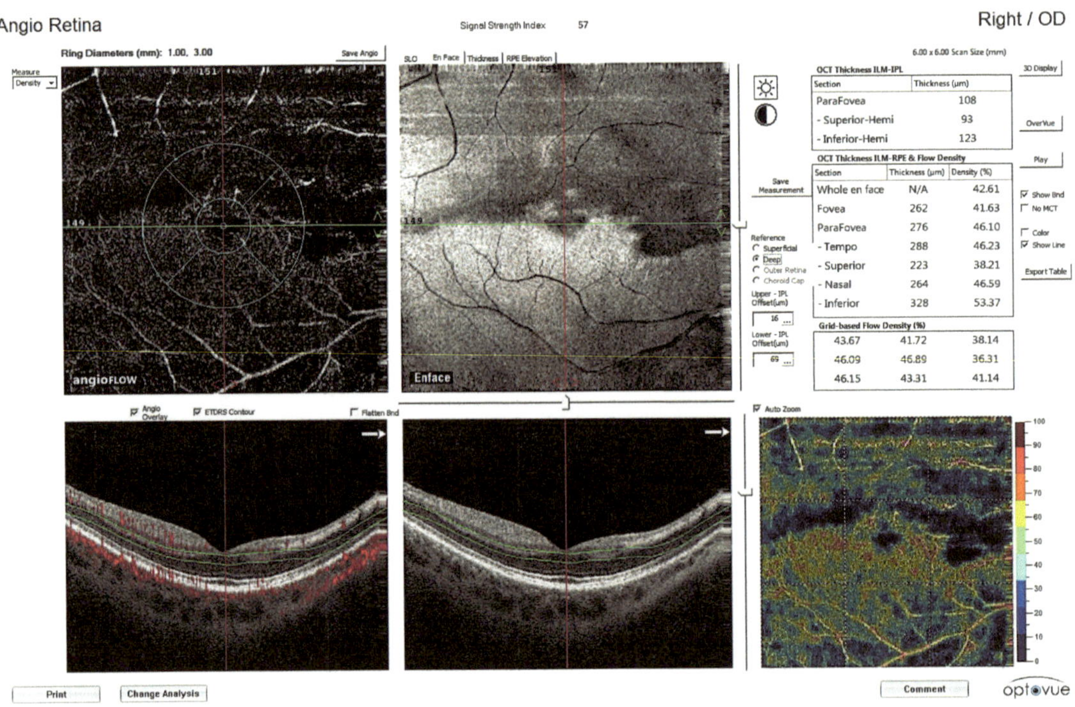

Fig. 3.22 Quantitative OCT angiography of branch artery occlusion. OCT angiogram (*upper left*) with en face OCT (*upper middle*). B-scan OCT with red flow lines (*lower left*) and color perfusion density map (*lower right*) showing extensive loss of blood flow (*blue*) in occluded capillary beds

References

Agemy S, Scipsemsa N, Shah C et al (2015) Retinal vascular perfusion density mapping using optical coherence tomography angiography in normals and diabetic retinopathy patients. Retina 31:2353–2363

Alkabes M, Salinas C, Vitale L et al (2011) En face optical coherence tomography of inner retinal defects after internal limiting membrane peeling for idiopathic macular hole. Invest Ophthalmol Vis Sci 52:8349–8355

Bradu A, Podoleanu AG (2014) Imaging the eye fundus with real-time en-face spectral domain optical coherence tomography. Biomed Opt Express 5:1233–1249

De Bats F, Wolff B, Vasseur V et al (2014) "En-face" spectral-domain optical coherence tomography findings in multiple evanescent white dot syndrome. J Ophthalmol 2014:928028

Flores-Moreno I, Arias-Barquet L, Rubio-Caso M, Ruiz-Moreno J, Duker J, Caminal J (2015) En face swept-source optical coherence tomography in neovascular age-related macular degeneration. Br J Ophthalmol 99:1260–1267

Ishibazawa A, Nagaoka T, Takahashi A et al (2015) Optical coherence tomography angiography in diabetic retinopathy: a prospective pilot study. Am J Ophthalmol 160:35–44

Nunes RP, Gregori G, Yehoshua Z et al (2013) Predicting the progression of geographic atrophy in age-related macular degeneration with SD-OCT en face imaging of the outer retina. Ophthalmic Surg Lasers Imaging Retina 44:344–359

Podoleanu A (2013) Clinical en face OCT atlas. Jaypee Brothers Medical Publishers, New Delhi

Podoleanu AG, Dobre GM, Webb DJ, Jackson DA (1997) Simultaneous en-face imaging of two layers in the human retina by low-coherence reflectometry. Opt Lett 22:1039–1041

Rispoli M, Le Rouic J, Lesnoni G et al (2012) Retinal surface en face optical coherence tomography: a new imaging approach in epiretinal membrane surgery. Retina 32:2070–2076

Rosen R, Hathaway M, Rogers J et al (2009) Multidimensional en-face OCT imaging of the retina. Opt Express 17:4112

van Velthoven ME, Vebraak FD, Garcia PM et al (2005) Evaluation of central serous retinopathy with en face optical coherence tomography. Br J Ophthalmol 89:1483–1488

Yali J, Ou T, Tokayer J et al (2012) Split-spectrum amplitude-decorrelation angiography with optical coherence tomography. Opt Express 20:4710–4725

Zhang K, Kang JU (2010) Real-time 4D signal processing and visualization using graphics processing unit on a regular nonlinear-k Fourier-domain OCT system. Opt Express 18:11772–11784

Swept-Source Optical Coherence Tomography

4

Colin S. Tan and SriniVas R. Sadda

Contents

C.S. Tan, MBBS,FRCSEd(Ophth),MMed(Ophth)
National Healthcare Group Eye Institute, Tan Tock Seng Hospital, Fundus Image Reading Center, National Healthcare Group Eye Institute, Singapore, Singapore

S.R. Sadda, MD (✉)
Doheny Eye Institute, David Geffen School of Medicine, University of California – Los Angeles, Los Angeles, USA
e-mail: ssadda@doheny.org

Abbreviations

AMD	Age-related macular degeneration
CNV	Choroidal neovascularization
FA	Fluorescein angiogram
ICGA	Indocyanine green angiogram
PED	Pigment epithelium detachment

C.H. Meyer et al. (eds.), *Spectral Domain Optical Coherence Tomography in Macular Diseases*,
DOI 10.1007/978-81-322-3610-8_4

SD-OCT Spectral domain optical coherence tomography
SS-OCT Swept-source optical coherence tomography

4.1 Introduction

In the two decades since optical coherence tomography (OCT) was first described (Huang et al. 1991), this technology has played essential roles in ophthalmology as well as other branches of medicine. The technology has been adapted to produce noninvasive, high-resolution images of both the anterior segment (cornea and structures at the angles) and posterior pole (retina, choroid, sclera, and optic disc).

Just as initial time domain OCT (TD-OCT) devices made way for spectral domain OCT (SD-OCT), advances in technology have now produced swept-source OCT (SS-OCT) devices which have even faster scanning speeds and less sensitivity roll-off. These features are crucial in allowing wider regions of the eye to be scanned and in visualizing more precise details of deeper structures such as the choroid and sclera (Fig. 4.1) (Adhi and Duker 2013; Mrejen and Spaide 2013). This chapter will explore the basics of SS-OCT and illustrate its utility in various conditions affecting both the anterior and posterior pole.

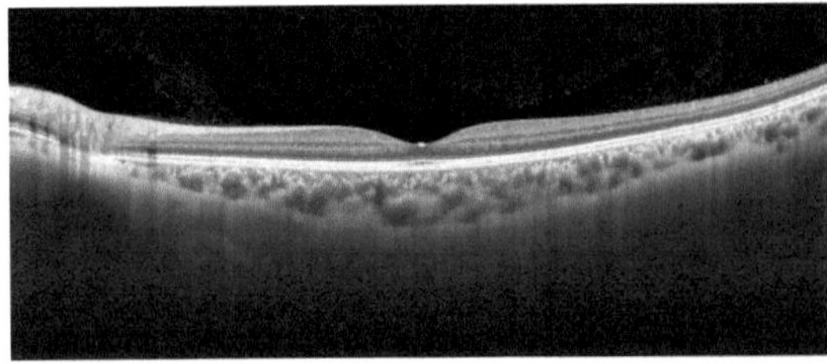

Fig. 4.1 SS-OCT image of a normal eye. In this 12 mm section, the structures within the retina and choroid are clearly visualized. Due to the reduced sensitivity roll-off, the vitreous is also clearly seen

4.2 Basics of Swept-Source Optical Coherence Tomography

In all its current iterations, OCT works by low-coherence interferometry, which involves an optical source directing a low-coherence light beam at a surface and detecting the reflected optical data. This data is then read by the interferometer as an interference pattern, and a depth profile is created (A-scan). By scanning along the sample in a linear fashion, a cross-sectional image (B-scan) is obtained. Combining multiple B-scans enable a three-dimensional (3D) or volume scan the tissue. Currently, OCT allows the imaging of tissue microstructure at micron-scale resolution, while the penetration depth of the scan is on the order of millimeters.

The first generation of OCT machines, known as "time domain" OCT, worked by using low-coherence light from a superluminescent diode and by mechanically translating the reference mirror axially to build up a depth scan. Three-dimensional volumes were then created by scanning the sample at various locations using scanning mirrors. However, TD-OCT was limited by the speed at which the reference mirror could be moved (a mechanical limitation), and A-scan rates were limited to 400 A-scans per second.

In SD-OCT, no moving reference mirrors were used. Instead, light from a fast sweeping laser was used together with a fixed reference mirror to generate a broadband interference pattern that was detected with spectrally separated detectors. A superluminescent diode or femtosecond laser is used as the broadband source, but a spectrometer was used instead of a photodetector.

In the latest generation of OCT, SS-OCT, the broadband source is a rapidly sweeping laser with a broad tuning bandwidth, typically centered on 1050 nm (Mansouri et al. 2013). Both SD-OCT and SS-OCT are based on spectral interferometry that uses Fourier transformation of the interference pattern to convert the signal to a depth profile. The advantages of this technology are that it is more sensitive (theoretically 20–30 dB better than TD-OCT) and is able to scan 100–1000 times faster than TD-OCT.

4.2.1 Capabilities and Advantages of Swept-Source Optical Coherence Tomography

Advances in technology have provided SS-OCT devices with several advantages compared to earlier SD-OCT:

1. *Faster scanning time*. By using a variety of laser tuning mechanisms, including rotating polygon mirrors, galvo-driven grating filters, and Fourier domain mode locking (FDML), higher scan speeds of 100,000 A-scans per second can be achieved. This reduces motion artifacts due to eye movements and loss of fixation (Drexler et al. 2014; Forte et al. 2009; Potsaid et al. 2010).
2. *Lower sensitivity roll-off* (Drexler et al. 2014; Potsaid et al. 2010).
3. *Deeper penetration* into the retina and choroid (Fig. 4.2) (Drexler et al. 2014; Potsaid et al. 2010).
4. The longer wavelength of the laser allows deeper penetration as there is less signal loss from melanin in the retinal pigment epithelium (RPE). This results in better signal-to-noise ratio.
5. *Longer imaging range* (both horizontally and vertically) as a result of the faster scanning time and lower sensitivity roll-off (Fig. 4.1).
6. *Higher detection efficiencies*, because there is no loss of signal from spectrometer grating (Drexler et al. 2014; Potsaid et al. 2010).

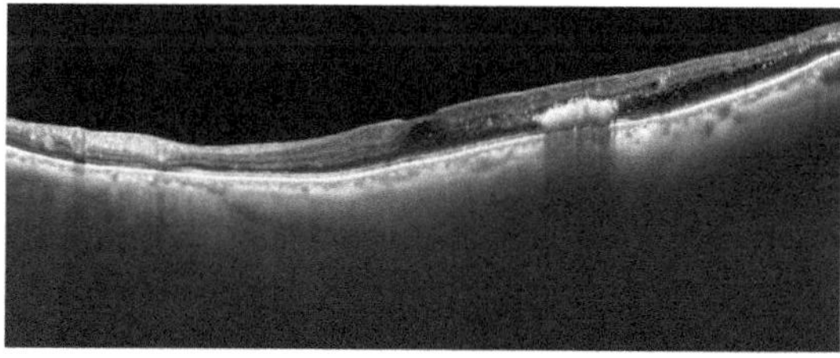

Fig. 4.2 Diabetic retinopathy. SS-OCT showing retinal thickening and intraretinal cysts. The hyperreflective area temporal to the fovea corresponds to hard exudates

4.2.2 Current Commercially Available Swept-Source Optical Coherence Tomography Devices

The *DRI OCT-1 Atlantis* (Topcon Corporation, Tokyo, Japan) is a SS-OCT device used for imaging of the posterior segment of the eye. The device uses a 1050 nm wavelength and is capable of scanning 100,000 A-scans per second. The faster scanning speed allows region areas of up to 12×9 mm to be imaged with a volume scan. The viewing software is capable of automated segmentation of various layers of the retina and choroid (Fig. 4.3).

The *SS-1000 CASIA Anterior Segment OCT* (Tomey Corporation, Nagoya, Japan) is a non-contact imaging system which uses a scanning light source centered on a wavelength of 1310 nm (Kawana et al. 2007). The device is capable of 30,000 A-scans per second, with resolution of up to 10 μm axially and 30 transversely (Liu et al. 2011). The SS-1000 CASIA produces cross-sectional images of the cornea and anterior segment and its structures within the angles.

With a wide scan length of 16 mm, the entire cross section of the anterior chamber can be imaged in a single B-scan. The device is able to produce volume scans consisting of 128 horizontal B-scans, each consisting of 512 A-scans. In addition, the SS-1000 CASIA allows 360-degree imaging of the scleral spur, trabecular meshwork, angle recess, and iris root (Kawana et al. 2007).

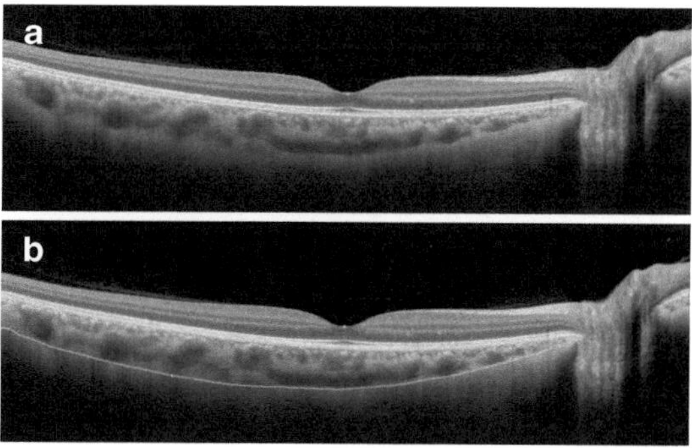

Fig. 4.3 Automated segmentation lines (in *green*) for the retina (**a**) and choroid (**b**) drawn by the imaging viewing software, allowing measurement of retinal and choroidal thickness, respectively

The *IOLMaster 700* (Carl Zeiss Meditec, Dublin, CA, USA) is a SS-OCT-based optical biometer.

4.3 Applications of Swept-Source Optical Coherence Tomography to Various Ocular Conditions

4.3.1 Age-Related Macular Degeneration

Age-related macular degeneration (AMD) is the commonest causes of visual loss in developed countries and the third commonest worldwide. Its prevalence is expected to increase as a result of the aging population trends observed in many parts of the world. OCT plays a crucial role in the diagnosis and monitoring of patients with AMD (Fig. 4.4). Quantitative assessments of retinal thickness or qualitative features such as the presence of retinal thickening and cysts and subretinal fluid and the presence of choroidal neovascularization (CNV) are criteria for initiation of treatment and are commonly used in both clinical practice and multicenter randomized controlled trials.

Since the pathology in AMD occurs in the deeper layers of the retina, with the CNV occurring either in the subretinal or sub-RPE space, SS-OCT will contribute greatly to our ability to visualize the pathology in these areas (Fig. 4.5). SS-OCT can be used to assess qualitative features and quantitative features such as choroidal thickness (Tan et al. 2015a, c and, with the use of OCT angiography, visualize the actual CNV lesion.

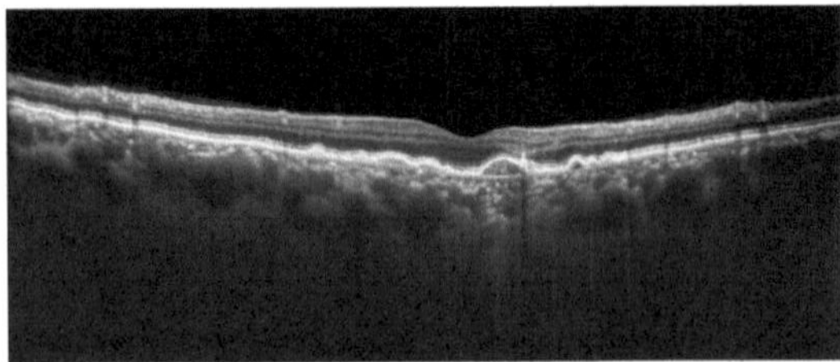

Fig. 4.4 Drusen. SS-OCT scan of an eye with drusen of various sizes. Bruch's membrane is clearly visualized beneath the drusen

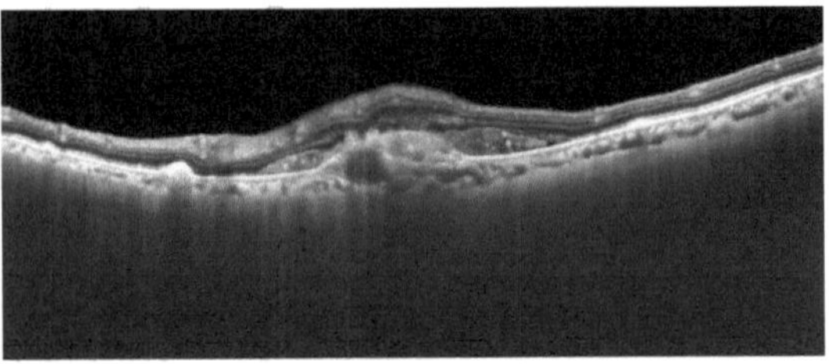

Fig. 4.5 Neovascular age-related macular degeneration. SS-OCT showing subretinal CNV and fluid. The choroid is relatively thin throughout this OCT B-scan

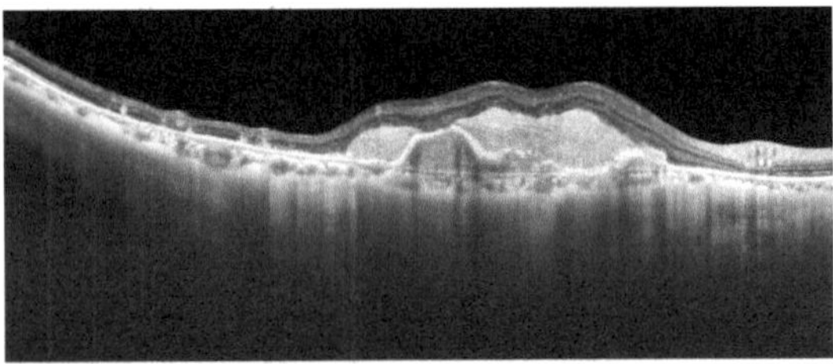

Fig. 4.6 Subretinal scar. SS-OCT showing subretinal scar resulting from neovascular AMD. The retinal pigment epithelium detachments are clearly seen beneath the scar, and Bruch's membrane forms a distinct line beneath the PED

It has been demonstrated that SS-OCT may be superior to SD-OCT in visualization of the deeper structures, including the sub-RPE space, Bruch's membrane, and the choroid (Figs. 4.6 and 4.7) (Tan et al. 2015a, c; Yasuno et al. 2009).

In a study by (Yasuno et al. 2009) comparing a prototype SS-OCT device with the Topcon 3D OCT-1000, 9 of 13 (69.2 %) eyes showed marked improvement in the qualitative image contrast of pathologic lesions beneath the RPE in SS-OCT images compared to SD-OCT images. SS-OCT enables better visualization of hyperreflective masses beneath the RPE, visualization of fibrin and structures beneath the CNV lesion, and visualization of Bruch's membrane as a separate line beneath a PED. In contrast, these structures were not as well seen on SD-OCT scans.

Another role of OCT in the evaluation of patients with AMD is the assessment of choroidal thickness. Various studies have reported that the choroid is thinner among patients with AMD compared to normal controls. Since differences in choroidal thicknesses may be affected by the

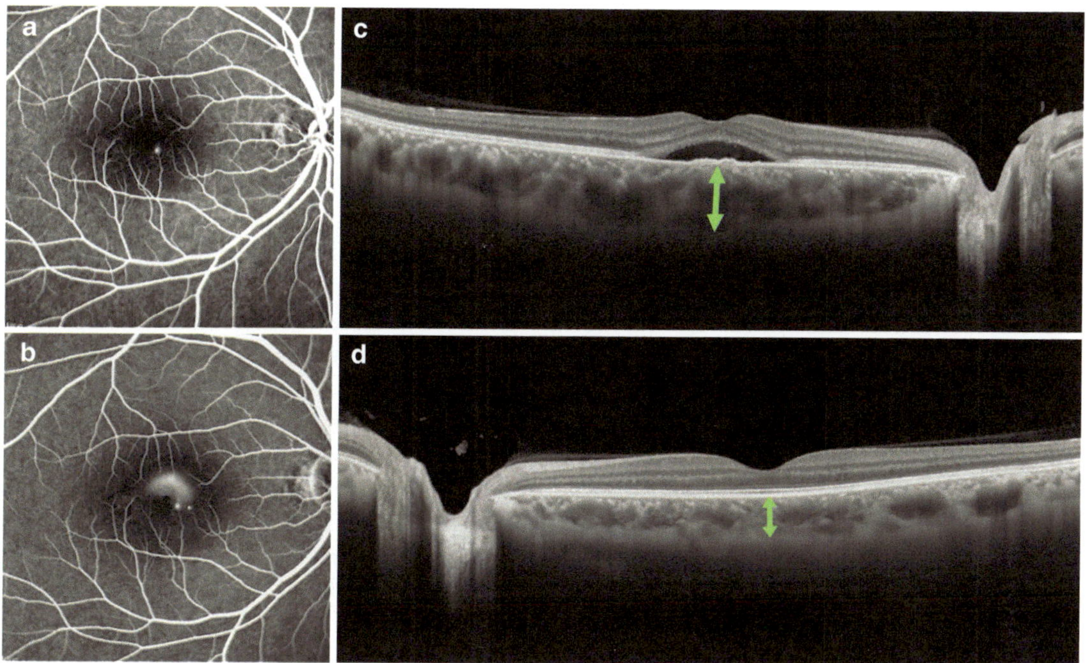

Fig. 4.7 Central serous chorioretinopathy. (**a**) Early FA with pinpoint hyperfluorescence. (**b**) FA illustrating a smoke stack pattern of leakage. (**c**) SS-OCT scan, showing subretinal fluid. There is slightly irregularity of the RPE, corresponding to the location of the leakage on fluorescein angiography. The choroid is also thickened (*green arrow*) relative to the choroid of fellow eye (**d**)

visualization of the choroid–scleral boundary, the image contrast of the OCT scan is of paramount importance. Several studies have found that the visualization of the choroid–scleral boundary is clearer when SS-OCT is used compared to SD-OCT (Tan et al. 2015c; Yasuno et al. 2009).

While many studies still use point thickness measurements subfoveally or at various points along a horizontal and/or vertical B-scan (Tan et al. 2012b, 2015c), these are limited by the fact that the choroid is a three-dimensional structure with considerable topographic variation (Tan and Cheong 2014; Tan et al. 2014a; Ouyang et al. 2011), and it has been suggested that evaluating the mean choroidal thickness in each sector of the ETDRS grid may give a more accurate representation of the variations in choroidal thickness in different diseases. The faster scanning speed and wider scan area of SS-OCT are an advantage in such studies. A study by Ueda-Arakawa et al. (2014) comparing choroidal thicknesses between patients with reticular drusen only or with neovascular AMD or geographic atrophy and normal controls found that the mean choroidal thickness and volume of each sector were significantly reduced in eyes with reticular drusen compared to normal controls.

The faster scanning speed of SS-OCT also makes this a useful modality for OCT angiography. While this is discussed in greater detail in another chapter, several authors have reported that OCT angiography allows noninvasive visualization of CNV lesions among AMD patients that correspond well to the size and location of the CNV seen on fluorescein angiography (FA) (Jia et al. 2014; Moult et al. 2014). In some cases, a feeder vessel can be identified. Other features such as reduced choroidal blood flow beneath and adjacent to regions of CNV have been reported (Jia et al. 2014; Moult et al. 2014).

4.3.2 Polypoidal Choroidal Vasculopathy

Polypoidal choroidal vasculopathy (PCV) is a disease characterized by the presence of abnormal vascular channels which supply the polyps. Currently, the gold standard for diagnosis of PCV is indocyanine green angiography (ICGA) (Lim et al. 2010; Tan et al. 2014c, 2015b). This modality, however, is costly and invasive, requiring an intravenous injection of the dye. The use of indocyanine green carries the risk of allergic reactions, especially among patients with known allergies to seafood and shellfish in particular. If OCT can be used to detect PCV, it would provide a fast, cheap, and noninvasive method of monitoring this condition.

SD-OCT devices use a light source with a wavelength of 840 nm, which is scattered at the level of the RPE. Since both the polyps and vascular channels that supply them are believed to lie beneath the RPE, visualization of these lesions on SD-OCT is difficult. In contrast, the longer wavelength of the SS-OCT would allow better visualization of structures located beneath the RPE. If the PCV lesion can consistently be visualized, SS-OCT can be used to detect the presence and level of activity and recurrence of PCV lesions.

Studies using SD-OCT and SS-OCT have reported the presence of hyperreflectivity beneath the RPE, which is presumed to correspond to the polyps (Fig. 4.8) (Yasuno et al. 2009).

Besides the traditional cross-sectional OCT B-scans, we are also able to visualize OCT scans using en face imaging. These allow visualization of lesions throughout the scan area at different planes of the retina, RPE, and choroid. Several papers have used this method on patients with PCV (Alasil et al. 2015; Sayanagi et al. 2015).

Sayanagi et al. (2015) reported the findings of en face SS-OCT on 19 eyes of 18 patients with PCV. Of 43 polypoidal lesions seen on ICGA in 14 eyes, 41 were detected using en face OCT. The polyps appeared as an RPE ring with inner reflectivity on slices obtained from the RPE layer. Within the RPE rings, the inner reflectivity manifested with either a mosaic (72 %) or homogenous (28 %) pattern. In most of the cases, the RPE rings were of the same size as the polypoidal lesions on ICGA, while in a minority, the rings were larger. In addition, en face OCT detected 15 of 17 eyes with a vascular network on ICGA. Using en face OCT, the networks appeared as a hyperreflective mesh-like configuration. Dilated choroidal vessels were seen beneath the RPE ring (the presumed polypoidal lesions) in 22 of 47 (47 %) RPE rings on en face images. These coincided with the dilated choroidal vessels seen on ICGA (Sayanagi et al. 2015).

Another paper by Alasil et al. (2015) demonstrated the relationship between the smaller PEDs that correlated with the polyps and the larger adjoining PEDs. Choroidal vascular abnormalities were detected in all eyes with PCV and included focal dilation, diffuse vascular dilation, and a branching vascular network (Alasil et al. 2015).

4.3.3 Deep Retinal and Choroidal Lesions

Due to the longer wavelength and greater penetration of its light source, it is not surprising that SS-OCT has been reported to be superior to SD-OCT and enhanced depth imaging OCT (EDI-OCT) for lesions deep to the RPE (Francis et al. 2015; Hayashi et al. 2014; Takahashi et al. 2013).

In a comparison of SS-OCT and EDI-OCT from 30 eyes with choroidal nevi (Francis et al. 2015), SS-OCT was found to be superior at visualizing intralesional vessels, intralesional granularity, and abnormal choriocapillaris in melanotic lesions. In contrast, EDI-OCT was found to be equivalent at identifying secondary retinal changes, distended bordering vessels, and visualization of the nevus–scleral interface with hyporeflective gradation beneath the lesion. The authors also found that the morphology of melanotic nevi was better visualized using SS-OCT compared to EDI-OCT (100 % with SS-OCT compared to 53 % with EDI-OCT), whereas both OCT modalities were equivalent in amelanotic lesions.

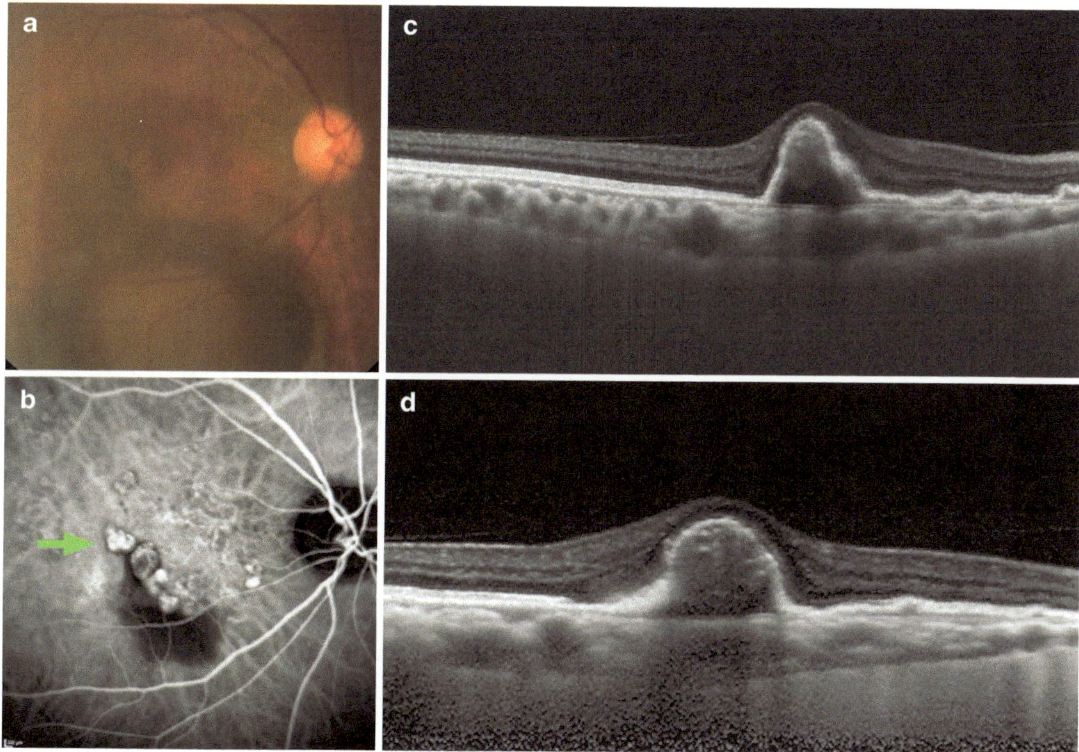

Fig. 4.8 Polypoidal choroidal vasculopathy. (**a**) Color fundus photograph illustrating extensive subretinal and sub-RPE hemorrhage with pigment epithelium detachments. (**b**) ICGA demonstrating multiple polyps (*green arrow*) with a branching vascular network supplying the polyps. (**c**) SS-OCT scan through one of the polyps. A round area of hyperreflectivity is seen beneath the retinal pigment epithelium detachment. (**d**) Corresponding SD-OCT scan through the same polyp

Hayashi et al. described the SS-OCT findings in two eyes with choroidal osteoma. Calcified regions appeared multilayered and spongelike, while a lamellar reflective pattern was noted in the decalcified regions. Hyperreflective moundlike areas with abnormal outer retinae were observed in both eyes. Of note, the chorioscleral border was visible in both cases.

Takahashi et al. described the OCT findings in a 60-year-old man with presumed retinal pigment epithelium hamartoma. Whereas standard SD-OCT demonstrated an elevation of the retina with complete shadowing of optical transmission, SD-OCT using the EDI setting and SS-OCT were able to image deeper structures within the pigmented lesion.

In a study by Sato et al., 26 eyes of 15 patients with optic disc drusen were evaluated using EDI-OCT and SS-OCT (Sato et al. 2013). EDI-OCT and SS-OCT both showed multiple optic disc drusen at different levels; most were located immediately anterior to the lamina cribrosa. The drusen appeared as ovoid regions of lower reflectivity that were bordered by hyperreflective material. In 12 eyes (46.2 %), there were internal hyperreflective foci. The mean diameter of the optic disc drusen was 686.8 μm (standard deviation ± 395.2 μm), and there was a significant negative correlation between the diameter of the optic disc drusen and the global retinal nerve fiber layer thickness ($r = -0.61$, $p = 0.001$).

4.3.4 Pathologic Myopia

SS-OCT has been reported to be useful for imaging of patients with pathologic myopia (Fig. 4.9). In a comparative observational case series of five patients with pathologic myopia (mean spherical equivalent, −16.00±4.70 D) (Lim et al. 2014), it was found that SS-OCT better visualized retinochoroidal structures. The choroid (SS-OCT 8/8 vs. SD-OCT 1/8), inner segment/outer segment line (SS-OCT 6/8 vs. SD-OCT 1/8), and external limiting membrane (ELM) (SS-OCT 7/8 vs. SD-OCT 2/8) were clearly seen in a higher proportion of SS-OCT compared to SD-OCT scans ($p < 0.01$ for all). In contrast, visualization of the sclera and retinal pigment epithelium (RPE) was similar using both OCT devices. The wider SS-OCT scan revealed additional pathology along the walls of the staphylomata, which were not visible using SD-OCT in 4/8 images. These included incomplete posterior vitreous detachment in one eye and peripheral retinoschisis in 3/8 eyes. Vitreoschisis was visible in 3/8 SS-OCT images but not in the SD-OCT images.

4.3.5 Dome-Shaped Macula

Using SS-OCT, Ellabban et al. described the tomographic features of dome-shaped macula (DSM) in 51 highly myopic eyes (35 patients). DSM was first described by Gaucher and associates as an inward convexity of the macula that occurred within the concavity of a posterior staphyloma in highly myopic eyes. In all reconstructed 3D images of the RPE, two outward concavities were seen within the posterior staphyloma, and a horizontal ridge was formed between these two concavities. In 42 of these eyes, this horizontal ridge was band shaped. The vertical OCT section through the fovea showed a convex configuration of RPE, but the horizontal section showed an RPE line that was almost flat. In nine eyes, 3D images showed a typical dome-shaped convexity within the staphyloma. OCT scans showed no outward protrusions in the external scleral surface, but marked scleral thinning was seen in the region of the two outward concavities of the RPE. The sclera of the fovea (518.6±97.6 μm) was significantly thicker than that in all four quadrants of the parafoveal area (range, 277.2–360.3 μm; $p < 0.001$). It has been suggested that dome-shaped macula is not related to the type of staphyloma, but rather is related to an anatomic or structural change within the sclera and can occur in eyes with any type of staphyloma (Ellabban et al. 2013a).

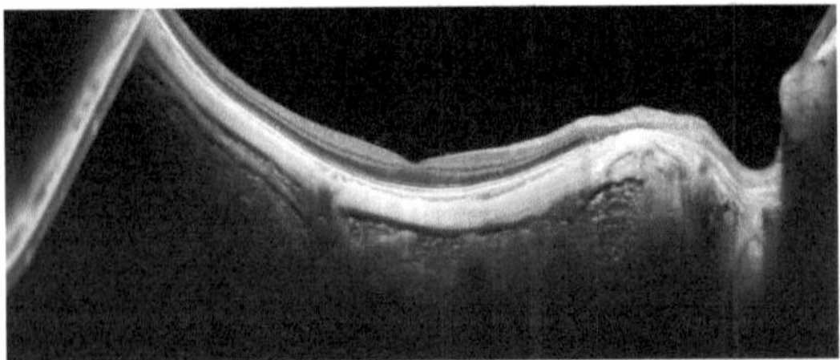

Fig. 4.9 High myopia. The choroid is significantly thinned, and the sclera can be seen clearly along the entire section of the OCT B-scan. Orbital connective tissue is seen external to the sclera. At the edge of the scan, the image is reflected due to the concavity of the myopic eye

4.3.6 Focal Scleral Ectasia

Pedinielli et al. described focal scleral ectasia in areas of macular/perimacular patchy chorioretinal atrophy secondary to pathologic myopia in 26 eyes of 13 patients on SS-OCT and 78 eyes of 39 patients on EDI-OCT (Pedinielli et al. 2013). Focal scleral ectasia is characterized by an abrupt posterior bowing of the sclera with different degrees of scleral schisis on its borders. It is noteworthy that the outer retina, the RPE, and the choroid were absent in areas of macular/perimacular patchy atrophy, as well as in focal scleral ectasia. The absence of these structures, together with the deep penetration OCT signal (both with EDI-OCT and SS-OCT), allowed visualization of retrobulbar vessels perforating the sclera at the borders or bottom of the focal scleral ectasia and running through the superficial scleral thickness for the whole extension of the atrophic area. These features were found in 12 out of 68 eyes (11 out of 39 consecutive patients, mean age 65.7 ± 11.9 years) with macular/perimacular patchy chorioretinal atrophy and were always observed inferior or temporal to the macula. The authors postulated that focal scleral ectasia in areas of macular/perimacular patchy atrophy may have developed from a scleral stretch-associated schisis, which is more pronounced inferiorly (possibly due to oculomotor, gravitational, and staphyloma-associated stretching forces), in areas of openings of anterior emissary for the short posterior ciliary arteries in the sclera. They are different from the recently described macular intrachoroidal cavitation. In focal scleral ectasia, the choroid, the RPE, and the outer retina are absent; there are various degrees of thinning/schisis of the inner retina, and there is an exaggerated focal scleral protrusion with an aspect of schisis on its borders.

4.3.7 Intrachoroidal Cavitations

Studies have described the use of SS-OCT to detect intrachoroidal cavitations in pathologic myopia (myopic spherical equivalent > −8 diopters). Ohno-Matsui et al. described patchy atrophy identified by funduscopy in macular intrachoroidal cavitation in 31 of 56 eyes (55.4 %) in the macular area and compared them to 68 consecutive patients with pathologic myopia without patchy atrophy (Ohno-Matsui et al 2013). The SS-OCT images showed that the sclera was bowed posteriorly in and around the patchy atrophy compared to neighboring sclera, whereas none of the 68 patients without patchy atrophy showed this finding. Macular intrachoroidal cavitation had OCT features similar to peripapillary intrachoroidal cavitation: the choroid in the macular intrachoroidal cavitation area appeared thickened, and the retina was caved into the cavitation. A direct communication between the vitreous cavity and intrachoroidal cavitation has been observed in some eyes. Retinoschisis was observed significantly more frequently in or around the patchy atrophy in eyes with macular intrachoroidal cavitation than in those without cavitation. The authors surmised that these findings suggest that patchy atrophy affects the scleral contour within posterior staphyloma beyond the funduscopically identified patchy atrophy by macular intrachoroidal cavitation. Such deformation of sclera may facilitate the development of retinoschisis in and around the patchy atrophy. Ohno-Matsui et al. also described the incidence of peripapillary intrachoroidal cavitation located temporal to the optic disc (defined as intrachoroidal cavitation located temporal to the optic disc seen in horizontal OCT section through the optic disc center) in 125 patients with pathologic myopia. In that series, 17 eyes of 16 patients had temporal intrachoroidal cavitation. All of the eyes had temporal or temporally wider annular conus. The intrachoroidal cavitation was observed temporal to the optic disc in 15 of 17 eyes, and two of the remaining eyes also had inferior intrachoroidal cavitation. Even in the two eyes with both temporal and inferior intrachoroidal cavitation, the temporal intrachoroidal cavitation was much wider than the inferior intrachoroidal cavitation. The average width of the temporal intrachoroidal cavitation in the horizontal OCT scan across the center of the optic disc was 1467.8 ± 1328.1 μm with a range of 442–6200 μm. In two eyes, the temporal intrachoroidal cavitation extended beyond the central fovea, and in one of these, the subfoveal choroidal thickness in the vertical OCT scan through the fovea appeared thickened because of a separation at the suprachoroidal space. Inner retinal defects at the border of the conus and temporal intrachoroidal cavitation were detected in two eyes. Although the authors postulated that the characteristics of temporal intrachoroidal cavitation did not provide clues on why they tend to be large, one possibility could be that the area temporal to the optic disc between the conus and central fovea might be the area where the mechanical tension is the highest in eyes with pathologic myopia. On the other hand, in eyes with an inferior intrachoroidal cavitation, the inferior edge of the staphyloma was generally close to the inferior border of the optic disc, and the inferior intrachoroidal cavitation did not appear to spread beyond the inferior edge of the staphyloma. The reason why the intrachoroidal cavitation develops temporal to the optic disc is not clear. All of the eyes with temporal intrachoroidal cavitation had a temporal or temporally wider annular conus. They suggested that the deformation of the posterior wall of the eye is more pronounced in the area of the conus because overlying layers are thinner than in the more normal regions temporal to the conus.

4.3.8 Optic Nerve and Peripapillary Pits

Ohno-Matsui et al. described the incidence and characteristics of pitlike structures around the optic disc and myopic conus in eyes with high myopia that were barely visible ophthalmoscopically but can be demonstrated by using SS-OCT (Ohno-Matsui et al. 2013). The authors evaluated 198 eyes of 119 patients with pathologic myopia and compared them to 32 eyes of 32 emmetropic subjects. Pitlike clefts were found at the outer border of the optic nerve or within the adjacent scleral crescent in 32 of 198 highly myopic eyes (16.2 %), but none were observed in the emmetropic eyes. The eyes with these pits were more myopic, had significantly longer axial lengths, and had significantly larger optic discs than the highly myopic eyes without pits. The pits were located in the optic disc area (optic disc pits) in 11 of 32 eyes and in the area of the conus outside the optic disc (conus pits) in 22 of 32 eyes. One eye had both optic disc pits and conus pits. The optic disc pits existed in the superior or inferior border of the optic disc. All but one eye with conus pits had a type IX staphyloma, and the location of the conus pits was present nasal to the scleral ridge or outside the ridge temporal to the nerve. The optic disc pits were associated with discontinuities of the lamina cribrosa, whereas the conus pits appeared to develop from a scleral stretch-associated schisis or to emissary openings for the short posterior ciliary arteries in the sclera. The nerve fiber tissue overlying the pits was discontinuous at the site of the pits. The authors hypothesized that the optic disc is first enlarged by a mechanical expansion of the papillary region in highly myopic eyes and becomes megalodisc-like. This mechanical expansion of the optic disc area results in stretching and expanding of the lamina cribrosa. Because of the mechanical tension on the lamina and surrounding peripapillary sclera, coupled with the myopic thinning of these structures, the lamina might dehisce from the peripapillary sclera, particularly at the superior and inferior poles, which are sites of decreased connective tissue support. This stage is observed by SS-OCT as a hyporeflective gap at the junction of the lamina cribrosa and the peripapillary sclera. Further increases of the gap seemed to be associated with disruption of the overlying nerve fibers or herniation of these fibers into the defect. The clinical importance of the pits lies in the disruption of the nerve fiber overlying the pits. In addition to the discontinuity of nerve fiber tissue overlying the pits, the lamina was dehisced from the peripapillary sclera at the site of optic disc pits. The dehisced lamina cribrosa due to optic disc pits and discontinuous peripapillary sclera due to conus pits could cause a condition similar to that of the material of a trampoline with its springs broken.

4.3.9 Tilted Disc Syndrome

Shinohara et al. described 38 eyes of 29 patients who were highly myopic, and 16 eyes of 15 patients were not highly myopic with tilted disc syndrome (TDS) (Shinohara et al. 2013). This has been thought to be a congenital anomaly caused by an incomplete closure of the fetal fissure of the eye, and it occurs in 1–2 % of the populations. The ophthalmic features of TDS include an inferonasal tilting of the optic disc, the presence of an inferior or inferonasal crescent, myopia, astigmatism, and an ectasia of the lower fundus or inferior staphyloma. The representative OCT findings of the optic disc were a sloping of the lamina cribrosa posteriorly from the upper part to the lower part, a protrusion of the upper edge of Bruch's membrane, and choroid. The distance and the depth of the most protruded point from the fovea (the most protruded point occurred along the vertical section across the fovea in 11 eyes and occurred 15° inferotemporal to the fovea in the remaining eyes) were significantly greater in the eyes with non-highly myopic TDS than those with highly myopic TDS ($P = 0.002$ for distance, $P = 0.03$ for depth). The average distance between the most protruded point and the fovea was 3497.4 ± 763.3 μm with a range of 2237–4473 μm in nine non-highly myopic eyes and 2451.2 ± 691.5 μm with a range of 1195–4290 μm in 15 highly myopic eyes. Similarly, the average depth of the most protruded point from the foveal plane was 935.8 ± 396.8 μm with a range of 537–1730 μm in the nine non-highly myopic eyes and 611.5 ± 284.4 μm with a range of 207–1100 μm in the 15 highly myopic eyes. The authors inferred from the similarities of the deformities in eyes with TDS and eyes with high myopia without TDS; the essential pathology of TDS might be a posterior bulge involving a wide area of inferior globe. The appearance of the optic disc might be influenced only by the relationship between the attachment site of the optic nerve and the upper edge of posterior bulge.

4.3.10 Vitreous Imaging

SS-OCT allows noninvasive, volumetric, and measurable in vivo visualization of the anatomic microstructural features of the posterior vitreous and vitreoretinal interface (Fig. 4.10). It is superior to SD-OCT for vitreous imaging, because it maintains high sensitivity over a much longer imaging range. In addition, the long wavelengths reduce artifacts caused by ocular opacities and induce less light scattering by the vitreous fibers. The high speed of SS-OCT combined with registration motion correction and merging enables volumetric imaging over a wider scan length and compensates for the movement of the vitreous fibers (Liu et al. 2015).

Enhanced vitreous imaging with SS-OCT may help in the assessment of the natural history and treatment response of various vitreoretinal interface diseases (Itakura and Kishi 2011; Itakura et al. 2013; Li et al. 2014; Liu et al. 2014; Spaide 2014; Stanga et al. 2014). The measurements and maps obtained using SS-OCT allow ophthalmologists to observe changes in vitreous detachment over time, perform preoperative planning, and assess treatment response to vitreous surgery or enzymatic vitreolysis.

A few studies have examined the vitreous with SS-OCT (Itakura and Kishi 2011; Itakura et al. 2013; Li et al. 2014; Liu et al. 2014; Spaide 2014; Stanga et al. 2014). The features which have been observed include the bursa premacularis (BPM), area of Martegiani, Cloquet's/BPM septum, Bergmeister papilla, posterior cortical vitreous (hyaloid) detachment, papillomacular hyaloid detachment, hyaloid attachment to retinal vessel(s), and granular opacities within vitreous cortex, Cloquet's canal, and BPM (Fig. 4.11).

The BPM is characterized as an optically empty space that is seen above the macula (Spaide 2014), while the area of Martegiani is a conical space above the optic nerve head. In some cases, the two areas are observed to be interconnected (Spaide 2014). Anterior to the premacular bursa is another lacuna, the supramacular bursa, which is distinct and separate from the premacular bursa. In some cases, both the supramacular and premacular bursas course anteriorly, and in 55.3 % of the eyes, they are observed to interconnect (Spaide 2014). A study by Itakura et al. confirmed the presence of BPM in individuals with a wide range of ages, ranging from 8 to 65 years. In addition, thickening of the vitreous cortex and perifoveal posterior vitreous detachment have been observed in older individuals more than 51 years of age.

Traditionally the vitreous is thought to be composed of liquid vitreous and vitreous gel, with the gel often defined by the presence of

Fig. 4.10 Vitreomacular traction. SS-OCT showing vitreous attachments to the retina

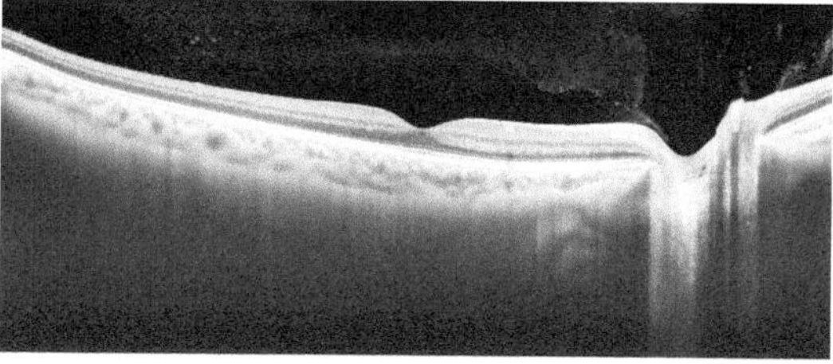

Fig. 4.11 SS-OCT scan showing clear spaces within the vitreous cavity. Note that the choroid–scleral boundary is also well visualized in this scan

collagen fibril (Sebag and Balazs 1985; Sebag and Balazs 1989). This presence of collagen fibrils was thought to play important roles in mitigating the mechanical stresses due to eye movement on the neuroretinal tissue. In a recent study, however, SS-OCT demonstrated the lack of fibrillar material in the bursal cavities (Spaide 2014). Spaide hypothesized that the viscoelasticity and the bursa in the vitreous could be the architectural features that mitigate the mechanical stresses on the neuroretinal tissue.

Posterior precortical vitreous pockets (PPVPs) are narrow liquefied spaces along the vitreoretinal interface in the macula (Li et al. 2014). There are significant correlations between the size of the PPVP and the patient's age, but the PPVP size does not appear to vary with refractive error. In a study of 73 subjects, the wall of the PPVP could not be visualized in all eyes. At around 3–4 years of age, the PPVP and Cloquet's canal (the remnant of the primary vitreous that arises from the optic disc, traverses the core vitreous, and ends in the retrolental space) have been reported to appear as separate spaces. Another study has also visualized the PPVPs as boat-shaped lacunae in the macular area bilaterally (Itakura and Kishi 2011). The posterior wall of the PPVP was reported to be a thin vitreous cortex, which is thinnest at the fovea.

4.4 Quantitative Measurements Using Swept-Source Optical Coherence Tomography

SS-OCT has been used in quantitative studies of choroidal and retinal thicknesses, which are used to diagnose the presence of diseases, monitor response to treatment, and prognosticate. The SS-OCT has a long-wavelength light source of 1050 nm and a tunable laser and has the potential for superior and simultaneous imaging of the retina and choroid because of the longer wavelength. Since SS-OCT has already been used in some clinical studies, the comparability of measurements obtained using SS-OCT with standard SD-OCT devices and the repeatability of its measurements are of interest to ophthalmologists. Determination of comparability and repeatability are prerequisites for quantifying a device's ability to separate real change from noise arising from machine- and observer-related differences.

4.4.1 Choroidal Thickness Measurements Using Swept-Source Optical Coherence Tomography

Deeper structures, such as the choroid–scleral interface (CSI), can be visualized more clearly with SS-OCT. In healthy eyes, it has been demonstrated that the SS-OCT visualizes the CSI in 100 % of eyes imaged compared with 68.4 % and 73.6 % of eyes imaged via non-enhanced depth imaging (EDI) and EDI-OCT, respectively (Adhi et al. 2014). While the clarity of the CSI has been found to be similar for SS-OCT compared with the Spectralis OCT and Cirrus HD-OCT among normal eyes, the median image quality score was significantly higher for the DRI OCT-1 compared with the Spectralis OCT in eyes with retinal diseases (Tan et al. 2015c). The image quality and clarity were noted to be affected by the presence of pathology, such as hard exudates or subretinal scars.

Several studies have compared point thickness measurements of subfoveal choroidal thickness (SFCT) and retinal thickness using SS-OCT and SD-OCT devices, although many of these studies were performed mostly on healthy eyes (Adhi et al. 2013, 2014; Copete et al. 2014; Ikuno et al. 2011; Matsuo et al. 2013; Tan et al. 2015c).

In general, the comparability of the SS-OCT with SD-OCT devices is good. The SFCT measurements from SS-OCT are generally slightly thicker compared with that from SD-OCT. The differences in SFCT range from 7.31 to 14.7 μm in healthy eyes (Adhi et al. 2013, 2014; Copete et al. 2014; Ikuno et al. 2011; Matsuo et al. 2013; Tan et al. 2015c). It has been reported that eyes with SFCT ≤200 μm had smaller differences between OCT devices compared with those with thicker choroids (mean 3.6 μm vs.

10.0 μm) (Tan et al. 2015c). It is possible that in eyes with thicker choroids, signal loss, artifacts, and shadows cast by the connective tissue between vessels might impair visualization of the CSI more in SD-OCT than in SS-OCT, thus accounting for the greater variability (Adhi et al. 2013; Copete et al. 2014; Ikuno et al. 2011; Matsuo et al. 2013; Tan et al. 2015c; Yamashita et al. 2012).

In diseased eyes, the SFCT measurements are still relatively comparable between SS-OCT and SD-OCT. In a study of 64 eyes with various retinal diseases, the mean difference in SFCT between SS-OCT and SD-OCT devices was 8.4 μm (Tan et al. 2015c). Another study performed on eyes with central serous chorioretinopathy (CSC) reported differences in SFCT of 4.6 μm (Hamzah et al. 2014).

4.4.2 Retinal Thickness Measurements Using Swept-Source Optical Coherence Tomography

At the point of writing, there has only been one report which compared retinal thicknesses between SS-OCT and SD-OCT devices (Tan et al. 2015a). In that study, the CRT measurements differed significantly among three OCT devices, with mean differences ranging from 15.6 to 37 μm. Intraclass correlation coefficients (ICCs) were at least 0.94 for any pair of machines. Similar results were observed in all nine ETDRS subfields. The differences likely arise from variation in the location of the lower segmentation boundary (Giani et al. 2010; Pierro et al. 2010; Tan et al. 2015a; Wolf-Schnurrbusch et al. 2009), i.e., at the second hyperreflective band for the DRI OCT-1, at the retinal pigment epithelium–Bruch's membrane complex for Spectralis, and above the third hyperreflective band for Cirrus. In general, the retinal thicknesses measured using different OCT devices are not comparable (Giani et al. 2010; Pierro et al. 2010; Tan et al. 2012a, 2014a, b, c; Wolf-Schnurrbusch et al. 2009), although several studies have reported methods to adjust segmentation lines or use regression equations to achieve comparability between SD-OCT devices (Tan et al. 2012a, 2014a, b, c).

The DRI OCT-1 produces retinal thickness maps from different scanning protocols. It has been found that in all ETDRS sectors, retinal thickness measurements obtained using the 3D and radial scans of the DRI OCT-1 were similar, with mean differences ranging from 0.7 to 3.8 μm (Tan et al. 2015a, c).

4.5 Scleral Imaging with Swept-Source Optical Coherence Tomography

The imaging of the sclera in vivo is possible with SS-OCT. The longer central wavelength allows improved penetration of tissue compared with SD-OCT devices, which enables the scleral boundaries to be visualized. Several studies have imaged the sclera using SS-OCT in eyes with high myopia (Ellabban et al. 2013b; Lopilly Park et al. 2014; Ohno-Matsui et al. 2012a). They reported that in between 57 and 68.4 % of subjects, the entire scleral layer was visualized by SS-OCT. However, the outer border of the sclera is difficult to detect in emmetropes (Liu et al. 2014) possibly as a result of the thicker choroid layer. In one study, the intra-observer reproducibility showed moderate to excellent measurement reproducibility, with an ICC of between 0.817 and 0.858 for the subfoveal scleral thickness. Interobserver reproducibility was good as well, with an ICC of 0.847 for the subfoveal scleral thickness (Lopilly Park et al. 2014).

The sclera is reported to be significantly thicker at the subfoveal and nasal regions compared with other regions (Ellabban et al. 2013b; Ohno-Matsui et al. 2012a). The degree of scleral thinning with time is asymmetrical throughout the posterior pole, with an estimated decrease per year of 5.6 μm at the foveal center, while the sclera thins at a rate of 12.1 μm per year at the inferior sectors. It has been speculated that this asymmetrical scleral thinning leads to the dome-shaped tomographic appearance (Ellabban et al. 2013a).

In myopia, the curvatures of the inner scleral surface of highly myopic eyes have been described to have several configurations: (1) sloping toward the optic nerve, (2) symmetrical and centered on the fovea, (3) asymmetrical, or (4) irregular (Ohno-Matsui et al. 2012a). Patients with irregular curvature were significantly older and had significantly longer axial lengths than those with other configurations. Eyes with irregular curvatures had more myopic fundus lesions. In addition, these eyes with irregular curvatures had temporally distorted shapes in the 3D MRI images. This is unlike eyes with symmetrical curvatures, which are reported to be symmetrical horizontally and sagittally in the MRI images. Among eyes with irregular curvatures, those with a pointed posterior pole were observed more frequently than those with the dull shape. It was speculated that the development and increase in depth of the staphylomas are the cause for the increased pointedness. Eyes in which the scleral curvatures sloped toward the optic nerve had nasally distorted shapes in the 3D MRI images (Ohno-Matsui et al. 2012a).

Studies have reported the morphology of intrascleral and retroscleral blood vessels in eyes with pathologic myopia and correlated these with ICGA (Ohno-Matsui et al. 2012a). The authors described that intrascleral and retrobulbar blood vessels were observed in the macular area of the highly myopic eyes. ICGA confirmed that these structures were the long posterior ciliary arteries (LPCAs) or the short posterior ciliary arteries (SPCAs) whose entry sites into the eye were displaced toward the temporal edge of the posterior staphyloma in 50 eyes. The authors also reported visualization of the intrascleral course of blood vessels, their cross sections, as well as the macular vortex veins and their exit from the sclera. In addition, retrobulbar blood vessels were observed posterior to the sclera in 26.7 % of eyes.

Recent studies have demonstrated the importance of the sclera in the pathogenesis of glaucoma. The mechanical influence of the peripapillary sclera on the lamina cribrosa is thought to be especially important. In one study, SS-OCT detected differences in the thicknesses of the posterior sclera between eyes with normotension glaucoma (497 μm) and eyes with primary open-angle glaucoma (671 μm) (Lopilly Park et al. 2014).

4.6 En Face Imaging Using Swept-Source Optical Coherence Tomography

SS-OCT can be used to produce en face images, which enables visualization of the macula at different depth levels. Due to its longer wavelength, reduced attenuation, and longer imaging range compared with SD-OCT, SS-OCT allows better en face imaging of the choroid and retina (Ferrara et al. 2014; Flores-Moreno et al. 2015). Characterization of the anatomy of the choroid and retina may help explain the pathophysiology of choroidal and retinal diseases.

En face SS-OCT can be useful in identifying choroidal neovascularization in neovascular AMD without the use of angiography. A study of 38 eyes with neovascular AMD demonstrated that the RPE and choriocapillaris are affected early in the disease process (Flores-Moreno et al. 2015). The neovascular complex was hyporeflective in 76.3 % of eyes, but was hyperreflective in the remaining 23.7 %. Hyporeflective changes were predominant at the level of the RPE, whereas hyperreflective changes were predominant at the level of the choriocapillaris and Sattler's and Haller's layers. In addition, in cases of neovascular AMD, the dye leakage in FA and ICGA is corresponded with the hyporeflective and hyperreflective changes seen on en face SS-OCT.

En face SS-OCT is also useful for observing eyes with PCV, since PCV lesions such as polyps and vascular networks exist beneath the RPE. A study demonstrated features including focal or diffuse choroidal vascular dilations (Alasil et al. 2015). Branching vascular networks were observed above and below Bruch's membrane and also in the choroidal vascular layer. Another study has described these networks as tortuous lines within a hyperreflective mesh (Sayanagi et al. 2015). En face imaging can demonstrate the extent of these lesions, so that it is possible to differentiate the vascular networks from other pathologies such as drusens. Notably, protrusions from the PED wall correspond with the polypoidal lesions seen on ICGA.

In reticular pseudodrusen, en face images through the choroid have revealed narrow and sparse choroidal vessels, which suggest choroidal involvement in its pathogenesis. The area of choroidal vasculature was also significantly reduced in eyes with reticular pseudodrusen compared with normal eyes (Ueda-Arakawa et al. 2014).

Ferrara and associates recently characterized chronic central serous chorioretinopathy (CSC) using en face SS-OCT (Ferrara et al. 2014). The en face image at the level of the RPE revealed the absence of signals corresponding to RPE detachment and/or loss. Focal and diffuse choroidal dilations were observed at the choriocapillaris and Sattler's and Haller's layers. In eyes with secondary choroidal neovascularization, hyporeflective signals at the choriocapillaris and throughout the choroid were observed. Other findings in CSC include focal choroidal excavations, and the en face scans highlighted the actual transverse shape of these excavations (Ellabban et al. 2013). The focal choroidal excavations were located within fluorescein leakage points and areas of choroidal hyperpermeability. It was hypothesized that these excavations may have formed from RPE retraction caused by focal scarring of choroidal connective tissue.

Lamina cribrosa structures can also be observed in vivo with en face SS-OCT (Takayama et al. 2013). In a study of 182 glaucomatous eyes, full-thickness focal defects near the margin of the lamina cribrosa were detected. These focal lamina cribrosa defects corresponded with neuroretinal rim thinning, concurrent or previous disc hemorrhages, abnormal circumpapillary retinal nerve fiber layer thickness, and visual field defects.

4.7 Applications of Anterior Segment Optical Coherence Tomography

In addition to scanning of the posterior pole, SS-OCT can also be used in imaging of structures in the anterior segment.

4.7.1 Identification and Quantification of Structures in the Angles

Anterior segment OCT has been used extensively to assess the angles of patients with glaucoma. The scleral spur is a key landmark in the angle of the eye, and successful identification of this structure using TD-OCT has been reported to vary from 64 to 80 % of patients, depending on the quadrant involved (Sakata et al. 2008). Among studies using SS-OCT, the sclera spur has been reported to be visualized in a higher proportion of eyes (typically in over 90 % of eyes) (Cumba et al. 2012; Liu et al. 2011; McKee et al. 2013; Tun et al. 2013). A paper by Liu et al. (2011) reported that the scleral spur was visible in over 90 % of eyes, although the advantage of SS-OCT varied with the scanning protocol and quadrant imaged. Tun et al. (2014) assessed the ability of SS-OCT to identify various structures in the angles of 148 subjects, which included 23 % with angle closure. Of the 592 quadrants assessed, identification of the scleral spur and Schwalbe's line was possible in 590 (99.7 %) and 585 (98.8 %) quadrants, respectively.

The scanning protocol that is used plays a role in determining the scleral spur visibility using SS-OCT. McKee et al. (2013) showed that using a low-density scan of 128 radial scans, each with 512 A-scans covering a distance of 16 mm across the anterior chamber, scleral spur visibility varied from 95 % nasally to 50 % inferiorly. When the scan density was increased to higher density – of 64 B-scans, each with 512 A-scans covering an area of 8×4 mm^2, with each of the four quadrants performed independently – the scleral spur visibility rose to 95 % inferiorly to 100 % in the temporal and superior quadrants.

The time required to produce a 360-degree scan is relatively short (typically under 3 s) and allows imaging of angle morphology with a high degree of accuracy. A study by Lai et al. (2013) has found good agreement between gonioscopy and SS-OCT in the identification of peripheral anterior synechiae (kappa = 0.79; 95 % CI, 0.67–0.91). More importantly, it has been reported that SS-OCT could be used to differentiate synechial closure from appositional closure with dynamic dark-light imaging and by observing the angle configuration (obtuse for synechial closure and acute for appositional closure).

SS-OCT can be used to discern the patency of sclerotomies following glaucoma filtration surgery (Lai et al. 2013). Analysis of the SS-OCT images allows measurement of the area of peripheral anterior synechiae and quantification of its involvement, and it has been suggested that this may be a vital tool for the assessment of the extent of peripheral anterior synechiae and its progression in glaucoma patients.

Quantification of various parameters in the angles, such as the angle opening distance, trabecular–iris space area, trabecular–iris angle, and iris volume, which are commonly used in the assessment of glaucoma patients using TD-OCT, can also be performed using SS-OCT (Liu et al. 2011). The iris volume has been suggested as a potential risk factor for angle closure in studies which used TD-OCT (Aptel and Denis 2010; Aptel et al. 2012). Mak et al. showed that the change in iris volume has a more substantive effect on the anterior chamber angle in eyes with a smaller ACV (Mak et al. 2013). This explains the increased predisposition of these eyes to develop angle closure. It has been suggested that the interplay between iris volume and anterior chamber volume is important for the investigation of the dynamics of primary angle closure since both ACV and iris volume were significant determinants of angle width.

A novel parameter – the iris–trabecular contact index (ITC index) – has been described using SS-OCT (Baskaran et al. 2013). This is a summary measure of the circumferential extent of angle closure and represents the extent of angle closure as a percentage. Inbuilt software of the OCT device analyzes the extent of iris–trabecular contact across 360° of the angle and calculates the extent of the angle closure as the ITC index. This has been found to compare favorably with gonioscopy, with area under the curve ranging from 0.83 to 0.91, depending on the definitions of gonioscopic angle closure which were used.

4.7.2 Biometry Using Swept-Source Optical Coherence Tomography

SS-OCT technology has been used to perform biometry and has shown comparable precision to current devices. Grulkowski et al. in 2013 reported strong correlations between the SS-OCT and the IOLMaster for axial length measurements ($r = 0.984$), with high intersession reproducibility of SS-OCT measurements (intraclass correlation coefficients >0.99).

The advantages of using SS-OCT include reduced scattering and attenuation from ocular opacities as a result of the longer wavelength (1065 nm). This may improve the accuracy of biometry in patients with severe cataracts, which currently present difficulty for devices such as the IOLMaster. All parameters, such as axial length, anterior chamber depth, central corneal thickness, keratometry, and white-to-white distance, can be obtained from a single data set, instead of using different instruments. The device is also able to produce basic images of the retina, allowing cataract surgeons to screen for obvious macular pathologies. The device is also noncontact, thus improving patient contact.

4.8 Limitations and Pitfalls of Swept-Source Optical Coherence Tomography

The limitations of SS-OCT include a small reduction in axial resolution due to the longer wavelength of the light source (Potsaid et al. 2010). However it is unlikely that this will have any clinical impact in the usual review of patients.

As there are currently only a few SS-OCT devices available commercially, this limits their application to standard clinical practice. Another consideration is the cost of the device (Srinivasan et al. 2007), which may make it difficult for ophthalmology clinics to acquire these devices. However, these limitations will likely be addressed in the future as SS-OCT devices become more readily available.

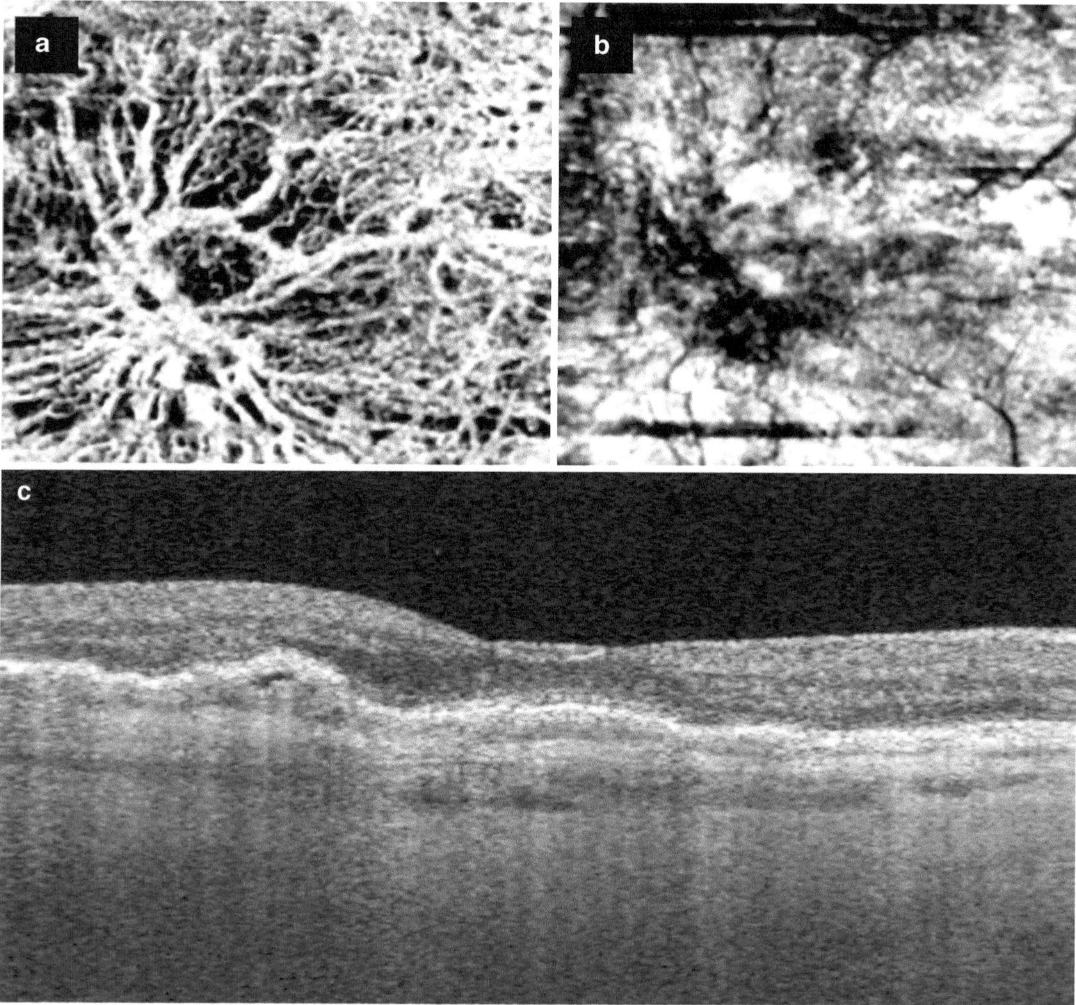

Fig. 4.12 OCT angiography of a patient with choroidal neovascularization secondary to age-related macular degeneration. (**a**) OCT angiogram showing the CNV net. (**b**) OCT structural projection image corresponding to the same region of the OCT angiogram. (**c**) Representative OCT B-scan of the CNV lesion (Acknowledgement: Topcon Advanced Biomedical Imaging Laboratory for its special assistance in developing the angiographic methodology and processing the data)

4.9 Future Developments of Swept-Source Optical Coherence Tomography

SS-OCT can be used for OCT angiography, which is covered in detail in another chapter. In brief, a 3×3 mm region of tissue can be scanned at a resolution of 5 μm within 4 s. The rapid scanning enables analysis of variation of reflectivity and phase shift, which is used to construct microvascular flow maps (Fig. 4.12). This allows the imaging of microvasculature of the retina and choriocapillaris without the use of intravenous dyes.

Conclusion

SS-OCT confers important advantages over earlier SD-OCT devices, among which are the faster scanning speed and the ability to image the deeper structures in the eye, thus allowing ophthalmologists to visualize the choroid and sclera in unprecedented detail. These have already presented important insights to ophthalmologists and will likely guide management of patients with ocular diseases in the years ahead.

References

Adhi M, Duker JS (2013) Optical coherence tomography-current and future applications. Curr Opin Ophthalmol 24:213–221

Adhi M, Liu JJ, Qavi AH et al (2013) Enhanced visualization of the choroido-scleral interface using swept-source OCT. Ophthalmic Surg Lasers Imaging Retina 44:S40–S42

Adhi M, Liu JJ, Qavi AH et al (2014) Choroidal analysis in healthy eyes using swept-source optical coherence tomography compared to spectral domain optical coherence tomography. Am J Ophthalmol 157: 1272–1281

Alasil T, Ferrara D, Adhi M et al (2015) En face imaging of the choroid in polypoidal choroidal vasculopathy using swept-source optical coherence tomography. Am J Ophthalmol 159:634–643

Aptel F, Denis P (2010) Optical coherence tomography quantitative analysis of iris volume changes after pharmacologic mydriasis. Ophthalmology 117:3–10

Aptel F, Chiquet C, Beccat S et al (2012) Biometric evaluation of anterior chamber changes after physiologic pupil dilation using Pentacam and anterior segment optical coherence tomography. Invest Ophthalmol Vis Sci 53:4005–4010

Baskaran M, Ho SW, Tun TA et al (2013) Assessment of circumferential angle-closure by the iris-trabecular contact index with swept-source optical coherence tomography. Ophthalmology 120:2226–2231

Copete S, Flores-Moreno I, Montero JA et al (2014) Direct comparison of spectral-domain and swept-source OCT in the measurement of choroidal thickness in normal eyes. Br J Ophthalmol 98:334–338

Cumba RJ, Radhakrishnan S, Bell NP et al (2012) Reproducibility of scleral spur identification and angle measurements using fourier domain anterior segment optical coherence tomography. J Ophthalmol 2012:487309

Drexler W, Liu M, Kumar A et al (2014) Optical coherence tomography today: speed, contrast, and multimodality. J Biomed Opt 19:071412

Ellabban AA, Tsujikawa A, Matsumoto A et al (2013a) Three-dimensional tomographic features of dome-shaped macula by swept-source optical coherence tomography. Am J Ophthalmol 155:320–328

Ellabban AA, Tsujikawa A, Ooto S et al (2013b) Focal choroidal excavation in eyes with central serous chorioretinopathy. Am J Ophthalmol 156:673–683

Ferrara D, Mohler KJ, Waheed N et al (2014) En face enhanced-depth swept-source optical coherence tomography features of chronic central serous chorioretinopathy. Ophthalmology 121:719–726

Flores-Moreno I, Arias-Barquet L, Rubio-Caso MJ et al (2015) En face swept-source optical coherence tomography in neovascular age-related macular degeneration. Br J Ophthalmol 99:306322

Forte R, Cennamo GL, Finelli ML et al (2009) Comparison of time domain Stratus OCT and spectral domain SLO/OCT for assessment of macular thickness and volume. Eye 23:2071–2078

Francis JH, Pang CE, Abramson DH et al (2015) Swept-source optical coherence tomography features of choroidal nevi. Am J Ophthalmol 159:169–176

Giani A, Cigada M, Choudhry N et al (2010) Reproducibility of retinal thickness measurements on normal and pathologic eyes by different optical coherence tomography instruments. Am J Ophthalmol 150:815–824

Grulkowski I, Liu JJ, Zhang JY et al (2013) Reproducibility of a long-range swept-source optical coherence tomography ocular biometry system and comparison with clinical biometers. Ophthalmology 120:2184–2190

Hamzah F, Shinojima A, Mori R et al (2014) Choroidal thickness measurement by enhanced depth imaging and swept-source optical coherence tomography in central serous chorioretinopathy. BMC Ophthalmol 14:145

Hayashi Y, Mitamura Y, Egawa M et al (2014) Swept-source optical coherence tomographic findings of choroidal osteoma. Case Rep Ophthalmol 5:195–202

Huang D, Swanson EA, Lin CP et al (1991) Optical coherence tomography. Science 254:1178–1181

Ikuno Y, Maruko I, Yasuno Y et al (2011) Reproducibility of retinal and choroidal thickness measurements in enhanced depth imaging and high-penetration optical coherence tomography. Invest Ophthalmol Vis Sci 52:5536–5540

Itakura H, Kishi S (2011) Aging changes of vitreomacular interface. Retina 31:1400–1404

Itakura H, Kishi S, Li D et al (2013) Observation of posterior precortical vitreous pocket using swept-source optical coherence tomography. Invest Ophthalmol Vis Sci 54:3102–3107

Jia Y, Bailey ST, Wilson DJ et al (2014) Quantitative optical coherence tomography angiography of choroidal neovascularization in age-related macular degeneration. Ophthalmology 121:1435–1444

Kawana K, Yasuno Y, Yatagai T et al (2007) High-speed, swept-source optical coherence tomography: a 3-dimensional view of anterior chamber angle recession. Acta Ophthalmol Scand 85:684–685

Lai I, Mak H, Lai G et al (2013) Anterior chamber angle imaging with swept-source optical coherence tomography: measuring peripheral anterior synechia in glaucoma. Ophthalmology 120:1144–1149

Li D, Kishi S, Itakura H et al (2014) Posterior precortical vitreous pockets and connecting channels in children on swept-source optical coherence tomography. Invest Ophthalmol Vis Sci 55:2412–2416

Lim TH, Laude A, Tan CS (2010) Polypoidal choroidal vasculopathy: an angiographic discussion. Eye 24:483–490

Lim LS, Cheung G, Lee SY (2014) Comparison of spectral domain and swept-source optical coherence tomography in pathological myopia. Eye 28:488–491

Liu S, Yu M, Ye C et al (2011) Anterior chamber angle imaging with swept-source optical coherence tomography: an investigation on variability of angle measurement. Invest Ophthalmol Vis Sci 52:8598–8603

Liu JJ, Witkin AJ, Adhi M et al (2014) Enhanced vitreous imaging in healthy eyes using swept source optical coherence tomography. PLoS One 9:e102950. doi:10.1371/journal.pone.0102950

Liu G, Tan O, Gao SS et al (2015) Postprocessing algorithms to minimize fixed-pattern artifact and reduce trigger jitter in swept source optical coherence tomography. Optics express 23:9824–34

Lopilly Park HY, Lee NY, Choi JA et al (2014) Measurement of scleral thickness using swept-source optical coherence tomography in patients with open-angle glaucoma and myopia. Am J Ophthalmol 157:876–884

Mak H, Xu G, Leung CK (2013) Imaging the iris with swept-source optical coherence tomography: relationship between iris volume and primary angle closure. Ophthalmology 120:2517–2524

Mansouri K, Nuyen B, Weinreb N (2013) Improved visualization of deep ocular structures in glaucoma using high penetration optical coherence tomography. Expert Rev Med Devices 10:621–628

Matsuo Y, Sakamoto T, Yamashita T et al (2013) Comparisons of choroidal thickness of normal eyes obtained by two different spectral-domain OCT instruments and one swept-source OCT instrument. Invest Ophthalmol Vis Sci 54:7630–7636

McKee H, Ye C, Yu M et al (2013) Anterior chamber angle imaging with swept-source optical coherence tomography: detecting the scleral spur, Schwalbe's Line, and Schlemm's Canal. J Glaucoma 22:468–472

Moult E, Choi W, Waheed NK et al (2014) Ultrahigh-speed swept-source OCT angiography in exudative AMD. Ophthalmic Surg Lasers Imaging Retina 45:496–505

Mrejen S, Spaide RF (2013) Optical coherence tomography: imaging of the choroid and beyond. Surv Ophthalmol 58:387–429

Ohno-Matsui K, Akiba M, Modegi T et al (2012a) Association between shape of sclera and myopic retinochoroidal lesions in patients with pathologic myopia. Invest Ophthalmol Vis Sci 53:6046–6061

Ohno-Matsui K, Akiba M, Moriyama M et al (2012b) Acquired optic nerve and peripapillary pits in pathologic myopia. Ophthalmology 119:1685–1692

Ohno-Matsui K, Akiba M, Moriyama M et al (2012c) Intrachoroidal cavitation in macular area of eyes with pathologic myopia. Am J Ophthalmol 154:382–393

Ohno-Matsui K, Shimada N, Akiba M et al (2013) Characteristics of intrachoroidal cavitation located temporal to optic disc in highly myopic eyes. Eye 27:630–638

Ouyang Y, Heussen FM, Mokwa N et al (2011) Spatial distribution of posterior pole choroidal thickness by spectral domain optical coherence tomography. Invest Ophthalmol Vis Sci 52:7019–7026

Pedinielli A, Souied EH, Perrenoud F et al (2013) In vivo visualization of perforating vessels and focal scleral ectasia in pathological myopia. Invest Ophthalmol Vis Sci 54:7637–7643

Pierro L, Giatsidis SM, Mantovani E et al (2010) Macular thickness interoperator and intraoperator reproducibility in healthy eyes using 7 optical coherence tomography instruments. Am J Ophthalmol 150: 199–204

Potsaid B, Baumann B, Huang D et al (2010) Ultrahigh speed 1050 nm swept source/Fourier domain OCT retinal and anterior segment imaging at 100,000 to 400,000 axial scans per second. Opt Express 18:20029–20048

Sakata LM, Lavanya R, Friedman DS et al (2008) Assessment of the scleral spur in anterior segment optical coherence tomography images. Arch Ophthalmol 126:181–185

Sato T, Mrejen S, Spaide RF (2013) Multimodal imaging of optic disc drusen. Am J Ophthalmol 156:275–282

Sayanagi K, Gomi F, Akiba M et al (2015) En-face high-penetration optical coherence tomography imaging in polypoidal choroidal vasculopathy. Br J Ophthalmol 99:29–35

Sebag J, Balazs EA (1985) Human vitreous fibres and vitreoretinal disease. Trans Ophthalmol Soc 104:123–128

Sebag J, Balazs EA (1989) Morphology and ultrastructure of human vitreous fibers. Invest Ophthalmol Vis Sci 30:1867–1871

Shinohara K, Moriyama M, Shimada N et al (2013) Analyses of shape of eyes and structure of optic nerves in eyes with tilted disc syndrome by swept-source optical coherence tomography and three-dimensional magnetic resonance imaging. Eye (Lond) 27:1233–1241

Spaide RF (2014) Visualization of the posterior vitreous with dynamic focusing and windowed averaging swept source optical coherence tomography. Am J Ophthalmol 158:1267–1274

Srinivasan VJ, Huber R, Gorczynska I et al (2007) High-speed, high-resolution optical coherence tomography retinal imaging with a frequency-swept laser at 850 nm. Opt Lett 32:361–363

Stanga PE, Sala-Puigdollers A, Caputo S et al (2014) In vivo imaging of cortical vitreous using 1050-nm swept-source deep range imaging optical coherence tomography. Am J Ophthalmol 157:397–404

Takahashi A, Ooto S, Yoshimura N (2013) High-penetration optical coherence tomography and enhanced depth imaging in presumed retinal pigment epithelial hamartoma. Retin Cases Brief Rep 7:179–182

Takayama K, Hangai M, Kimura Y et al (2013) Three-dimensional imaging of lamina cribrosa defects in glaucoma using swept-source optical coherence tomography. Invest Ophthalmol Vis Sci 54: 4798–4807

Tan CS, Cheong KX (2014) Macular choroidal thicknesses in healthy adults--relationship with ocular and demographic factors. Invest Ophthalmol Vis Sci 55:6452–6458

Tan CS, Li KZ, Lim TH (2012a) A novel technique of adjusting segmentation boundary layers to achieve comparability of retinal thickness and volumes between spectral domain and time domain optical coherence tomography. Invest Ophthalmol Vis Sci 53:5515–5519

Tan CS, Ouyang Y, Ruiz H et al (2012b) Diurnal variation of choroidal thickness in normal, healthy subjects measured by spectral domain optical coherence tomography. Invest Ophthalmol Vis Sci 53:261–266

Tan CS, Cheong KX, Lim LW et al (2014a) Topographic variation of choroidal and retinal thicknesses at the macula in healthy adults. Br J Ophthalmol 98:339–344

Tan CS, Li KZ, Lim TH (2014b) Calculating the predicted retinal thickness from spectral domain and time domain optical coherence tomography – comparison of different methods. Graefes Arch Clin Exp Ophthalmol 252:1491–1499

Tan CS, Ngo WK, Lim LW et al (2014c) A novel classification of the vascular patterns of polypoidal choroidal vasculopathy and its relation to clinical outcomes. Br J Ophthalmol 98:1528–1533

Tan CS, Chan JC, Cheong KX et al (2015a) Comparison of retinal thicknesses measured using swept-source and spectral-domain optical coherence tomography devices. Ophthalmic Surg Lasers Imaging Retina 46:172–179

Tan CS, Ngo WK, Chen JP et al (2015b) EVEREST study report 2: imaging and grading protocol, and baseline characteristics of a randomised controlled trial of polypoidal choroidal vasculopathy. Br J Ophthalmol 99:624–628

Tan CS, Ngo WK, Cheong KX (2015c) Comparison of choroidal thicknesses using swept source and spectral domain optical coherence tomography in diseased and normal eyes. Br J Ophthalmol 99:354–358

Tun TA, Baskaran M, Zheng C et al (2013) Assessment of trabecular meshwork width using swept source optical coherence tomography. Graefes Arch Clin Exp Ophthalmol 251:1587–1592

Tun TA, Baskaran M, Perera SA et al (2014) Sectoral variations of iridocorneal angle width and iris volume in Chinese Singaporeans: a swept-source optical coherence tomography study. Graefes Arch Clin Exp Ophthalmol 252:1127–1132

Ueda-Arakawa N, Ooto S, Ellabban AA et al (2014) Macular choroidal thickness and volume of eyes with reticular pseudodrusen using swept-source optical coherence tomography. Am J Ophthalmol 157:994–1004

Wolf-Schnurrbusch UE, Ceklic L, Brinkmann CK et al (2009) Macular thickness measurements in healthy eyes using six different optical coherence tomography instruments. Invest Ophthalmol Vis Sci 50:3432–3437

Yamashita T, Yamashita T, Shirasawa M et al (2012) Repeatability and reproducibility of subfoveal choroidal thickness in normal eyes of Japanese using different SD-OCT devices. Invest Ophthalmol Vis Sci 53:1102–1107

Yasuno Y, Miura M, Kawana K et al (2009) Visualization of sub-retinal pigment epithelium morphologies of exudative macular diseases by high-penetration optical coherence tomography. Invest Ophthalmol Vis Sci 50:405–413

Normal Choroidal Morphology

5

Daniela Ferrara, Andre Romano, and Jay S. Duker

Contents

D. Ferrara, MD, PhD (✉)
Tufts University School of Medicine,
Boston, MA, USA
e-mail: daniela@ferrara.md

A. Romano, MD, PhD
Department of Ophthalmology, Federal University
Sao Paulo, Sao Paulo, Brazil

University of Miami, Miller School of Medicine,
Miami, FL, USA

Neovista Eye Center, Americana, Brazil

J.S. Duker, MD
Tuft Medical Center, Tufts University School of
Medicine, Boston, MA, USA

5.1 Introduction

Recent technological advances in ophthalmic imaging, especially those in optical coherence tomography (OCT), revealed morphological changes of the choroid related to a wide number of pathological chorioretinal conditions, indicating a pivotal role in underlying disease mechanisms, in natural history of diseases, and also in response to therapeutic interventions.

OCT now permits the acquisition of high-speed, high-resolution imaging that generates tridimensional, depth-resolved optical reconstruction of the choroid. The ability to better characterize the in vivo morphology of the normal choroid is of fundamental importance to understand the role of the choriocapillaris and choroidal vasculature in physiological and pathological states of the eye.

5.2 Optical Coherence Tomography as a Valuable Tool to Investigate the Choroid

5.2.1 Fourier-Domain Optical Coherence Tomography Technologies

The physics of the OCT device plays a key role when investigating the choroid on OCT. Spectral-domain (SD)-OCT is the standard for diagnosis

C.H. Meyer et al. (eds.), *Spectral Domain Optical Coherence Tomography in Macular Diseases*,
DOI 10.1007/978-81-322-3610-8_5

and management of chorioretinal disorders in the clinical practice, but the documentation of the choroid may be compromised by limited depth of penetration (~850 nm), even when applying the enhanced depth imaging (EDI) method (Adhi et al. 2014; Spaide et al. 2008). The EDI-OCT is an acquisition technique that generally exhibits better quality of the choroid and choroidal-scleral interface, because the peak sensitivity is displaced posteriorly. By placing the zero-delay line toward the sclera, rather than at the level of the posterior vitreous, the roll-off sensitivity does not compromise the tomographic registration (Spaide et al. 2008; Spaide 2010). Although valuable to investigate the choroid in full thickness, this technique does not contribute significantly to documentation of the choriocapillaris given its proximity to the retinal pigment epithelium (RPE) (Spaide 2009).

Swept-source (SS)-OCT is a modified Fourier-domain and depth-resolved technology that offers potential advantages over SD-OCT, including reduced sensitivity roll-off with imaging depth, higher detection efficiencies, improved imaging range, adaptability to longer imaging wavelengths of ~1050 nm that improve penetration of the choroid, and higher image acquisition speeds (Unterhuber et al. 2005). SS-OCT employs a wavelength sweeping laser light source and a photodiode detector that records the interference of the backscattered light from the retina, while in SD-OCT a broadband light source is used, and a spectrometer and line scan camera record the interference (Potsaid et al. 2010). The improved performance of SS-OCT enables higher density raster scan protocols and deeper image penetration, contributing to better visualization of the choriocapillaris and choroidal vessels (Adhi et al. 2015; Ferrara et al. 2014; Montaghiannezam et al. 2012; Sohrab et al. 2012; Srinivasan et al. 2008).

Despite potential advantages of SS-OCT in comparison to SD-OCT to investigate the choroid, the differences between the two technologies are related to the qualitative assessment. Quantitative observations seem to be significantly correlated and highly reproducible, assuming that retinochoroidal and choroidal-scleral interfaces are clearly visible (Branchini et al. 2012; Copete et al. 2014; Ellabban et al. 2012; Hirata et al. 2011; Matsuo et al. 2013; Tan et al. 2015; Yamashita et al. 2012).

5.2.2 Structural Optical Coherence Tomography

Cross-sectional OCT imaging is widely used in the clinical ophthalmological practice and has been considered a fundamental tool in the diagnosis and management of chorioretinal diseases. The integrity of the RPE/Bruch's membrane/choriocapillaris complex and the subfoveal total choroidal thickness are among the features of fundamental importance for clinical interpretation. Cross-sectional OCT, however, has limited ability to document in details the choriocapillaris and individual choroidal layers, even in normal eyes with preserved anatomy. Some studies have assessed in conjunction the choriocapillaris and medium-size choroidal vessels when using cross-sectional OCT (Adhi et al. 2013; Branchini et al. 2013).

En face OCT imaging is generated by successive alignment of multiple adjacent B-scans rendering a tridimensional dataset. It allows high-definition depth-resolved reconstruction of the choroidal tissue in a plane parallel to the anatomic structures, rather than in a perpendicular plane. En face OCT documents details of the choroid not readily appreciated on cross-sectional OCT, besides offering ideal correlation with other imaging modalities. Nonetheless, for optimal interpretation, both cross-sectional and en face OCT images should be analyzed in conjunction, in a multidimensional assessment. Although the identification of feeder arterioles and draining venules is limited even on en face OCT, choriocapillaris and medium-size and large-size choroidal vessels can be clearly identified (Adhi et al. 2015; Ferrara et al. 2014; Montaghiannezam et al. 2012; Sohrab et al. 2012; Srinivasan et al. 2008). For such, post-acquisition image processing and registration is of fundamental importance. OCT image quality can be improved to correct eye movements, tilting, illumination, and image noise, for example. Another major aspect to properly evaluate the choroid on en face OCT is image registration using the RPE or Bruch's membrane as a reference surface. This digital processing compensates the natural curvature of the back of the eye and, in result, permits documentation of each individual choroidal layer in one distinct plan (Figs. 5.1, 5.2, and 5.3).

5.2.3 Optical Coherence Tomography Angiography

OCT angiography is a recently developed technology that allows noninvasive documentation of vascular structures and is a useful investigative tool of the choriocapillaris and choroidal microvasculature in physiological and pathological conditions. The basic principle of OCT angiography assumes that all other elements remaining static, the only difference between sequential OCT scans in a given location of the tissue is caused by the motion of erythrocytes within the vessels. It can be obtained with several different technologies, classified into two major groups: amplitude based and phase based. Important examples of amplitude-based technologies are the split-spectrum amplitude-decorrelation angiography (SSADA), scattering OCT, and speckle variance (Jia et al. 2012), while examples of phase-based technologies are phase-variance OCT and Doppler OCT (Fingler et al. 2007; Kim et al. 2011). All of these can be implemented in high-speed Fourier-domain OCT, either SD-OCT or SS-OCT systems.

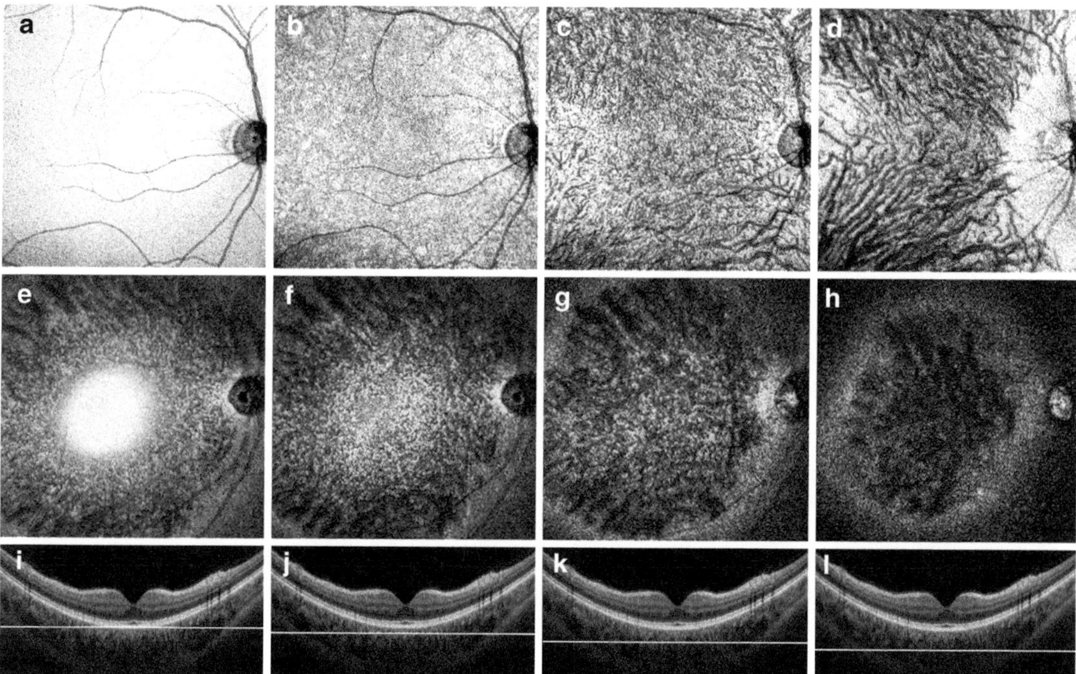

Fig. 5.1 Structural en face optical coherence tomography (OCT) of normal eyes obtained with swept-source OCT. In the *upper row*, en face OCT was registered taking the Bruch's membrane as a reference surface to compensate the natural curvature of the eye. Each scan documents an individual choroidal layer, as follows: retinal pigment epithelium (RPE) (**a**), choriocapillaris (**b**), inner choroid (**c**), and outer choroid (**d**). Note at the level of the outer choroid (**d**) a peripapillary area without choroidal vessels, correspondent to the so-called watershed zone. In the *middle row*, original en face OCT scans without registration. Each scan documents multiple choroidal layers; the following levels are documented in the center of the scans: RPE (**e**), choriocapillaris (**f**), inner choroid (**g**), and outer choroid (**h**). In the *lower row*, cross-sectional OCT centered at the fovea. Individual choroidal layers are not readily appreciated. The horizontal lines indicate the level of en face scans, as follows: RPE (**i**), choriocapillaris (**j**), inner choroid (**k**), and outer choroid (**l**)

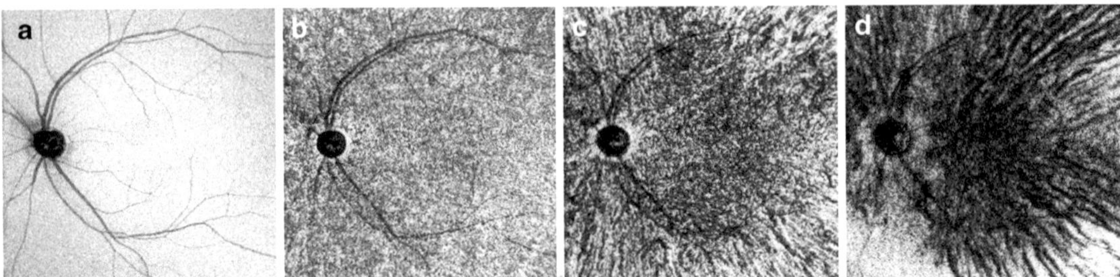

Fig. 5.2 Structural en face optical coherence tomography (OCT) of normal eye obtained with swept-source OCT. Images were registered taking the Bruch's membrane as a reference surface to compensate the natural curvature of the eye. En face OCT at the level of the retinal pigment epithelium (**a**) is characterized by homogeneous hyperreflective layer. The only hyporeflective structures are the optic disc and the shadowing artifact of overlying retinal vessels. En face OCT at the level of the choriocapillaris (**b**) shows homogeneous reticular pattern throughout the scan. En face OCT at the level of the inner choroid (**c**) shows in the macular area a complex, interwoven network of short and relatively thin vascular segments crossing over each other and homogeneously distributed, while in extramacular areas the vessels are fewer in number. En face OCT scans at the level of the outer choroid (**d**) show wider vessels, interwoven in the center of the macula but assuming a distinct radial distribution beyond the macular area toward the equator

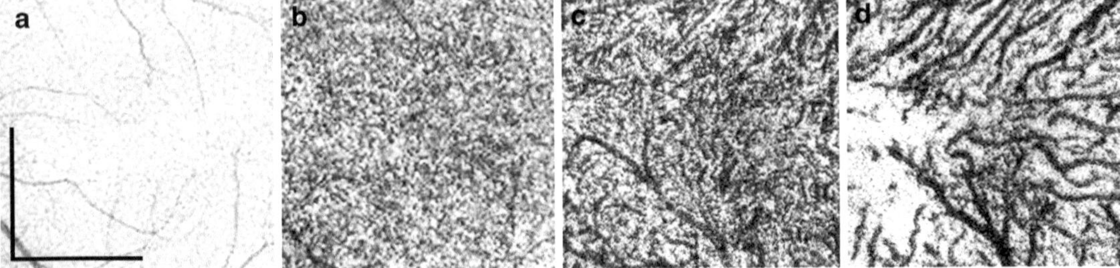

Fig. 5.3 Structural en face optical coherence tomography (OCT) of normal eye obtained with a swept-source OCT prototype operating at 1050 nm. Images were registered taking the Bruch's membrane as a reference surface to compensate the natural curvature of the eye. Magnified fields show details of the individual layers as follows: retinal pigment epithelium (**a**), choriocapillaris (**b**), inner choroid (**c**), and outer choroid (**d**). Vertical and horizontal scale bars measuring 1.5 mm

OCT angiography has fundamental differences when compared to standard fluorescein angiography or indocyanine green angiography; direct comparison between these methods is not always feasible and should be taken with caution. The proper interpretation of OCT angiography must consider the physical principles of imaging acquisition: images do not change throughout the acquisition process, and since no exogenous dye is used, leakage, staining, or pooling is not documented. On the other hand, it is subject to specific artifacts mostly related to the optical reconstruction of vascular tissues. One important limitation is the fact that OCT angiography identifies the vascular flow within a limited dynamic range. There is a sensitivity limit, which is the slowest detectable flow determined by the elapsed time between sequential scans. There is also a saturation limit, which is the fastest detectable flow that is differentiated by the decorrelation signal. All these considerations are relevant when interpreting OCT angiography of the choroidal vasculature. Although the choroid has the highest blood flow per unit weight tissue in the human body (Alm and Bill 1973), the blood flow in the choriocapillaris and choroidal vasculature may occasionally be too slow or too fast to be documented by this imaging method.

5.3 Normal Choroidal Thickness on Structural Optical Coherence Tomography

While choroidal thinning on OCT has been associated with various pathological conditions such as AMD, age-related choroidal atrophy, and high myopia, it is important to note that the total choroidal thickness also varies widely in the normal population at both the subfoveal and the extramacular locations (Branchini et al. 2013; Flores-Moreno et al. 2013; Kim et al. 2011; Spaide 2009; Wei et al. 2013). Variability related with gender, age, axial length, and refractive error has been reported (Barteselli et al. 2012; Margolis and Spaide 2009; Sanchez-Cano et al. 2014). It may be challenging, therefore, to establish normative values or to identify a clear threshold between normal and pathological choroidal thickness in the clinical setting.

The subfoveal total choroidal thickness has been found to correlate significantly with age, and progressive subfoveal total choroidal thinning occurs in normal aging eyes (Fujiwara et al. 2009; Ikuno and Tano 2009; Ikuno et al. 2010; Manjunath et al. 2010; Margolis and Spaide 2009; Hirata et al. 2011; Ooto et al. 2015). Subfoveal choroidal thickness was also found to be negatively correlated with axial length (Benavente-Perez et al. 2010; Esmaeelpour et al. 2010; Hirata et al. 2011; Li et al. 2011; Ooto et al. 2015) and positively correlated with refractive error (Fujiwara et al. 2009; Ikuno and Tano 2009; Ikuno et al. 2010). Diurnal variations on the same individuals were also reported (Brown et al. 2009; Ikuno et al. 2010; Tan et al. 2012) and seem to correlate with diurnal variations of the ocular axial length (Chakraborty et al. 2011).

Progressive choroidal thinning in normal aging eyes was documented in both *post-mortem* histopathological studies and in vivo investigations, using either cross-sectional OCT or en face OCT (Adhi et al. 2015; Ferrara et al. 2016; Ikuno et al. 2010; Manjunath et al. 2011; Margolis and Spaide 2009; McLeod and Lutty 1994; Spaide 2009; Wei et al. 2013). Investigations on en face OCT suggested that the proportion between individual choroidal layers may also change in older individuals, and it is possible that in normal aging eyes, the choriocapillaris loss may be relatively more significant than loss of medium-size and large-size choroidal vessels. Morphological changes in the choriocapillaris and choroidal vasculature patterns have not been correlated so far with the normal aging process (Ferrara et al. 2016).

Caution is needed when comparing choroidal thickness measurements reported in different studies available in the literature, because variations in demographic or clinical characteristics may preclude a direct correlation between different cohorts. In one of the first attempts to obtain normative values for the normal population using SD-OCT, the mean subfoveal total choroidal thickness in a small group of patients, mean age of 50 years, was found to be 287 μm, which was found to decrease approximately 15 μm for each decade of life (Margolis and Spaide 2009). Subfoveal total choroidal thickness seems to decrease especially after the age of 40 (Ferrara et al. 2016); Ruiz-Medrano et al. 2014). In another cohort, the following measurements were found on SS-OCT for each age range: 325.6 ± 51.1 μm (0–10 years), 316.7 ± 90.1 μm (11–20 years), 313.9 ± 80.3 μm (21–40 years), 264.6 ± 79.3 μm (41–60 years), and 276.3 ± 88.8 μm (older than 60 years), in addition to different choroidal thickness profiles for each age group with greater variations in the temporal quadrant of the fundus (Ruiz-Medrano et al. 2014). Several other studies have reported highly variable values for mean subfoveal total choroidal thickness, investigating cohorts of different demographic characteristics (Benavente-Perez et al. 2010; Hirata et al. 2011). As a gross estimate, in vivo subfoveal total choroidal thinning was considered to progress 1.56 μm per year, which is higher than 1.1 μm per year estimated from *post-mortem* specimens (Margolis and Spaide 2009). Although several aspects can justify such difference, to some extent it may be related to the lack of blood flow in histological examination (Feeney-Burns et al. 1990; Ramrattan et al. 1994; Sarks 1976).

In addition, normal variations of the choroidal-scleral contour also contribute to the variability in total choroidal thickness measurements, which vary throughout the fundus (Adhi et al. 2014;

Branchini et al. 2013). In normal eyes the choroid is thickest under the fovea, showing marked thinning toward the periphery in all four quadrants – nasal, temporal, superior, and inferior (Esmaeelpour et al. 2010; Hirata et al. 2011; Ikuno et al. 2010; Manjunath et al. 2010). The peripapillary total choroidal thickness was found to be the thinnest inferiorly to the optic disk (Ho et al. 2011; Tanabe et al. 2012).

The suprachoroidal layer is not commonly observed on OCT in normal eyes. It is estimated to be documented on cross-sectional OCT in only 5 % of healthy emmetropic eyes as two distinct bands: an upper hyperreflective band corresponding to the suprachoroidal layer and a lower hyporeflective band supposedly corresponding to the suprachoroidal space, which in vivo was previously visualized only in eyes with choroidal effusion (Michalewska et al. 2015).

5.4 Normal Choroidal Morphology on Structural En Face Optical Coherence Tomography

The normal choroid has been investigated on recent research using depth-resolved en face OCT, extracted from tridimensional datasets, which is strikingly superior than cross-sectional OCT for this matter. Most of these recent studies use SS-OCT, since it documents deeper structures better than SD-OCT (Adhi et al. 2015; Ferrara et al. 2014; Ferrara et al. 2016; Montaghiannezam et al. 2012; Sohrab et al. 2012; Sohrab and Fawzi 2013; Srinivasan et al. 2008). The morphological features of the choroid do not seem to present qualitative changes during normal aging, although quantitative changes are typically observed, as discussed above (Ferrara et al. 2016).

Structural en face OCT of the RPE in normal eyes is regularly homogeneous and hyperreflective throughout the scan, including the macular and peripapillary areas. The only hyporeflective elements correspond to the optic disk and to the tomographic shadowing artifact of the overlying normal retinal vessels (Ferrara et al. 2016). These references are important for the proper interpretation of the image, because this artifact is transmitted on en face layers throughout the volumetric dataset and should not be confounded with actual choroidal vessels.

Structural en face OCT of the choriocapillaris and choroidal microvasculature are challenging to be obtained, even in normal eyes, because of the small caliper and complexity of the vascular network. No distinct capillary vessels can be readily identified on en face OCT, with the current available technology. Instead, they appear as homogeneous reticular pattern throughout the scan, including the macular and peripapillary areas, lying at a level external to the RPE and internal to the choroidal vasculature. Microvascular choroidal anastomoses between the choriocapillaris and terminal arterioles or venules from the inner choroid are also present at this level. However, since both choriocapillaris and microvascular anastomosis appear on en face OCT as a reticular pattern, no tomographic distinction can be made between them (Ferrara et al. 2016) (Fig. 5.4).

Structural en face OCT of the inner and outer choroid in normal eyes has distinct characteristics, depending on the area of the fundus and on the level of the scan. In the macular area, choroidal vessels appear on en face OCT as highly complicated, interwoven, short vascular segments crossing over each other. In en face scans of extramacular areas, choroidal vessels are straighter and fewer in number representing a radial distribution outward from the center of the macula toward the equator (Ferrara et al. 2016). En face scans at the level of the inner choroid present thinner vessels, homogeneously distributed in the macular area through the topography of the retinal vascular arcades. En face scans at the level of the outer choroid present wider vessels, interwoven in the center of the macula but assuming clear radial distribution beyond the macular area toward the equator (Montaghiannezam et al. 2012; Sohrab et al. 2012). No distinct anatomic boundary can be determined between inner and outer choroid, since vessel caliber and distribution change in a progressive gradient. Also, arteries and veins cannot be differentiated based on tomographic features (Ferrara et al. 2016).

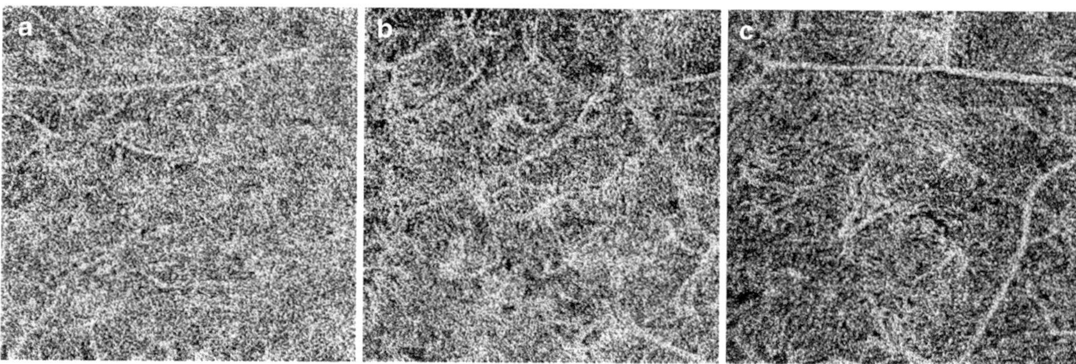

Fig. 5.4 Optical coherence tomography (OCT) angiography of a normal eye obtained with ultrahigh speed swept-source OCT prototype operating at 1060 nm (Choi et al. 2013). Scans document the choriocapillaris in different sectors of the fundus. In the center of the macula (**a**), the choriocapillaris shows dense reticular appearance, while it shows less dense appearance in the mid-periphery (**b**) and a lobular appearance toward the equator (**c**)

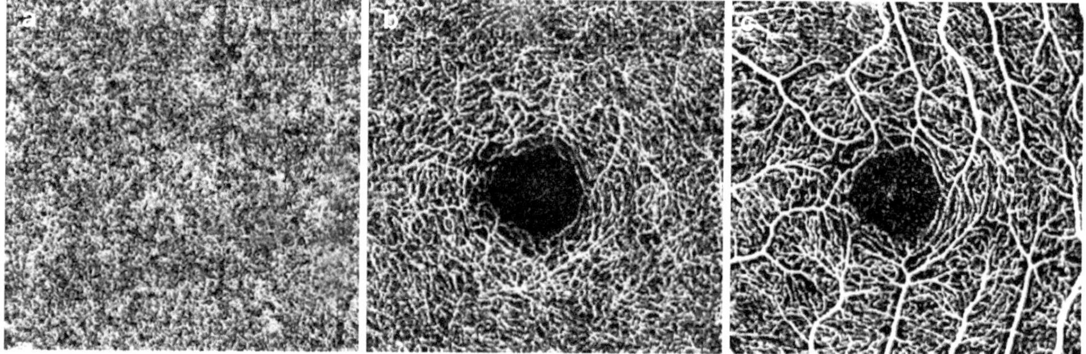

Fig. 5.5 Optical coherence tomography (OCT) angiography of a normal eye obtained with a commercially available spectral-domain OCT. OCT angiography documents the choriocapillaris (**a**) in the center of the macular area. OCT angiography of the retinal circulation is also shown in comparison with the choroidal circulation, at the level of the deep retinal plexus (**b**) and superficial retinal plexus (**c**)

A peripapillary area of preserved choriocapillaris but absent medium-size and large-size choroidal vessels, corresponding to the angiographic description of the so-called watershed zone (Hayreh 1975; Hayreh 1990), can be documented on en face OCT (Fig. 5.5).

5.5 Normal Choroidal Morphology on Optical Coherence Tomography Angiography

OCT angiograms can be generated by tridimensional rendering from cross-sectional images of the speckle decorrelation between sequential scans, repeatedly acquired on the same position, as discussed above. Assuming the documented tissue remains static, all scans will be identical, except where there is erythrocyte motion within the blood vessels. This motion results in local oscillation of backscattered light intensity, which can be calculated by comparing each pixel on the scans and results in a motion contrast. A volumetric dataset documenting the tissue on OCT angiography can be obtained by performing this operation for all transverse positions of the scan (Choi et al. 2013).

As a general rule discussed above, it is important to take into account artifacts for proper interpretation of the OCT images. Therefore, the choroidal vasculature should not be confounded with the shadowing artifact from large retinal blood vessels, which have lower signal levels and more rapidly fluctuating speckle pattern to occur below them (Choi et al. 2013).

OCT angiogram of the choriocapillaris documents distinct capillary density and pattern depending on the location in the fundus, in agreement with previous characterization on histopathological studies (McLeod and Lutty 1994; Olver 1990; Yoneya 1987; Zhang 1994). In the center of the macula, the choriocapillaris exhibits dense reticular or honeycomb appearance, while it has less dense and lobular structure toward the equator. OCT angiography may be a better tool to differentiate choriocapillaris from feeding arterioles and draining vessels, in comparison to structural en face OCT, because the speckle decorrelation is related to the erythrocyte speed. Nonetheless, the differentiation between arterioles and venules on OCT angiography has been attempted but is still challenging (Choi et al. 2013). The same agreement between in vivo and post-mortem spatial characterization of the choroidal vessels was observed on OCT angiography of the inner choroid (Choi et al. 2013). Larger choroidal vessels have higher flow rates and therefore can only be visualized with en face OCT intensity images, which generates contrast from light scattering and fringe washout effects instead of speckle decorrelation.

References

Adhi M, Brewer E, Waheed NA, Duker JS (2013) Analysis of morphological features and vascular layers of choroid in diabetic retinopathy using spectral-domain optical coherence tomography. JAMA Ophthalmol 131:1267–1274

Adhi M, Liu JJ, Qavi AH, Grulkowski I, Lu CD, Mohler KJ, Ferrara D, Kraus MF, Baumal CR, Witkin AJ, Waheed NK, Hornegger J, Fujimoto JG, Duker JS (2014) Choroidal analysis in healthy eyes using swept source optical coherence tomography compared with spectral domain optical coherence tomography. Am J Ophthalmol 157:1272–1281

Adhi M, Ferrara D, Mullins RF, Baumal CR, Mohler KJ, Kraus MF, Liu J, Badaro E, Alasil T, Hornegger J, Fujimoto JG, Duker JS, Waheed NK (2015) Characterization of choroidal layer in normal aging eyes using enface swept-source optical coherence tomography. PLoS One 10:e0133080

Alm A, Bill A (1973) Ocular and optic nerve blood flow at normal and increased intraocular pressures in monkeys (Macaca irus): a study with radioactively labelled microspheres including flow determinations in brain and some other tissues. Exp Eye Res 15:15–19

Barteselli G, Chhablani J, El-Emam S, Wang H, Chuang J, Kosak I, Cheng L, Bartsch DU, Freeman WR (2012) Choroidal volume variations with age, axial length, and sex in healthy subjects: a three-dimensional analysis. Ophthalmology 119:2572–2578

Benavente-Perez A, Hosking SL, Logan NS, Bansal D (2010) Reproducibility-repeatability of choroidal thickness calculation using optical coherence tomography. Optom Vis Sci 87:867–872

Branchini L, Regatieri CV, Flores-Moreno I, Baumann B, Fujimoto JG, Duker JS (2012) Reproducibility of choroidal thickness measurements across three spectral domain optical coherence tomography systems. Ophthalmology 119:119–123

Branchini LA, Adhi M, Regatieri CV, Nandakumar N, Liu JJ, Laver N, Fujimoto JG, Duker JS (2013) Analysis of choroidal morphologic features and vasculature in healthy eyes using spectral-domain optical coherence tomography. Ophthalmology 120:1901–1908

Brown JS, Flitcroft DI, Ying GS, Francis EL, Schmid GF, Quinn GE, Stone RA (2009) In vivo human choroidal thickness measurements: evidence for diurnal fluctuations. Invest Ophthalmol Vis Sci 50:5–12

Chakraborty R, Read SA, Collins MJ (2011) Diurnal variations in axial length, choroidal thickness, intraocular pressure, and ocular biometrics. Invest Ophthalmol Vis Sci 52:5121–5134

Choi W, Mohler K, Potsaid B, Lu CD, Liu JJ, Jayaraman V, Cable AE, Duker JS, Huber R, Fujimoto JG (2013) Choriocapillaris and choroidal microvasculature imaging with ultrahigh speed OCT angiography. PLoS One 8:e81499

Copete S, Flores-Moreno I, Montero JA, Duker JS, Ruiz-Moreno JM (2014) Direct comparison of spectral-domain and swept-source OCT in the measurement of choroidal thickness in normal eyes. Br J Ophthalmol 98:334–338

Ellabban AA, Tsujikawa A, Matsumoto A, Ogino K, Hangai M, Ooto S, Yamashiro K, Akiba M, Yoshimura N (2012) Macular choroidal thickness and volume in eyes with angioid streaks measured by swept source optical coherence tomography. Am J Ophthalmol 153:1133–1143

Esmaeelpour M, Povazay B, Hermann B, Hofer B, Kajic V, Kapoor K, Sheen NJ, North RV, Drexler W (2010) Three-dimensional 1060-nm OCT: choroidal thickness maps in normal subjects and improved posterior segment visualization in cataract patients. Invest Ophthalmol Vis Sci 51:5260–5266

Feeney-Burns L, Burns RP, Gao CL (1990) Age-related macular changes in humans over 90 years old. Am J Ophthalmol 109:265–278

Ferrara D, Mohler KJ, Waheed N, Adhi M, Liu JJ, Grulkowski I, Kraus MF, Baumal C, Hornegger J, Fujimoto JG, Duker JS (2014) En face enhanced-depth swept-source optical coherence tomography features of chronic central serous chorioretinopathy. Ophthalmology 121:719–726

Ferrara D, Waheed NK, Duker JS (2016) Investigating the choriocapillaris and choroidal vasculature with new optical coherence tomography technologies. Prog Retin Eye Res 52:130–155

Fingler J, Scwartz D, Yang C, Fraser SE (2007) Mobility and transverse flow visualization using phase variance contrast with spectral domain optical coherence tomography. Opt Express 15:12636–12653

Flores-Moreno I, Lugo F, Duker JS, Ruiz-Moreno JM (2013) The relationship between axial length and choroidal thickness in eyes with high myopia. Am J Ophthalmol 155:314–319

Fujiwara T, Imamura Y, Margolis R, Slakter JS, Spaide RF (2009) Enhanced depth imaging optical coherence tomography of the choroid in highly myopic eyes. Am J Ophthalmol 148:445–450

Hayreh SS (1975) Segmental nature of the choroidal vasculature. Br J Ophthalmol 59:631–648

Hayreh SS (1990) In vivo choroidal circulation and its watershed zones. Eye (Lond) 4:273–289

Hirata M, Tsujikawa A, Matsumoto A, Hangai M, Ooto S, Yamashiro K, Akiba M, Yoshimura N (2011) Macular choroidal thickness and volume in normal eyes measured by swept-source optical coherence tomography. Invest Ophthalmol Vis Sci 52:4971–4978

Ho J, Branchini L, Regatieri C, Krishnan C, Fujimoto JG, Duker JS (2011) Analysis of normal peripapillary choroidal thickness via spectral domain optical coherence tomography. Ophthalmology 118:2001–2007

Ikuno Y, Kawaguchi K, Nouchi T, Yasuno Y (2010) Choroidal thickness in healthy Japanese subjects. Invest Ophthalmol Vis Sci 51:2173–2176

Ikuno Y, Tano Y (2009) Retinal and choroidal biometry in highly myopic eyes with spectral-domain optical coherence tomography. Invest Ophthalmol Vis Sci 50:3876–3880

Jia Y, Tan O, Tokayer J, Potsaid B, Wang Y, Liu JJ, Kraus MF, Subhash H, Fujimoto JG, Hornegger J, Huang D (2012) Split-spectrum amplitude-decorrelation angiography with optical coherence tomography. Opt Express 20:4710–4725

Kim SW, Oh J, Kwon SS, Yoo J, Huh K (2011) Comparison of choroidal thickness among patients with healthy eyes, early age-related maculopathy, neovascular age-related macular degeneration, central serous chorioretinopathy, and polypoidal choroidal vasculopathy. Retina 31:1904–1911

Li XQ, Larsen M, Munch IC (2011) Subfoveal choroidal thickness in relation to sex and axial length in 93 Danish university students. Invest Ophthalmol Vis Sci 52:8438–8441

Manjunath V, Taha M, Fujimoto JG, Duker JS (2010) Choroidal thickness in normal eyes measured using Cirrus HD optical coherence tomography. Am J Ophthalmol 150:325–329

Manjunath V, Goren J, Fujimoto JG, Duker JS (2011) Analysis of choroidal thickness in age-related macular degeneration using spectral-domain optical coherence tomography. Am J Ophthalmol 152:663–668

Margolis R, Spaide RF (2009) A pilot study of enhanced depth imaging optical coherence tomography of the choroid in normal eyes. Am J Ophthalmol 147:811–815

Matsuo Y, Sakamoto T, Yamashite T, Tomita M, Shirasawa M, Terasaki H (2013) Comparisons of choroidal thickness of normal eyes obtained by two different spectral-domain OCT instruments and one swept-source OCT instrument. Invest Ophthalmol Vis Sci 54:7630–7636

McLeod DS, Lutty GA (1994) High-resolution histologic analysis of the human choroidal vasculature. Invest Ophthalmol Vis Sci 35:3799–3811

Michalewska Z, Michalewski J, Nawrocka Z, Dulczewska-Cichecka K, Nawrocki J (2015) Suprachoroidal layer and suprachoroidal space delineating the outer margin of the choroid in swept-source optical coherence tomography. Retina 35:244–249

Montaghiannezam R, Schwartz DM, Fraser SE (2012) In vivo human choroidal vascular pattern visualization using high-speed swept-source optical coherence tomography at 1060 nm. Invest Ophthalmol Vis Sci 53:2337–2348

Mullins RF, Johnson MN, Faidley EA, Skeie JM, Huang J (2011) Choriocapillaris vascular dropout related to density of drusen in human eyes with early age-related macular degeneration. Invest Ophthalmol Vis Sci 52:1606–1612

Olver JM (1990) Functional anatomy of the choroidal circulation: methyl methacrylate casting of human choroid. Eye 4:262–272

Ooto S, Hangai M, Yoshimura N (2015) Effects of sex and age on the normal retinal and choroidal structures on optical coherence tomography. Curr Eye Res 40:213–225

Potsaid B, Baumann B, Huang D, Barry S, Cable AE, Schuman JS, Duker JS, Fujimoto JG (2010) Ultrahigh speed 1050 nm swept source/fourier domain OCT retinal and anterior segment imaging at 100,000 to 400,000 axial scans per second. Opt Express 18:20029–20048

Ramrattan RS, van der Schaft TL, Mooy CM, de Bruijn WC, Mulder PG, de Jong PT (1994) Morphometric analysis of Bruch membrane, the choriocapillaris, and the choroid in aging. Invest Ophthalmol Vis Sci 35:2857–2864

Ruiz-Medrano J, Flores-Moreno I, Pena-Garcia P, Montero JA, Duker JS, Ruiz-Moreno JM (2014) Macular choroidal thickness profile in a healthy population measured by swept-source optical coherence tomography. Invest Ophthalmol Vis Sci 55: 3532–3542

Sanchez-Cano A, Orduna E, Segura F, Lopez C, Cuenca N, Abecia E, Pinilla I (2014) Choroidal thickness and volume in healthy young white adults and the relationships between them and axial length, ammetrophy and sex. Am J Ophthalmol 158:574–583

Sarks SH (1976) Ageing and degeneration in the macular region: a clinic-pathological study. Br J Ophthalmol 60:324–341

Sohrab MA, Fawzi AA (2013) Review of en-face choroidal imaging using spectral-domain optical coherence tomography. Med Hypothesis Discov Innov Ophthalmol 2:69–73

Sohrab M, Wu K, Fawzi AA (2012) A pilot study of morphometric analysis of choroidal vasculature in vivo, using en face optical coherence tomography. PLoS One 7:e48631

Spaide RF (2009) Age related choroidal atrophy. Am J Ophthalmol 147:801–810

Spaide RF (2010) Choroidal imaging with optical coherence tomography. In: Holz FG, Spaide RF (eds) Medical retina focus on retinal imaging. Springer, Berlin, pp 169–190

Spaide RF, Koizumi H, Pozzoni MC (2008) Enhanced depth imaging spectral-domain optical coherence tomography. Am J Ophthalmol 146:496–500

Srinivasan VJ, Adler DC, Chen Y, Gorczynska I, Huber R, Duker JS, Schuman JS, Fujimoto JG (2008) Ultrahigh-speed optical coherence tomography for three-dimensional and en face imaging of the retina and optic nerve head. Invest Ophthalmol Vis Sci 49:5103–5110

Tan CS, Ngo WK, Cheong KX (2015) Comparison of choroidal thickness using swept-source and spectral domain optical coherence tomography in diseased and normal eyes. Br J Ophthalmol 99:354–358

Tan CS, Ouyang Y, Ruiz H, Sadda SR (2012) Diurnal variation of choroidal thickness in normal, healthy subjects measured by spectral domain optical coherence tomography. Invest Ophthalmol Vis Sci 53:261–266

Tanabe H, Ito Y, Terasaki H (2012) Choroid is thinner in inferior region of optic disks of normal eyes. Retina 32:134–139

Unterhuber A, Považay B, Hermann B, Sattmann H, Chavez-Pirson A, Drexler W (2005) In vivo retinal optical coherence tomography at 1040 nm – enhanced penetration into the choroid. Opt Express 13: 3252–3258

Wei WB, Xu L, Jonas JB, Shao L, Du KF, Wang S, Chen CX, Wang YX, Zhou JQ, You QS (2013) Subfoveal choroidal thickness: the Beijing Eye Study. Ophthalmology 120:175–180

Yamashita T, Shirasawa M, Arimura N, Terasaki H, Sakamoto T (2012) Repeatability and reproducibility of subfoveal choroidal thickness in normal eyes of Japanese using different SD-OCT devices. Invest Ophthalmol Vis Sci 53:1102–1107

Yoneya STMM (1987) Angioarchitecture of the human choroid. Arch Ophthalmol 105:681–687

Zhang H (1994) Scanning electron-microscopic study of corrosion casts on retinal and choroidal angioarchitecture in man and animals. Prog Retin Eye Res 13:243–270

6 Optical Coherence Tomography Angiography

Masanori Hangai

Contents

M. Hangai, MD PhD (✉)
Department of Ophthalmology, Saitama Medical University, Saitama, Japan

Department of Ophthalmology, Doheny Eye Institute, University of Southern California, Los Angeles, CA, USA
e-mail: hangainori@gmail.com

6.1 Introduction

Various techniques to image retinal, choroidal, and optic disc microvascular networks have been developed for research purposes and clinical tests in the diagnosis and monitoring of fundus diseases. Color fundus photography, fluorescein angiography (FA), and indocyanine green angiography (ICGA) have become standard methods required for fundus disease management. However, some disadvantages remain with these conventional methods. FA and ICGA require exogenous dye injection into the systemic circulation, which carries the risk of allergic side effects. This risk has limited the use of FA and ICGA, particularly in private eye clinics. The second is the inability to show three-dimensional (3D) vascular networks. Vessels, particularly capillary networks, of the retina, choroid, and optic disc have 3D layered structures, but it has been difficult to focus on layer levels on which pathological lesions are present.

C.H. Meyer et al. (eds.), *Spectral Domain Optical Coherence Tomography in Macular Diseases*,
DOI 10.1007/978-81-322-3610-8_6

Optical coherence tomography (OCT) is an imaging technology based on the principle of low-coherence interferometry and does not require the use of exogenous agents or an eye contact lens. In addition to its noninvasive nature, this technology offers depth-resolved structural information with micrometer-scale depth resolution. OCT has become the most commonly used imaging modality for fundus disease and glaucoma. It enables cross-sectional (B-scan) imaging of the retina/choroid and optic nerve head. High-speed imaging with spectral-domain and swept-source OCT technologies enables 3D imaging, which allows for *en face* visualization of the fundus structure. Conventional B-scan OCT images are comprised of serial A-scans, each of which is constructed according to the intensity of light reflected back from the tissue at each depth. OCT angiography is based on the same technology as conventional OCT imaging, but selectively detects signals associated with motion corresponding to blood flow in the fundus. Thus, OCT angiography noninvasively visualizes 3D retinal and choroidal vascular networks and enables visualization of these networks in *en face* sections, as in FA and ICGA. Increasing attention has been paid to potential clinical applications of this technology in retinal ischemic diseases, macular diseases, and glaucoma. The promising advantages and current technical limitations of OCT angiography technology are discussed in this chapter to enhance the clinical use of this technology and resolve limitations in the future.

6.2 Optical Coherence Tomography Angiography Technology

Reflected OCT probe light not only includes reflectivity intensity information from the tissue but also other signals associated with motion, such as Doppler frequency shifts, speckle variance, phase variance, and decorrelation signal (differences in backscattered OCT signal intensity or amplitude) (Mahmud et al. 2013). In the fundus, these signals are generated by flowing blood in the retinal and choroidal circulations. Thus, detection of these signals enables the visualization of vascular networks, including arteries, veins, and capillaries. Because motion-related signals change with time, repeated volumetric raster scans (3D scans) (Fig. 6.1) allow us to obtain information about the locations of motion-related signals. Here, it is technically important to repeat several volumetric raster scans at a precisely identical location of interest. Involuntary eye movement during fixation, particularly in patients with visual acuity loss, decreases accuracy. To overcome this problem, the application of an eye tracking system is useful. Registering and merging horizontal and vertical scans to obtain a single motion-corrected 3D data cube is another useful method. In any event, these OCT angiography scans are enabled by the high imaging speeds achieved through Fourier-domain OCT technology.

An *en face* view of motion-related signals provides OCT angiography images, the same as fundus photography, FA, and IA. Here, both reflectivity intensity-based and OCT angiographic images are obtained together and correspond spatially (Fig. 6.2, a prototype OCT angiography for RS-3000 Advance [NIDEK CO., LTD, Gamagori, Japan]). OCT reflectivity intensity-based images can be used as a topographical map for OCT angiographic images.

6.3 Is Optical Coherence Tomography Angiography an Alternative to Dye Angiography?

Because OCT angiography does not require the use of exogenous dye, physicians may expect this new method to be an alternative to dye angiography. Although the visualization of retinal capillaries as seen in OCT angiography appears to be similar to that of FA, there are some essential differences in the resulting clinical information between the methods. In OCT angiography, dye leakage and pooling, which correspond to blood plasma leakage and pooling, cannot be detected. This is a critical disadvantage of OCT angiography, because dye

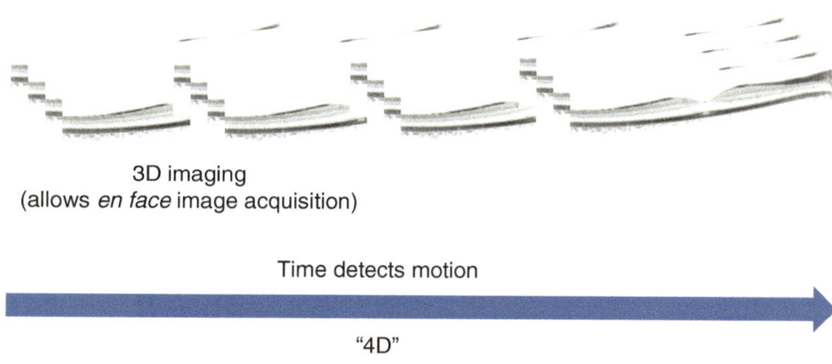

Fig. 6.1 Repeated raster scans at the same location of interest for OCT angiography imaging

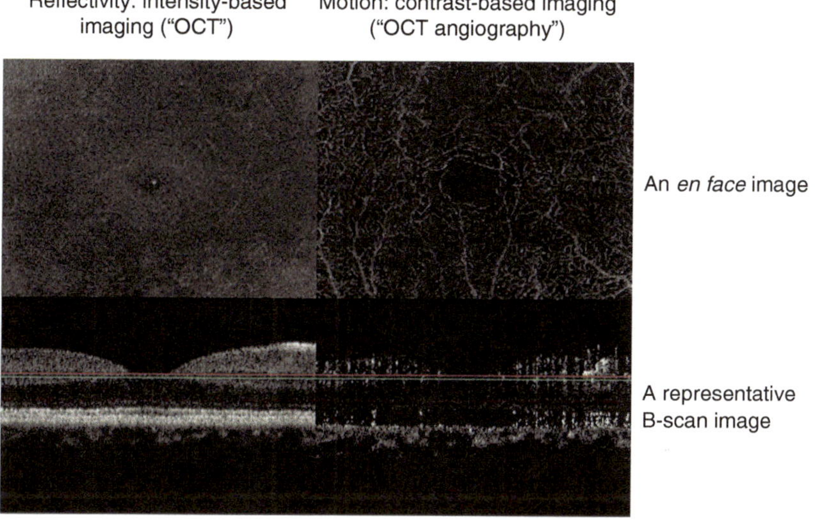

Fig. 6.2 Perifoveal capillary imaging

leakage and pooling are clinically important findings to detect macular edema and active retinal and choroidal neovascularization (CNV) in the diagnosis and management of retinal and macular diseases. Thus, OCT angiography alone cannot be an alternative to dye angiography. However, serial OCT B-scans (a reflectivity intensity image) allow for the detection of intraretinal cystoid spaces and serous retinal detachment. Therefore, the use of angiographic OCT images taken together with OCT B-scan images enables us to manage retinal and macular diseases, even without FA or IA. OCT angiography allows for the depth resolution of vascular structures, which is not feasible in FA. This is expected to be a potentially powerful advantage of OCT angiography, as discussed in the next section. Importantly, because OCT angiography does not require the use of exogenous agents, it can be performed at every visit without the risk of allergic side effects. OCT angiography can provide additive clinical information that conventional angiography cannot; thus, it is recommended that OCT angiography be used in combination with conventional angiography for an accurate diagnosis, particularly for the diagnosis of rare diseases. However, the use of both reflectivity and angiographic OCT imaging may be enough to manage well-defined common pathologies, such as macular edema and serous retinal detachment, in eyes with diabetic maculopathy and retinal vein occlusive diseases.

6.4 Advantages of Optical Coherence Tomography Angiography Over Dye Angiography

The most powerful advantage of OCT angiography technology is the capability to resolve a 3D capillary network. The retinal capillary network is comprised of four layers: the retinal nerve fiber layer (RNFL), and the superficial, intermediate, and deep capillary plexus layers (Iwasaki and Inomata 1986; Snodderly and Weinhaus 1990; Snodderly et al. 1992). It is possible that the formation of retinal capillary pathologies in each layer, such as capillary non-perfusion and microaneurysms, differs among cases, and these differences may influence visual prognosis and response to treatment. In fact, retinal artery occlusive diseases reportedly showed different and variable involvement of the superficial and intermediate/deep capillary plexus layers (Yu et al. 2015). In particular, 22 % of eyes with retinal artery occlusive diseases had isolated deep capillary ischemia producing paracentral acute middle maculopathy while sparing the superficial capillary plexus, but the fluorescein angiographic appearance was normal (Yu et al. 2015). Although these findings were obtained from the increased reflectivity in each retinal layer as an indirect sign of ischemia, OCT angiography enables the direct observation of capillary perfusion and non-perfusion.

We have tried to resolve each of the four retinal capillary plexus layers based on a retinal layer segmentation method (Figs. 6.3 and 6.4). A raster scan for 3D OCT imaging can provide both reflectivity intensity and motion contrast signals that correspond to each other spatially. A segmentation algorithm to detect layer boundaries on reflectivity intensity B-scans allows for the determination of boundaries between the RNFL and ganglion cell layer (GCL), between the inner plexiform layer (IPL) and inner nuclear layer (INL), and between the INL and outer plexiform layer (OPL). Angiographic images between the posterior boundary of the RNFL and the line of *x*-pixels (1 pixel = 31.4 μm) anterior to the RNFL are defined as the RNFL capillary plexus (RNFLP) (Fig. 6.3). Angiographic images

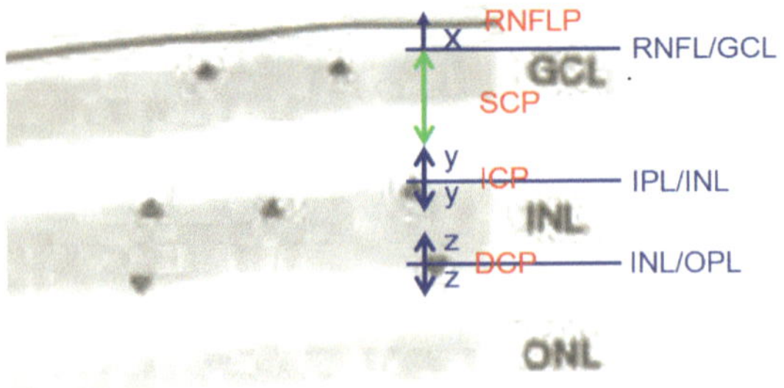

Fig. 6.3 A schema showing the capillary layer segmentation method in which four retinal capillary plexus layers were defined based on layer boundary segmentations of reflectivity intensity optical coherence tomography B-scans. In the retinal nerve fiber layer (*RNFL*), the capillary plexus (*RNFLP*), superficial capillary plexus (*SCP*), intermediate capillary plexus (*ICP*), and deep capillary plexus (*DCP*) are present within the RNFL, from the ganglion cell layer (*GCL*) to the RNFL, along the anterior boundary of the inner nuclear layer (*INL*), and along the posterior boundary of the INL, respectively. Each capillary plexus was defined using the segmentation boundaries

between the two lines of *y*-pixels anterior and posterior to the anterior boundary of the INL are defined as the intermediate capillary plexus (ICP). Angiographic images between the two lines of *z*-pixels anterior and posterior to the posterior boundary of the INL are defined as the deep capillary plexus (DCP). Angiographic images between the RNFLP and ICP are defined as the superficial capillary plexus (SCP). Capillary patterns on *en face* images were compared by changing the numbers of *x*, *y*, and *z* pixels.

Figure 6.4 presents *en face* images of the four retinal capillary plexus layers when *x*, *y*, and *z* were set to 5. The RNFL appearance shows a striated pattern of capillaries along the retinal nerve fiber bundles. The SCP, ICP, and DCP images each show different capillary network patterns. We found two major problems in depicting each of the four retinal capillary plexus layers. One was that the RNFLP around the fovea and temporal raphe could not be depicted. Figure 6.5 indicates that visualization of RNFLP appearance is improved when the value of *x* in Fig. 6.3 is changed from 1 to 6. At least 3 pixels are necessary to depict the RNFLP. However, even if the *x* value is increased to 6, the RNFLP around the

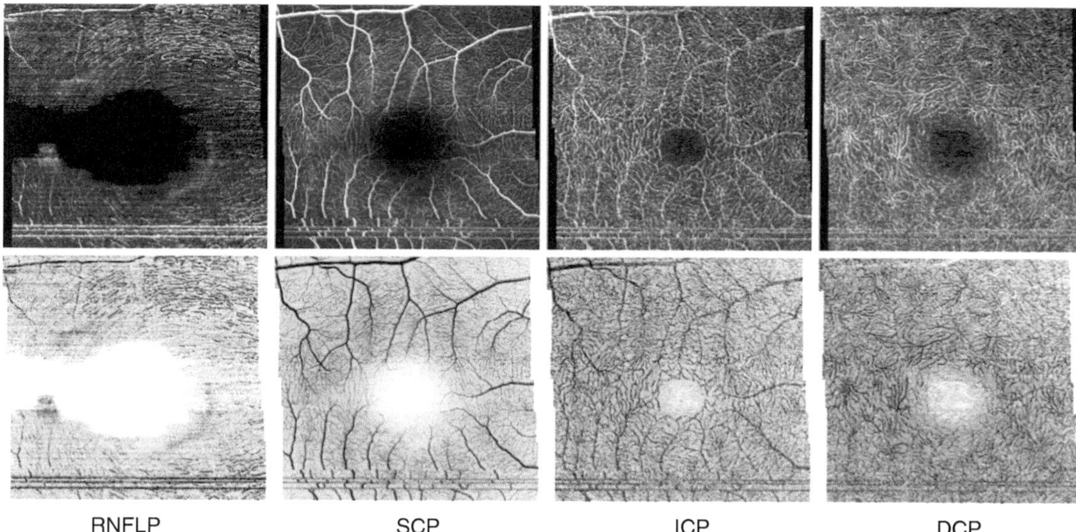

Fig. 6.4 Four retinal capillary plexus images acquired by OCT angiography. OCT angiographic signals are shown as *white* (*upper column*) and *black* (*lower column*). *RNFLP* retinal nerve fiber layer capillary plexus, *SCP* superficial capillary plexus, *ICP* intermediate capillary plexus, *DCP* deep capillary plexus

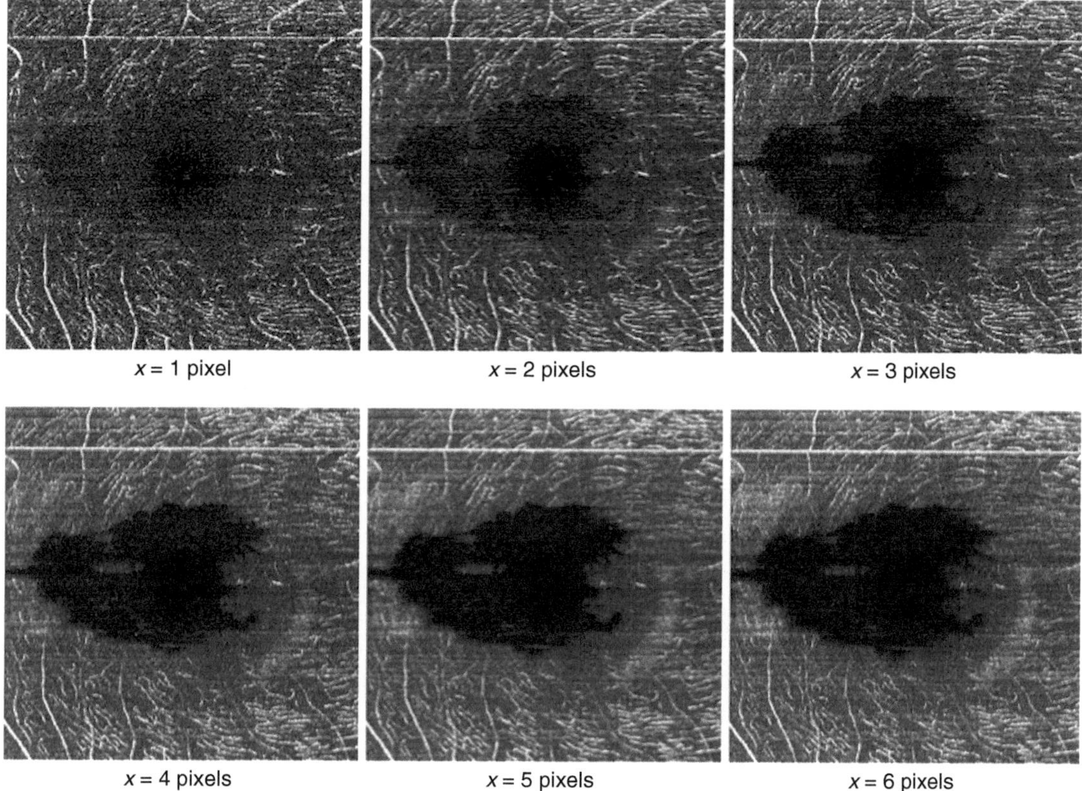

Fig. 6.5 Retinal nerve fiber layer capillary plexus appearance when the value of "x" in Fig. 6.3 is changed from 1 to 6

temporal raphe cannot be visualized. This problem is likely attributable to the difficulty in segmenting the very thin RNFL around the fovea and temporal raphe (Fig. 6.6).

The second problem was a partial overlap of capillary patterns between the SCP and ICP (Fig. 6.7). This overlap is seen in and outside the fovea. This problem may be attributable to the anatomy of the retinal capillary plexus and the failure to detect motion-related signals in each layer selectively. The perifoveal capillary ring, as indicated by blue arrows in Fig. 6.7, is continuously connected with the SCP and ICP; that is, the perifoveal capillary network is not clearly shown to have four layers, and perifoveal capillaries are shared by the SCP and ICP. This anatomical overlap should be taken into consideration when the segmentation results are interpreted. The capillaries indicated by red arrows in Fig. 6.7 demonstrate that capillaries in the SCP are projected onto ICP images, regardless of how completely the SCP and ICP are separated spatially in the segmented volume. This problem may be a methodological failure in the OCT angiography algorithm. These overlaps could not be deleted by changing the value of y in Fig. 6.3 (Figs. 6.8 and 6.9). Appropriate values of y range from 1 to 5 for SCP imaging and from 5 to 11 for ICP imaging. We subtracted ICP signals at $y=1$, 3, 5, 7, and 9 from those at $y=3$, 5, 7, 9, and 11, respectively (Fig. 6.10). The subtracted images showed an SCP pattern when the subtraction was performed from ICP signals at $y=7$ or more, suggesting that ICP images at $y=7$ or more include SCP signals. Thus, the best value for y for both SCP and ICP imaging seems to be 5 for our algorithm. However, the current algorithm in our OCT angiography technique could not completely delete the partial signal overlap, even when the segmentation volume was changed. It appears that a z-value of at least 5 is required for clear DCP imaging (Fig. 6.11) that does not include an overlap with the ICP.

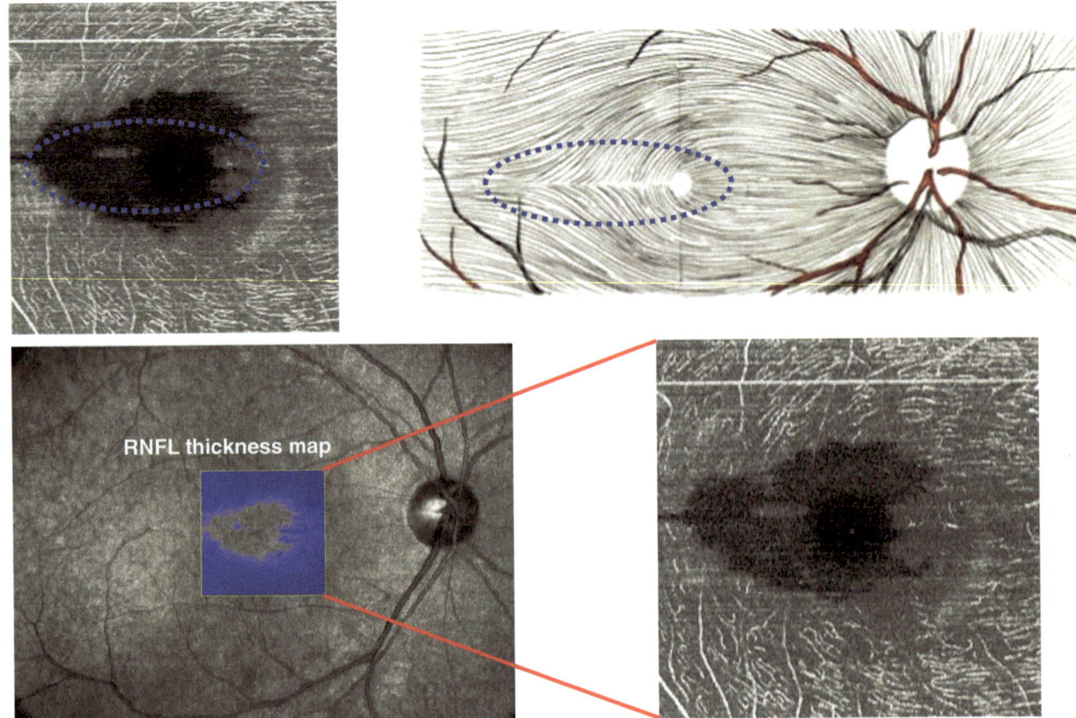

Fig. 6.6 An absence of capillary signal around the fovea and temporal raphe is associated with areas of segmentation failure on the RNFL thickness map. The *blue dotted circle* indicates the area without OCT angiographic signals, which corresponds to the fovea and temporal raphe

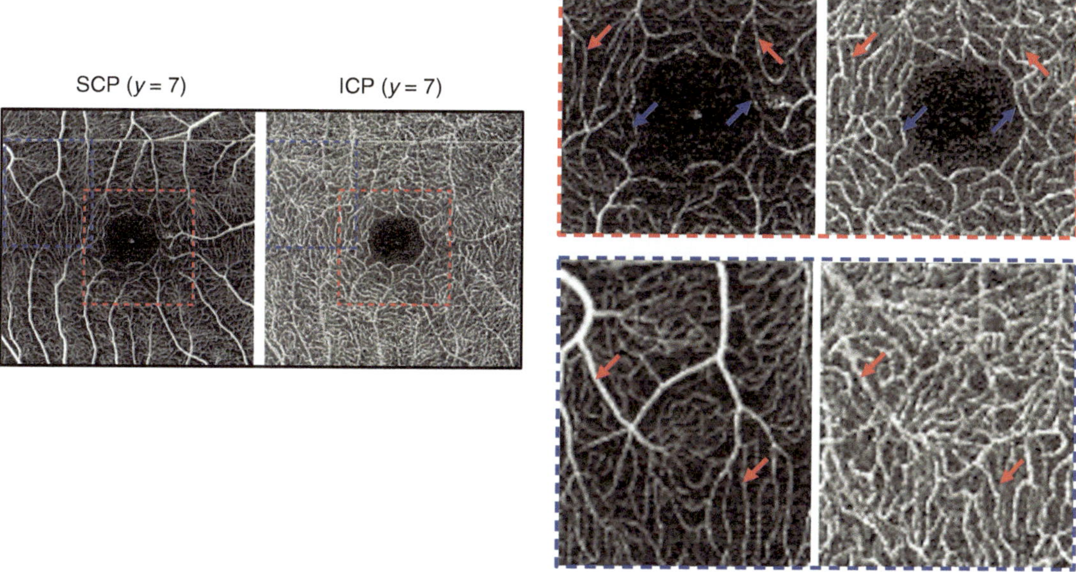

Fig. 6.7 An example showing a partial overlap of capillary patterns between SCP and ICP. *En face* images in which $y = 7$ are shown. Enlarged images of the *red* and *blue dashed squares* are shown on the right side. The *red arrows* indicate the vessels that can be seen both in SCP and ICP

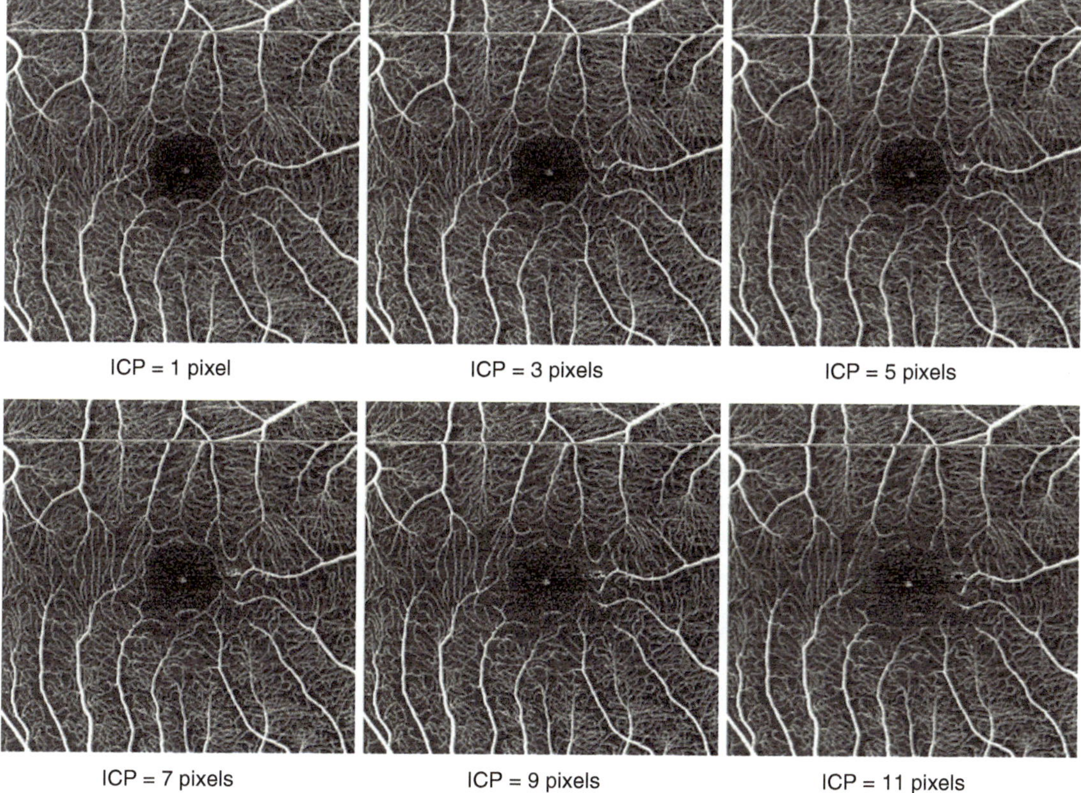

Fig. 6.8 Superficial capillary plexus appearances when the value of "y" in Fig. 6.3 is changed from 1 to 11

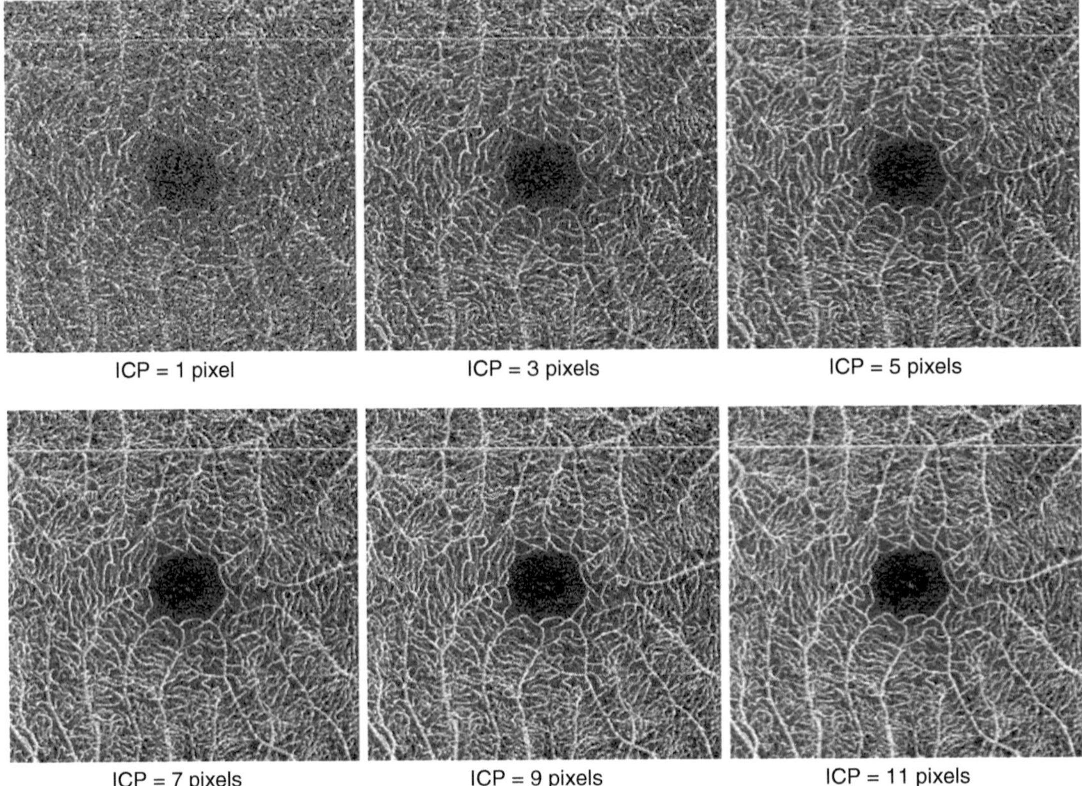

Fig. 6.9 Intermediate capillary plexus appearances when the value of "y" in Fig. 6.3 is changed from 1 to 11

6.5 Clinical Applications: Retinopathy

OCT angiography allows for the visualization of major pathological vascular features, including microaneurysms and capillary non-perfusion, in various retinal diseases such as diabetic retinopathy, retinal vein occlusion, and macular telangiectasia (MacTel) (Ishibazawa et al. 2015; Jia et al. 2015). A major interest is differences in the imaging of these features between FA and OCT angiography.

6.5.1 Microaneurysm Imaging

The retinal capillary pattern appears similar on OCT angiography and FA in eyes with diabetic maculopathy (Fig. 6.12). OCT angiography shows microaneurysms as highly reflective dots, which indicates that there is some flow within the microaneurysms. However, interestingly, some microaneurysms detected on FA were not seen on OCT angiography (Fig. 6.12, red arrows), and some highly reflective dots on OCT angiography did not correspond to microaneurysms on FA (Fig. 6.12, yellow arrows) (Jia et al. 2015). Microaneurysms that were undetected by OCT angiography may have less flow than those detectable by FA. If this is true, OCT angiography is useful in discriminating active microaneurysms from inactive microaneurysms. Further studies are required to determine the phenomenon that underlies the disagreement. OCT angiography is also able to show the disruption of perifoveal capillaries. OCT angiography images do not depict leakage and pooling exactly but show diffuse signals in areas with perifoveal cystoid spaces (Fig. 6.12, red arrowheads). It is not certain whether these signals correspond to flow within the cystoid spaces or are imaging artifacts.

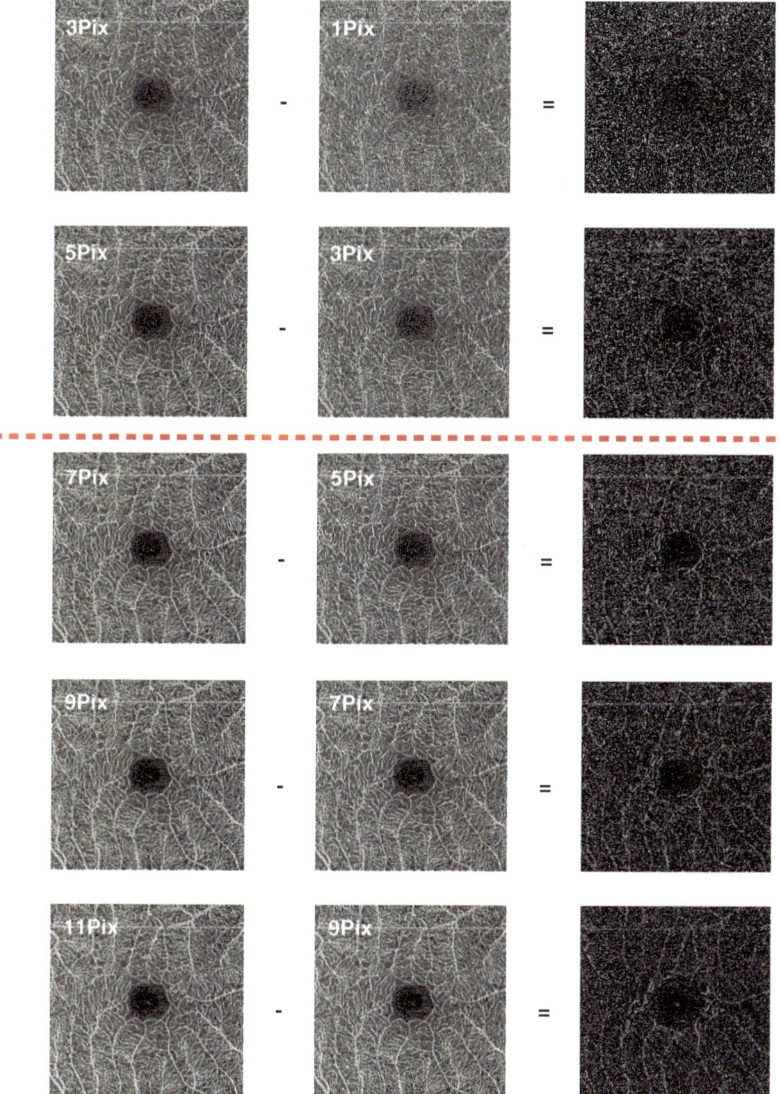

Fig. 6.10 Subtraction of intermediate capillary plexus images for different values of "y"

6.5.2 Capillary Layer Levels of Microaneurysms, Capillary Dilation, and Capillary Non-perfusion

OCT angiography can demonstrate the capillary layer levels of microaneurysms and capillary non-perfusion (Jia et al. 2015). It has been difficult to determine capillary layer levels where microaneurysms are formed in FA. Figure 6.13 shows that a microaneurysm is present in an eye with early diabetic retinopathy in the deep capillary plexus layer, as determined by OCT angiography. Figure 6.14 shows the presence of microaneurysms and capillary dilation in an eye with MacTel type 1 in the superficial, intermediate, and deep capillary plexus layers, as found by OCT angiography. In contrast to FA, leakage from capillaries cannot be detected on OCT angiography, which helped the observation of the actual dilation of capillary vessels as in early-phase FA. Such information is useful to deepen our understanding of vascular complications associated with various retinal diseases.

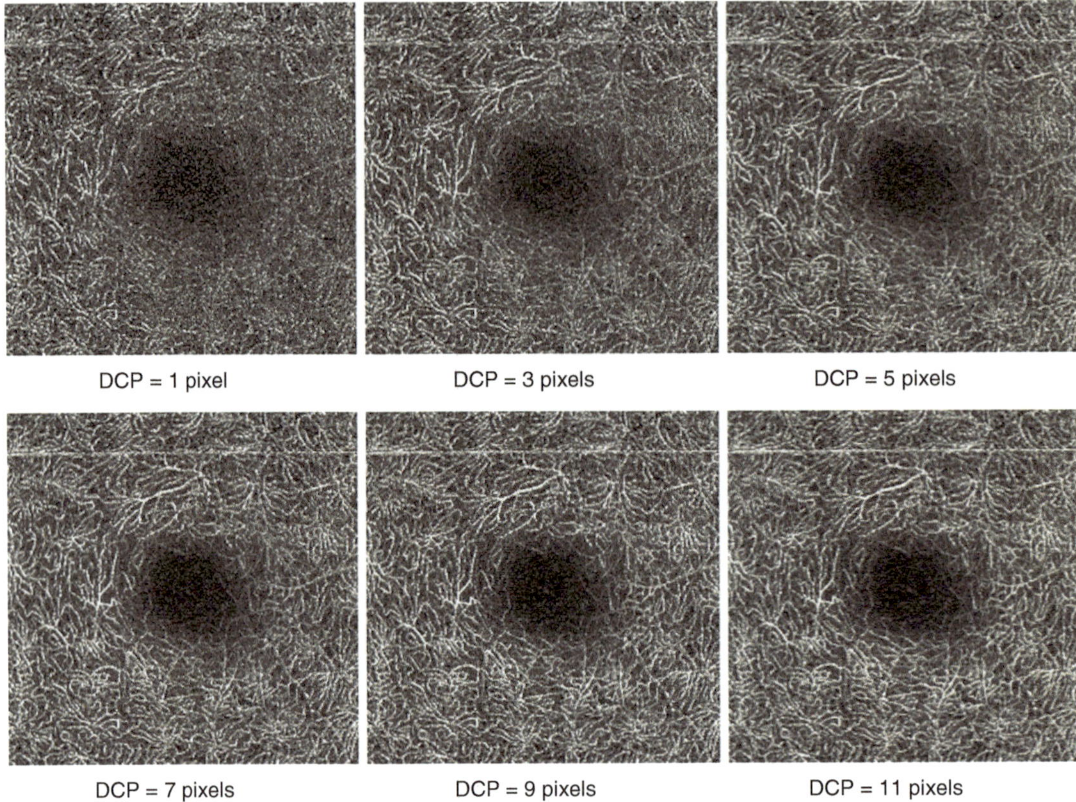

Fig. 6.11 Deep capillary plexus appearances when the value of "z" in Fig. 6.3 is changed from 1 to 11

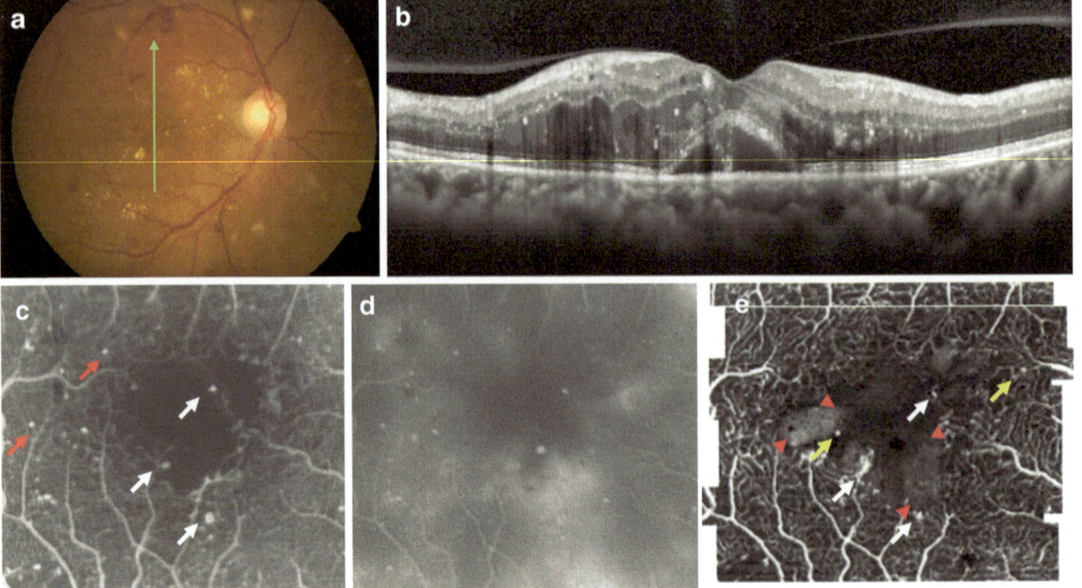

Fig. 6.12 The right eye of a patient with diabetic macular edema. (**a**) A color fundus photograph. The *green arrow* indicates a scan line of the optical coherence tomography (OCT) B-scan in (b). (**b**) A vertical OCT B-scan. (**c**) An enlarged image from early-phase (23 s) fluorescein angiography (FA). (**d**) An enlarged image from late-phase (12 min) FA. (**e**) An *en face* OCT angiography image

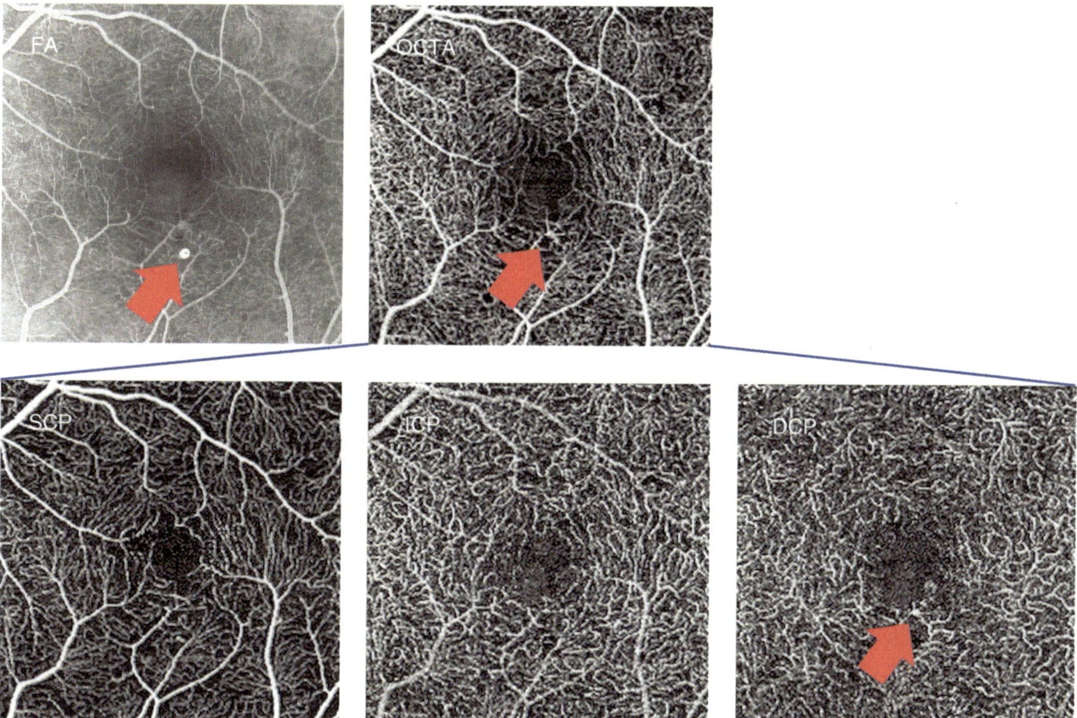

Fig. 6.13 Capillary layer levels with microaneurysms in the left eye of a patient with early diabetic retinopathy as determined by optical coherence tomography angiography (*OCTA*). In this case, the OCTA layer images show that a parafoveal microaneurysm (*red arrow*) is present in the deep capillary plexus (*DCP*) layer. *FA*, fluorescein angiography; *SCP*, superficial capillary plexus; *ICP*, intermediate capillary plexus

6.5.3 Blood Plasma Filling in Cystoid Macular Edema

Unexpectedly, blood plasma filling in cystoid macular edema is observable on OCT angiography (Figs. 6.12 and 6.14). It is possible that OCT angiography detects motion driven by blood plasma leakage into cystoid spaces. It is mandatory to determine the differences in cystoid space visualization between FA and OCT angiography.

6.6 Clinical Applications: Choroidal Neovascularization

An increasing number of studies have reported that OCT angiography can visualize CNV in eyes with age-related maculopathy, polypoidal choroidal vasculopathy, and retinal angiomatous proliferation. Importantly, OCT angiography allows the acquisition of depth-resolved information about CNV networks and the time course after treatment (Dansingani et al. 2015; Huang et al. 2015; Inoue et al. 2015; Jia et al. 2014a, 2015; Palejwala et al. 2015). In Fig. 6.15, the OCT angiography image in the segmented choroidal depth (violet color) demonstrates abnormally coiled newly formed vessels in regions corresponding to those with hyperfluorescence on FA. CNV is more clearly depicted by OCT angiography than by ICGA. A recent study reported that OCT angiography revealed the presence of a distinct CNV corresponding to IA hyperpermeability and small undulations in slight retinal pigment epithelium (RPE) detachment in chronic central serous chorioretinopathy (Quaranta-El Maftouhi et al. 2015). Thus, it is possible that OCT angiography can detect CNV undetectable on conventional dye angiography.

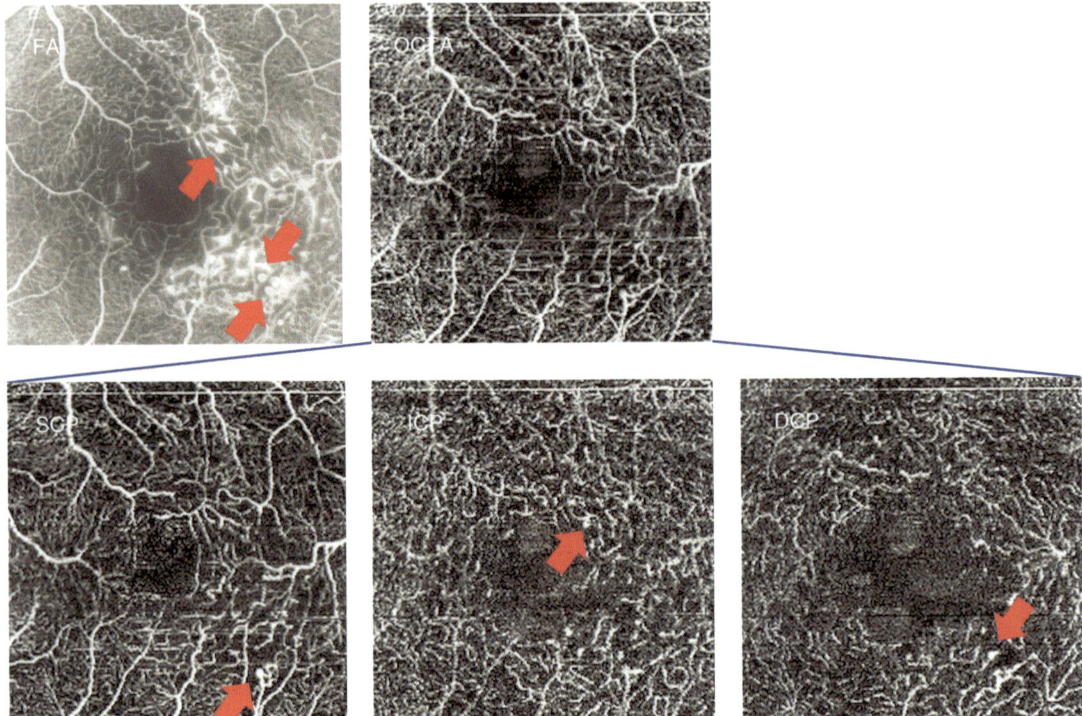

Fig. 6.14 Capillary layer levels with microaneurysms and capillary dilation in the left eye of a patient with macular telangiectasia type 1 as determined by optical coherence tomography angiography (*OCTA*). In this case, microaneurysms (*red arrows*) and capillary dilation are seen throughout the capillary layers in the OCTA layer images. *FA*, fluorescein angiography; *SCP*, superficial capillary plexus; *ICP*, intermediate capillary plexus; *DCP*, deep capillary plexus

6.7 Clinical Applications: Glaucoma

6.7.1 Radial Peripapillary Capillary Network Imaging

Glaucoma is a progressive disease in which the death of retinal ganglion cells (RGCs) occurs faster than age-dependent loss following RGC axonal injury within the optic disc lamina cribrosa. The loss of RGCs appears clinically as thinning of the optic disc neuroretinal rim and RNFL defects. Because the RNFL is rich in capillaries, forming a radial peripapillary capillary network (Fig. 6.16), glaucomatous RNFL thinning may appear as a loss of capillary density, as seen in Fig. 6.16. An RNFL defect, which is simply a decrease in RNFL reflectivity, is known as an early sign of glaucoma. A recent study reported that reduced peripapillary retinal perfusion in glaucomatous eyes can be visualized as focal defects and quantified using the peripapillary flow index and peripapillary vessel density with high repeatability and reproducibility (Liu et al. 2015). A research issue of interest is whether the losses of peripapillary capillary flow and density as measured by OCT angiography are accurate indicators of early glaucoma.

6.7.2 Optic Disc Capillary Imaging

OCT angiography also allows for the evaluation of optic disc capillary perfusion. It was reported recently that a dense microvascular network was observed in normal optic discs on OCT angiography and was visibly decreased in eyes with glaucoma (Jia et al. 2014a, b). The disc flow index was highly correlated with the visual field pattern standard deviation and showed complete

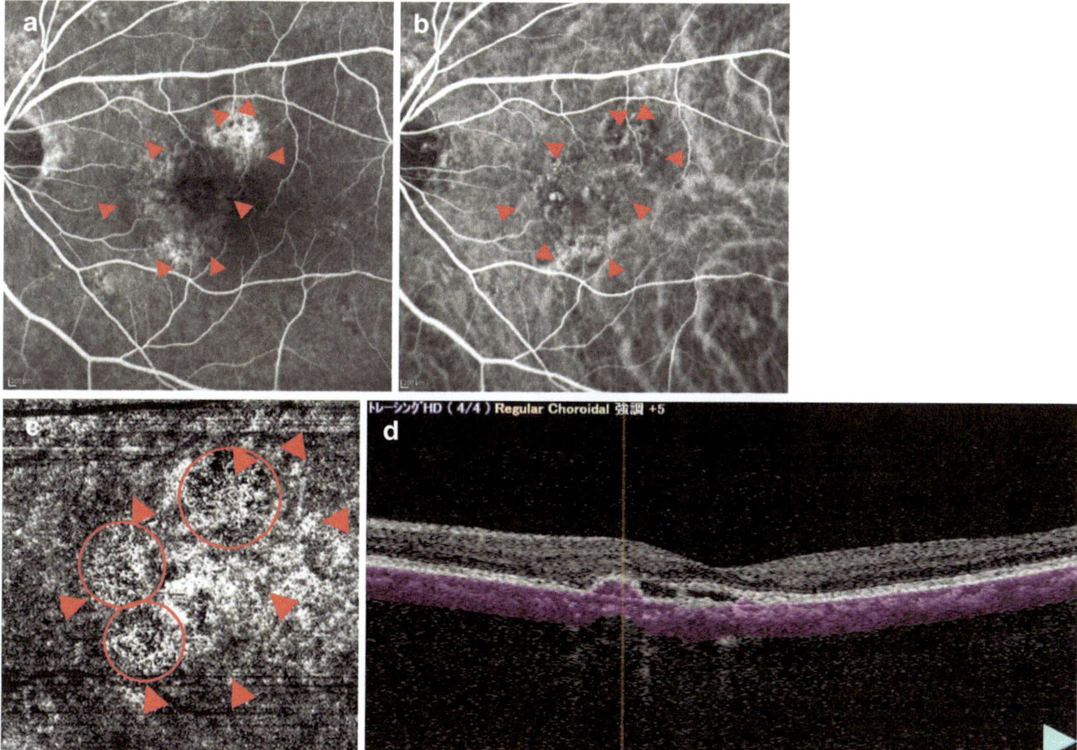

Fig. 6.15 Detection of choroidal neovascularization by using optical coherence tomography angiography. The left eye of a 65-year-old man with unilateral polypoidal choroidal vasculopathy. (**a**, **b**) Fluorescein and indocyanine green angiography (43 s after dye injection). (**c**) An *en face* image from optical coherence tomography (OCT) angiography. (**d**) An OCT B-scan in which the *violet color* indicates the segmentation depth of the choroid. A region surrounded by *Red arrowheads* indicates the region where a branching vascular network (type 1 choroidal neovascularization) and polypoidal lesions are present. *Red circles* indicate the area of type 1 choroidal neovascularization

sensitivity and specificity in discrimination between normal and glaucomatous eyes (Jia et al. 2014a, b). This is an interesting result suggesting that a decrease in optic disc perfusion as measured by OCT angiography is a highly accurate discriminator of glaucoma.

Another important target of OCT angiography in glaucoma is the lamina cribrosa, which is believed to be a principal site of glaucomatous injuries to RGC axons. The lamina cribrosa consists of laminar beams of scleral collagenous tissue and occasional elastic fibers, which generate laminar pores through which bundles of RGC axons leave the eye. Thus, the lamina cribrosa is likely a supporting structure for unmyelinated RGC axons. The lamina cribrosa suffers from age-dependent remodeling and shows characteristic atrophic changes in glaucoma such as thinning, posterior bowing, and posterior migration. Most recently, it was reported that the lamina cribrosa showed focal defects associated with visual field defects, neuroretinal rim thinning, and RNFL defects (Kiumehr et al. 2012; Takayama et al. 2013; Tatham et al. 2014). Thus, structural changes in laminar structures characteristic of glaucoma may underlie the pathological mechanism by which glaucomatous optic neuropathy commences and progresses.

Each laminar beam includes a single capillary. However, FA is not effective for the observation of laminar capillaries. Optic disc circulation is comprised of four components, including RNFL capillaries, prelaminar capillaries, laminar capillaries, and retrolaminar capillaries. Although FA is able to visualize a gross view of optic disc circulation, it is unable to distinguish laminar

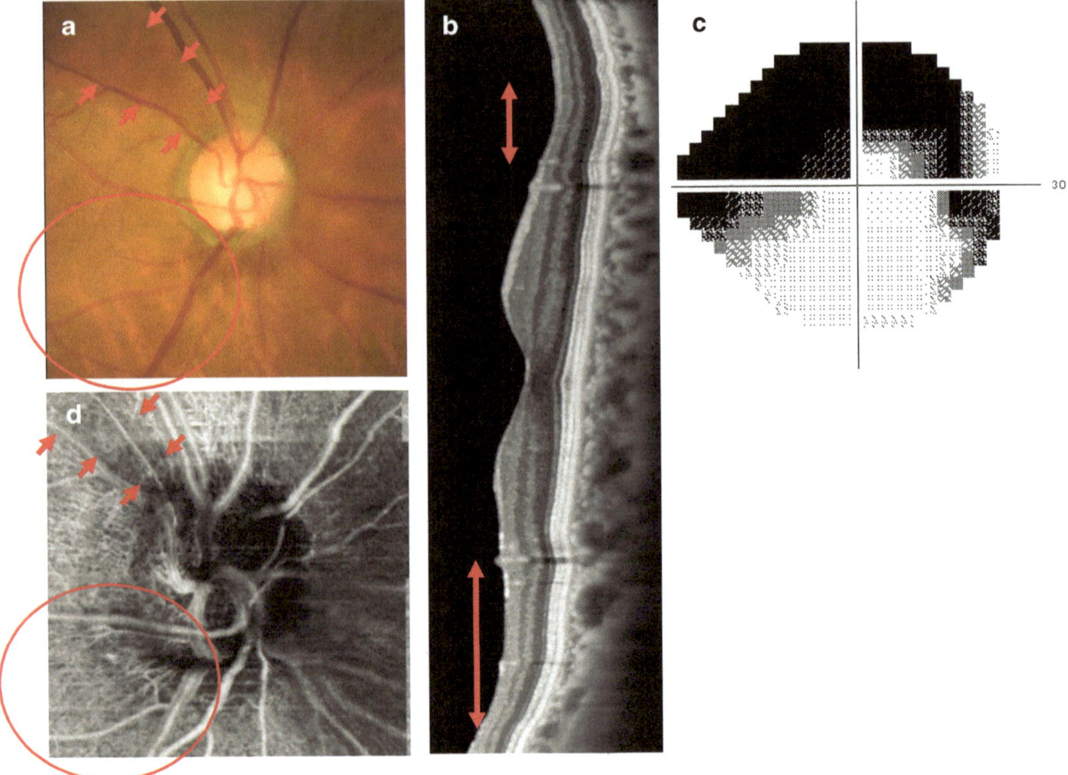

Fig. 6.16 Radial peripapillary capillary imaging by using optical coherence tomography angiography as an indicator of glaucomatous optic neuropathy. (**a**) Color fundus photography. (**b**) Vertical optical coherence tomography (OCT) B-scan. (**c**) Grayscale map from a standard automated perimetry 24-2 program. (**d**) An *en face* OCT angiography image. *Red arrows* indicate a relatively narrow retinal nerve fiber layer (RNFL) defect that corresponds with the lower nasal step visual field defect. *Dotted circles* indicate the diffuse RNFL defect corresponding with the large visual field defect in the upper panel. *Double arrows* indicate regions with RNFL thinning on OCT B-scan images

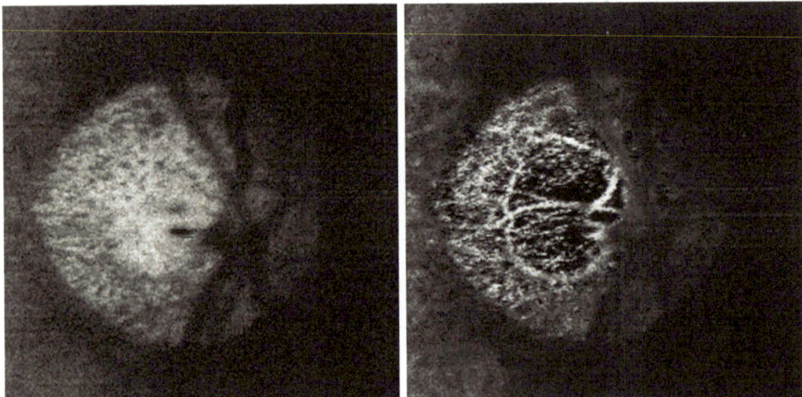

Fig. 6.17 An *en face* enhanced depth imaging optical coherence tomography (EDI-OCT) angiography image of the laminar capillary plexus in a normal eye. An *en face* reflectivity intensity-based OCT image (*left column*) depicts laminar beams and pores, and a corresponding *en face* EDI-OCT angiography image (*right column*) depicts laminar capillaries within the laminar beams. The laminar capillaries are dense throughout the lamina cribrosa

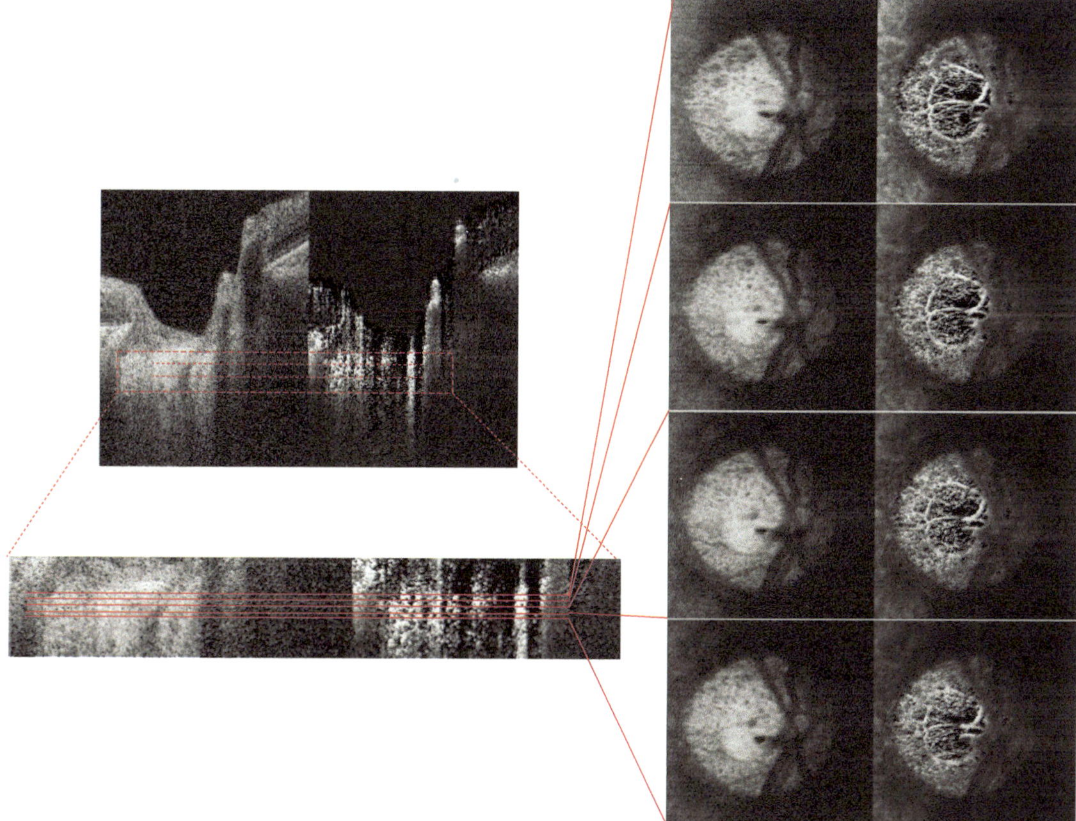

Fig. 6.18 Serial *en face* optical coherence tomography angiography images of a normal eye. The laminar capillaries are dense throughout the lamina cribrosa at all laminar depths

capillaries from the rest of the optic disc capillary components. OCT angiography allows for the selective visualization of the laminar capillary network and the observation of capillaries at arbitrary depths (Figs. 6.17, 6.18, and 6.19). It has been shown that the enhanced depth imaging (EDI)-OCT method allows for improved visualization of the lamina cribrosa structure. Therefore, the use of EDI-OCT mode is likely more effective in visualizing laminar capillaries than conventional OCT mode. Importantly, OCT angiography is able to depict laminar capillaries selectively and at arbitrary depths. When observed on EDI-OCT angiography, the lamina cribrosa shows a laminar dense capillary plexus associated with laminar beams throughout the laminar depth in normal eyes. By contrast, laminar capillary signals were apparently defective at all laminar depths in an eye with glaucoma (Fig. 6.19). This finding in our pilot study proposes the hypothesis that the lamina cribrosa in eyes with glaucoma lacks a healthy capillary circulation and consequently loses its normal remodeling response to mechanical injuries, thus becoming susceptible to glaucomatous injuries.

6.8 Limitations of the Current Optical Coherence Tomography Angiography Method

A limitation of current OCT angiography technology is that imaging is limited to a small area when obtaining high-contrast capillary images. The wider the imaging area, the less clear OCT angiography images become (Figs. 6.20 and 6.21). A pixel spacing of at least 12 μm is required

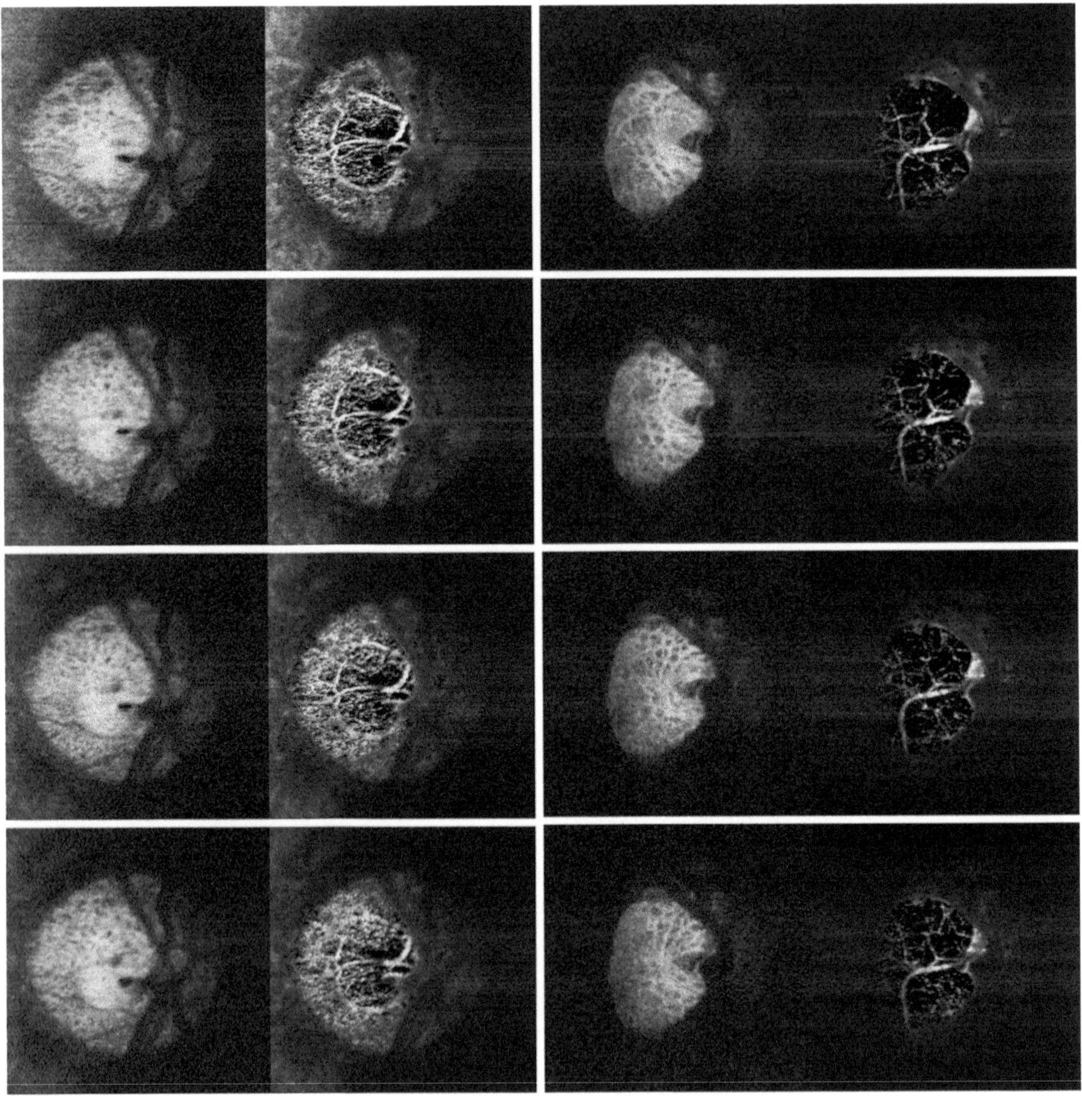

Fig. 6.19 A comparison of laminar capillary plexus images as detected by optical coherence tomography (OCT) angiography. The *left columns* show serial *en face* OCT angiography images of a normal eye, which demonstrate dense laminar capillaries throughout the lamina cribrosa at all laminar depths. The *right column* shows serial *en face* OCT angiography images of a glaucomatous eye, which demonstrate defects in OCT angiography signals throughout the laminar depths

to visualize each of the retinal capillaries clearly (Fig. 6.21). Therefore, when the OCT imaging speed is 5300 rpm, a 3 mm×3 mm square is the largest area in which OCT angiography achieves acceptably clear capillary visualization. Unfortunately, this area is smaller than a clinically useful size, such as the macular and posterior pole areas. An increase in imaging speed will allow for wider areas of clear capillary imaging. Currently, a montage of single OCT angiography images over a wider area is a possible solution to obtain clear OCT angiography images of larger regions (Fig. 6.22).

Another limitation is that OCT angiography signals are blocked by retinal lesions such as retinal hemorrhage, hard exudates, and cystoid

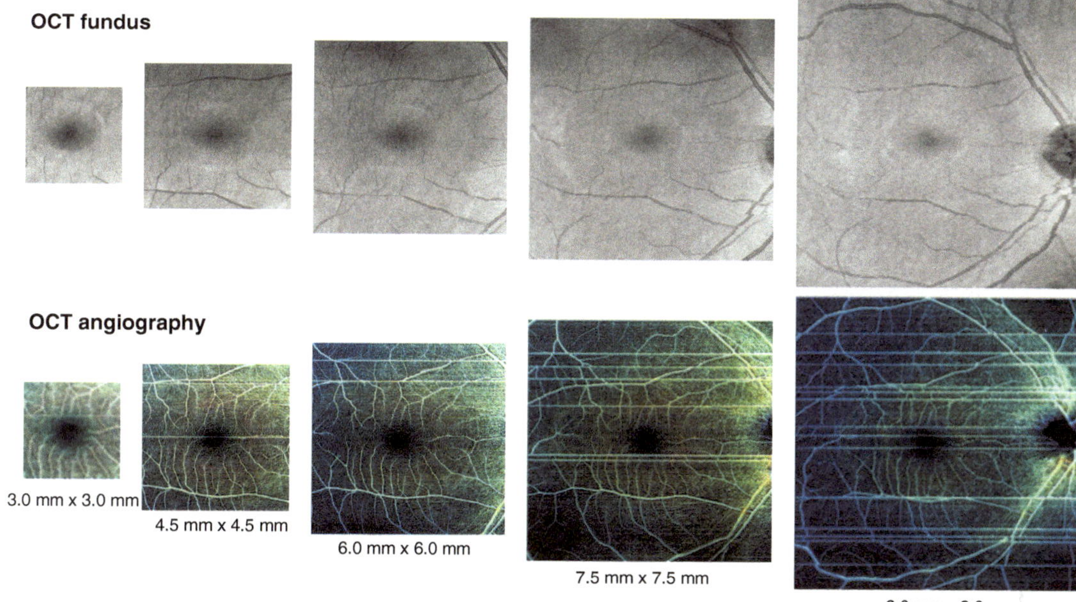

Fig. 6.20 Quality of optical coherence tomography (*OCT*) angiography images and scanning area. The numbers of A-scans and B-scans were fixed at 256 and 256, respectively, and only the scan area was changed. The wider the scan area, the more unclear the OCT angiography image becomes

spaces, as well as by reflectivity intensity-based OCT signals. A perifoveal capillary abnormality in central retinal vein occlusion and branch retinal occlusion is an interesting issue; however, fresh retinal hemorrhage, hard exudates, and cystoid spaces often accompany a macular lesion and almost totally block OCT angiographic signals (Fig. 6.23). When retinal hemorrhages are not as dense, capillary signals in the SCP are well-visualized, but those in deeper layers are almost undetectable. The use of an EDI-OCT method or a 1-μm probe light source may only slightly decrease the signal blockade.

6.9 Future Advances

Regardless of the current limitations of OCT angiography and OCT hardware, OCT angiography will become an increasingly useful tool for clinical and research purposes. This is because this method does not require exogenous dye injection and provides different clinical information than dye angiography. Higher imaging speeds will enable the acquisition of clear OCT angiography images in wider areas. In the near future, an increase in scanning speed will allow ultra-wide field OCT angiography as wide as UWF™ (Optos plc, Queensferry House, Scotland, UK), which enables us to determine retinal non-perfusion areas fully in eyes with diabetic retinopathy and vein occlusive disease. Alternatively, automated montages may also provide an ultra-wide field OCT angiography image. Almost all OCT companies will introduce an OCT angiography function in their instruments. Thus, OCT angiography will be clinically accepted as a useful additive method to reflectivity intensity based-OCT.

Acknowledgement All of the OCT angiography images used in this chapter were obtained by the prototype OCT angiography software developed for RS-3000 Advance (NIDEK CO., LTD, Gamagori, Japan), and the OCT device was provided by the NIDEK. The author appreciates his collaborators, Mrs. Masaaki Hanebuchi (NIDEK) and Yasuhiro Furuuchi (NIDEK) for their help in the preliminary experiments. The research was partially supported by a Grant-in-Aid for Scientific Research (15K10845) from the Japan Society for the Promotion of Science (JSPS) KAKENHI.

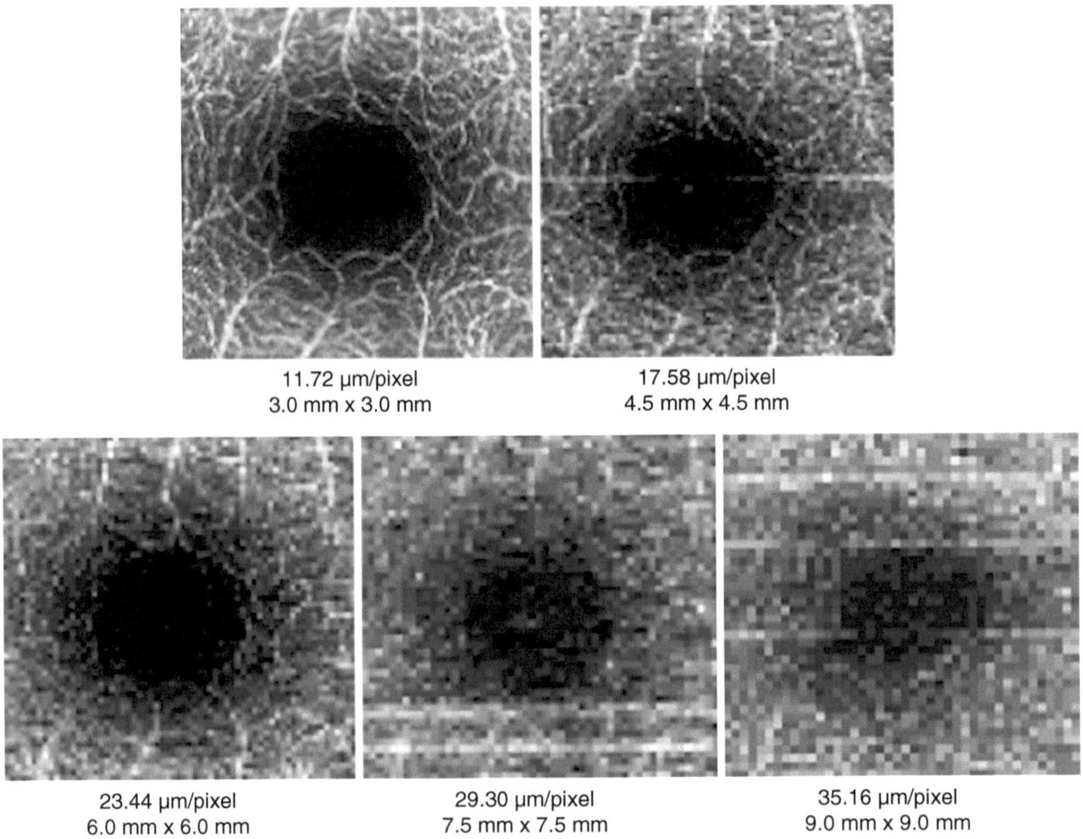

11.72 μm/pixel
3.0 mm x 3.0 mm

17.58 μm/pixel
4.5 mm x 4.5 mm

23.44 μm/pixel
6.0 mm x 6.0 mm

29.30 μm/pixel
7.5 mm x 7.5 mm

35.16 μm/pixel
9.0 mm x 9.0 mm

Fig. 6.21 Quality of perifoveal capillary imaging in optical coherence tomography angiography. The numbers of A-scans and B-scans were fixed at 256 and 256, respectively, and only the scan area was changed. The wider the scan area, the more obscure the perifoveal capillary plexus becomes

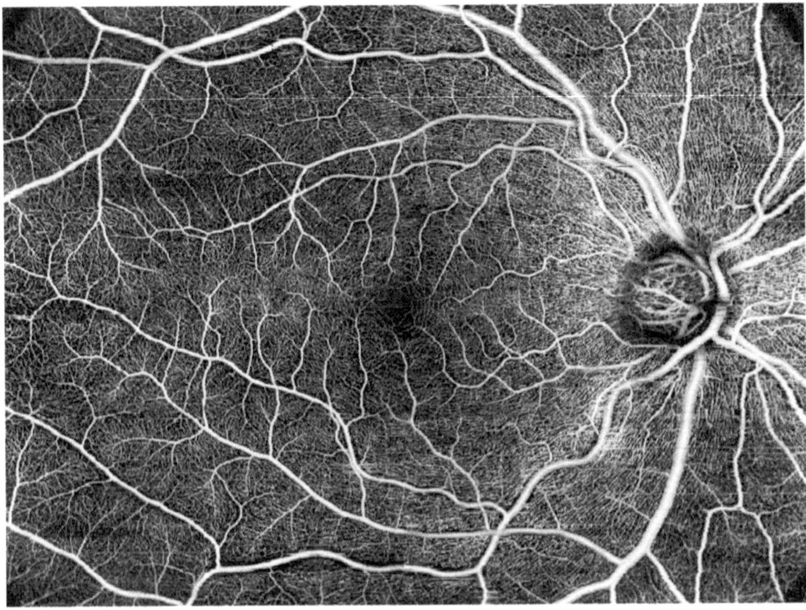

Fig. 6.22 A montage of single *en face* optical coherence tomography images over the posterior pole of a normal eye

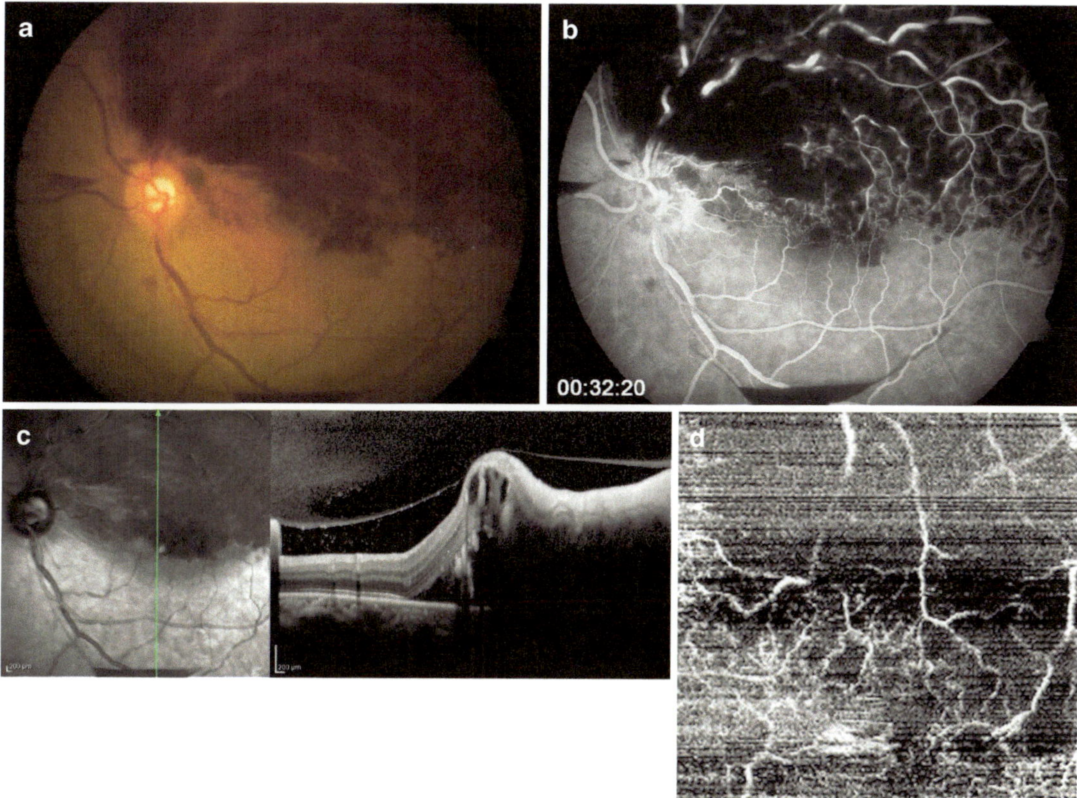

Fig. 6.23 A case of branch retinal vein occlusion showing blocked optical coherence tomography angiography signals. (**a**) Color fundus photography. (**b**) Fluorescein angiography (32.2 s). (**c**) Vertical optical coherence tomography (OCT) B-scan. The *green arrow* indicates the scan line for the OCT B-scan. (**d**) *En face* OCT angiography image

References

Dansingani KK, Balaratnasingam C, Klufas MA et al (2015) Optical coherence tomography angiography of shallow irregular pigment epithelial detachments in pachychoroid spectrum disease. Am J Ophthalmol 160:1243–1254. doi:10.1016/j.ajo.2015.08.028

Huang D, Jia Y, Rispoli M et al (2015) Optical coherence tomography angiography of time course of choroidal neovascularization in response to anti-angiogenic treatment. Retina 35:2260–2264

Inoue M, Balaratnasingam C, Freund KB (2015) Optical coherence tomography angiography of polypoidal choroidal vasculopathy and polypoidal choroidal neovascularization. Retina 35:2265–2274

Ishibazawa A, Nagaoka T, Takahashi A et al (2015) Optical coherence tomography angiography in diabetic retinopathy: a prospective pilot study. Am J Ophthalmol 160:35–44.e1

Iwasaki M, Inomata H (1986) Relation between superficial capillaries and foveal structures in the human retina. Invest Ophthalmol Vis Sci 27:1698–1705

Jia Y, Bailey ST, Hwang TS et al (2015) Quantitative optical coherence tomography angiography of vascular abnormalities in the living human eye. Proc Natl Acad Sci U S A 112:E2395–E2402

Jia Y, Bailey ST, Wilson DJ et al (2014a) Quantitative optical coherence tomography angiography of choroidal neovascularization in age-related macular degeneration. Ophthalmology 121:1435–1444

Jia Y, Wei E, Wang X et al (2014b) Optical coherence tomography angiography of optic disc perfusion in glaucoma. Ophthalmology 121:1322–1332

Kiumehr S, Park SC, Syril D et al (2012) In vivo evaluation of focal lamina cribrosa defects in glaucoma. Arch Ophthalmol 130:552–559

Liu L, Jia Y, Takusagawa HL et al (2015) Optical coherence tomography angiography of the peripapillary retina in glaucoma. JAMA Ophthalmol 133:1045–1052

Mahmud MS, Cadotte DW, Vuong B et al (2013) Review of speckle and phase variance optical coherence tomography to visualize microvascular networks. J Biomed Opt 18:50901

Palejwala NV, Jia Y, Gao SS et al (2015) Detection of non-exudative choroidal neovascularization in age-related macular degeneration with optical coherence tomography angiography. Retina 35:2204–2211

Quaranta-El Maftouhi M, El Maftouhi A, Eandi CM (2015) Chronic central serous chorioretinopathy imaged by optical coherence tomographic angiography. Am J Ophthalmol 160:581–587

Snodderly DM, Weinhaus RS (1990) Retinal vasculature of the fovea of the squirrel monkey, Saimiri sciureus: three-dimensional architecture, visual screening, and relationships to the neuronal layers. J Comp Neurol 297:145–163

Snodderly DM, Weinhaus RS, Choi JC (1992) Neural-vascular relationships in central retina of macaque monkeys (Macaca fascicularis). J Neurosci 12: 1169–1193

Takayama K, Hangai M, Kimura Y et al (2013) Three-dimensional imaging of lamina cribrosa defects in glaucoma using swept-source optical coherence tomography. Invest Ophthalmol Vis Sci 54: 4798–4807

Tatham AJ, Miki A, Weinreb RN et al (2014) Defects of the lamina cribrosa in eyes with localized retinal nerve fiber layer loss. Ophthalmology 121:110–118

Yu S, Pang CE, Gong Y et al (2015) The spectrum of superficial and deep capillary ischemia in retinal artery occlusion. Am J Ophthalmol 159:53–63

7 Spectral Domain Optical Coherence Tomography-Based Imaging Biomarkers and Hyperspectral Imaging

Surabhi Ruia and Sandeep Saxena

Contents

S. Ruia, MS • S. Saxena, MS,FRCSEd,FRCS, FRCOphth,FAICO (✉)
Department of Ophthalmology, King George's Medical University, Lucknow, UP, India
e-mail: sandeepsaxena2020@gmail.com

7.1 Introduction

"Biomarker", a merged word of "biological marker", refers to a broad subcategory of medical signs that objectively indicate the state of health and well-being of an individual. These can be anatomical, biochemical, molecular parameters or imaging features. They are measurable by laboratory assay, physical examination or medical imaging. In clinical practice, they are useful in the refinement of diagnosis, measuring disease progression or predicting and monitoring effects of therapeutic interventions. Their source can be tissue or body fluid such as plasma, urine, synovial fluid or tissue biopsy (Strimbu and Tavel 2010). Imaging biomarkers target the diseased organ or tissue and are hence specific indicators. The biochemical biomarkers, in contrast, tend to integrate information from the entire body. Biomarkers hold great promise for customization of treatment for the individual as information gained from diagnostic or progression markers would result in a highly efficient intervention in the disease process. With the introduction of imaging biomarkers, improved imaging technologies are being used for detection of molecules, biochemical processes in the retina. These will facilitate in early detection, assessment and monitoring of retinal pathologies. Hyperspectral imaging, a novel technology, collects information from across the electromagnetic spectrum for every pixel in an image. Spectral imaging

C.H. Meyer et al. (eds.), *Spectral Domain Optical Coherence Tomography in Macular Diseases*, DOI 10.1007/978-81-322-3610-8_7

techniques facilitate higher signal-to-noise ratio and lower light intensity at the retina in comparison with Fourier transform approach.

7.2 Biomarkers as Surrogate End points

Biomarkers are often used as surrogate end points in clinical trials. They act as surrogates or substitutes for clinically meaningful end points. Clinical end points are variables that represent a study subject's health and well-being from the subject's perspective. These end points have the potential to definitively demonstrate whether interventions in a trial are effective or ineffective, as well as safe or unsafe. For example "survival" is considered the gold-standard clinical end point for most HIV trials. To be considered a surrogate end point, there must be solid scientific evidence (epidemiological, therapeutic and/or pathophysiological) that a biomarker consistently and accurately predicts a clinical outcome (Strimbu and Tavel 2010). This requires the determination of relevance and validity. Relevance refers to a biomarker's ability to appropriately provide clinically relevant information to the public, the healthcare providers, or the health policy officials. Validity refers to the need to characterize a biomarker's effectiveness or utility as a surrogate end point. The biomarker proposed as a surrogate should be capable of being measured objectively, accurately, precisely and reproducibly. Biomarkers are also important in the development of new drug therapies through identification of drug targets. They also serve as "progression" markers to delineate the development and course of a disease. The changes in these progression markers can be used to understand the effect of therapy in altering the disease process.

7.3 Biomarkers of Imaging in Ocular Diseases

Spectral domain optical coherence tomography (SD-OCT) with its high-resolution in vivo imaging has proven to be useful in identifying various imaging biomarkers in a range of ocular diseases. These include age-related macular degeneration, retinitis pigmentosa, diabetic retinopathy and epiretinal membrane. SD-OCT-based imaging parameters have also been documented as prognostic biomarkers in neurological diseases like spinocerebellar ataxia, Huntington's disease, Parkinson's disease and systemic lupus nephritis.

7.3.1 Age-Related Macular Degeneration

Age-related macular degeneration (AMD) is a progressive degenerative disorder leading to gradual deterioration of central vision. One of the early clinical features in AMD is the appearance of drusen. It has been shown histologically that photoreceptors overlying and distal to drusen undergo degeneration. Ability to use imaging biomarkers for detection of cases which are likely to progress rapidly will benefit from early preventative interventions. SD-OCT and adaptive optics have been used to monitor drusen over time, for their progression in terms of size and their direct effect on the overlying photoreceptor layers (Godara et al. 2010). With the use of microperimetry, functional data of photoreceptors can be obtained to correlate with the high-resolution structural imaging information. These qualitative imaging-based biomarkers provide a valuable tool for detecting the earlier stages of the disease, tracking progression and monitoring treatment response.

SD-OCT has also been used for imaging morphology, reflectivity properties of drusen, quantifying their number and monitoring the longitudinal evolution in these characteristics. Area, volume, height and reflectivity of drusen are informative features useful for estimating the likelihood of progression to exudative AMD from an early or intermediate stage (Folgar et al. 2016).

High-density SD-OCT macular volumes have been documented to have a potential role in the prediction of disease progression risk in cases of intermediate AMD (de Sisternes et al. 2014).

The novel measures of retinal pigment epithelium-drusen complex (RPEDC) are obtained by high-density SD-OCT. The RPEDC abnormal thickening (OCT drusen) and RPEDC abnormal thinning volumes are generated by semiautomated segmentation of total RPEDC within a 5-mm-diameter macular field. OCT drusen volume changes predict progression to advanced AMD with choroidal neovascularization. The alteration in RPEDC thinning volume predicts progression to geographic atrophy. These quantitative SD-OCT biomarkers predict 2-year AMD progression and may serve as useful biomarkers for future clinical trials.

7.3.2 Diabetic Retinopathy

A new parameter, "parallelism", has been projected to evaluate retinal layer integrity using SD-OCT. OCT images are skeletonized, and the orientation of segmented lines in the image is termed "parallelism". The orientation of photoreceptor layer status at the fovea has been categorized, including continuity of the external limiting membrane (ELM) band, inner segment ellipsoid zone and the presence of hyperreflective foci in the outer retinal layers. Parallelism was observed to be significantly lower in eyes with diabetic macular edema (DME) in comparison with normal eyes. A positive correlation with visual acuity was also documented. Eyes with an intact inner segment ellipsoid zone or ELM band had significantly better visual acuity and higher parallelism, than eyes with a discontinuous or absent inner segment ellipsoid zone or ELM band. Significantly higher parallelism and better visual acuity were observed in the group without hyperreflective foci in the outer retinal layers. This novel image parameter, "parallelism", serves as a potential biomarker to prognosticate visual outcome in DME (Uji et al. 2014a).

Three different phenotypes have been recently characterized in diabetic retinopathy to stratify risk of progression to vision-threatening complications. Microaneurysm turnover has been validated as a prognostic biomarker of the development of DME (Cunha-Vaz et al. 2014). SD-OCT for identification of subclinical macular oedema and multifocal electroretinogram for providing functional data appear to be good candidates for organ-specific biomarkers for diabetic retinopathy. Disorganization of the foveal retinal inner layers and photoreceptor ELM disruption have also been documented as robust SD-OCT-based imaging biomarkers for predicting visual outcome in eyes with center involving DME (Sun et al. 2014).

Recently, certain biomolecules have been documented to have an association with disease severity and structural alteration in the retina. These have the potential to serve as biomarkers to prognosticate the visual outcome. An increase in serum levels of vascular endothelial growth factor (VEGF) and intercellular adhesion molecule-1 (ICAM-1) has been found to be associated with an increase in the severity of diabetic retinopathy. Further, increase in serum levels of these two molecules was also observed to be associated with disruption of photoreceptor ELM and inner segment ellipsoid zone in diabetic retinopathy (Jain et al. 2013). Anti-myeloperoxidase antibody (anti-MPO) is a valid, sensitive and specific marker for measuring the activity of the enzyme myeloperoxidase in serum. Myeloperoxidase enzyme has been proposed to be one of the mediators of the inflammatory process in diabetic retinopathy. A recent study has documented anti-MPO as a biomarker for progression of diabetic retinopathy (Sinha et al. 2016). The role of SD-OCT-based imaging of retinal nerve fiber layer (RNFL) thinning has also been documented as a biomarker for disease progression in diabetic retinopathy (Srivastav et al. 2015). SD-OCT-based macular thickness parameters central subfield and cube average thickness have been documented to serve as surrogate markers for prognosticating the disease severity. Targeted screening of DME serves as a significant indicator for progression of disease process within the grade of retinopathy, which may not be clinically evident (Ruia and Saxena 2016; Ruia et al. 2016). Thiobarbituric acid reactive substance and nitric oxide have also been documented to serve as potential biochemical biomarkers (Ruia et al. 2016).

7.3.3 Epiretinal Membrane

"Parallelism" has also been projected to evaluate retinal layer integrity in individuals with epiretinal membrane. The more parallel the retinal layers, the better the visual acuity of the individual. Parallelism is documented to significantly correlate with metamorphosia and visual acuity in eyes with ERM (Uji et al. 2014b).

7.3.4 Retinitis Pigmentosa

Spectral domain optical coherence tomography line scans serve as a tool for structural biomarkers, and full-field standard automated perimetry serve as functional biomarkers in patients with autosomal dominant retinitis pigmentosa. The total photoreceptor layer and the photoreceptor ellipsoid zone width have been documented to have a significant correlation with the functional biomarker of visual sensitivity obtained on automated perimetry (Smith et al. 2016).

7.4 Spectral Domain Optical Coherence Tomography Retinal Imaging Biomarkers for Neurological Diseases

7.4.1 Neuromyelitis Optica

SD-OCT-based peripapillary RNFL thickness and macular ganglion cell complex thickness have been proposed to serve as biomarkers for differentiating neuromyelitis optica spectrum disorder, multiple sclerosis and healthy controls. Visual acuity, contrast vision acuity and expanded disability status scale score are other biomarkers that have been documented. Temporal peripapillary RNFL atrophy has been observed to be more severe in patients with multiple sclerosis without episode of optic neuritis. Patients with neuromyelitis optica have been observed to show retinal degeneration independent of optic neuritis when compared to healthy controls (Outteryck et al. 2015).

7.4.2 Huntington's Disease

Enhanced depth imaging SD-OCT has been used to image changes in retinal and choroidal structure in Huntington's disease and to evaluate any potential correlation with the stage of the disease. Both the choroidal and retinal macula are altered in Huntington's disease and serve as potential biomarkers for monitoring neurodegeneration in this disease. No difference was observed in peripapillary choroidal and RNFL thickness (Andrade et al. 2016).

7.4.3 Parkinson's Disease

SD-OCT and confocal scanning laser ophthalmoscopy have been used to analyse the morphological changes in the retina of patients with Parkinson's disease. Peripapillary RNFL thickness and macular thickness and volume are measured by SD-OCT. Stereometric parameters of the optic disc are acquired by Heidelberg Retina Tomograph. The macular region and especially the foveola with the highest density of photoreceptor cells were observed to be more sensitive biomarkers (Bittersohl et al. 2015).

7.4.4 Systemic Lupus Erythematosus

Macular volume and thickness and peripapillary RNFL thickness using SD-OCT have been proposed as biomarkers for diagnosing and monitoring neuropsychiatric involvement in SLE. No significant difference in retinal thickness or macular volume was observed between neuropsychiatric SLE patients and non-neuropsychiatric SLE patients. However, SLE patients as a whole have been observed to show significant RNFL and macular thinning compared to controls. Temporal superior and temporal inferior RNFL thickness have been found to correlate with scores of test for assessing complex attention. These findings suggest that OCT measurements may be indicative of neurodegeneration in SLE and may be a useful biomarker for early cognitive impairment in SLE (Liu et al. 2015).

7.5 Hyperspectral Imaging

Hyperspectral imaging is a novel imaging tool that collects and processes information from across the electromagnetic spectrum. The recorded spectra have fine wavelength resolution and cover a wide range of wavelengths. The goal of hyperspectral imaging of the retina is to obtain the spectrum for each pixel in the image with the purpose of identifying materials or detecting biochemical and metabolic processes within the retina. Pupillary aperture and the radiant power at the retina are the two limitations during application of any imaging technique for retinal pathology. Spectral imaging techniques facilitate higher signal-to-noise ratio and lower light intensity at the retina in comparison with Fourier transform approach (Harvey et al. 2002).

Hyperspectral computed tomographic spectroscopy provides a feasible method for measurement and analysis of vascular oxygen content in the healthy and diseased retina. The images obtained clearly distinguish between oxygenated and deoxygenated hemoglobin. This serves as a potentially useful measure of vascular functions enabling early detection of various retinopathies. Recent studies have documented the use of this technique for measuring intravascular oxygen saturation (oximetry) in cases with diabetic retinopathy. In subjects with proliferative diabetic retinopathy, oxygen saturation was found to be significantly lower in the arteries, whereas it was significantly higher in the veins in comparison with controls (Kashani et al. 2014).

Studies on experimental animals have used oximetry measurements to study the variation during an acute retinal vein occlusion. Retinal oximetry measurements, 1 h after induction of retinal vein occlusion, revealed a statistically significant reduction in the intravascular oxygen saturation. This decrease was reversible in animals that spontaneously re-cannulated the vein occlusion (Jaime et al. 2012).

Hyperspectral mapping of macular pigment in vivo has been proposed to play a useful role in the assessment of subjects with age-related macular degeneration. Non-negative matrix factorization is used for analyzing the three-dimensional full spatial-spectral data cube, wherein the data is decomposed to give spectral signatures and spatial distribution, in search for the macular pigment absorbance spectrum. Snapshot hyperspectral imaging in combination with advanced mathematical analysis provides a simple cost-effective approach for macular pigment mapping in vivo (Fawzi et al. 2011).

The utility of hyperspectral imaging has also been studied for the assessment and management of primary open-angle glaucoma. A significant association between neuroretinal rim differential light absorption (a measure of spectral absorption properties) and visual field sensitivity has been observed (Denniss et al. 2011).

Amyloidopathic disorders such as Alzheimer's disease present with symptoms years after significant neurodegeneration. Accumulation of pathologic amyloid-β peptides causes neuronal death. Direct identification and quantitation of soluble amyloid aggregates using spectrophotometric technique have been evaluated to aid in early detection of amyloidopathy in Alzheimer's disease. The technique has been found to be useful for monitoring retinal and brain amyloidopathy in studies on experimental animal. With retinal amyloidopathy occurring well before that in the brain, translation of noninvasive retinal-plaque imaging to humans has the potential to facilitate early and accurate amyloidopathic disorder diagnosis and therapy assessment (Koronyo et al. 2012).

References

Andrade C, Beato J, Monteiro A et al (2016) Spectral-domain optical coherence tomography as a potential biomarker in Huntington's disease. Mov Disord 31(3):377–383

Bittersohl D, Stemplewitz B, Keserü M et al (2015) Detection of retinal changes in idiopathic Parkinson's disease using high-resolution optical coherence tomography and heidelberg retina tomography. Acta Ophthalmol 93:578–584

Cunha-Vaz J, Ribeiro L, Lobo C (2014) Phenotypes and biomarkers of diabetic retinopathy. Prog Retin Eye Res 41:90–111

Denniss J, Schiessl I, Nourrit V et al (2011) Relationships between visual field sensitivity and spectral absorption properties of the neuroretinal rim in glaucoma by multispectral imaging. Invest Ophthalmol Vis Sci 52:8732–8738

Fawzi AA, Lee N, Acton JH et al (2011) Recovery of macular pigment spectrum in vivo using hyperspectral image analysis. J Biomed Opt 16:106008

Folgar FA, Yuan EL, Sevilla MB et al, Study A.R.E.D. and Group S (2016) Drusen volume and retinal pigment epithelium abnormal thinning volume predict 2-year progression of age-related macular degeneration. Ophthalmology 123:39–50

Godara P, Siebe C, Rha J et al (2010) Assessing the photoreceptor mosaic over drusen using adaptive optics and SD-OCT. Ophthalmic Surg Lasers Imaging Retina 41:104–108

Harvey AR, Lawlor J, McNaught AI et al (2002) Hyperspectral imaging for the detection of retinal disease. In: International symposium on optical science and technology. International Society for Optics and Photonics

Jaime GRL, Kashani AH, Saati S et al (2012) Acute variations in retinal vascular oxygen content in a rabbit model of retinal venous occlusion. PLoS One 7: 50179

Jain A, Saxena S, Khanna VK et al (2013) Status of serum VEGF and ICAM-1 and its association with external limiting membrane and inner segment-outer segment junction disruption in type 2 diabetes mellitus. Mol Vis 19:1760–1768

Kashani AH, Lopez Jaime GR, Saati S et al (2014) Noninvasive assessment of retinal vascular oxygen content among normal and diabetic human subjects: a study using hyperspectral computed tomographic imaging spectroscopy. Retina 34:1854–1860

Koronyo Y, Salumbides BC, Black KL et al (2012) Alzheimer's disease in the retina: imaging retinal aβ plaques for early diagnosis and therapy assessment. Neurodegener Dis 10:285–293

Liu GY, Utset TO, Bernard JT (2015) Retinal nerve fiber layer and macular thinning in systemic lupus erythematosus: an optical coherence tomography study comparing SLE and neuropsychiatric SLE. Lupus 24:1169–1176

Outteryck O, Majed B, Defoort-Dhellemmes S et al (2015) A comparative optical coherence tomography study in neuromyelitis optica spectrum disorder and multiple sclerosis. Mult Scler J 21:1781–1793

Ruia S, Saxena S (2016) Targeted screening of macular edema by spectral domain optical coherence tomography for progression of diabetic retinopathy. Indian J Ocular Biol 1:102

Ruia S, Saxena S, Prasad S et al (2016) Correlation of biomarkers thiobarbituric acid reactive substance, nitric oxide and central subfield and cube average thickness in diabetic retinopathy: a cross-sectional study. Int J Retina Vitreous 2:1

Sinha S, Saxena S, Das S et al (2016) Antimyeloperoxidase antibody is a biomarker for progression of diabetic retinopathy. Journal of diabetes and its complications 30:700–704

de Sisternes L, Simon N, Tibshirani R et al (2014) Quantitative SD-OCT imaging biomarkers as indicators of age-related macular degeneration progression predicting AMD progression using SD-OCT features. Invest Ophthalmol Vis Sci 55:7093–7103

Smith TB, Parker M, Steinkamp PN et al (2016) Structure-function modeling of optical coherence tomography and standard automated perimetry in the retina of patients with autosomal dominant retinitis pigmentosa. PLoS One 11(2):e0148022

Srivastav K, Saxena S, Mahdi AA et al (2015) Increased serum urea and creatinine levels correlate with decreased retinal nerve fibre layer thickness in diabetic retinopathy. Biomarkers 20:470–473

Strimbu K, Tavel JA (2010) What are biomarkers? Curr Opin HIV AIDS 5:463

Sun JK, Lin MM, Lammer J et al (2014) Disorganization of the retinal inner layers as a predictor of visual acuity in eyes with center-involved diabetic macular edema. JAMA Ophthalmol 132:1309–1316

Uji A, Murakami T, Unoki N et al (2014a) Parallelism for quantitative image analysis of photoreceptor–retinal pigment epithelium complex alterations in diabetic macular edema parallelism in DME. Invest Ophthalmol Vis Sci 55:3361–3367

Uji A, Murakami T, Unoki N et al (2014b) Parallelism as a novel marker for structural integrity of retinal layers in optical coherence tomographic images in eyes with epiretinal membrane. Am J Ophthalmol 157:227–236

Part II
Medical Retina

Diabetic Macular Edema

8

Zachary M. Bodnar, Ankit Desai, and Levent Akduman

Contents

Z.M. Bodnar, MD • L. Akduman, MD (✉)
Department of Ophthalmology, Saint Louis University, Saint Louis, MO, USA
e-mail: akdumanlevent@gmail.com

A. Desai, MD
Department of Ophthalmology, Henry Ford Hospital, Detroit, MI, USA

8.1 Introduction

Diabetic maculopathy is the most common cause of visual impairment in diabetic retinopathy and is manifested most frequently as diabetic macular edema (DME) (Williams et al. 2004). The three primary tools used by ophthalmologists in the evaluation of diabetic macular edema are slit-lamp biomicroscopy, fluorescein angiography, and macular optical coherence tomography (OCT). The Early Treatment in Diabetic Retinopathy Study (ETDRS) established recommendations for the treatment of DME by defining clinically significant diabetic macular edema (CSDME) as one or more of the following:

1. Retinal thickening within 500 μ of the macular center
2. Hard exudates within 500 μ of the macular center with adjacent retinal thickening
3. Retinal thickening one optic disc area or larger in size within one disc diameter of the macular center

The ETDRS showed that CSDME leads to moderate vision loss in one out of four patients within 3 years and that this risk is halved by focal laser photocoagulation (from approximately 26 to 13 %) (ETDRS 1991). Clinicians are now increasingly adopting the use of intravitreal anti-angiogenic agents for the treatment of CSDME,

C.H. Meyer et al. (eds.), *Spectral Domain Optical Coherence Tomography in Macular Diseases*, DOI 10.1007/978-81-322-3610-8_8

which indeed has become the standard of care in most parts of the world.

Criteria for CSDME established by the ETDRS are based solely on observation by slit-lamp biomicroscopy and/or stereo fundus photography as this study took place before OCT was available for clinical use (ETDRS 1991). Fluorescein angiography has been in use for over half a century and can identify vascular abnormalities including microaneurysms, neovascularization, intraretinal microvascular abnormalities, capillary non-perfusion and leakage. However, leakage detected by fluorescein angiography does not necessarily correspond to macular edema (Bhagat et al. 2009). Only OCT can measure macular thickness objectively. This is important because no observation correlates better with visual acuity in DME than axial retinal thickening, although the degree to which retinal thickening corresponds to visual acuity depends on the pattern of DME seen (Network et al. 2007; Nussenblat et al. 1987; Shimura et al. 2011). Additionally, OCT is the best modality for visualizing and evaluating pathology of the vitreomacular interface, including epiretinal membranes (ERM) and vitreomacular traction (VMT), which may contribute to the persistence of DME after focal laser photocoagulation or intravitreal pharmacotherapy with anti-VEGF, and it can also identify patients who may benefit from pars plana vitrectomy (PPV) and membrane peel (MP) (Ghazi et al. 2007; Capone 2000). Finally, unlike FA and fundus photography, OCT can provide both objective and quantitative assessment of the retina in DME. Thus, it plays a central role in the evaluation of DME.

8.2 Optical Coherence Tomography Findings in Diabetic Macular Edema

Several morphologic patterns of DME have been identified using OCT. Several authors have described three basic patterns: sponge-like retinal thickening, cystoid macular edema, and serous retinal detachment (Baskin 2010; Panozzo et al. 2002). Kim et al. proposed an extended classification of five patterns (Kim et al. 2006):

1. Diffuse retinal thickening (Fig. 8.1)
2. Cystoid macular edema (Fig. 8.2)
3. Serous retinal detachment (Fig. 8.3)
4. Posterior hyaloidal traction (Fig. 8.4)
5. Posterior hyaloidal traction with tractional retinal detachment (Fig. 8.5)

Of these, the most common pattern is diffuse retinal thickening (39.5 %), and the least common are posterior hyaloidal traction (12.7 %) and tractional retinal detachment (2.9 %) (Ahmadpour-Baghdadabad et al. 2013; Kim et al. 2006; Otani et al. 1999). The other patterns typically do not appear in isolation, with the most common combination being diffuse retinal thickening and CME (29.0 %). Serous retinal detachment is more common in males and patients with a serum triglyceride ≥200 mg/dL (Ahmadpour-Baghdadabad et al. 2013). Patterns that are significantly associated with a decrease in visual acuity are diffuse retinal thickening, CME, and posterior hyaloidal traction. Some studies have suggested that the greatest decrease in vision occurs in the presence of CME and posterior hyaloidal traction, but others indicate that the degree of visual loss may not necessarily correlate with the type of pattern seen (Ahmadpour-Baghdadabad et al. 2013; Shimura et al. 2011). While the relationship between retinal thickening and decreased visual acuity is a characteristic of DME, it is not observed in macular edema secondary to other diseases, including CRVO, Irvine-Gass syndrome, posterior uveitis, and retinitis pigmentosa (Catier et al. 2005).

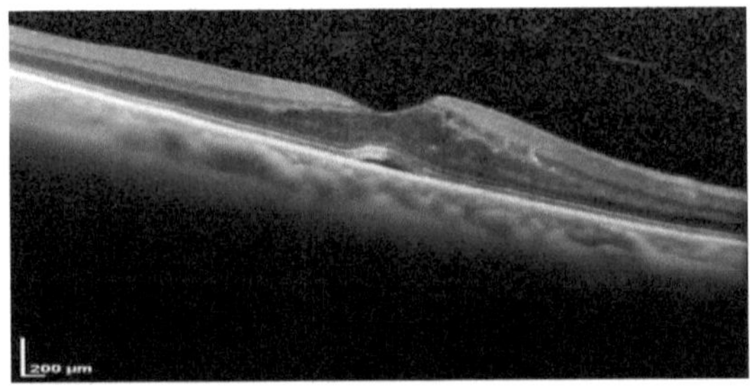

Fig. 8.1 Diffuse retinal thickening. SD-OCT showing sponge-like swelling, low reflective, expanded and irregular areas of the retina, and small amount of subfoveal fluid

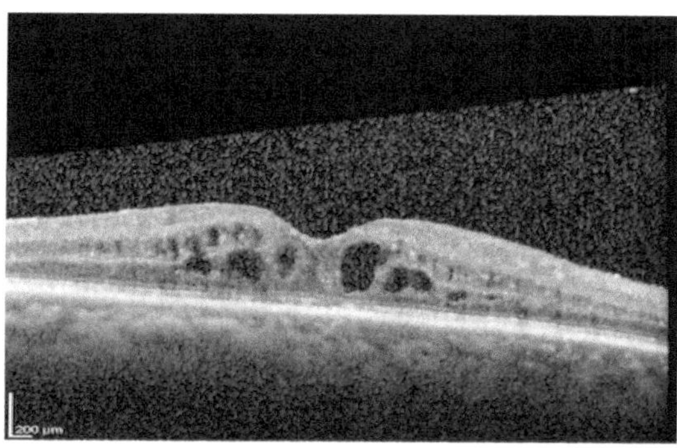

Fig. 8.2 Cystoid macular edema. SD-OCT showing hypo-reflective fluid-filled cystic cavities within the outer retinal layers, separated by hyper-reflective septae of neuroretinal tissue

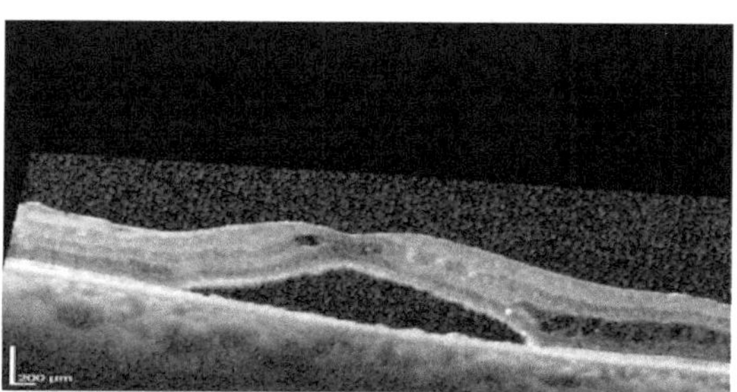

Fig. 8.3 Serous retinal detachment. SD-OCT showing fluid accumulation between the detached retinal pigment epithelium and neurosensory retina

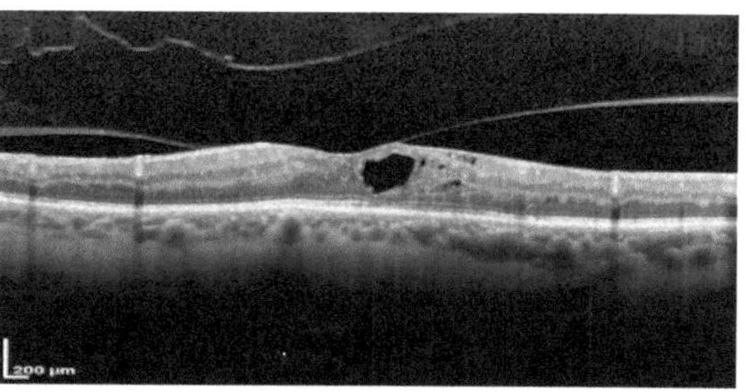

Fig. 8.4 Posterior hyaloidal traction. SD-OCT showing attached posterior hyaloid inducing some tractional effect possibly exacerbating the underlying edema. The hyper-reflective foci with posterior shadowing represent small exudates

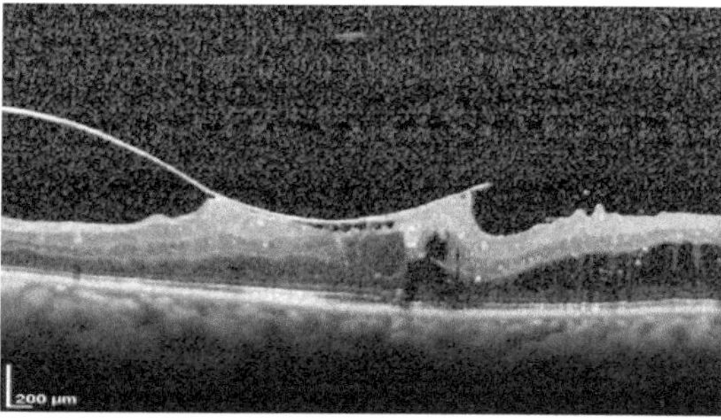

Fig. 8.5 Posterior hyaloidal traction (more severe form)

Soliman et al. investigated the morphological patterns of DME and identified what they believed to be progressive stages. In their scheme, stage 1 consists of leakage on FA without any changes visible via OCT. Stage 2 consists of thickening of the outer nuclear layer (ONL) and/or Henle's layer. Stage 3 includes the morphological changes of stage 2 plus cystic changes of the ONL and/or Henle's layer. Stage 4 is similar to stage 3 but also includes cystic changes of the inner nuclear layer (INL). Stage 5 has the appearance of stage 4 plus serous retinal detachment. Solimon correlated increasing central macular thickness as well as decreased BCVA with each successive stage (Soliman et al. 2007).

Kim et al. investigated the response to focal laser photocoagulation in eyes with DME and diffuse retinal thickening, CME, and/or vitreomacular interface abnormalities and found that all patterns showed a significant decrease in thickening after treatment. Eyes with DME had a greater reduction in thickening and improvement in visual acuity after treatment than eyes with either CME or vitreomacular interface disease, and persistent edema after laser treatment was more common in the CME and vitreoretinal interface anomaly groups (Kim et al. 2009).

While the ETDRS established focal laser photocoagulation as the gold standard of treatment for CSDME more than 30 years ago, clinicians have been increasingly exploring the use of anti-VEGF agents for the treatment of DME. Shimura et al. followed 143 eyes with DME without any history of prior treatment for 12 weeks after a single intravitreal injection of 1.25 mg of bevacizumab. Eyes with vitreomacular interface abnormalities were excluded from the study, but eyes with diffuse macular thickening, CME, as well as serous retinal detachment all experienced a decrease in foveal thickness after injection. The percentage of improvement was significantly greater in the CME and diffuse retinal thickening eyes than in the eyes with serous retinal detachment. Similarly, the visual acuity improved in all patterns after injection, but the effect was significantly more pronounced in the CME and diffuse retinal thickening eyes than in the eyes with serous retinal detachment. The foveal thickness decreased gradually after injection and reached its nadir at approximately 8 weeks in all groups, after which thickening began to recur. The magnitude of improvement in foveal thickening was inversely proportional to the duration of diabetes in CME and diffuse retinal thickening groups, but not in the serous retinal detachment group. Additionally, for unclear reasons, the CME eyes appeared to cluster into two groups: a high-sensitivity group with a greater than 40 % maximal reduction in foveal thickness and a low-sensitivity group with a less than 30 % maximal reduction (Shimura et al. 2013).

Cheema et al. found a positive treatment effect in terms of improved BCVA at 6-month follow-up after a mean of 2.05 intravitreal injections of bevacizumab in patients with focal cystoid edema, which they defined as limited retinal thickening with cyst formation and preservation of the macular contours; they found no significant improvement in BCVA in eyes with diffuse DME, typical CME, or SRF despite significant decreases in central macular thickness. Eyes with vitreomacular interface abnormalities were excluded from analysis (Cheema et al. 2014).

While the above studies suggest that different patterns of DME as determined by OCT may respond differently to intravitreal bevacizumab, conflicting data exists. A retrospective study by Koytak et al. found no variation in improvement in BCVA after a single injection of bevacizumab between eyes with diffuse retinal thickening, CME, or serous retinal detachment. However, in this study, eyes were classified by the predominant OCT pattern of macular edema (Koytak et al. 2013). Regardless, some variability may exist in the way different authors sort OCT images into different patterns of macular edema. A well-designed clinical trial might help to clarify the responses of different OCT patterns of macular edema to anti-VEGF therapy and improve our understanding of appropriate dosing intervals.

Intravitreal corticosteroids have also been used in the treatment of DME. Shimura et al. investigated whether the effectiveness of intravitreal triamcinolone acetonide depended on the pattern of DME as determined by OCT. They found that while there was no difference in baseline visual acuity between the groups, and all groups experienced an improvement in BCVA after treatment with triamcinolone, the improvement was much better in eyes with diffuse retinal thickening and CME as compared to eyes with serous retinal detachment. Intravitreal triamcinolone had no significant effect in eliminating subretinal fluid in this study (Shimura et al. 2011).

8.3 Macular Thickening

The average retinal thickness in an area 500 μ in diameter centered on the fovea is 174 ± 18 μ, in healthy individuals and almost never exceeds 216 μ. Central foveal thickness in healthy patients is, on average, 152 ± 21 μ. In contrast, a central foveal thickness of 200–250 μ or more is considered by many authors to signify the presence of edema (Kim et al. 2009). Figure 8.6 demonstrates diffuse retinal thickening with loss of the foveal contour and epiretinal membrane formation. Sánchez-Tocino et al. found a maximal foveal thickness of 180 μ in normal subjects. They calculated a sensitivity of 93 % and specificity of

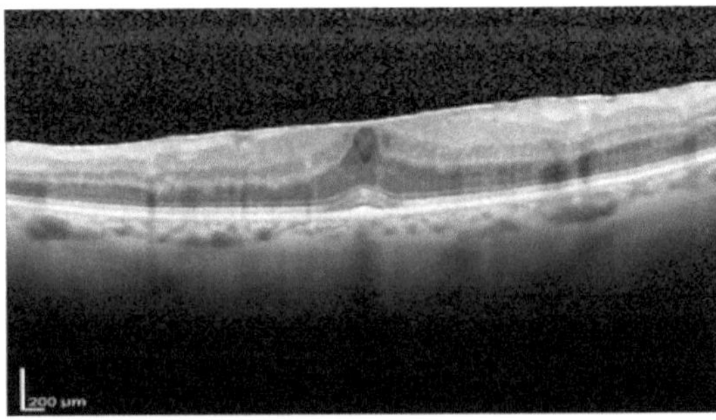

Fig. 8.6 Diffuse retinal thickening with epiretinal retinal membrane. SD-OCT showing complete loss of the foveal contour with hyper-reflective signal seen just anterior to the neurosensory retina

75 % for detecting CSDME when using this number as threshold for measurements made via the manual caliper tool on Zeiss OCT machine, as compared to the gold standard ETDRS methods (Sánchez-Tocino et al. 2002).

As subtle or focal macular thickening can be challenging to see with slit-lamp ophthalmoscopy; the assessment of macular thickness by OCT can be an effective screening tool for the detection of DME. Goebel and Kretzchmar-Gross compared foveal macular thickness as measured by OCT vs standard ETDRS methods for the diagnosis of CSDME and determined that OCT has a sensitivity of 89 % and specificity of 96 % (Goebel and Kretzchmar-Gross 2002). Most commercial OCT devices produce a macular thickness map with measurements at the central fixation point (Panozzo et al. 2002) and ETDRS-like macular areas, making correlation with clinical observations according to the ETDRS protocol straightforward. Figure 8.7 is an example report from a Stratus OCT device. Macular thickening correlates with a decrease in visual acuity in eyes with diffuse retinal thickening and CME, but not in eyes with subretinal fluid (Shimura et al. 2011).

8.4 Limitations

Measurements of retinal thickening will differ between OCT machines of different manufacture due to dissimilarities in their algorithms for segmentation. In particular, while all devices identify the vitreomacular interface as the inner retinal border, they may differ on the signal used to delimit the outer retinal boundary. For example, the older versions of the RTVue software treat the IS/OS junction as the outer retinal border, while newer updates of the RTVue software, the Cirrus HD-OCT and the Spectralis, use a band corresponding to the RPE/Bruch's membrane/choriocapillaris complex (Hee et al. 1995). One practical implication of this is that sequential measurements of macular thickness in the same eye made with different OCT implementations are not directly comparable. Also, different OCT devices will have different, proprietary normative databases for age, sex, and race (Sikorski et al. 2013).

An additional consideration is that signal strength, artifacts, and other imaging defects may introduce errors in image segmentation that impact the measurement of macular thickness. These types of errors include failure to identify the inner or outer retinal boundaries, truncation of the image due to inappropriate depth, and incorrect localization of the foveal center. The clinician must be cognizant of these factors when interpreting OCT measurements and assessing imaging quality. Manual correction of many of these types of errors is possible on most commercial OCT platforms. The savvy clinician may use false color images to examine subtle retinal structures, but should be aware that false color may also introduce image artifacts (Sikorski et al. 2013).

OCT of the macula in DME best serves the retinal physician as an adjective study besides careful clinical observation, fundus photography, and FA. A Cochrane review designed to evaluate the diagnostic accuracy of OCT for detecting CSDME concluded that OCT is not sufficiently accurate to diagnose the central type of macular edema (Wolf-Schnurrbusch et al. 2009).

8.5 Cystoid Macular Edema

Persistent macular edema leads to the formation of cystoid spaces consisting of septate pockets of fluid, primarily in the Henle's layer and the outer plexiform layer, but can sometimes also be found in the inner plexiform layer. Perifoveal cysts tend to localize mainly to the outer retinal layers (Otani et al. 1999). They appear on OCT as areas of hypo-reflectivity. Figure 8.8 shows typical CME with larger cysts in the outer retinal layers and the beginnings of small cyst formation in the inner layers.

Ex vivo histological specimens of a small number of patients with DME and early OCT-based studies lead to the hypothesis that cystoid macular edema results from long-standing cytoplasmic swelling of the Muller cells, leading to their necrosis and the formation of the

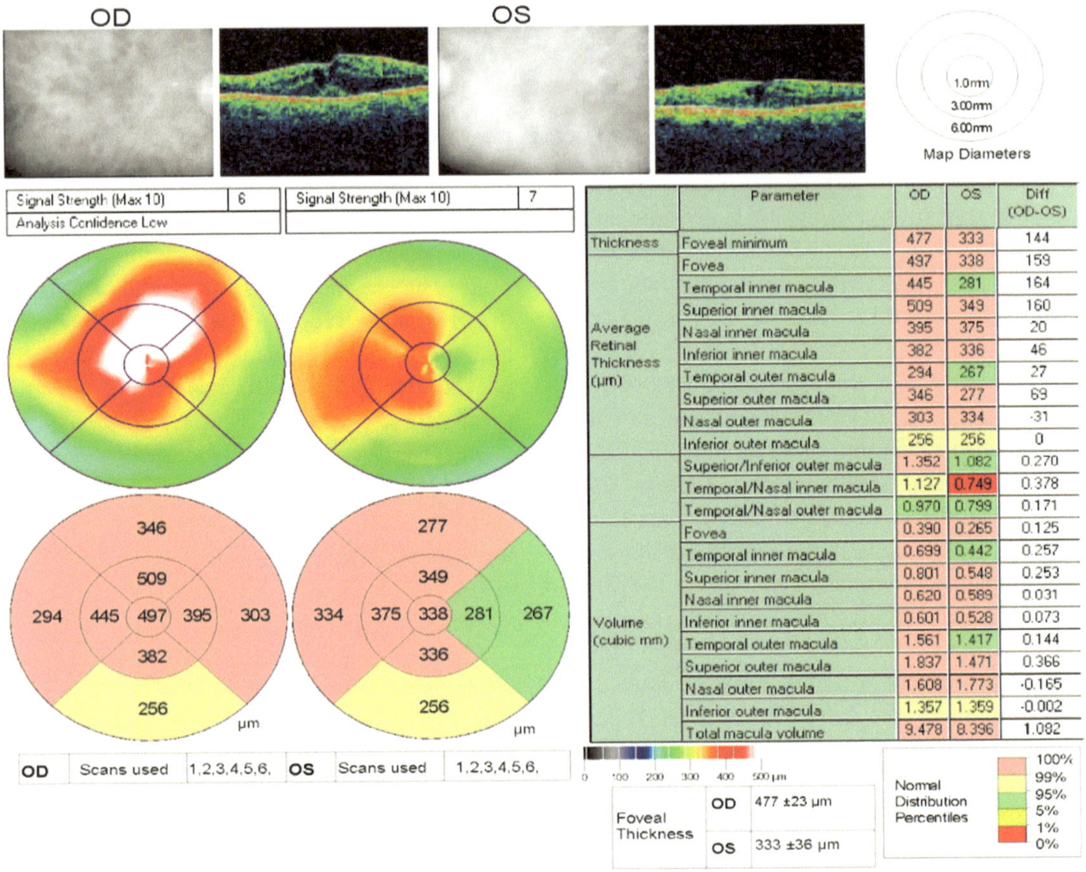

OD
OS
1.0mm
3.00mm
6.00mm
Map Diameters
Signal Strength (Max 10) 6
Analysis Confidence Low
Signal Strength (Max 10) 7
346
509
294 445 497 395 303
382
256
µm
277
349
334 375 338 281 267
336
256
µm
OD Scans used 1,2,3,4,5,6,
OS Scans used 1,2,3,4,5,6,
Parameter OD OS Diff (OD-OS)
Thickness Foveal minimum 477 333 144
Average Retinal Thickness (µm)
Fovea 497 338 159
Temporal inner macula 445 281 164
Superior inner macula 509 349 160
Nasal inner macula 395 375 20
Inferior inner macula 382 336 46
Temporal outer macula 294 267 27
Superior outer macula 346 277 69
Nasal outer macula 303 334 -31
Inferior outer macula 256 256 0
Superior/Inferior outer macula 1.352 1.082 0.270
Temporal/Nasal inner macula 1.127 0.749 0.378
Temporal/Nasal outer macula 0.970 0.799 0.171
Volume (cubic mm)
Fovea 0.390 0.265 0.125
Temporal inner macula 0.699 0.442 0.257
Superior inner macula 0.801 0.548 0.253
Nasal inner macula 0.620 0.589 0.031
Inferior inner macula 0.601 0.528 0.073
Temporal outer macula 1.561 1.417 0.144
Superior outer macula 1.837 1.471 0.366
Nasal outer macula 1.608 1.773 -0.165
Inferior outer macula 1.357 1.359 -0.002
Total macula volume 9.478 8.396 1.082
0 100 200 300 400 500 µm
Foveal Thickness
OD 477 ±23 µm
OS 333 ±36 µm
Normal Distribution Percentiles
100%
99%
95%
5%
1%
0%

Fig. 8.7 Stratus OCT report. This OCT device produces a macular thickness map and reports the average thickness in each of nine ETDRS-like regions of the macula. Average thickness measurements at various points, including the fovea, are tabulated and compared to an age-matched normative database. Macular volume is also quantified

200 µm

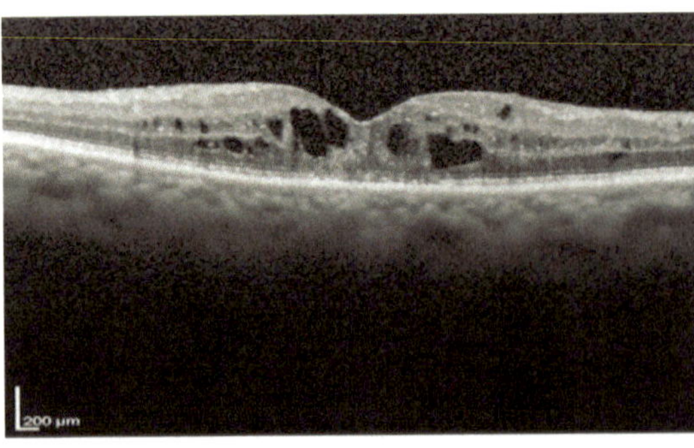

Fig. 8.8 Cystoid macular edema. SD-OCT showing large perifoveal cysts in the outer retinal layers. Small cysts are seen in the inner rental layers

cystic cavities (Fine and Brucker 1981; Yanoff et al. 1984). More recent high-definition OCT studies suggest that the fluid collection may in fact be extracellular. Regardless, cellular dysfunction and eventual death does result.

In long-standing macular edema, the cystic cavities may coalesce into one large foveal cavity (Fig. 8.9). Secondarily, these changes may produce OCT findings consisting of obscuration of the normal laminar structure, flattening of the foveal depression, and retinal thickening. Cysts may enlarge in size to span the full thickness of the retina which may lead to atrophy and profound loss of vision. Figure 8.10 shows such an eye with severe CME and disruption of the outer segments. Fluid can be seen underneath the neurosensory retina in some cases (Koleva-Georgieva and Sivkova 2009). Cystoid

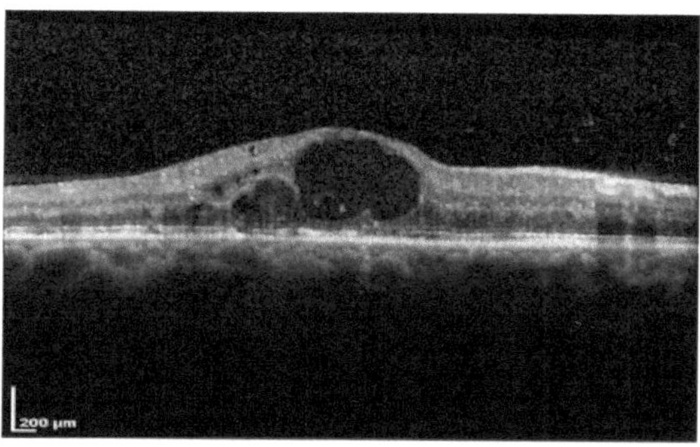

Fig. 8.9 Cystoid macular edema. SD-OCT showing small cysts that have coalesced to form one large cyst

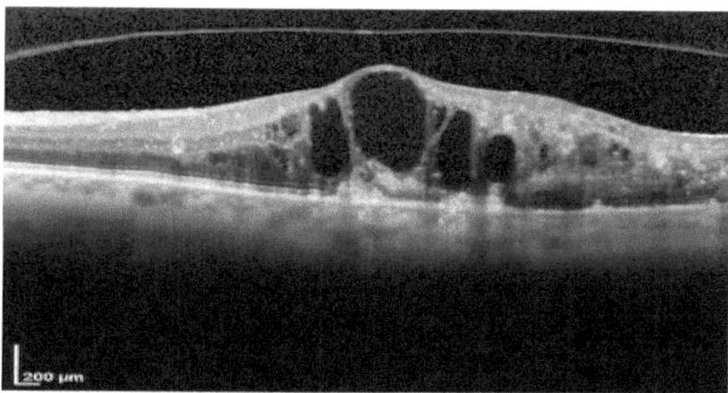

Fig. 8.10 Severe cystoid macular edema. SD-OCT showing cystic cavities that have expanded to involve the full thickness of the retina. Concomitant disruption of the outer segments can be seen

changes are less common in macular edema secondary to ERM alone than it is in DME (Otani et al. 2010).

8.6 Disruption of the Outer Retinal Layers

The external limiting membrane (ELM) and the junction between the photoreceptor inner and outer segments (IS/OS junction), recently know the ellipsoid zone, are well visualized as hyper-reflective lines within the outer retina on OCT. It has been shown that disruption of these layers is associated with poorer visual acuity as well as decreased sensitivity by microperimetry in DME (Brar et al. 2010; Hatef et al. 2011; Maheshwary et al. 2010; Otani et al. 2010; Pendergast et al. 2000; Yohanan et al. 2013). Unsurprisingly, final visual acuity correlates with status of the photoreceptor layer. Figure 8.11 depicts an atrophic retina with loss of the outer segments due to macular ischemia from chronic DME.

8.7 Abnormalities of the Vitreomacular Interface

The presence of vitreomacular traction provides a stronger indication for surgery vs pharmacologic therapy or laser treatment in patients with DME. The Diabetic Retinopathy Clinical Research Network Writing Committee (DRCR.net) has shown positive treatment effects of vitrectomy on DME in eyes with vitreomacular traction (DRCR.net 2010). The precise role of vitreomacular traction in the pathogenesis of DME is unclear, but Nasrallah et al. have noted that macular edema is more commonly present when the overlying posterior hyaloid is attached (Nasrallah et al. 1988). Pendergast et al. suggested that vitrectomy with removal of the posterior hyaloid face was beneficial in some eyes that were unresponsive to laser therapy with diffuse diabetic macular edema and a taut posterior hyaloid (Pendergast et al. 2000). In the context of the present discussion, however, it is important to note that OCT was used neither in the evaluation of the vitreomacular interface nor in macular edema in this study; evaluation was performed with slit-lamp biomicroscopy (Capone 2000). OCT has been shown to be more sensitive at the detection of posterior vitreous detachment than slit-lamp exam, so it is possible that had OCT been used in this study that the results may have been less pronounced (Akiyama et al. 2015). Indeed, a recent study using swept-source OCT actually revealed a strong correlation between CME and PVD (Abe et al. 2013). Another work indicates that subtle tractional effects that may be invisible on cross-sectional OCT can become apparent as fine folds when viewed using three-dimensional OCT. Abe et al. found that such eyes had improvement in macular edema after internal limiting membrane (ILM) peeling, but clinical significance of this is unclear; ILM peeling is known to improve edema, but some studies have

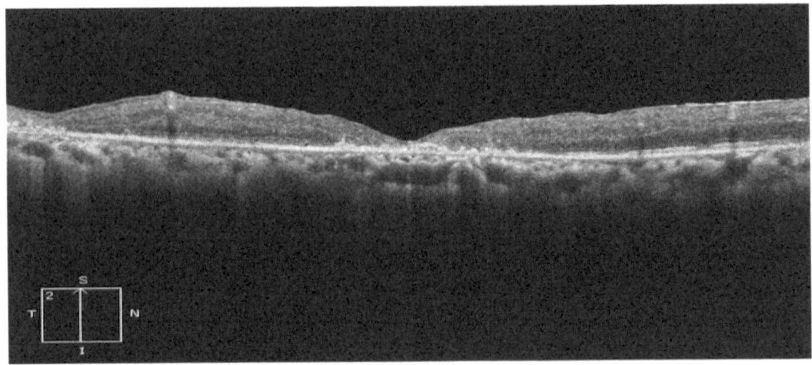

Fig. 8.11 Macular atrophy. SD-OCT showing macular ischemia secondary to diabetic macular edema. There is atrophy of the retina with loss of the outer segments

shown no impact on long-term outcomes, and others have indicated potentially deleterious effects including dissociation of the NFL and weakening of the b-wave on ERG (Mitamura and Ohtsuka 2005; Terasaki et al. 2003).

8.8 Other Findings

The dilated lumen of retinal microaneurysms can clearly be seen on high-definition OCT as a moderately reflective area circumscribed by more reflective walls. The anterior and posterior vessel walls usually appear hyper-reflective relative to the lateral walls, which is most likely due to a higher axial than transverse resolution, but may also be secondary to scattering from the blood accumulated in the microaneurysms (Bolz et al. 2009b).

Intraretinal and vitreous hemorrhages are hyper-reflective and may produce posterior shadowing (Akiyama et al. 2015). Similarly, hard exudates appear on OCT as small foci of hyper-reflectivity accompanied by posterior shadowing (Fig. 8.12) (Akiyama et al. 2015; Otani et al. 1999; Sull et al. 2009). These can be found in both the foveal and extrafoveal regions, most commonly in the outer plexiform and outer nuclear layers (Hatef et al. 2011; Otani et al. 1999). Actually, tiny reflective foci can be seen in all layers of the retina in all eyes with clinically significant DME. They are found in all layers of the retina and not visible by FA, infrared imaging, fundus biomicroscopy, or fundus photography. In fact, they are seen only in gray-scale cross-sectional images and are obfuscated by false color. Bolz et al. postulate that these well-demarcated foci represent small proteinaceous or lipid deposits and, when they become confluent, can be appreciated as hard exudates (Bolz et al. 2009b).

8.9 Correlation with Fluorescein Angiography

Several leakage patterns in FA of DME correspond to patterns of edema or morphologic changes that can be seen on OCT images. While leakage on FA is not necessary to make the diagnosis of CSDME, it has been used to identify sites of anomalous vascular permeability within the fundus that can be targeted with focal or grid laser photocoagulation. Understanding the corresponding changes in OCT images can further help the clinician plan and administer treatment.

The severity of leakage on FA is correlated both with the severity of outer retinal thickening and cystic changes of the inner and outer retina. Capillary non-perfusion on FA is associated with loss of the inner retinal layers on OCT (Fig. 8.11) (Sull et al. 2009). Large foveal cysts on OCT correspond to a petaloid leakage pattern

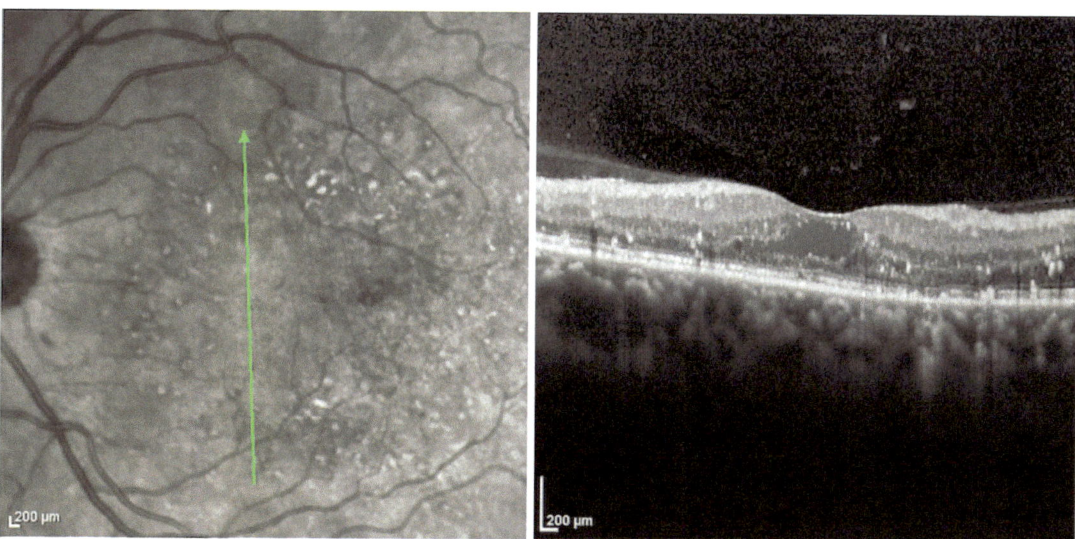

Fig. 8.12 Hard exudates. SD-OCT showing pinpoint hyper-reflective foci in these en face and cross-sectional images. *Green arrow* shows the cross-section of image taken

on late-phase FA. A honeycomb-like appearance of leakage is produced by smaller perifoveal cysts (Otani 2007; Yeung et al. 2009). Cross-sectional OCT imaging reveals that the large cyst in the petaloid leakage pattern exists within the ONL and OPL and may be associated with subretinal fluid in 30 % of cases, while the smaller cysts of the honeycomb pattern may be found in ONL, OPL, INL, and IPL (Bolz et al. 2009a). It is hypothesized that the petaloid pattern of cyst formation in the center of macula is due to oblique aligned fibers of the outer plexiform layer in this area; the honeycomb pattern in the surrounding area occurs where the fibers become arranged more vertically. In a study by Ikeda et al., the honeycomb pattern occurred only in eyes with an attached posterior hyaloid. They concluded that traction of the macula by the posterior hyaloid membrane may distort the tissue and decrease retinal tissue pressure, which combined with the increased vascular permeability of diabetic retinopathy and produce the honeycomb pattern on FA (Ikeda et al. 1999).

In contrast, there is no association between serous retinal detachment as detected by OCT and any leakage pattern on FA (Yeung et al. 2009). Similarly diffuse hyperfluorescence is associated with a number of morphological patterns on OCT and does not correlate any specific OCT findings (Bolz et al. 2009a).

8.10 Conclusions

OCT has provided new insights into the pathoanatomy of CSDME at the tissue level. It reveals that several patterns of diabetic macular edema exist. This may have prognostic implications in terms of visual outcomes and responses to treatment, in particular, antiangiogenic agents and intravitreal corticosteroids. OCT is far more sensitive than clinical examination at identifying abnormalities of the vitreomacular interface, and this can help the retinal physician identify good candidates for surgery. OCT is the only modality available for accurately measuring the macular thickness, which is a sensitive parameter for identifying diabetic macular edema and has a strong correlation with visual acuity, in certain patterns of edema. OCT, in conjunction with FA and slit-lamp biomicroscopy, is thus an essential tool for the evaluation and treatment of diabetic macular edema in the modern era.

References

Abe S et al (2013) Three-dimensional imaging of the inner limiting membrane folding on the vitreomacular interface in diabetic macular edema. Jpn J Ophthalmol 57:553–562

Ahmadpour-Baghdadabad M, Manaviat M, Shojaodiny-Ardekani A (2013) Optical corehence tomography in diabetic macular edema: patterns and related risk factors. Nepal J Ophthalmol 5:190–194

Akiyama H, Itakura H, Kashima T, Danjie L, Shimoda Y (2015) Observation of the vitreous in diabetic macular edema using swept-source OCT. Adv Ophthalmol Vis Syst 2:00037

Baskin DE (2010) Optical coherence tomography in diabetic macular edema. Curr Opin Ophthalmol 21:172–177

Bhagat N, Grigorian RA, Tutela A, Zarbin MA (2009) Diabetic macular edema: pathogenesis and treatment. Surv Ophthalmol 54:1–32

Bolz M, Ritter M, Schneider M, Simader C, Scholda C, Schmidt-Erfurth U (2009a) A systematic correlation of angiography and high-resolution optical coherence tomography in diabetic macular edema. Ophthalmology 116:66–71

Bolz M, Schmidt-Erfurth U, Deak G, Mylonas G, Kreichbaum K, Scholda C (2009b) Optical coherence tomographic hyperreflective foci. Ophthalmology 116:914–920

Brar M, Yuson R, Kozak I, Mojana F, Cheng L, Barsch DU, Oster SF, Freeman WR (2010) Correlation between morphologic features on spectral-domain optical coherence tomography and angiographic leakage patterns in macular edema. Retina 30:383

Capone A (2000) Vitrectomy for refractory diabetic macular edema. Semin Ophthalmol 15:78–80

Catier A, Tadayoni R, Paques M, Erginay A, Haouchine B, Gaudric A, Massin P (2005) Characterization of macular edema from various etiologies by optical coherence tomography. Am J Ophthalmol 140:200–206

Cheema HR, Al Habash A, Al-Askar E (2014) Improvement of visual acuity based on optical coherence tomography patterns following intravitreal bevacizumab treatment in patients with diabetic macular edema. Int J Ophthalmol 7:251–255

Diabetic Retinopathy Clinical Research Network Writing Committee on behalf of the DRCR.net (2010) Vitrectomy outcomes in eyes with diabetic macular edema and vitreomacular traction. Ophthalmology 117:1087–1093

Early Treatment Diabetic Retinopathy Study design and baseline patient characteristics (1991) ETDRS report number 7. Ophthalmology 98:741–756

Fine BS, Brucker AJ (1981) Macular edema and cystoid macular edema. Am J Ophthalmol 92:466–481

Ghazi NG, Ciralsky JB, Shah SM et al (2007) Optical coherence tomography findings in persistent diabetic macular edema: the vitreomacular interface. Am J Ophthalmol 144:747–754

Goebel W, Kretzchmar-Gross T (2002) Retinal thickness in diabetic retinopathy: a study using optical coherence tomography (OCT). Retina 22:759–767

Hatef E, Colantuoni E, Wang J, Ibrahim M, Shulman M, Adhi F, Sepah YJ, Channa R, Khwaja A, Nguyen QD, Do DV (2011) The relationship between macular sensitivity and retinal thickness in eyes with diabetic macular edema. Am J Ophthalmol 152:400–405

Hee MR, Puliafito CA, Wong C, Duker J, Reichel E, Rutlege B, Schuman J, Swanson E, Fujimoto J (1995) Quantitative assessment of macular edema with ocular coherence tomography. Arch Ophthalmol 113: 1019–1029

Ikeda T, Sato K, Katano T, Hayashi Y (1999) Attached posterior hyaloid membrane and the pathogenesis of honeycombed cystoid macular edema in patients with diabetes. Am J Ophthalmol 127:478–479

Kim NR, Kim YJ, Chin HS, Moon YS (2009) Optical coherence tomographic patterns in diabetic macular oedema: prediction of visual outcome after focal laser photocoagulation. Br J Ophthalmol 93:901–905

Kim BY, Smith SD, Kaiser PK (2006) Optical coherence tomographic patterns of diabetic macular edema. Am J Ophthalmol 142:405–412

Koleva-Georgieva D, Sivkova N (2009) Assessment of serous macular detachment in eyes with diabetic macular edema by use of spectral-domain optical coherence tomography. Graefes Arch Clin Exp Ophthalmol 247:1461–1469

Koytak A, Altinisik M, Sari ES, Artunay O, Akkan JCU, Tuncer K (2013) Effect of a single intavitreal bevacizumab injection on different optical coherence tomographic patterns of diabetic macular oedema. Eye 27:716–721

Maheshwary AS, Oster SF, Yuson RM, Cheng L, Mojana F, Freeman WR (2010) The association between percent disruption of the photoreceptor inner segment-outer segment junction and visual acuity in diabetic macular edema. Am J Ophthalmol 150:63–67

Mitamura Y, Ohtsuka K (2005) Relationship of dissociated optic nerve fiber layer appearance to internal limiting membrane peeling. Ophthalmology 112:1766–1770

Nasrallah F, Jalkh AE, VanCoppenolle F et al (1988) The role of the vitreous in diabetic macular edema. Ophthalmology 9:1335–1339

Network DRCR, Browning DJ, Glassman AR et al (2007) Relationship between optical coherence tomography-measured central retinal thickness and visual acuity in diabetic macular edema. Ophthalmology 114: 525–536

Nussenblat RB, Kaufman SC, Palestine AG, Davis MD, Ferris FL (1987) Macular thickening and visual acuity. Ophthalmology 94:1134–1139

Otani T (2007) Correlation between optical coherence tomography and fluorescein angiography findings in diabetic macular edema. Ophthalmology 114:104–107

Otani T, Kishi S, Maruyama Y (1999) Patterns of diabetic macular edema with optical coherence tomography. Am J Ophthalmol 127:688–693

Otani T, Yamaguchi Y, Kishi S (2010) Correlation between visual acuity and foveal microstructural changes in diabetic macular edema. Retina 30:774–780

Panozzo G, Gusson E, Parolini B, Mercanti A (2002) Role of OCT in the diagnosis and follow up of diabetic macular edema. Semin Ophthalmol 17:1–7

Pendergast SD, Hassan TS, Williams GA, Cox MS, Margherio RR, Ferrone PJ, Garretson BR, Trese MT (2000) Vitrectomy for diffuse diabetic macular edema associated with a taut premacular posterior hyaloid. Am J Ophthalmol 130:178–186

Sánchez-Tocino H, Alvarez-Vidal A, Maldonado MJ, Morano-Montñés J, García-Layana A (2002) Retinal thickness study with optical coherence tomography in patients with diabetes. Invest Ophthalmol Vis Sci 43:1588–1594

Shimura M, Yasuda K, Nakazawa T, Hirano Y, Sakamoto T, Ogura Y, Shiono T (2011) Visual outcome after intravitreal triamcinalone acetonide depends on optical coherence tomographic patterns in patients with diffuse diabetic macular edema. Retina 31:748–754

Shimura M, Yasuda K, Yasuda M, Nakazawa T (2013) Visual outcome after intravitreal bevacizumab depends on the optical coherence tomographic patterns of patients with diffuse diabetic macular edema. Retina 33:740–747

Sikorski BL, Malukiewicz G, Stafiej J, Lesiewska-Junk H, Raczynska D (2013) The diagnostic function of OCT in diabetic maculopathy. Mediators Inflamm 2013:434560

Soliman W, Sander B, Jørgensen TM (2007) Enhanced optical coherence patterns of diabetic macular oedema and their correlation with the pathophysiology. Acta Ophthalmol Scand 85:613–617

Sull A, Vuong L, Price L et al (2009) Comparison of spectral/Fourier domain optical coherence tomography instruments for assessment of normal macular thickness. Retina 30:235–245

Terasaki H, Kojima T, Niwa H, Piao CH, Ueno S, Kondo M et al (2003) Changes in focal macular electroretinograms and foveal thickness after vitrectomy for diabetic macular edema. Invest Ophthalmol Vis Sci 44:4465–4472

Wolf-Schnurrbusch UEK, Ceklic L, Brinkmann CK et al (2009) Macular thickness measurements in healthy eyes using six different optical coherence tomography instruments. Invest Ophthalmol Vis Sci 50:3432–3437

Williams R, Airey M, Baxter H, Forrester J, Kennedy-Martin T, Girach A (2004) Epidemiology of diabetic retinopathy and macular oedema: a systematic review. Eye 18:963–983

Yanoff M, Fine BS, Brucker AJ, Eagle RC (1984) Pathology of human cystoid macular edema. Surv Ophthalmol 28:505–511

Yeung L, Garcia P, Landa G, Rosen RB (2009) Correlation between spectral domain optical coherence tomography findings and fluorescein angiography patterns in diabetic macular edema. Ophthalmology 116:1158–1167

Yohanan J, Bittencourt M, Sepah YJ, Hatef E, Sophie R, Moradi A, Liu H, Ibrahim M, Do DV, Coulantouni E, Nguyen QD (2013) Association of retinal sensitivity to integrity of photoreceptor inner/outer segment junction in patients with diabetic macular edema. Ophthalmology 120:1254–1261

9 Retinal Photoreceptor Ellipsoid Zone Integrity in Diabetic Macular Edema

Sandeep Saxena, Khushboo Srivastav, Surabhi Ruia, Prateep Phadikar, and Levent Akduman

Contents

9.1 Introduction

Diabetes mellitus is attaining epidemic magnitudes worldwide (Bjork et al. 2003). Diabetic macular edema (DME) is the most common cause of vision loss in diabetic retinopathy (Sharma et al. 2005). A good correlation between macular thickness parameters, assessed by spectral domain optical coherence tomography (SD-OCT), and visual acuity has been observed by several studies (Kim et al. 2006; Martidis et al. 2002; Strom et al. 2002; Yamamoto et al. 2001). However, recent reports show only a weak correlation between central retinal thickness and visual acuity in DME (Nunes et al. 2010). This is suggestive of a role of disruption of the microstructural architecture of retina for impairment of visual acuity.

The optical biopsy of the foveal region, with ultrahigh resolution SD-OCT, identified four distinct bands in the outer retina. An international panel (Staurenghi et al. 2014) for consensus on the nomenclature of structures visible on OCT has brought an end to disputed anatomic attributions. The panel has ascribed the term *band* to the retinal layers signifying their three-dimensional structure. The term *zone* has been ascribed to the tissue structures whose anatomic correlate cannot be clearly delineated. The innermost of the four distinct bands in the outer retina is designated to be the external limiting membrane (ELM), a linear confluence of junctional complexes between Muller cells and photoreceptors. The second hyperreflective layer correlates to the inner segment ellipsoid zone (EZ) of photoreceptors (Fig. 9.1). The third layer correlates to the interdigitation zone between cone outer segment tips and apical processes of the retinal pigment epithelium (RPE). The outermost highly reflective zone represents the retinal pigment epithelium (RPE)/Bruch's complex.

S. Saxena, MS,FRCSEd,FRCS,FRCOphth,FAICO (✉)
K. Srivastav, MS • S. Ruia, MBBS • P. Phadikar, MBBS
Department of Ophthalmology, King George's Medical University, Lucknow, UP, India
e-mail: sandeepsaxena2020@gmail.com

L. Akduman, MD
Department of Ophthalmology, Saint Louis University, Saint Louis, MO, USA

C.H. Meyer et al. (eds.), *Spectral Domain Optical Coherence Tomography in Macular Diseases*, DOI 10.1007/978-81-322-3610-8_9

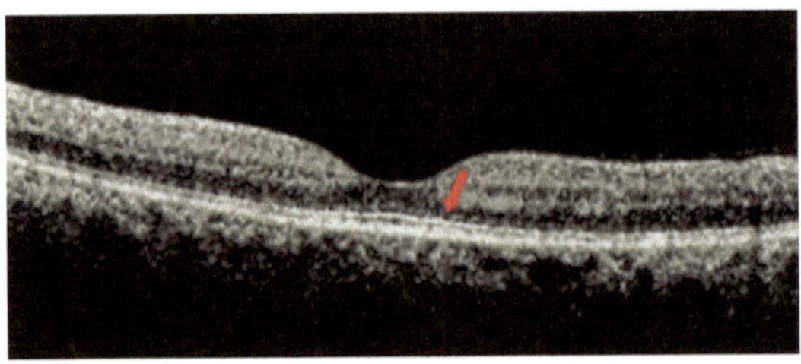

Fig. 9.1 SD-OCT showing intact inner segment ellipsoid zone (*red arrow*)

Using ultrahigh resolution SD-OCT images of human foveal cone photoreceptors, Fernandez et al. in 2008 identified the ellipsoid and myoid segments of the inner segment of photoreceptors. Spaide and Curcio in 2011 studied a model drawing of the outer retina (drawn to scale) based on published histology and concluded that the second band initially ascribed as inner segment-outer segment (IS-OS) junction of photoreceptor was essentially the EZ of the photoreceptor (Srinivasan et al. 2006). Lu et al. in 2012 seconded this concept by using an anatomical model of the outer retina from the leopard frog to correlate the second band to EZ.

With the cellular level resolution obtained by SD-OCT, multivariate analysis demonstrated a statistically significant relationship between visual acuity and percentage disruption of EZ. Recently, a significant correlation between macular thickness parameter and disruption of EZ with increasing severity of diabetic retinopathy has also been documented (Saxena et al. 2015).

9.2 Classification Systems for Ellipsoid Zone Disruption

A. Maheshwary et al. evaluated the EZ on horizontal and vertical scans of SD-OCT images in patients with DME. Disruption of EZ within 500 microns of the fovea was assessed and graded from 0 to 2 as follows:
   - Grade 0: Intact EZ
   - Grade 1: Focal EZ disruption of 200 microns or less in length
   - Grade 2: EZ disruption greater than 200 microns in length

   A statistically significant correlation between percentage disruption of the EZ and visual acuity was found. A convincing trend suggesting a decrease in visual acuity with increasing macular volume was documented. Percentage disruption of the EZ was recognized as an important predictor of visual acuity among DME patients (Maheshwary et al. 2010).

B. Jain et al. gave the grading system of disruption of ELM and EZ in patients with diabetic retinopathy. The occurrence of disruption of the ELM prior to disruption of the photoreceptor EZ was pointed out for the first time. This was based on the grounds of work done by Omri et al. in 2010, who lay emphasis on ELM being considered as a third retinal barrier. They reported that the RPE cell barrier junctions and ELM share common proteins like occludin. Decrease in the content of occludin at the level of ELM along with swelling of Muller cells is responsible for cyst formation in DME. The shortening of the photoreceptor EZ was documented to be a secondary consequence of the fragmented ELM by Mehalow et al. in 2003.

EZ and ELM band disruption were graded as follows (Jain et al. 2013):

- Grade 0: No disruption of ELM and EZ
- Grade 1: ELM disruption, intact EZ
- Grade 2: Both ELM and EZ disrupted

Several studies have concluded that the status of ELM and EZ is closely associated with visual acuity in diabetic retinopathy (Chhablani et al. 2012; Ito et al. 2013; Ko et al. 2004; Otani et al. 2010; Shin et al. 2012). Yamauchi et al. proposed that the origin of the EZ and ELM was related to the biological activities of the photoreceptor cells. They studied the ELM and EZ in brown Norwegian rats and found that the EZ and ELM disappeared after euthanasia (Yamauchi et al. 2011). Increase in the level of severity of diabetic retinopathy results in decreased biological activity of the ELM and EZ, which in turn results in the disruption of these layers and a decrease in visual acuity.

C. Sharma et al. put forward a simplified, comprehensive, and physician-friendly approach to grading EZ disruption based on OCT imaging of macula:
   - Grade 0: Intact EZ
   - Grade 1: Focal disruption (localized, subfoveal EZ disruption)
   - Grade 2: Global disruption (generalized EZ disruption throughout the macular cube)

The grade of subfoveal ELM and EZ disruption was associated with an increase in the severity of diabetic retinopathy and a decrease in visual acuity (Fig. 9.2). Global EZ disruption was associated with marked decrease in visual acuity as compared to "focal" disruption (Sharma et al. 2014).

Although the pathogenesis of diabetic retinopathy is not completely understood, several risk factors have been established. These include poor glycemic control, dyslipidemia, alteration in levels of serum urea, and serum creatinine (Ashakiran et al. 2010; Bloomgarden 2007). A number of interconnecting biochemical pathways have been proposed as potential links between hyperglycemia and diabetic retinopathy. These include increased expression of biomolecules such as vascular endothelial growth factor (VEGF), accelerated formation of advanced glycation end products (AGEs) like N-carboxy methyl lysine (N-CML), increase in oxidative stress markers, and leukostasis (Moore et al. 2003; Murata et al. 1995; Sebekova et al. 2002; Zong et al. 2011). VEGF is known to induce retinal expression of intercellular adhesion molecule-1 (ICAM-1) in turn initiating retinal leukocyte adhesion and blood-retinal barrier breakdown (Lu et al. 1999). Studies have documented a strong correlation between disruption of EZ and increase in levels of these biomolecules in diabetic retinopathy. A positive association between increasing serum levels of N-CML, VEGF, and ICAM and disruption of EZ has been reported by Saxena et al. in 2014. Disruption of EZ and ELM has been documented to have a positive association with serum levels of VEGF and ICAM by Jain et al. in 2013. Recently, a significant association between disruption of ELM and EZ with increased levels of serum cholesterol, low-density lipoprotein, and triglycerides has also been determined (Jain et al. 2015). Sharma et al. in 2015 ascertained a significant correlation between increased severity of retinopathy and increase in oxidative stress. Oxidative stress was indicated by an increase in lipid peroxidase, decrease in glutathione, and

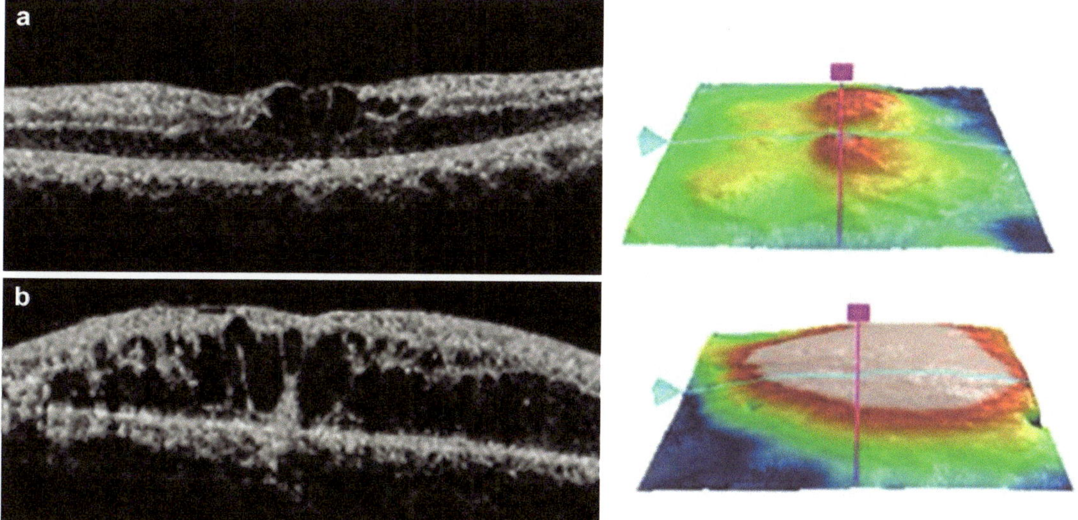

Fig. 9.2 SD-OCT showing (**a**) focal and (**b**) global disruption of inner segment ellipsoid zone with corresponding retinal thickness segmentation maps

increase in nitrosative stress parameters. These studies have increased the understanding of the structural and functional alterations of the retina in diabetic retinopathy.

D. Helmy et al. put forward a new classification system for DME, utilizing the ratio between the vertical height of the largest macular cyst and the maximum measured macular thickness, as observed on OCT imaging (Helmy and Atta Allah 2013). The four classification groups were as follows:
   CME I – Cysts less than 30 % of macular thickness
   CME II – Cysts between 30 and 60 % of macular thickness
   CME III – Cysts between 60 and 90 % of macular thickness
   CME IV – Cyst more than 90 % of macular thickness

Each grade was then subdivided according to certain morphologic features using labels "A," "B," "C," and "D."

A – Cysts without any disruption to the ELM or EZ
B – Cysts with ELM disruption
C – Cysts with EZ disruption
D – Cysts with disruption of both ELM and EZ

Presence of hyperreflective foci in the outer retinal layers from the ELM to the RPE within the 1 mm of fovea was designated with "+" signs. These hyperreflective foci represent tiny intraretinal protein and/or lipid deposits (Bolz et al. 2009). Inclusion of hyperreflective foci provide valuable information on the degree of blood-retinal barrier breakdown and its influence on visual acuity.

E. Another classification system was proposed to overcome the limitation of variability in the reflectivity levels of continuous EZ seen on SD-OCT. For this, transverse length of each disrupted EZ was quantified. Classifications were as follows:
   - Intact line – highly reflective and continuous line (physiologic)
   - Faint line – presence of a continuous line with lower reflectivity (less than half of the OCT reflectivity of the RPE)
   - Disrupted line – absent or discontinuous line

SD-OCT reflectivity of the ELM band was similarly analyzed. Relatively homogeneous and continuous ELM bands were described as *intact*. Absent or discontinuous ELM bands were described as *disrupted* (Murakami et al. 2012).

9.3 Integrity of Ellipsoid Zone and Pharmacological/Surgical Intervention

Few interventional studies have evaluated the role of the integrity of ELM and EZ on SD-OCT as a prognostic factor for visual outcome post-pharmacologic and surgical intervention. A statistically significant association was found between visual acuity and intact ELM and EZ post-pars plana vitrectomy with internal limiting membrane peel for DME (Yanyali et al. 2011).

Restoration of EZ and ELM was evaluated in patients with DME who were successfully treated with intravitreal triamcinolone. The integrity of EZ was found to correlate well with final visual acuity post-intervention. On multivariate analysis, the mean length of disrupted EZ and ELM band showed greater correlation to visual acuity than the length of either disrupted EZ or ELM band taken alone. The initial visual acuity (prior to treatment) and photoreceptor status both were found to assist in predicting the posttreatment recovery of EZ and subsequent visual recovery (Shin et al. 2012).

In a study by Chung et al. pre- and post-intervention assessment of visual acuity, fundus autofluorescence (FAF), and SD-OCT imaging of patients with DME who received intravitreal bevacizumab were performed. Foveal FAF was graded on a scale of 1–4. Better preinjection visual acuity and intact EZ and ELM band were associated with better visual acuity after treatment. Significantly increased FAF was seen in DME associated with disruption of EZ. It was concluded that correlation of FAF with SD-OCT and visual acuity can help predict the restoration of the integrity of EZ (Chung et al. 2012).

Wakabayashi retrospectively reviewed 41 eyes of 41 patients with DME who underwent vitrectomy. Associations between axial length, postoperative visual acuity, and visibility of EZ on SD-OCT were studied. Wakabayashi observed that median axial length was longer in those with a visible EZ at 12 months after surgery and that longer axial length predicted better visual outcomes after vitrectomy in patients with DME (Wakabayashi et al. 2013). The mechanism of this protective effect was not fully elucidated, but a similar relationship has been established between axial length and DME, as well as diabetic retinopathy itself (Man et al. 2012). This protective effect is presumed to be secondary to an inverse relationship between axial length and ocular blood flow, a parameter attributed to stretch-induced microvascular anatomical changes, such as vessel thinning, that appear to result in diminished pressure against the vascular wall, and a resultant decrease in microvascular leakage and damage to retinal microstructure (Quigely and Cohen 1999).

References

Ashakiran S, Krishnamurthy N, Navin S et al (2010) Behaviour of serum uric acid and lipid profile in relation to glycemic status in proliferative and non-proliferative diabetic retinopathy. Curr Neurobiol 2:57–61

Bjork S, Kapur A, King H et al (2003) Global policy: aspects of diabetes in India. Health Policy 66:61–72

Bloomgarden ZT (2007) Screening for and managing diabetic retinopathy: current approaches. Am J Health Syst Pharm 64:S8–S14

Bolz M, Schmidt-Erfurth U, Deak G et al (2009) Optical coherence tomographic hyper-reflective foci: a morphologic sign of lipid extravasation in diabetic macular edema. Ophthalmology 116:914–920

Chhablani JK, Kim JS, Cheng L et al (2012) External limiting membrane as a predictor of visual improvement in diabetic macular edema after pars plana vitrectomy. Graefes Arch Clin Exp Ophthalmol 250:1415–1420

Chung H, Park B, Shin HJ (2012) Correlation of fundus autofluorescence with spectral-domain optical coherence tomography and vision in diabetic macular edema. Ophthalmology 119:1056–1065

Fernandez EJ, Hermann B, Povazay B et al (2008) Ultrahigh-resolution optical coherence tomography and pancorrection for cellular imaging of the living human retina. Opt Express 16:11083–11094

Helmy YM, Atta Allah HRA (2013) Optical coherence tomography classification of diabetic cystoid macular edema. Clin Ophthalmol 7:1731–1737

Ito S, Miyamoto N, Ishida K et al (2013) Association between external limiting membrane status and visual acuity in diabetic macular edema. Br J Ophthalmol 97:228–232

Jain A, Saxena S, Khanna VK et al (2013) Status of serum VEGF and ICAM-1 and its association with external limiting membrane and inner segment-outer segment junction disruption in type 2 diabetes mellitus. Mol Vis 19:1760–1768

Jain A, Saxena S, Ruia S et al (2015) Altered lipid profile is associated with external limiting membrane and inner segment ellipsoid band disruption in type 2 diabetes mellitus: a preliminary study. Open Sci J Clin Med 3:37–41

Kim BY, Smith SD, Kaiser PK (2006) Optical coherence tomographic patterns of diabetic macular edema. Am J Ophthalmol 142:405–412

Ko TH, Fujimoto JG, Duker JS et al (2004) Comparison of ultrahigh- and standard-resolution optical coherence tomography for imaging macular hole pathology and repair. Ophthalmology 111:2033–2043

Lu M, Perez VL, Ma N et al (1999) VEGF increases retinal vascular ICAM-1 expression in vivo. Invest Ophthalmol Vis Sci 40:1808–1812

Lu RW, Curcio CA, Zhang Y et al (2012) Investigation of the hyper-reflective inner/outer segment band in optical coherence tomography of living frog retina. J Biomed Opt 17:060504

Maheshwary AS, Oster SF, Yuson RM et al (2010) The association between percent disruption of the photoreceptor inner segment-outer segment junction and visual acuity in diabetic macular edema. Am J Ophthalmol 150:63–67

Man RE, Sasongko MB, Sanmugasundram S et al (2012) Longer axial length is protective of diabetic retinopathy and macular edema. Ophthalmology 119:1754–1759

Martidis A, Duker JS, Greenberg PB et al (2002) Intravitreal triamcinolone for refractory diabetic macular edema. Ophthalmology 109:920–927

Mehalow AK, Kameya S, Smith RS et al (2003) CRB1 is essential for external limiting membrane integrity and photoreceptor morphogenesis in the mammalian retina. Hum Mol Genet 12:2179–2189

Moore TC, Moore JE, Kaji Y et al (2003) The role of advanced glycation end products in retinal microvascular leukostasis. Invest Ophthalmol Vis Sci 44:4457–4464

Murakami T, Nishijima K, Akagi T et al (2012) Optical coherence tomographic reflectivity of photoreceptors beneath cystoid spaces in diabetic macular edema. Invest Ophthalmol Vis Sci 53:1506–1511

Murata T, Ishibashi T, Khalil A et al (1995) Vascular endothelial growth factor plays a role in hyperpermeability of diabetic retinal vessels. Ophthalmic Res 27:48–52

Nunes S, Pereira I, Santos A et al (2010) Central retinal thickness measured with HD-OCT shows a weak correlation with visual acuity in eyes with CSME. Br J Ophthalmol 94:1201–1204

Omri S, Omri B, Savoldelli M et al (2010) The outer limiting membrane (OLM) revisited: clinical implications. Clin Ophthalmol 4:183–195

Otani T, Yamaguchi Y, Kishi S (2010) Correlation between visual acuity and foveal microstructural changes in diabetic macular edema. Retina 30:774–780

Quigely M, Cohen S (1999) A new pressure attenuation index to evaluate retinal circulation. A link to protective factors in diabetic retinopathy. Arch Ophthalmol 117:84–89

Saxena S, Mishra N, Khanna V et al (2014) Increased serum N-CML, VEGF and ICAM-1 is associated with photoreceptor inner segment ellipsoid disruption in diabetic retinopathy. JSM Biotechnol Bioeng 2:1039

Saxena S, Srivastav K, Akduman L (2015) Spectral domain optical coherence tomography based alterations in macular thickness and inner segment ellipsoid are associated with severity of diabetic retinopathy. Int J Ophthalmol Clin Res 2:007

Sebekova K, Kupcova V, Schinzel R et al (2002) Markedly elevated levels of plasma advanced glycation end products in patients with liver cirrhosis – amelioration by liver transplantation. J Hepatol 36:66–71

Sharma S, Oliver-Fernandez A, Liu W et al (2005) The impact of diabetic retinopathy on health-related quality of life. Curr Opin Ophthalmol 16:155–159

Sharma S, Saxena S et al (2015) Nitric oxide levels in diabetic retinopathy and its association with disruption of photoreceptor IS-OS junction and topographic alterations in retinal pigment epithelium. Clin Exp Ophthalmol. doi:10.1111/ceo.12506

Sharma SR, Saxena S, Mishra N et al (2014) The association of grades of photoreceptor inner segment-ellipsoid band disruption with severity of retinopathy in type 2 diabetes mellitus. J Case Rep Stud 2:205

Shin HJ, Lee SH, Chung H et al (2012) Association between photoreceptor integrity and visual outcome in diabetic macular edema. Graefes Arch Clin Exp Ophthalmol 250:61–70

Spaide RF, Curcio CA (2011) Anatomical correlates to the bands seen in the outer retina by optical coherence tomography: literature review and model. Retina 31:1609–1619

Srinivasan VJ, Ko TH, Wojtkowski M et al (2006) Noninvasive volumetric imaging and morphometry of the rodent retina with high-speed, ultrahigh-resolution optical coherence tomography. Invest Ophthalmol Vis Sci 47:5522–5528

Staurenghi G, Sadda S, Chakravarthy U et al (2014) for the International Nomenclature for Optical Coherence Tomography (IN_OCT) Panel. Proposed lexicon for anatomic landmarks in normal posterior segment spectral-domain optical coherence tomography. Ophthalmology 21:1572–1578

Strom C, Sander B, Larsen N et al (2002) Diabetic macular edema assessed with optical coherence tomography and stereo fundus photography. Invest Ophthalmol Vis Sci 43:241–245

Wakabayashi Y, Kimura K, Muramatsu D et al (2013) Axial length as a factor associated with visual outcome after vitrectomy for diabetic macular edema. Invest Ophthalmol Vis Sci 54:6834–6840

Yamamoto S, Yamamoto T, Hayashi M et al (2001) Morphological and functional analyses of diabetic macular edema by optical coherence tomography and multifocal electroretinograms. Graefes Arch Clin Exp Ophthalmol 239:96–101

Yamauchi Y, Yagi H, Usui Y et al (2011) Biological activity is the likely origin of the intersection between the photoreceptor inner and outer segments of the rat retina as determined by optical coherence tomography. Clin Ophthalmol 5:1649–1653

Yanyali A, Bozkurt KT, Macin A et al (2011) Quantitative assessment of photoreceptor layer in eyes with resolved edema after pars plana vitrectomy with internal limiting membrane removal for diabetic macular edema. Ophthalmologica 226:57–63

Zong H, Ward M, Stitt AW (2011) AGEs, RAGE, and diabetic retinopathy. Curr Diab Rep 11:244–252

Effect of Therapy on Diabetic Macular Oedema

10

Samia Fatum, Elizabeth Pearce, and Victor Chong

Contents

S. Fatum, MD • V. Chong, MD, FRCS, FRCOphth (✉)
Oxford Eye Hospital, Oxford University Hospitals, Oxford, UK
e-mail: victor@eretina.org

E. Pearce, MD
Department of Optometry, Moorfields Eye Hospital, London, UK

10.1 Introduction

Anti-vascular endothelial growth factor (VEGF) therapies have changed the dynamics in the management of patients with diabetic macular oedema (DME); increasingly it is the treatment of choice when there is extensive oedema in foveal-involving DME. The role of laser in the anti-VEGF era has to be re-examined. Despite the efficacy of laser, the mechanism of laser treatment remains unclear. Armed with extensive clinical trial data and the experience of using anti-VEGF agents for DME, retinal specialists have found that a significant number of patients do not respond to anti-VEGF agents or require continuous monthly dosing. In these patients, steroids may be useful as an alternative or as adjunct therapy. Less than 10 years ago, we only had to decide whether to laser or not. At the time of writing in late 2015, we have three anti-VEGF agents in common use, two approved steroids, and several different new laser modalities as well as our old friend conventional laser. We should also not forget that vitrectomy may be useful in some cases, and pharmaceutical agent to release vitreomacular adhesion may be worth consideration in a few cases.

10.2 Laser Photocoagulation

When laser was first introduced for DME, we were taught to "shoot at the red dots". The red dots are microaneurysms, and shooting at them

C.H. Meyer et al. (eds.), *Spectral Domain Optical Coherence Tomography in Macular Diseases*,
DOI 10.1007/978-81-322-3610-8_10

directly suggests that laser works by direct coagulation. Over the years, physicians have noticed that oedema may improve even if they missed the microaneurysms. Now we have a better understanding of the absorption of the laser energy. With the commonly used argon laser at the time with a blue-green wavelength, the majority of the energy is absorbed by the retinal pigment epithelium (RPE). The blood (oxyhaemoglobin) inside the microaneurysms (red dots) is not well absorbed by the laser, and hence the concept of direct coagulation has been brought into doubt. Furthermore, clinical studies of treatment of DME, comparing argon green and krypton red (which are not absorbed by blood) (Olk 1990), showed no differences in efficacy. Therefore, it is unlikely that direct coagulation is needed to reduce oedema.

10.2.1 Subthreshold Conventional Laser as Endpoint Management

Bandello and colleagues (Bandello et al. 2005) suggested "light" laser is as effective as "classic" laser treatment. Since we now know that laser scars (Fig. 10.1) are not needed, as anti-VEGF does not create any laser scars, yet it is effective in reducing oedema in DME, the concept of moving to lighter treatment is not new.

Recently, endpoint management (Lavinsky et al. 2014) proposed that it can reduce collateral damage and can still be effective. The concept is to reduce the energy, so it is just not visible in colour photos, but mild changes appear in optical coherent topography (OCT). So far, there is no prospective randomised controlled trial to suggest that it is effective; however, there is a similar study to suggest that it might not be more effective than modified Early Treatment Diabetic Retinopathy Study (ETDRS) laser. The Diabetic Retinopathy Clinical Research Network (DRCR.net) (Fong et al. 2007) compared mild macular grid laser (MMG) with modified ETDRS laser treatment, citing the latter as the most commonly used method in performing laser for DME at the time of the study among the network investigators.

MMG burns are located over the entire posterior pole from 500 to 3000 microns from the centre of the macula, without burns within 500 microns of the optic disc. The burn intensity of the grid laser is barely visible (light grey); 200–300 burns in total are distributed evenly over the treatment area (approx. 2–3 burn widths apart). The MMG burns are lighter and more diffuse in nature and are distributed over the whole macula in both areas of thickened and unthickened retina. Microaneurysms are not directly photocoagulated. In contrast, the modified ETDRS laser comprised of treating only areas of thickened retina (and areas of retinal non-perfusion) and leaking microaneurysms. MMG did not show any superiority over modified ETDRS laser treatment. However, MMG did work in reducing oedema.

10.2.2 Subthreshold Micropulse Laser

The concept of micropulse laser is to deliver more energy to the RPE cells without the collateral damage to the neurosensory retina. Laser energy is delivered in pulses. For example, using a 5 % duty cycle at 200 ms duration, there is a very short active (ON) energy (0.1 ms) followed by a period of no (OFF) energy (1.9 ms). With each "burn" of 200 ms duration, there would be 100 of these short pulses. The OFF period allows the tissue to cool off, and hence more energy can be delivered to the targeted tissue (RPE) without heating the surrounding neurosensory retina.

We have published one of the first prospective randomised controlled trials to suggest that micropulse laser is as good as modified ETDRS treatment but with less scarring (Figueira et al. 2009) (Fig. 10.2).

Vujosevic and colleagues (Vujosevic et al. 2010) confirmed our findings but also showed that retinal sensitivity is significantly better in patients treated with micropulse laser. Furthermore, not only were the laser scars not visible on clinical examination, fundus autofluorescence did not change in the micropulse diode laser group even after retreatment. Once we understand that micropulse laser works through

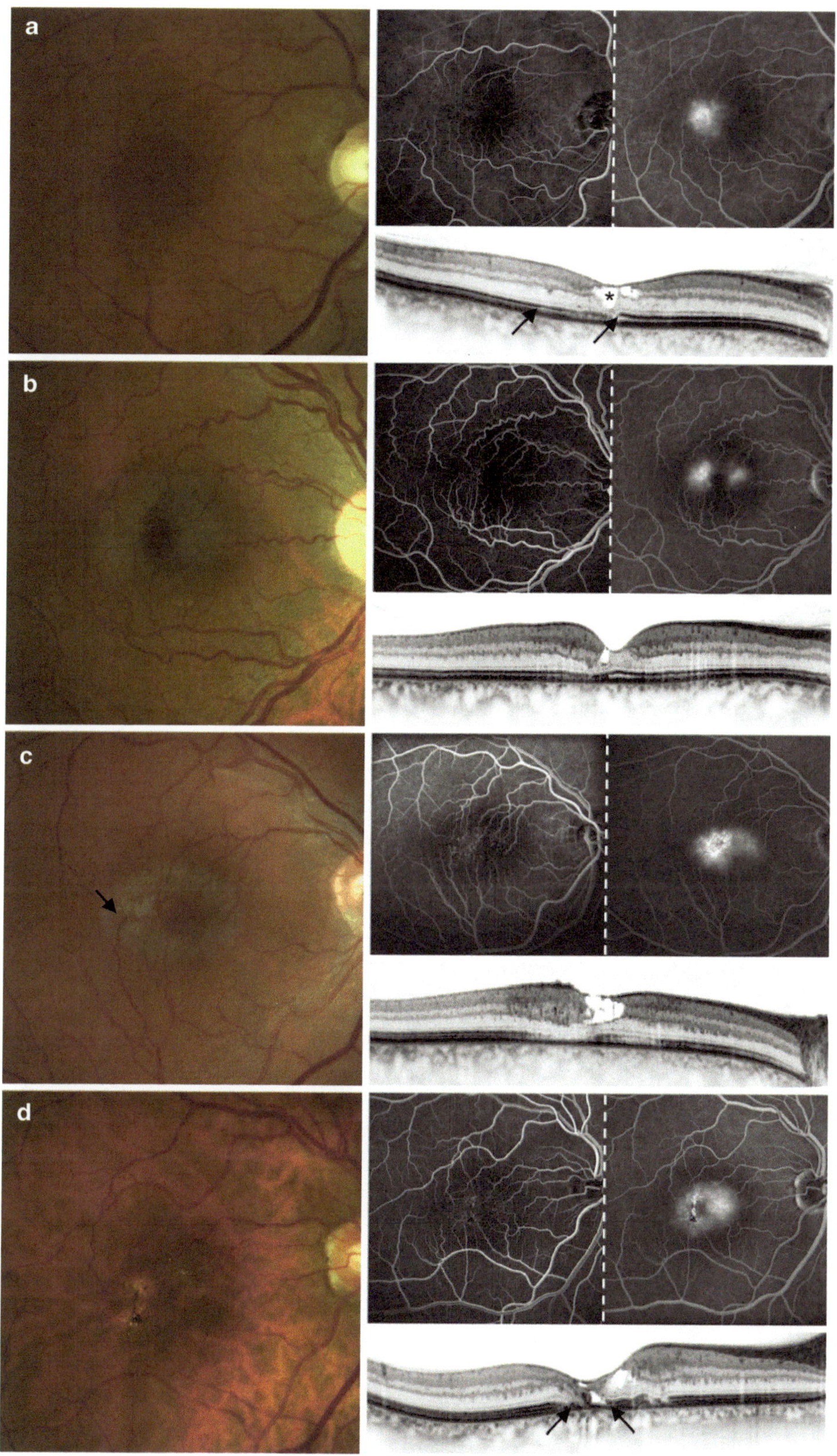

Fig. 10.1 Laser scar. SD-OCT showing retinal pigmented epithelial loss and outer retinal disorganisation corresponding to conventional laser scar. (**a**–**b**) Different examples of conventional laser scars

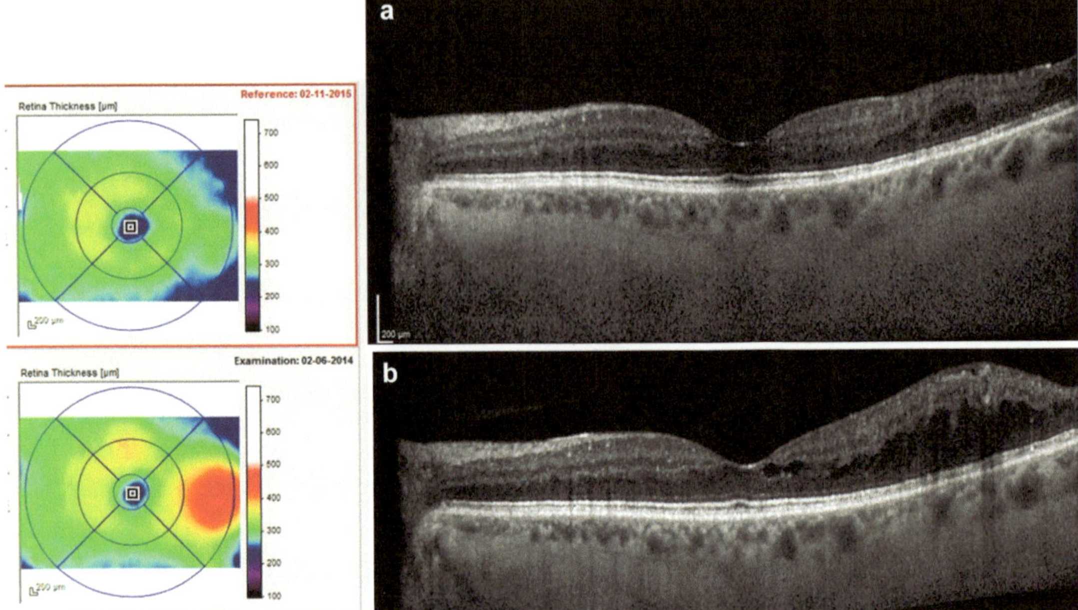

Fig. 10.2 Micropulse treatment. (**a**) SD-OCT post-micropulse laser treatment without any visible laser scar. (**b**) Baseline SD-OCT with diabetic macular oedema

activation of the RPE cells and it does not cause any visible collateral damage, it seems to make sense to remove the spacing between laser “burns”. This was confirmed in a prospective randomised controlled trial that high-density treatment is more effective (Lavinsky et al. 2011) than low density and modified ETDRS treatment.

10.3 Anti-VEGF Agents

Several pivotal trials have shown that anti-VEGF agents are superior to laser (Korobelinik et al. 2014; Nguyen et al. 2012). In a recent head to head comparison of three commonly used anti-VEGF agents, bevacizumab, ranibizumab and aflibercept (DRCR.net Protocol T) were able to improve visual acuity with 9.7 letters, 11.8 letters and 13.3 letters, respectively. When the vision was less than 69 letters (approximately 20/50) at baseline, the visual-acuity gain was 11.8 letters, 14.2 letters and 18.9 letters for bevacizumab, ranibizumab and aflibercept, respectively ($P<0.001$ for aflibercept vs. bevacizumab, $P=0.003$ for aflibercept vs. ranibizumab and $P=0.21$ for ranibizumab vs. bevacizumab) (Wells et al. 2015).

Furthermore, the central subfield thickness on OCT decreased, on average by 101 ± 121 microns, 147 ± 134 microns and 169 ± 138 microns, with bevacizumab, ranibizumab and aflibercept, respectively. As it is a single study and also the treatment protocol was different from that recommended by the dosology of the approved drugs, it is unclear how the drug would compare with the recommended dosology. Furthermore, the dosage of ranibizumab was 0.3 mg, the approved dose in the USA for DME, rather than 0.5 mg commonly used for AMD and the approved dose for DME in most of the world. The latter might not be particularly meaningful as the head to head of 0.3 mg vs. 0.5 mg did not show any meaningful differences between the two dosages (Nguyen et al. 2012).

Nevertheless, the treatment protocol used in Protocol T was pragmatic and can be easily implemented. The study drugs were injected into the study eyes at baseline and then every 4 weeks unless visual acuity was 20/20 or better with a central subfield thickness below the eligibility threshold, and there was no improvement or worsening in response to the past two injections. Improvement was considered to be an increase in the visual-acuity letter score of five or more (approximately 1 Snellen line) or a decrease in the central subfield thickness of 10% or more; worsening was considered to be a decrease in the visual-acuity letter score of five or more or an increase in the central subfield thickness of 10% or more.

Starting at the 24-week visit, irrespective of visual acuity and central subfield thickness, an injection was withheld if there was no improvement or worsening after two consecutive injections, but treatment was reinitiated if the visual-acuity letter score or the central subfield thickness worsened.

Laser photocoagulation therapy (focal, grid or both) was initiated at or after the 24-week visit for persistent diabetic macular oedema, defined on the basis of protocol-specified criteria. Treatment for diabetic macular oedema other than the randomly assigned anti-VEGF agent or laser therapy was permitted if a study eye met the criteria for treatment failure.

10.3.1 Subgroup Analysis Based on Baseline OCT

As mentioned previously, anti-VEGF agents were superior to laser treatment overall; however, anti-VEGF agents are not suitable for everyone. In some cases, it is due to the cost of the drug, in others the frequency of the follow up or the concern over the associated adverse events of the treatment. Hence, it may be useful to consider whether in some circumstances, laser might be an alternative.

Based on the RESTORE study (Mitchell et al. 2011), using time-domain OCT, if the central subfield thickness (CST) is less than 300 microns, there were no significant differences in efficacy between laser and ranibizumab treatment groups. Bearing in mind, if using most spectral-domain (SD) OCT, the value should be near 340–350 microns, as most SD-OCT measured a CST about 40–50 microns more. Furthermore, even for those between 300 and 400 microns on time-domain OCT (i.e. 340–440 microns in SD-OCT), the visual gain was about seven letters compared with four letters. It is statistically significant but might be less clinically meaningful. In particular, in clinical settings, the number of injections tends to be lower than in clinical trials.

10.3.2 Patterns of Anti-VEGF Responses

Undoubtedly the overall results of anti-VEGF are good; however, as noted in Protocol T, there is a big variation in OCT responses. For instance, even in the aflibercept group, which showed the best response, the average reduction of retinal thickness was 169 ± 138 microns; the variation is almost as big as the average reduction. Furthermore, if one is looking at the bevacizumab group (probably the most commonly used anti-VEGF worldwide), the average reduction of retinal thickness was 101 ± 121 microns; the variation is larger than the reduction. This suggests a big variation in individual responses.

In DRCR.net Protocol I, one of the earlier studies, DRCR.net analysed 37 baseline demographic, systemic, ocular, OCT, and fundus photographic variables that were assessed for association with change in visual acuity or OCT between baseline and 1 year. After adjusting for baseline visual acuity, a larger visual-acuity treatment benefit was associated with younger age ($P<0.001$), less severe diabetic retinopathy on clinical exam ($P=0.003$), and the absence of surface wrinkling retinopathy ($P<0.001$). CST evolution during the first treatment year also predicted better vision outcomes ($P<0.001$). After adjusting for baseline CST, lipid was associated with more favourable OCT improvement ($P=0.004$) (Bressler et al. 2012).

CST evolution can be summarised into four groups as shown in Table 10.1 (Bressler et al. 2012). One could argue that about two thirds of the patients have early response and good vision gain, confirming the first-line role of anti-VEGF agents. The late responders may be treated with anti-VEGF if there were no other treatments available. However, with steroid approved for DME, it is reasonable to wait for the late responders to respond, or one should consider changing therapy earlier. Finally about a quarter of the patients did not respond anatomically, and the vision gain was no different from the laser monotherapy arm. It is important to identify this group of patients earlier and offer alternative therapies or surgery (Figs. 10.3, 10.4, 10.5 and 10.6).

Table 10.1 Central subfield thickness evolution in DRCR.net Protocol I ranibizumab-treated patients

OCT-CST	Week 16	Week 32	1 year	N	%	Vision gain
Early and consistent	+	+	+	143	49.7	12
Early but inconsistent	+	–	–	43	14.9	11
Late responders	–	±	±	36	12.5	8
Nonresponders	–	–	–	66	22.9	4

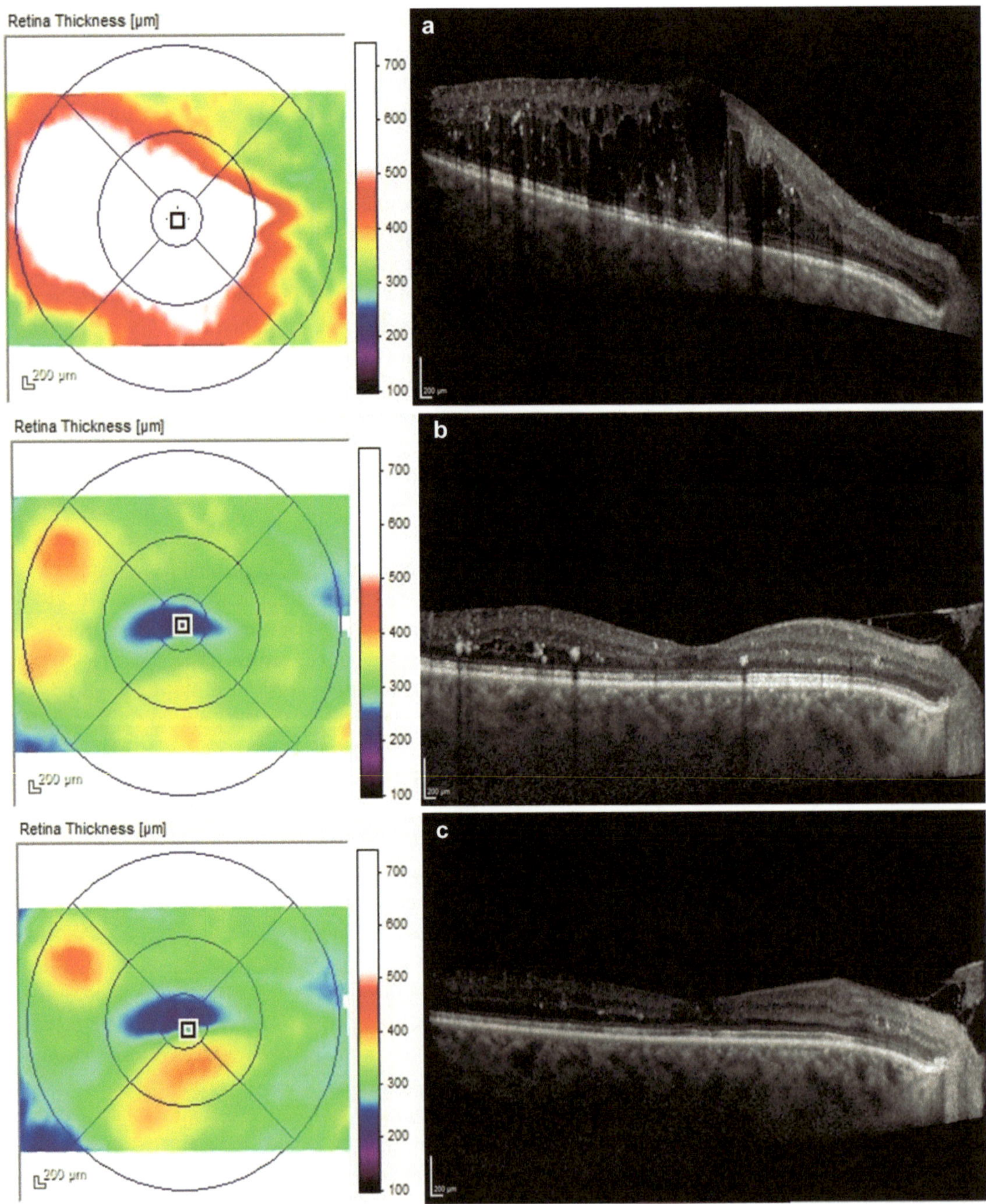

Fig. 10.3 Early and consistent response with anti-VEGF therapy. (**a**) Baseline SD-OCT showing significant diabetic macular oedema. (**b**) After three ranibizumab injections with significant improvement. (**c**) After another three ranibizumab injections showing consistent effect

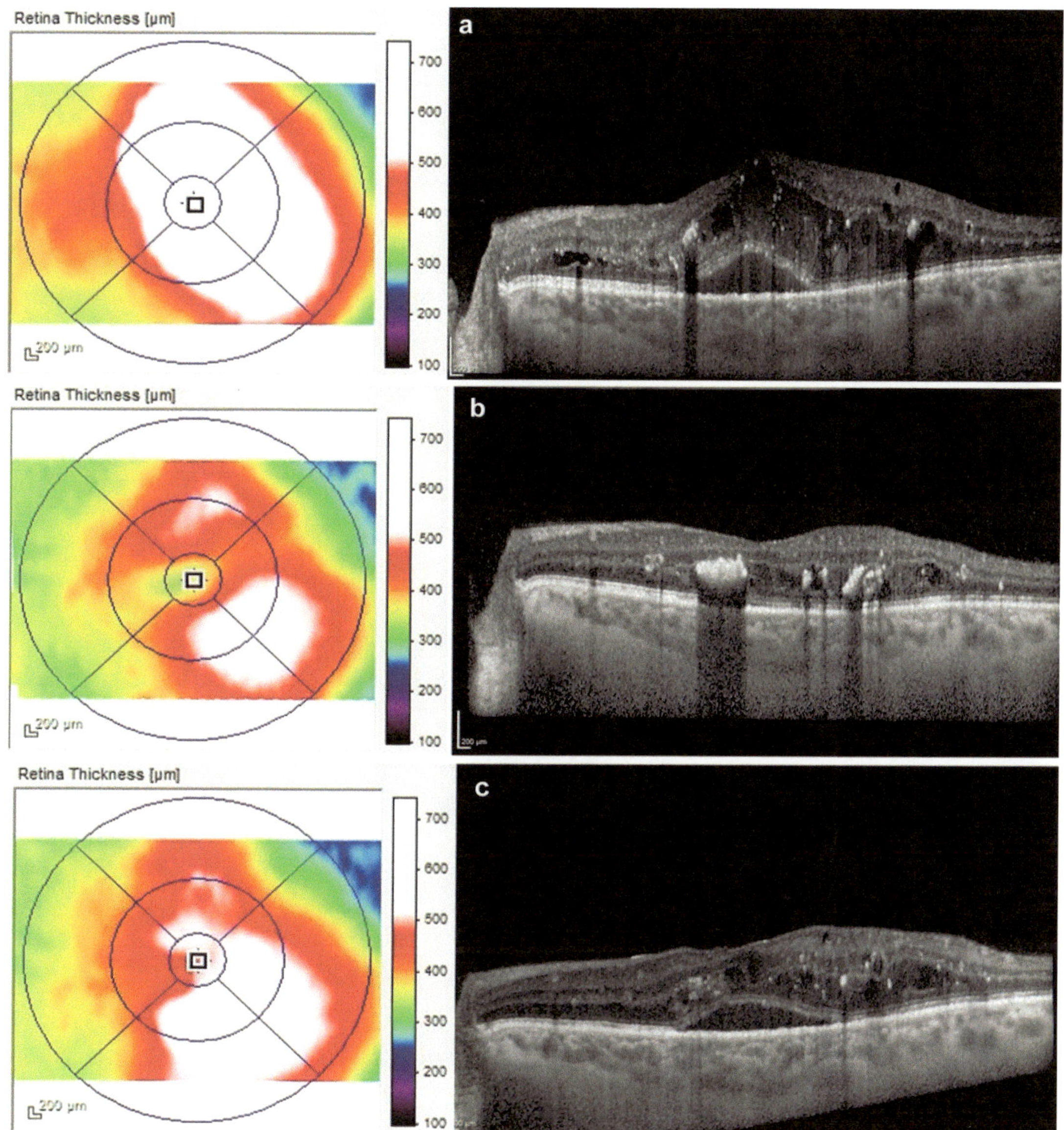

Fig. 10.4 Early but inconsistent response after anti-VEGF therapy. (**a**) Baseline SD-OCT showing significant diabetic macular oedema. (**b**) After three ranibizumab injections with significant improvement. (**c**) After another three ranibizumab injections showing deterioration towards baseline

10.4 Steroids

The pathophysiology of macular oedema is complex (Scholl et al. 2011). In view of the nonresponders to anti-VEGF-treated DME patients, including steroid therapy in the treatment paradigm of DME is essential (Stewart 2012). There are now two steroids that have been approved for the treatment of DME based on the pivotal trial data (Boyer et al. 2014; Campochiaro et al. 2012). Cataract and increased intraocular pressure (IOP) are the most common adverse events with steroid. The former is almost universal after 1 year of treatment, so the authors would only consider steroid as a long-term treatment in pseudophakic patients or in those who would be happy to have

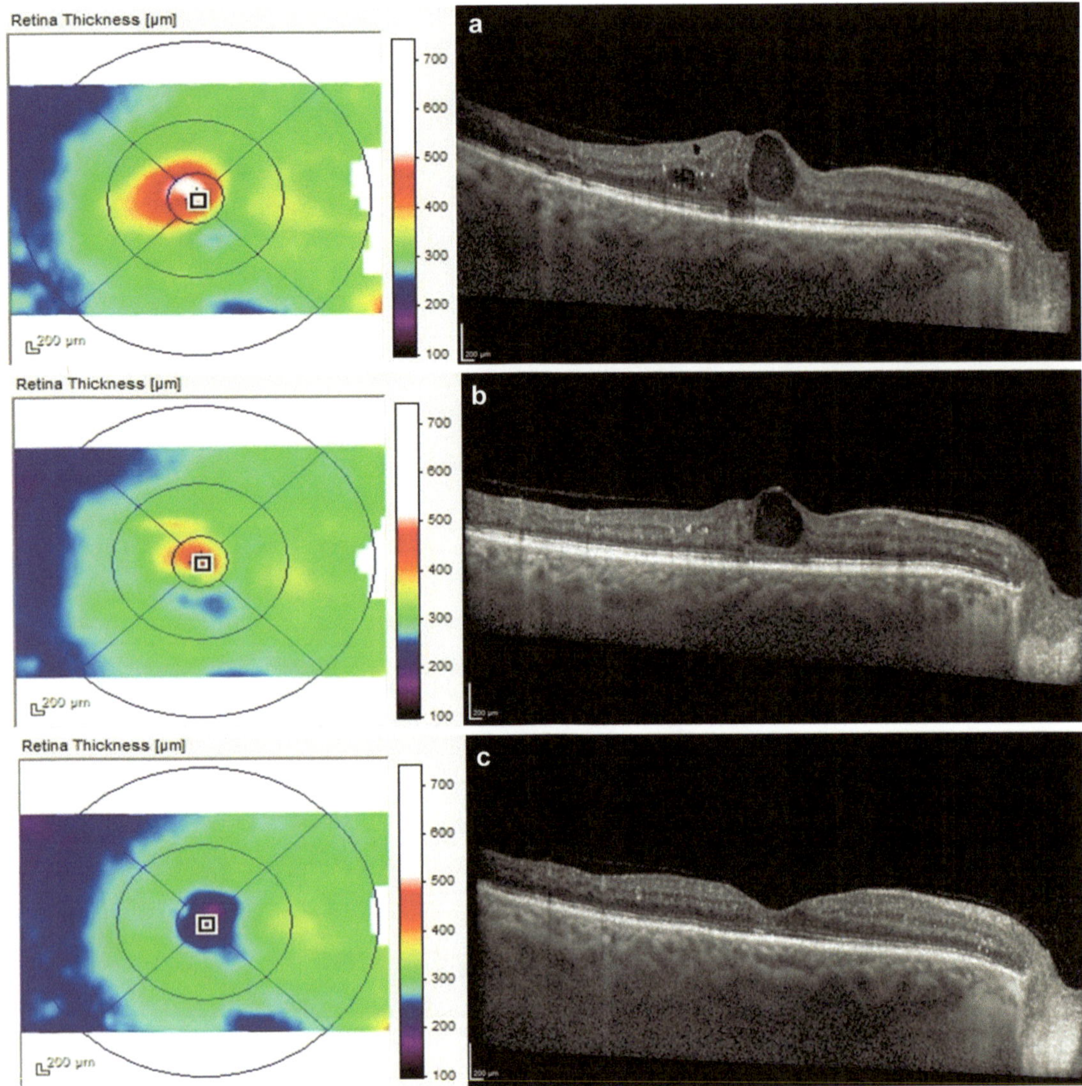

Fig. 10.5 Late responder after anti-VEGF therapy. (**a**) Baseline SD-OCT showing significant diabetic macular oedema. (**b**) After three ranibizumab injections with slight improvement. (**c**) After another three ranibizumab injections showing significant improvement

cataract surgery if needed. The reported rate of increase of IOP varies, but in most cases it is manageable (Boyer et al. 2014; Campochiaro et al. 2012). In diabetic retinopathy, the retina is already compromised; the increase in IOP may be more clinically important. Even when the IOP appears to be controlled by anti-glaucoma drops, the long-term compliance of patients is often in doubt.

There might be a case for vitrectomised pseudophakic eye to use steroids as the first-line therapy (Boyer et al. 2011). Although the DRCR.net suggested that there were no meaningful differences in the response to ranibizumab in vitrectomised and non-vitrectomised (Bressler et al. 2015), many retinal specialists have found that ranibizumab does not appear to last as long in vitrectomised eye. There is also animal experimental support that there are no differences in the intraocular pharmacokinetics of ranibizumab (Ahn et al. 2014) (Fig. 10.7).

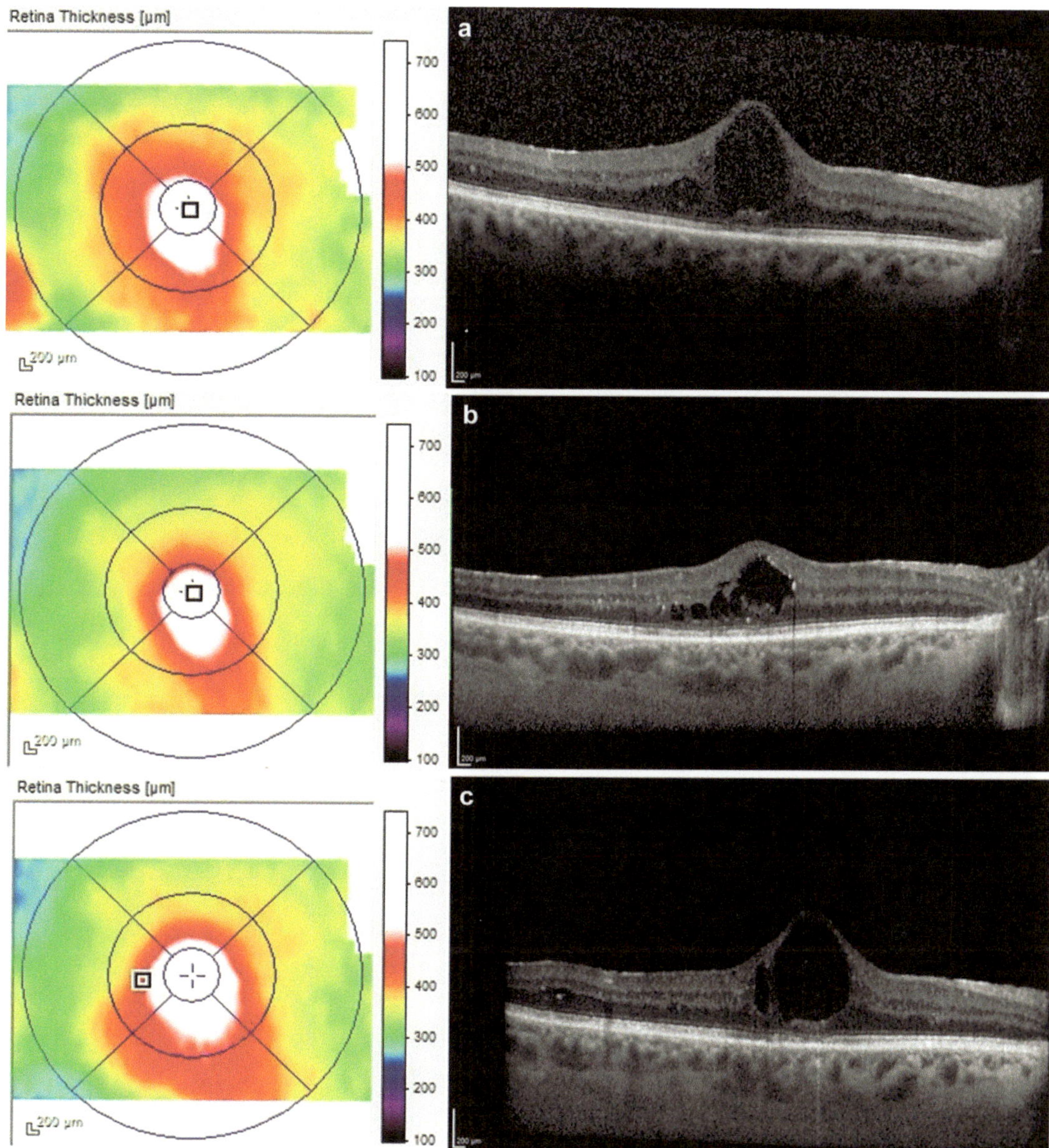

Fig. 10.6 Nonresponder after anti-VEGF therapy. (**a**) Baseline SD-OCT showing significant diabetic macular oedema. (**b**) After three ranibizumab injections with no improvement. (**c**) After another three ranibizumab injections still showing no improvement

10.5 Pharmacologic Vitreolysis

The presence of a posterior vitreous detachment (PVD) reduces the risk of developing of DME. Pharmacologic vitreolysis such as ocriplasmin might be useful in some patients. However, current data shows ocriplasmin does not manage to achieve a PVD with a single injection (de Smet and Castilla 2013). There are also some suggestions that the efficacy in patients with established DME is worse than in those without (Fig. 10.8).

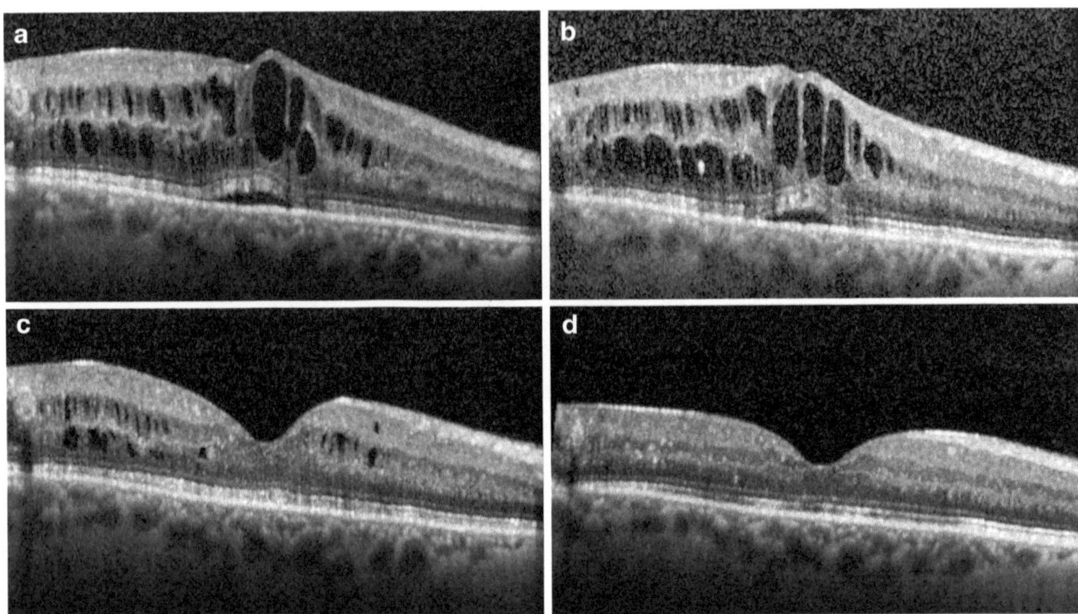

Fig. 10.7 Dexamethasone implant. (**a**) Baseline SD-OCT in a vitrectomised pseudophakic eye with diabetic macular oedema. (**b**) After three ranibizumab injections showing no improvement. (**c**) After 18 monthly ranibizumab injections showing significant improvement but not completely "dry". (**d**) After a single dexamethasone implant, the retina remained "dry" for over 12 months

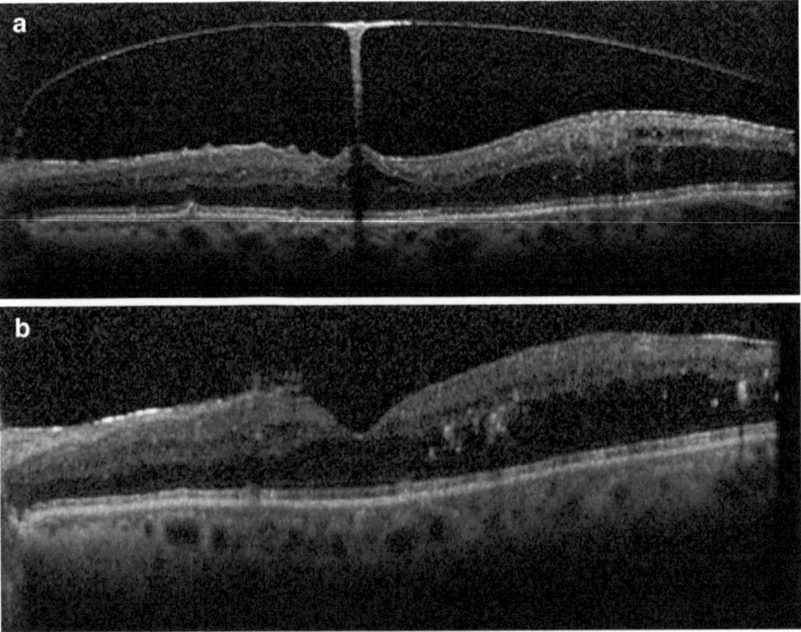

Fig. 10.8 Ocriplasmin injection. (**a**) Diabetic macular oedema patient with vitreomacular traction, after six ranibizumab injections showing residual macular oedema. (**b**) After ocriplasmin injection, the traction was released, and the oedema disappeared without any further ranibizumab injection

10.6 Vitrectomy

There were numerous studies to suggest vitrectomy is useful in DME. However, the recently published systematic review did not show a benefit over laser in DME patients without epiretinal membrane or vitreomacular traction (Simunovic et al. 2014). Nonetheless, DME patients with epiretinal membrane, even those without significant traction, are more likely to be nonresponsive to anti-VEGF agents. It might be still worthwhile starting with anti-VEGF agents in these patients, but vitrectomy should be considered earlier in the treatment course.

References

Ahn SJ, Ahn J, Park S, Kim H, Hwang DJ, Park JH, Park JY, Chung JY, Park KH, Woo SJ (2014) Intraocular pharmacokinetics of ranibizumab in vitrectomized versus nonvitrectomized eyes. Invest Ophthalmol Vis Sci 55:567–573

Bandello F, Polito A, DelBorrello M, Zemella N, Isola M (2005) "Light" versus "classic" laser treatment for clinically significant diabetic macular oedema. Br J Ophthalmol 89:864–870

Boyer DS, Faber D, Gupta S, Patel SS, Tabandeh H, Li XY, Liu CC, Lou J, Whitcup SM, Ozurdex CHAMPLAIN Study Group (2011) Dexamethasone intravitreal implant for treatment of diabetic macular edema in vitrectomized patients. Retina 31:915–923

Boyer DS, Yoon YH, Belfort R Jr, Bandello F, Maturi RK, Augustin AJ, Li XY, Cui H, Hashad Y, Whitcup SM, Ozurdex MEAD Study Group (2014) Three-year, randomized, sham-controlled trial of dexamethasone intravitreal implant in patients with diabetic macular edema. Ophthalmology 121:1904–1914

Bressler SB, Qin H, Beck RW, Chalam KV, Kim JE, Melia M et al (2012) Factors associated with changes in visual acuity and central subfield thickness at 1 year after treatment for diabetic macular edema with ranibizumab. Arch Ophthalmol 130:1153–1161

Bressler SB, Melia M, Glassman AR, Almukhtar T, Jampol LM, Shami M, Berger BB, Bressler NM, Diabetic Retinopathy Clinical Research Network (2015) Ranibizumab plus prompt or deferred laser for diabetic macular edema in eyes with vitrectomy before anti-vascular endothelial growth factor therapy. Retina 35:2516–2528

Campochiaro PA, Brown DM, Pearson A, Chen S, Boyer D, Ruiz-Moreno J, Garretson B, Gupta A, Hariprasad SM, Bailey C, Reichel E, Soubrane G, KapikB BK, Kane FE, Green K, FAME Study Group (2012) Sustained delivery fluocinolone acetonide vitreous inserts provide benefit for at least 3 years in patients with diabetic macular edema. Ophthalmology 119:2125–2132

de Smet MD, Castilla M (2013) Ocriplasmin for diabetic retinopathy. Expert Opin Biol Ther 13:1741–1747

Figueira J, Khan J, Nunes S, Sivaprasad S, Rosa A, de Abreu JF, Cunha-Vaz JG, Chong NV (2009) Prospective randomised controlled trial comparing subthreshold micropulse diode laser photocoagulation and conventional green laser for clinically significant diabetic macular oedema. Br J Ophthalmol 93:1341–1344

Fong DS, Strauber SF, Aiello LP, Beck RW, Callanan DG, Danis RP, Writing Committee for the Diabetic Retinopathy Clinical Research Network et al (2007) Comparison of the modified Early Treatment Diabetic Retinopathy Study and mild macular grid laser photocoagulation strategies for diabetic macular edema. Arch Ophthalmol 125:469–480

Korobelinik JF, Do DV, Schmidt-Erfurth U, Boyser DS, Holz FG, Heier JS et al (2014) Intravitreal aflibercept for diabetic macular edema. Ophthalmology 232:2247–2254

Lavinsky D, Cardillo JA, Melo LA Jr, Dare A, Farah ME, Belfort R Jr (2011) Randomized clinical trial evaluating mETDRS versus normal or high-density micropulse photocoagulation for diabetic macular edema. Invest Ophthalmol Vis Sci 52:4314–4323

Lavinsky D, Sramek C, Wang J, Huie P, Dalal R, Mandel Y, Palanker D (2014) Subvisible retinal laser therapy: titration algorithm and tissue response. Retina 34:87–97

Mitchell P, Bandello F, Schmidt-Erfurth U, Lang GE, Massin P, Schlingemann RO et al (2011) The RESTORE study: ranibizumab monotherapy or combined with laser versus laser monotherapy for diabetic macular edema. Ophthalmology 118:615–625

Nguyen QD, Brown DM, Marcus DM, Boyer DS, Patel S, Feiner L et al (2012) Ranibizumab for diabetic macular edema: results from 2 phase III randomized trials: RISE and RIDE. Ophthalmology 119:789–801

Olk RJ (1990) Argon green (514 nm) versus krypton red (647 nm) modified grid laser photocoagulation for diffuse diabetic macular edema. Ophthalmology 97:1101–1112

Scholl S, Augustin A, Loewenstein A, Rizzo S, Kupperman B (2011) General pathophysiology of macular edema. Eur J Ophthalmol 6:S10–S19

Simunovic MP, Hunyor AP, Ho IV (2014) Vitrectomy for diabetic macular edema: a systematic review and meta-analysis. Can J Ophthalmol 49:188–195

Stewart MW (2012) Corticosteroid use for diabetic macular edema: old fad or new trend? Curr Diab Rep 12:364–375

Vujosevic S, Bottega E, Casciano M, Pilotto E, Convento E, Midena E (2010) Microperimetry and fundus autofluorescence in diabetic macular edema: subthreshold micropulse diode laser versus modified early treatment diabetic retinopathy study laser photocoagulation. Retina 30:908–916

Wells JA, Glassman AR, Ayala AR, Jampol LM, Aiello LP, Antoszyk AN et al (2015) Aflibercept, bevacizumab or ranibizumab for diabetic macular edema. N Eng J Med 372:1192–1203

11 Retinal Vein Occlusion

Ute E.K. Wolf-Schnurrbusch

Contents

11.1 Background

Central retinal vein occlusion (CRVO) and branch retinal vein occlusion (BRVO) are retinal vascular diseases that may cause significant ocular morbidity and vision loss (David et al. 1988; Rogers et al. 2010). It commonly affects men and women equally and occurs predominantly in the age of 65 years (Lang and Handel 1992; Noma et al. 2005 and 2008; Chen et al. 1995; Iturralde et al. 2006). Younger individuals which present with a clinical picture of CRVO may have an underlying inflammatory etiology (Fekrat and Finkelstein 1999). Most common risk factors associated with CRVO and BRVO are systemic hypertension, diabetes, hyperlipidemia, glaucoma, carotid insufficiency, smoking, and age-related atherosclerosis (Noma et al. 2005; Sunness et al. 1991). Other associated factors are listed in Table 11.1.

U.E.K. Wolf-Schnurrbusch, PD MD
Department of Ophthalmology, University Hospital Bern, Inselspital, University Bern, Bern, Switzerland
e-mail: Ute.Wolf@insel.ch

11.2 Clinical Features

Retinal vein occlusion presents as a sudden painless loss of vision, but it may also present with a history of a gradual decline of vision which may correlate with less severe occlusions. The typical clinical constellation in CRVO includes superficial flame-shaped and deep blot-type retinal hemorrhages from the optic nerve head in all four quadrants of the fundus ("blood and thunder" appearance). Often there is a marked dilated, tortuous retinal venous system in combination with optic nerve head swelling. Cotton-wool spots, splinter hemorrhages, and macular edema (ME) are present to varying degrees.

Generally, the described intraretinal hemorrhages are less marked in BRVO and if the occlusion is perfused or nonischemic and is much more marked if the occlusion is non-perfused or ischemic and associated with retinal capillary non-perfusion. The localization of the venous

C.H. Meyer et al. (eds.), *Spectral Domain Optical Coherence Tomography in Macular Diseases*,
DOI 10.1007/978-81-322-3610-8_11

Table 11.1 Risk factors for retinal vascular diseases like CRVO and BRVO

Systemic vascular alterations	Diabetes mellitus, systemic hypertension, carotid insufficiency, age-related atherosclerosis
Ocular diseases	Open-angle glaucoma, ischemic optic neuropathy, pseudotumor cerebri, tilted optic nerve heads, optic nerve head drusen
Hematologic alterations/hyperviscosity syndromes	Dysproteinemias, blood dyscrasias, elevated plasma homocysteine, factor XII deficiency, antiphospholipid antibody syndrome, activated protein C resistance, protein C and protein S deficiency
Autoimmune vasculitis	Systemic lupus erythematosus
Medications	Oral contraceptive, diuretics, hepatitis B vaccine
Infectious vasculitis	HIV, syphilis, herpes zoster, sarcoidosis
Other conditions	Pregnancy, after retrobulbar block, smoking

block determines the hemorrhage distribution. If in BRVO the venous obstruction is at the optic nerve head, two quadrants of the fundus may be involved, whereas if the occlusion is peripheral to the disc, one quadrant or less may be involved with retinal hemorrhages.

11.3 Pathogenesis

The clinical picture of a CRVO may be explained by the occlusion of the main trunk of the central retinal vein; however, the pathophysiology is still not clearly understood. Histopathologic studies of enucleated eyes showed a thrombus occluding the lumen of the central retinal vein at or proximal to the lamina cribrosa (Green et al. 1981). This finding suggests that the anatomic variations at the level of the lamina cribrosa may be an important pathogenic point.

The interruption of venous flow in BRVO eyes almost always occurs at retinal intersections. Histopathologically, the retinal artery and vein share a common adventitial sheath. Especially in BRVO the lumen of the vein may be compressed up to one third at the crossing side (Bandello et al. 1998). This and also the vitreous may play important roles in compression of the susceptible arteriovenous crossing sites as evidenced by studies demonstrating that eyes with decreased axial length and a likelihood of vitreo-macular attachment at the crossing are at increased risk of BRVO. The resulting venous obstruction leads to elevation of venous pressure that may overload the collateral drainage capacity and lead to ME and ischemia by mechanisms that are still under investigation.

11.4 Treatment Strategies

The vision loss is mostly caused by ME due to reduced blood perfusion and subsequent retinal hypoxia. The ME may also lead to additional reduction in visual acuity that often exceeds the primary ischemic damage and thus represents an important target for therapeutically intervention.

Treatment strategies for ME comprise focal laser photocoagulation (The Branch Vein Occlusion Study Group 1984; Central Retinal Vein Occlusion Study Group 1993; Klein and Finkelstein 1989), intravitreal steroids (Jonas et al. 2005), surgical procedures (Berker and Batman 2008), and, most recently, injection of anti-vascular endothelial derived growth factor protein (VEGF) compounds (Costa et al. 2007; Priglinger et al. 2007).

11.5 Imaging

At the time of initial presentation, a careful assessment of both eyes, including abnormal VA, iris stromal vessels, pupillary reaction, intraocular

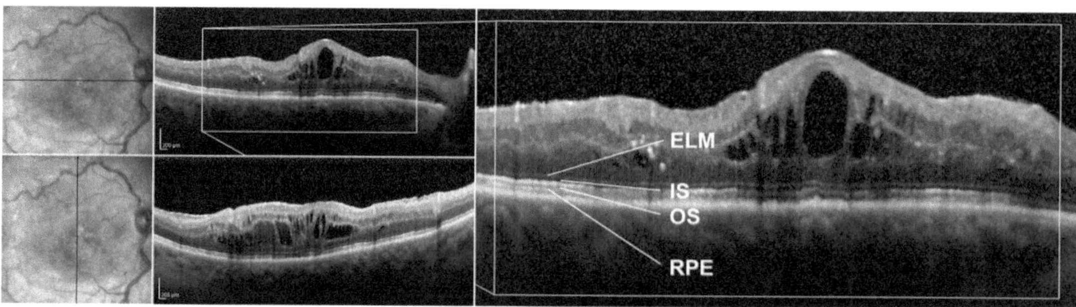

Fig. 11.1 Female patient (TK, 69 years) OD with cystoid edema due to CRVO. BCVA was 33 letters at baseline. Spectralis OCT images show intact external limiting membrane (*ELM*), intact photoreceptor inner segments (*IS*) and outer segments (*OS*), and intact retinal pigment epithelium (*RPE*) in the horizontal (B) and vertical (C) scan. This patient was included into group 1 because of the intact outer retina complex

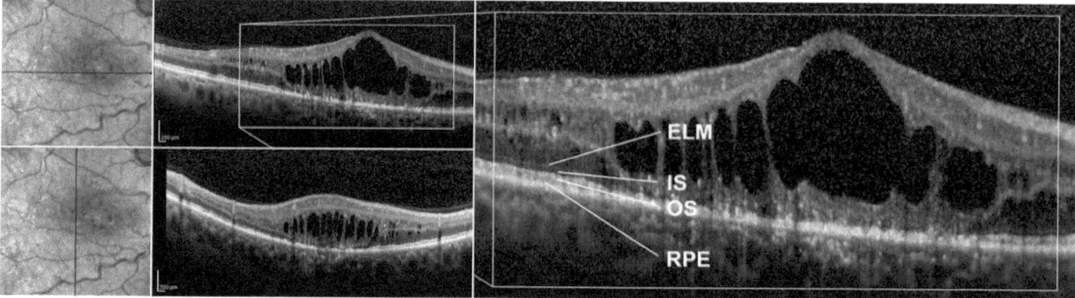

Fig. 11.2 Female patient (JP, 59 years) OD with hard exudates and cystoid edema due to CRVO. BCVA was 22 letters at baseline. Spectralis OCT images show cystoid edema, disturbances in the outer retina complex with involvement of ELM, and irregular RPE in the horizontal (B) and vertical (C) scan. This patient was included into group 2 because of disturbances in the outer retina complex

pressure, as well as history of the duration and the degree of the retinal ischemia, will determine treatment options and an individualized follow-up schedule. Fluorescein and ICG angiography could be useful for the evaluation of treatment options.

Spectral domain OCT (SD-OCT) offers new insight into retinal structures and their alterations especially regarding the integrity of the retinal layers in the fovea. So some interesting factors with predictive value were detected for a favorable short-term visual outcome after anti-VEGF treatment for ME secondary to CRVO (Wolf-Schnurrbusch et al. 2011). One important factor is the presence and integrity of the external limiting membrane (ELM) (Fig. 11.1). It is a bad prognostic sign for the short-term recovery of visual acuity of the ELM if the foveal region is "disturbed" and if we were not able to follow the hyper-reflective band of the ELM in the horizontal or in the vertical SD-OCT scans (Fig. 11.2). Patients with ME in whom SD-OCT images demonstrate an intact outer limiting membrane have a better outcome after intravitreal anti-VEGF therapy than patients with severely compromised outer retinal structures. The integrity of the photoreceptor inner segments (IS) and outer segments (OS) and the retinal pigment epithelium (RPE) is easily assessable, as well as the presence of subretinal and intraretinal fluid accumulation.

Central retinal thickness (CRT) could be analyzed from the volume scan and monitored over time. Attention should be paid to segmentation errors which were obvious if the single scans (which were used for the volume calculation) were carefully checked.

References

Bandello F, Tavola A, Pierro L (1998) Axial length and refraction in retinal vein occlusions. Ophthalmologica 212:133–135

Berker N, Batman C (2008) Surgical treatment of central retinal vein occlusion. Acta Ophthalmol 86:245–252

Central Retinal Vein Occlusion Study Group (1993) Central vein occlusion study of photocoagulation therapy. Baseline findings. Central Vein Occlusion Study Group. Online J Curr Clin Trials Doc No 95.

Chen JC, Klein ML, Watzke RC, Handelman IL, Robertson JE (1995) Natural course of perfused central retinal vein occlusion. Can J Ophthalmol 30:21–24

Costa RA, Jorge R, Calucci D, Melo LA Jr, Cardillo JA, Scott IU (2007) Intravitreal bevacizumab (avastin) for central and hemicentral retinal vein occlusions: IBeVO study. Retina 27:141–149

David R, Zangwill L, Badarna M, Yassur Y (1988) Epidemiology of retinal vein occlusion and its association with glaucoma and increased intraocular pressure. Ophthalmologica 197:69–74

Fekrat S, Finkelstein D (1999) Venous occlusive disease. In: Regillo CD, Brown GC, Flynn HW (eds) Vitreoretinal disease: the essentials, 1st edn. Thieme, New York

Green W, Chan C, Hutchins G (1981) Central retinal vein occlusions: a prospective histopathologic study of 29 eyes in 28 cases. Retina 1:27–55

Iturralde D, Spaide RF, Meyerle CB (2006) Intravitreal bevacizumab (Avastin) treatment of macular edema in central retinal vein occlusion: a short-term study. Retina 26:279–284

Jonas JB, Akkoyun I, Kamppeter B, Kreissig I, Degenring RF (2005) Intravitreal Triamcinolone acetonide for treatment of central retinal vein occlusion. Eur J Ophthalmol 15:751–758

Klein ML, Finkelstein D (1989) Macular grid photocoagulation for macular edema in central retinal vein occlusion. Arch Ophthalmol 107:1297–1302

Lang GE, Handel A (1992) Clinical and fluorescein angiography changes in patients with central retinal vein occlusion. A unicenter study of 125 patients. Klin Monbl Augenheilkd 201:302–308

Noma H, Funatsu H, Yamasaki M et al (2005) Pathogenesis of macular edema with branch retinal vein occlusion and intraocular levels of vascular endothelial growth factor and interleukin-6. Am J Ophthalmol 140: 256–261

Noma H, Funatsu H, Mimura T, Hori S (2008) Changes of vascular endothelial growth factor after vitrectomy for macular edema secondary to retinal vein occlusion. Eur J Ophthalmol 18:1017–1019

Priglinger SG, Wolf AH, Kreutzer TC (2007) Intravitreal bevacizumab injections for treatment of central retinal vein occlusion: six-month results of a prospective trial. Retina 27:1004–1012

Rogers S, McIntosh RL, Cheung N et al (2010) The prevalence of retinal vein occlusion: pooled data from population studies from the United States, Europe, Asia, and Australia. Ophthalmology 117:313–319

Sunness JS, Gass JDM, Singerman U (1991) Retinal and choroidal changes in pregnancy. In: Singerman U, Jampol LM (eds) Retinal and choroidal manifestations of systemic disease. Baltimore, Wiliams & Wiliams

The Branch Vein Occlusion Study Group (1984) Argon laser photocoagulation for macular edema in branch vein occlusion. The Branch Vein Occlusion Study Group. Am J Ophthalmol 98:271–282

Wolf-Schnurrbusch UEK, Ghanem R, Rothenbuehler SP, Enzmann V, Framme C, Wolf S (2011) Predictors of short-term visual outcome after anti-VEGF therapy of macular edema due to central retinal vein occlusion. Invest Ophthalmol Vis Sci 52:3334–3337

12 Retinal Artery Occlusion

Weng Onn Chan, Jagjit S. Gilhotra, Ghazal Ismail, and Sandeep Saxena

Contents

12.1 Introduction

Acute retinal arterial obstruction presents as a sudden, painless monocular loss of vision and/or visual field defect due to involvement of either the central retinal artery, central retinal artery occlusion (CRAO), or an arterial branch, branch retinal artery occlusion (BRAO) (von Graefes 1859). CRAO occurs at the rate of 1 per 10,000 outpatient visits in the United States, of which 1–2 % cases are bilateral (Rumelt et al. 1999). Multiple etiologies have been undermined for this condition. Systemic hypertension and valvular heart disease in adults and coagulation defects in young are important causes of embolism causing retinal vasculature obstruction (Augsburger and Magargal 1980; Pfaffenbach and Hollenhorst 1972; Rumelt et al. 1999; Savino et al. 1977).

Disturbance in the blood supply to the inner layers of the retina is the underlying cause of loss of vision in CRAO. An anatomical variant of short posterior ciliary artery, the cilioretinal artery, occurs in approximately 14 % of the population and gives additional supply to the macula from the choroidal circulation (Justice and Lehmann 1976). Occlusion of the central retinal artery due to any cause will give rise to oedema in the inner retinal layers and pyknosis of the ganglion cell nuclei, resulting in ischaemic necrosis. The retina, hence, opacifies and appears yellowish-white which resolves in 4–6 weeks. However, the foveola assumes a cherry-red spot because of two reasons: firstly, the intact underlying retinal pigment epithelium and choroid and, secondly, foveolar supply by the choriocapillaris (Fig. 12.1). In eyes with cilioretinal artery, supply to the papillomacular bundle is spared, and hence they have better visual prognosis (Justice and Lehmann 1976). Fundus fluorescein angiography (FFA) shows delay in arteriovenous transit time as well as delayed retinal arterial and subsequent

W.O. Chan, MB, ChB, MPhil • J.S. Gilhotra, MBBS, FRANZCO (✉)
South Australian Institute of Ophthalmology, Royal Adelaide Hospital, Adelaide, Australia
e-mail: jsgilhotra@gmail.com

G. Ismail, MS • S. Saxena, MS,FRCSEd,FRCS, FRCOphth,FAICO
Department of Ophthalmology, King George's Medical University, Lucknow, UP, India

C.H. Meyer et al. (eds.), *Spectral Domain Optical Coherence Tomography in Macular Diseases*, DOI 10.1007/978-81-322-3610-8_12

choroidal filling (Beatty and Au Eong 2000) (Fig. 12.2). Also, narrowing of arteries with normal fluorescein transit has been observed after recanalisation.

12.2 Optical Coherence Tomography Findings in Retinal Artery Occlusion

In the acute phase following retinal artery occlusion, there is an isolated increase in the inner retinal thickness and hyper-reflectivity. Importantly, there is an absence of hyporeflective cystic spaces from fluid accumulation that differentiates retinal oedema from retinal artery occlusion from other vascular causes (Rodrigues 2013). This is because oedema from retinal artery occlusion is due to cytoplasmic swelling from coagulation necrosis rather than extracellular fluid accumulation (Coady et al. 2015; Chu et al. 2013). The area of retinal swelling is typically well demarcated and corresponds to the area subserved by the occluded artery (Mathew et al. 2010). Shadowing of underlying structures can mask the outer retinal layers that

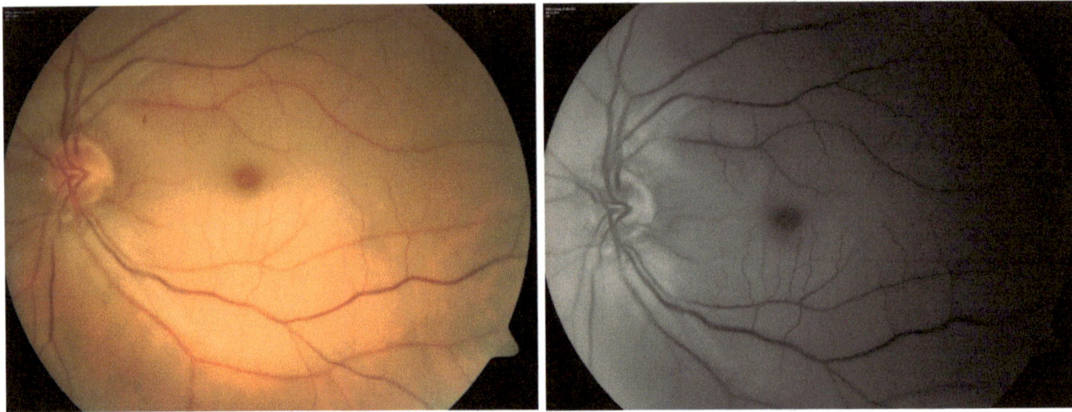

Fig. 12.1 Central retinal arterial occlusion. Fundus photograph showing diffusely pale retina with a cherry-red spot at the fovea without cilioretinal artery sparing

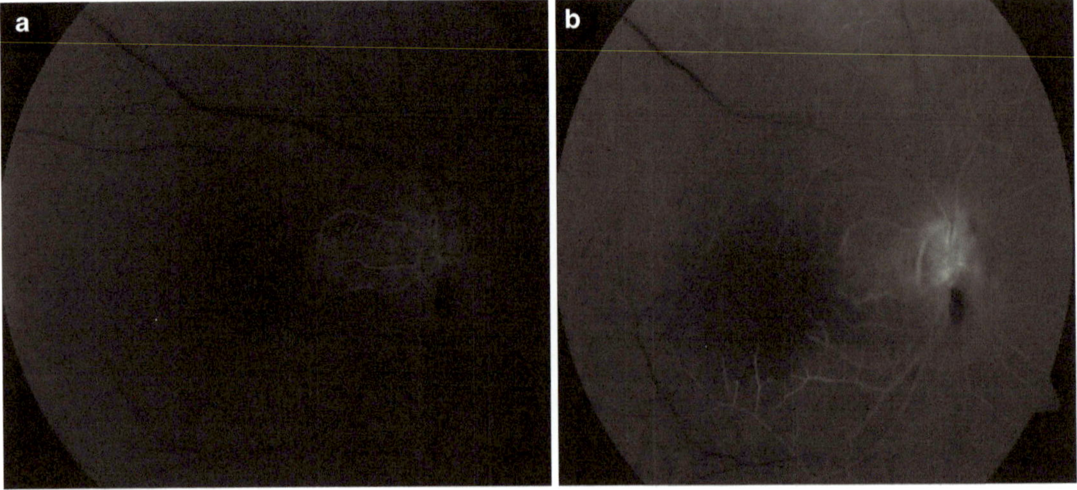

Fig. 12.2 Central retinal arterial occlusion. (**a**). Fundus fluorescein angiography showing early perfusion of the cilioretinal artery (**b**). Delayed arteriovenous transit and late staining of the disc seen in late phase

lead to the layers appearing hyporeflective or widened (Rodrigues 2013; Mathew et al. 2010) (Fig. 12.3).

In BRAO, the OCT findings associated with ischaemia are striking when contrasted to the adjacent perfused retina. The temporal changes are similar to what is seen in CRAO (Ritter et al. 2012). While differentiating the types of retinal emboli is clinical in nature, OCT has been used to demonstrate complete occlusion of an obstructed artery (Shah et al. 2010) and can be used to show recanalisation (Fig. 12.4). Prominence of middle limiting membrane has been described as a reliable indicator of acute retinal ischaemia. Histologically, it is thought to correspond to cytoplasmic swelling of bipolar cell synapses in the inner OPL (Chu et al. 2013). Figure 12.5 contrasts the presence of p-MLM in the affected retina to the normal retina (Fig. 12.6).

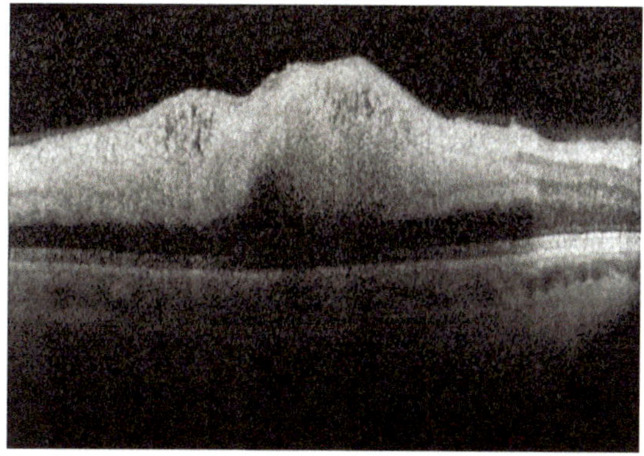

Fig. 12.3 Branched retinal arterial occlusion. SD-OCT showing grossly thickened and increase hyper-reflectivity of the inner retinal layers with resultant optical shadowing of the outer retinal layers. Note normal retina nasally for comparison

In the chronic phase, there will be isolated inner retinal thinning with the absence of stratification of the inner retinal layers. The outer retinal layers are always spared (Cruz-Villegas et al. 2004; Ghazi et al. 2010; Rodrigues 2013). Normal foveal depression is lost as the thinned retina extends up to the level of foveal depression (Ghazi et al. 2010). The inner retinal atrophy is coupled with increase outer retinal reflectivity and better visualisation of the outer choroid and large choroidal vessels (Ghazi et al. 2010). The presence of aforementioned features is important in distinguishing post-acute retinal artery occlusion from non-acute optic neuropathy

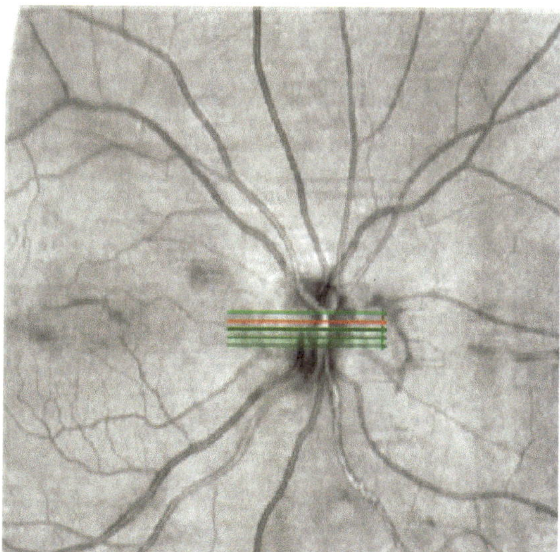

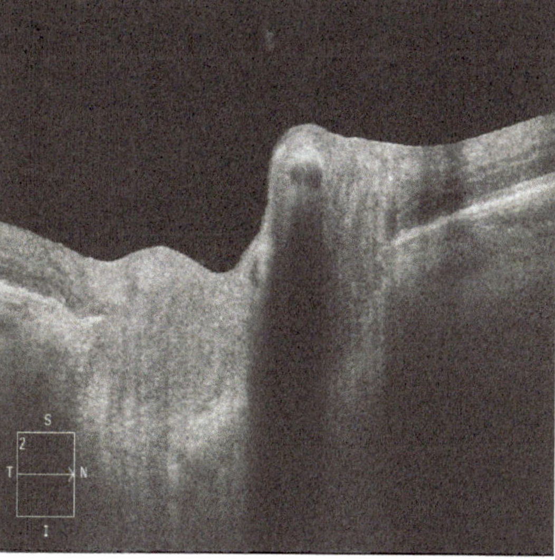

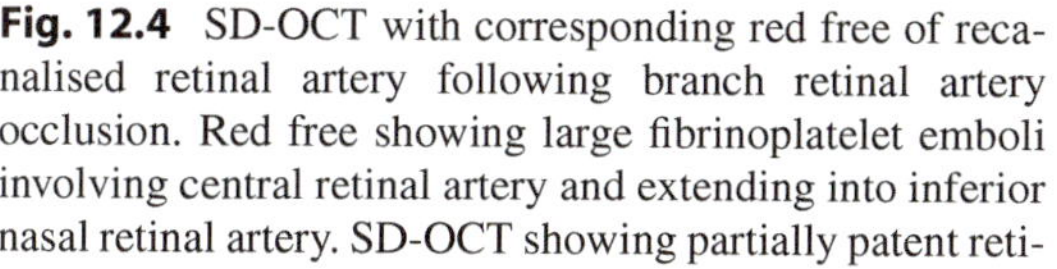

Fig. 12.4 SD-OCT with corresponding red free of recanalised retinal artery following branch retinal artery occlusion. Red free showing large fibrinoplatelet emboli involving central retinal artery and extending into inferior nasal retinal artery. SD-OCT showing partially patent retinal artery with superior semicircular hyper-reflective emboli (Images courtesy of Prof. J. E. Craig and Miss. A Chappell, Department of Ophthalmology Flinders Medical Centre, South Australia)

(Ghazi et al. 2010). While retinal thinning occurs with non-acute optic neuropathy, the thinning is limited to nerve fibre and ganglion cell layers, and the thinning is significantly less severe and spares the foveal depression (Ghazi et al. 2010) (Fig. 12.7).

Several studies have documented the temporal change of OCT findings in retinal artery occlusion (Asefzadeh and Ninyo 2008; Leung et al. 2007; Ritter et al. 2012; Saxena et al. 2013).

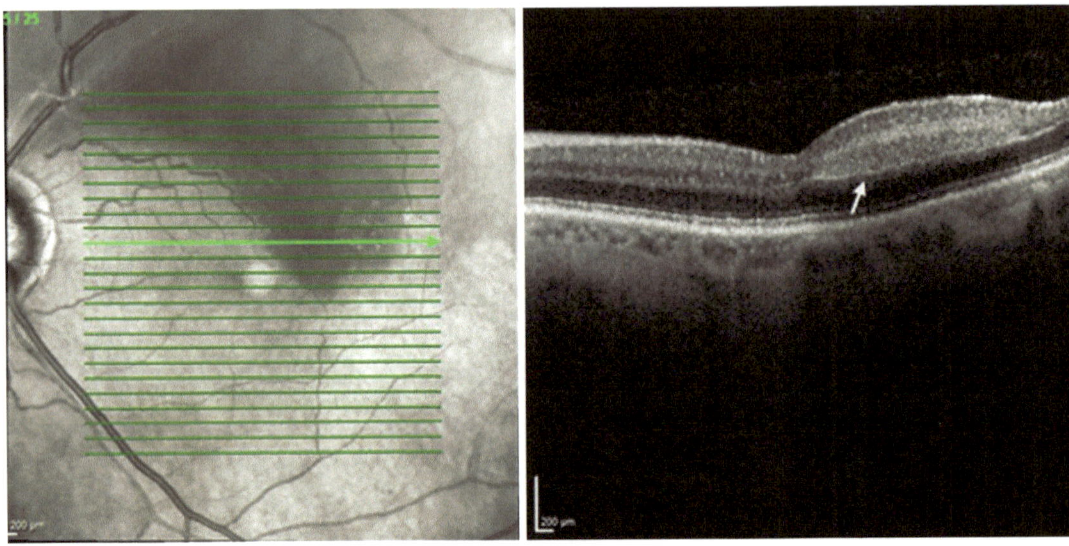

Fig. 12.5 Branched retinal arterial occlusion. SD-OCT with corresponding red free showing superior BRAO. The involved retina temporally has thickened and hyper-reflective inner retinal layers in contrast to the unaffected retina. Note the prominent middle limiting membrane separating the inner and outer retinal layer (*white arrow*)

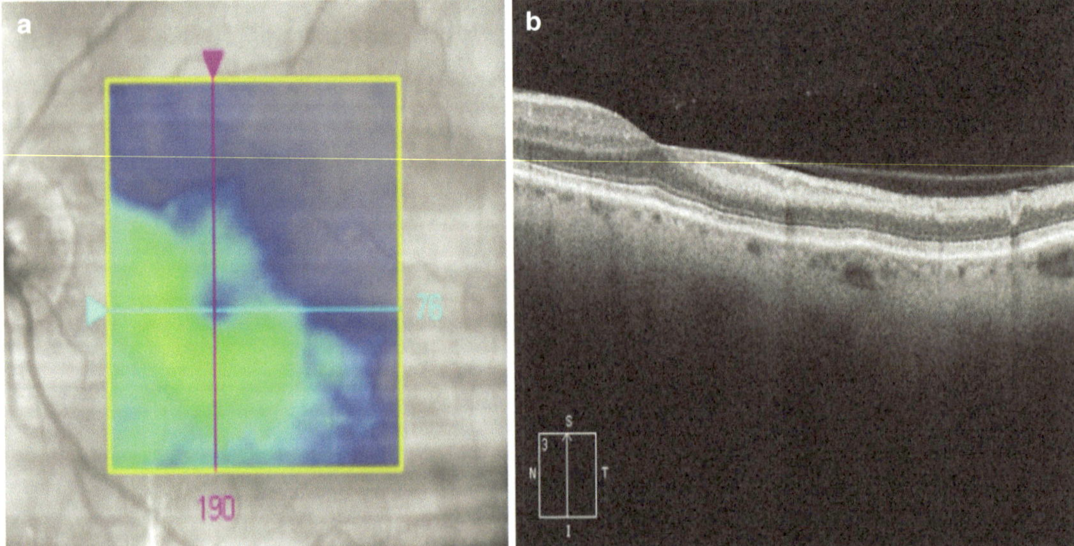

Fig. 12.6 Old superior branched retinal arterial occlusion. (**a**) SD-OCT contrasting superior and inferior retina in a patient with old superior BRAO. The inferior retina has normal thickness and preserved architecture while superior retina showing significant thinning of inner retinal layers but preserved outer retinal layers. (**b**) Thickness map showing corresponding decrease in overall retinal thickness in superior retina subserved by the occluded artery

Study	OCT findings	Days from onset
	Inner retinal swelling	0–3
	Decreasing retinal swelling	7
	Pseudo normalisation	28
	Gross inner retinal thinning and stability	From 90 days

In CRAO, Saxena et al. observed an initial increased inner retinal swelling. This is followed by gradual decrease in the retinal swelling which is indicative of reperfusion acute oxidative injury leading to acute damage and cell death. Values of average retinal nerve fibre layer (RNFL) thickness improve in a month indicating 'pseudo normalisation' which occurs with the restoration of blood supply and washout of free radicals and other oxidative stress mediators. Marked atrophic changes are observed by the end of three months with noticeable diminution of average RNFL thickness (Saxena et al. 2013). Ritter et al. documented similar temporal relationship of OCT changes in BRAO (Ritter et al. 2012). Figures 12.8

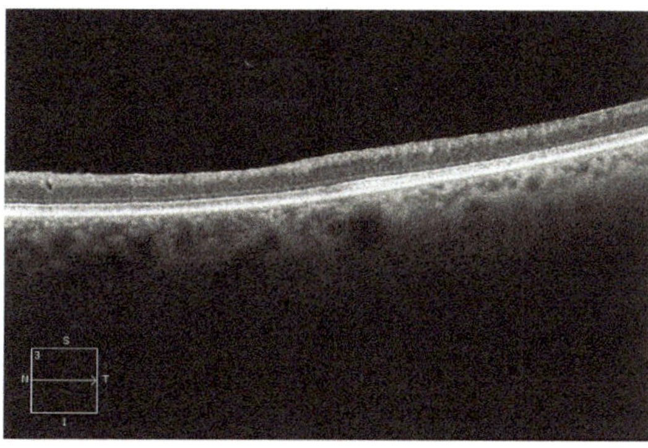

Fig. 12.7 SD-OCT of CRAO at day 90 following occlusion. Note overall decrease in retinal thickness and poorly defined inner retinal layers but intact outer retinal layers

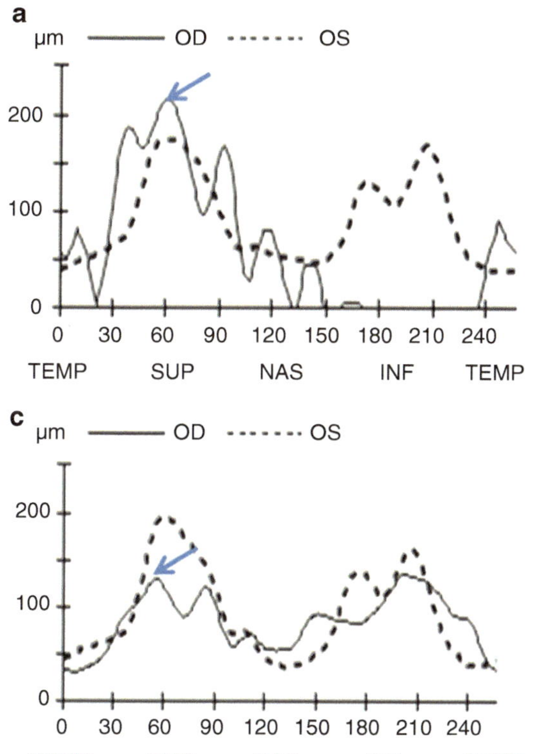

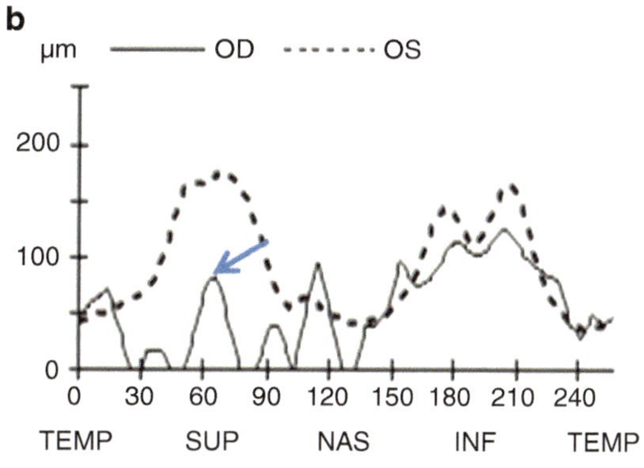

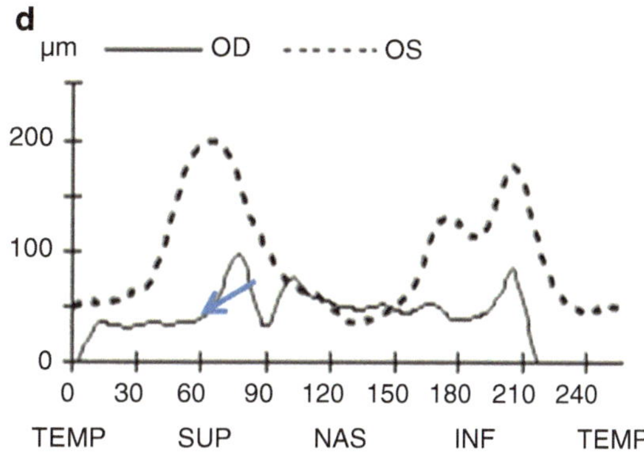

Fig. 12.8 Retinal nerve fibre layer (RNFL) thickness profiles of normal (OS) and CRAO-affected eye (OD) show initial rise due to retinal oedema on day 3 (**a**) followed by marked decrease on day 7 (**b**) suggestive of acute reperfusion injury. Nearly normal values on day 30 (**c**) due to return of circulation and washout of reperfusion stress mediators. Marked decrease in the value of average RNFL thickness can be noted by day 90 due to setting in of atrophy

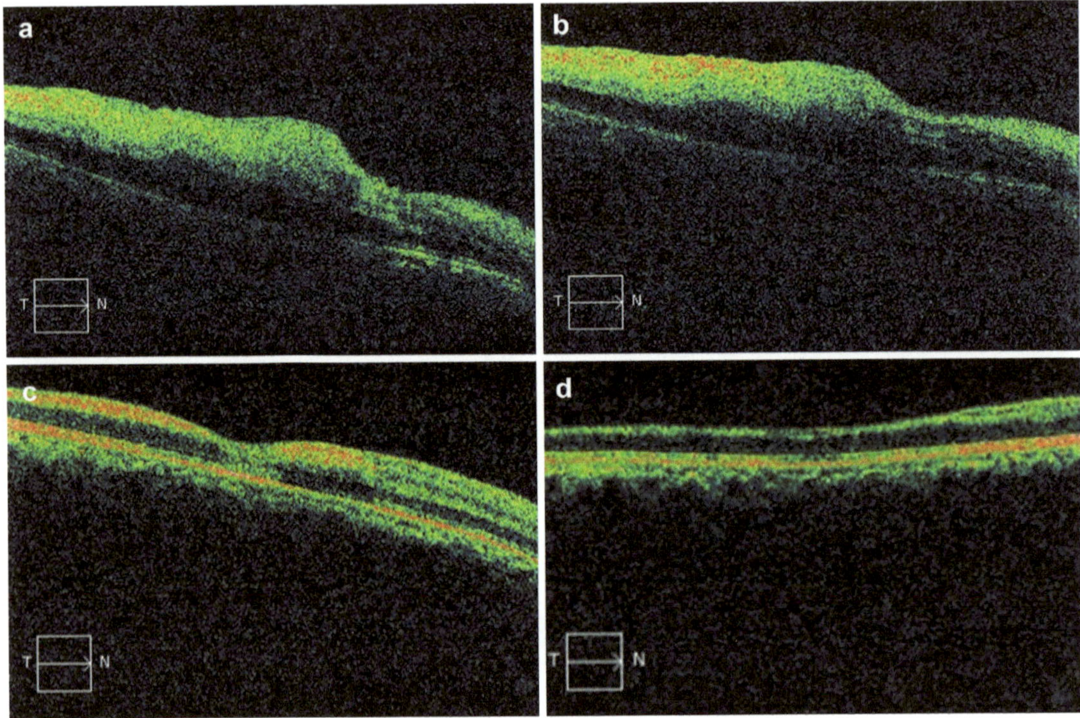

Fig. 12.9 OCT images show increased hyper-reflectivity and thickness of inner retinal layer with low reflectivity of outer retinal layer in CRAO-affected eye. Progressive decrease in hyper-reflectivity of inner layers is seen with time (**a** day 3, **b** day 7, **c** day 30, **d** day 90)

and 12.9 highlight the temporal changes following CRAO.

Prognostically, Ahn reported worse final BCVA with greater retinal thickening on presentation, while Leung et al. reported a worse functional outcome with greater degree of retinal thickening (Ahn et al. 2015; Leung et al. 2007). Cho et al. also reported better BCVA in patients with preserved foveal and outer nuclear layer thickness following BRAO (Cho et al. 2010). In contrast to this, Saxena et al. found that visual outcome was not directly related to the degree of macular thickness and peripapillary RNFL thickness. Even with 'pseudo normalisation' of thickness of nerve fibre layer and macular thickness, there is no gain in visual acuity (Saxena et al. 2013).

Thus the SD-OCT is an invaluable tool for not only monitoring retinal changes with time but also for guiding the corrective measures for salvaging vision in RAO.

References

Ahn SJ, Woo SJ, Park KH, Jung C, Hong JH, Han MK (2015) Retinal and choroidal changes and visual outcome in central retinal artery occlusion: an optical coherence tomography study. Am J Ophthalmol 159:667–676. doi:10.1016/j.ajo.2015.01.001

Asefzadeh B, Ninyo K (2008) Longitudinal analysis of retinal changes after branch retinal artery occlusion using optical coherence tomography. Optometry 79:85–89. doi:10.1016/j.optm.2007.08.021

Augsburger J, Magargal L (1980) Visual prognosis following treatment of acute central retinal artery obstruction. Br J Ophthalmol 64:913–917

Beatty S, Au Eong KG (2000) Acute occlusion of the retinal arteries: current concepts and recent advances in diagnosis and management. J Accid Emerg Med 17:324–329

Cho HJ, Kim CG, Kim JW, Lee JH (2010) The relationship between the visual prognoses of branch retinal artery obstruction and foveal thickness on OCT. Korean J Ophthalmol 24:297–301. doi:10.3341/kjo.2010.24.5.297

Chu YK, Hong YT, Byeon SH, Kwon OW (2013) In vivo detection of acute ischemic damages in retinal arterial occlusion with optical coherence tomography: a "prominent middle limiting membrane sign". Retina 33:2110–2117. doi:10.1097/IAE.0b013e3182899205

Coady PA, Cunningham ET Jr, Vora RA, McDonald HR, Johnson RN, Jumper JM, Fu AD, Haug SJ, Williams SL, Lujan BJ (2015) Spectral domain optical coherence tomography findings in eyes with acute ischaemic retinal whitening. Br J Ophthalmol 99:586–592. doi:10.1136/bjophthalmol-2014-304900, Epub 2014 Jul 3

Cruz-Villegas V, Puliafito CA, Fujimoto JG (2004) Retinal vascular diseases. In: Optical coherence tomography of ocular diseases. Thorofare, NJ: Slack. pp 103–110

Ghazi NG, Tilton EP, Patel B, Knape RM, Newman SA (2010) Comparison of macular optical coherence tomography findings between post acute retinal artery occlusion and non acute optic neuropathy. Retina 30:578–585. doi:10.1097/IAE.0b013e3181bf5fd5

Justice J, Lehmann RP (1976) Cilioretinal arteries: a study based on review of stereo fundus photographs and fluorescein angiographic findings. Arch Ophthalmol 94:1355

Leung CK, Tham CC, Mohammed S, Li EY, Leung KS, Chan WM, Lam DS (2007) In vivo measurements of macular and nerve fibre layer thickness in retinal arterial occlusion. Eye (Lond) 21:1464–1468

Mathew R, Papavasileiou E, Sivaprasad S (2010) Autofluorescence and high-definition optical coherence tomography of retinal artery occlusions. Clin Ophthalmol 4:1159–1163. doi:10.2147/OPTH.S13592

Pfaffenbach D, Hollenhorst R (1972) Morbidity and survivorship of patients with embolic cholesterol crystals in the ocular fundus. Trans Am Ophthalmol Soc 70:337

Ritter M, Sacu S, Deák GG, Kircher K, Sayegh RG, Pruente C, Schmidt-Erfurth UM (2012) In vivo identification of alteration of inner neurosensory layers in branch retinal artery occlusion. Br J Ophthalmol 96:201–207. doi:10.1136/bjo.2010.198937

Rodrigues IA (2013) Acute and chronic spectral domain optical coherence tomography features of branch retinal artery occlusion. BMJ Case Rep. doi:10.1136/bcr-2013-009007

Rumelt S, Dorenboim Y, Rehany U (1999) Aggressive systematic treatment for central retinal artery occlusion. Am J Ophthalmol 128:733–738

Savino PJ, Glaser JS, Cassady J (1977) Retinal stroke: is the patient at risk? Arch Ophthalmol 95:1185

Saxena S, Mishra N, Meyer CH et al (2013) Ischaemia reperfusion injury in CRAO. BMJ Case Rep. doi:10.1136/bcr-2013-201415

Shah VA, Wallace B, Sabates NR (2010) Spectral domain optical coherence tomography findings of acute branch retinal artery occlusion from calcific embolus. Indian J Ophthalmol 58:523–524. doi:10.4103/0301-4738.71703

vonGraefes A (1859) Ueber Embolie der Arteria centralis retinae alsUrsacheplotzlicherErblindung. Arch Ophthalmol 5:136–157

Drusen Secondary to Age-Related Macular Degeneration

13

Karen B. Schaal and Philip J. Rosenfeld

Contents

13.1 Introduction

Drusen are one of the earliest signs of age-related macular degeneration (AMD). They can be classified based on their fundus appearance as distinct or indistinct, hard or soft, and small (<63 μm), medium (≥63 <125μm), or large (≥125 μm) depending on their greatest linear dimension. These drusen characteristics, combined with the presence of any pigmentary abnormalities, are important risk factors for disease progression and staging of disease severity (Davis et al. 2005; Klein et al 2002; Wang et al. 2003). The most recent classification system separates AMD into three distinct stages: early (medium-sized drusen), intermediate (medium-sized drusen with pigmentary abnormalities or large drusen with or without pigmentary abnormalities), and late (macular neovascularization (MNV) and/or any geographic atrophy (GA)) (Ferris et al. 2013).

Histologically, drusen are focal accumulations of extracellular material (mainly lipids and proteins) and are typically located between the basal lamina of the retinal pigment epithelium (RPE) and the inner collagenous layer of Bruch's membrane (BM). On color fundus imaging, drusen appear as yellow-white accumulations, whereas on spectral domain-optical coherence tomography (SD-OCT), drusen are defined by an elevation of the overlaying RPE above a certain threshold. One of the advantages of using SD-OCT imaging for measuring and following drusen over time is the capability of capturing the two- and three-dimensional features

K.B. Schaal, MD • P.J. Rosenfeld, MD, PhD (✉)
Bascom Palmer Eye Institute, Miami, FL, USA
e-mail: prosenfeld@med.miami.edu

C.H. Meyer et al. (eds.), *Spectral Domain Optical Coherence Tomography in Macular Diseases*,
DOI 10.1007/978-81-322-3610-8_13

of drusen using cross-sectional B-scans, en face topological maps, and drusen volume and area measurements.

13.2 Drusen as Risk Factors for Predicting the Progression to Late Age-Related Macular Degeneration

Manual grading of stereoscopic color fundus images was the gold standard for many years when classifying the stages of AMD, particularly in large epidemiologic studies such as Age-Related Eye Disease Study (AREDS 2001). Drusen characteristics were manually evaluated using a grid composed of circles with different radii with radial lines dividing the circles into subsections. These grids were overlaid on color fundus images. Different classification and grading systems used different grids, and drusen classifications were correlated with disease progression. Grading systems for drusen quantification used in large clinical trials were the Wisconsin Age-Related Maculopathy Grading System (Klein et al. 1991), the International Classification and Grading System for Age-Related Maculopathy and AMD (Bird et al. 1995) (as well as a modified version), the Age-Related Macular Disease Study Classification System used in the AREDS, and the Clinical Age-Related Maculopathy Study Staging System (CARMS) (Bartlett and Eperjesi 2007). Reproducibility of grading was difficult to achieve even for experienced graders who were challenged by the variability of drusen appearance, inter-patient variability in fundus pigmentation, media opacities, and variable image quality. This led to the introduction of semiautomated and automated algorithms for drusen quantitation using digital fundus photos (Bartlett and Eperjesi 2007; Friberg et al. 2007; Smith et al. 2005). Overall, none of these automated techniques gained widespread acceptance due to their variable degrees of robustness and accuracy.

13.3 Drusen Quantitation Using SD-OCT Imaging Versus Color Fundus Photos

On color fundus images, drusen are defined based on pigmentary changes in the macula, which are clinically detectable once they reach 25–30 μm in diameter (Sarks et al. 1999). As a planar image modality, color fundus imaging cannot provide any information about three-dimensional morphology of drusen, such as volume, or the location of pigmentary abnormalities relative to the RPE, such as whether they are above or below the RPE. SD-OCT provides high-speed, high-resolution, and high-density scans of the macula, which can be evaluated in three dimensions. When using cross-sectional B-scans, the integrity of the RPE and the photoreceptors overlying drusen can be visualized in great detail. SD-OCT images can show structural changes predictive of disease progression to late AMD, such as the intra- or subretinal fluid indicative of neovascular AMD, hyper-reflective foci overlying drusen, subsidence of the outer retina, and heterogenous internal reflectivity of drusenoid lesions indicative of nascent GA (nGA) (Wu et al. 2014) (Fig. 13.1), and choroidal thickness measurements below drusen of <135 μm (Ouyang et al. 2013), which is indicative of evolving GA.

The algorithm developed at the Bascom Palmer Eye Institute (BPEI) for SD-OCT imaging (Cirrus, Carl Zeiss Meditec, Dublin, CA) defines typical drusen as accumulations of material below the RPE, which leads to an elevation of the overlying RPE (Gregori et al. 2011). Once drusen lead to an RPE elevation above a minimal threshold, SD-OCT can provide reliable volume measurements (Gregori et al. 2011; Gregori et al. 2014). This algorithm can therefore distinguish between typical drusen, which elevate the RPE, and subretinal drusenoid deposits (SDD), which are located above the RPE and underneath the retina (Curcio et al 2013; Zweifel et al. 2010). Due to

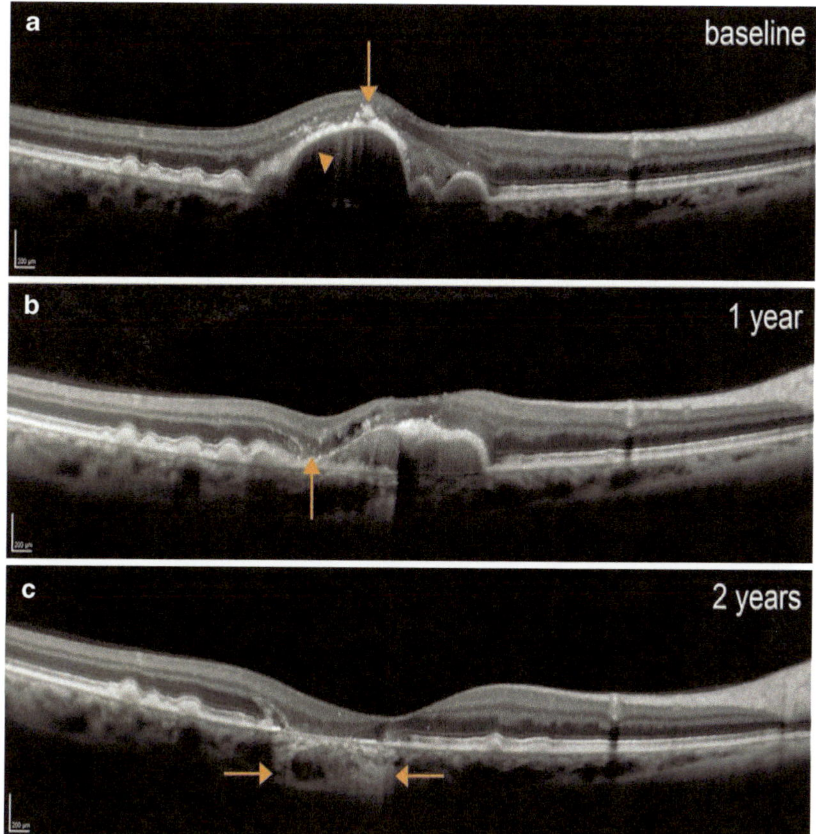

Fig. 13.1 Cross-sectional SD-OCT B-scans through the fovea of a 61-year-old man (*right eye*) with intermediate AMD followed for over 2 years. (**a**) Baseline visit shows a large drusenoid retinal pigment epithelial detachment (PED) with signs predictive for pending atrophy such as hyper-reflective foci (*arrow*) and hyper-transmissions within the PED (*arrowhead*), presumably due to RPE breakdown. (**b**) After 1 year the large drusenoid PED has partially collapsed with an adjacent area of outer retinal subsidence (*arrow*), a sign for nascent geographic atrophy (nGA). (**c**) Two years after baseline the PED has completely collapsed, leaving drusen-associated atrophy with the characteristic hyper-transmission into the choroid (*area between arrows*) resulting from loss of the RPE, photoreceptor, and choriocapillaris

the selected threshold, this SD-OCT algorithm does not include small, shallow drusen or SDDs, which might be apparent on color fundus imaging. This could explain why there was only fair agreement between drusen area measurements obtained from color fundus photos and the SD-OCT algorithm, with the SD-OCT algorithm missing the small, flat drusen resulting in smaller drusen area measurements compared with manual color fundus measurements (Yehoshua et al. 2013). However, this SD-OCT algorithm does reliably measure the more clinically meaningful medium and large drusen, which are widely acknowledged risk factors for disease progression. Moreover, when comparing the change in drusen area assessed by SD-OCT and color fundus photos longitudinally, the two image modalities showed a good correlation. This suggests that both imaging modalities essentially captured the same changes. SD-OCT imaging has the added advantage that it can measure changes in drusen volume, which is a far more sensitive technique for measuring changes in drusen size compared with area measurements. For example, drusen volume can decrease by more than 50 % of the cube root volume without any apparent change in drusen area on the corresponding color fundus photo (Yehoshua et al. 2011b). The reason why drusen volume was found to be a more sensitive indicator of drusen growth compared with area measurements is because area measurements tended to plateau, while drusen volume continued to increase over time. Based on these findings, SD-OCT imaging is currently the most reliable strategy for following drusen morphology and progression over time and has replaced color fundus imaging for clinical trials.

13.4 SD-OCT Algorithms to Quantify Drusen Load

Different research groups have developed SD-OCT algorithms for quantifying drusen in the macula and monitoring their morphological changes over time (Chen et al. 2014; Folgar et al. 2016; Gregori et al. 2011; Schlanitz et al. 2015). The algorithm developed at BPEI is fully automated, FDA approved, and commercially available on the Cirrus SD-OCT instrument (Carl Zeiss Meditec Inc, Dublin, CA). This algorithm calculates the difference between the elevation of the RPE (caused by drusen) and a virtual RPE floor free of deformations (called the RPE fit) (Gregori et al. 2011). The difference between the RPE and the RPE fit results in reproducible measurements of drusen area and volume (Gregori et al. 2011, 2014) (Fig. 13.2).

The minimum detectable RPE elevation was chosen to be 19 μm (10 pixels) to minimize the contribution of noise that accompanies any measurement technique. A significant deviation from the RPE fit would therefore be any RPE elevation greater than 19 μm, which would subsequently be counted as a druse. The preferred pattern for measuring drusen is the 200 × 200 scan pattern (200 A-scans per B-scan and 200 B-scans in each cube), which consists of 40,000 A-scans with a uniform spacing of 30 μm between each A-scan and each B-scan. This scan pattern covers a 6 mm×6 mm area centered on the fovea.

Another SD-OCT algorithm for drusen segmentation was developed by a research group at Duke University (Chiu et al. 2012; Jain et al. 2010). This algorithm segments the retina into three retinal boundaries: inner aspect of the inner limiting membrane (ILM), inner aspect of the RPE-drusen complex, and outer aspect of Bruch's membrane. The spacing between adjacent B-scans was 66 μm, which might explain why this algorithm had difficulty detecting small drusen. Any hyper-reflective material contiguous with the RPE, such as SDDs, is segmented and included into the analysis as well, which is a unique feature of this algorithm. This algorithm segments at the inner border of the RPE band rather than the outer border and can therefore capture diffuse RPE thickening even before drusen form. However, this algorithm was designed for the Bioptigen system and is not currently commercially available.

Another drusen segmentation strategy is based on polarization-sensitive OCT (PS-OCT), which segments the RPE based on its depolarizing properties and allows quantitative drusen area and volume assessment (Baumann et al. 2010; Gotzinger et al. 2008; Sugita et al. 2013). After the actual position of the RPE is located based on its polarization uniformity (DOPU) value, drusen are segmented by calculating the difference between the actual RPE position and a virtual RPE position free of any deformations. However, this segmentation strategy is experimental and not widely available at this time.

The performance characteristics of commercially available algorithms for drusen detection were compared between three different SD-OCT instruments. Drusen segmentation results were compared between the Cirrus instrument (Carl Zeiss Meditec, Dublin, CA), the 3D OCT-1000 device (Topcon, Tokyo, Japan), and the Spectralis instrument (Heidelberg Engineering, GmbH, Heidelberg, Germany) (Schlanitz et al. 2010). Overall, the Cirrus drusen segmentation algorithm made

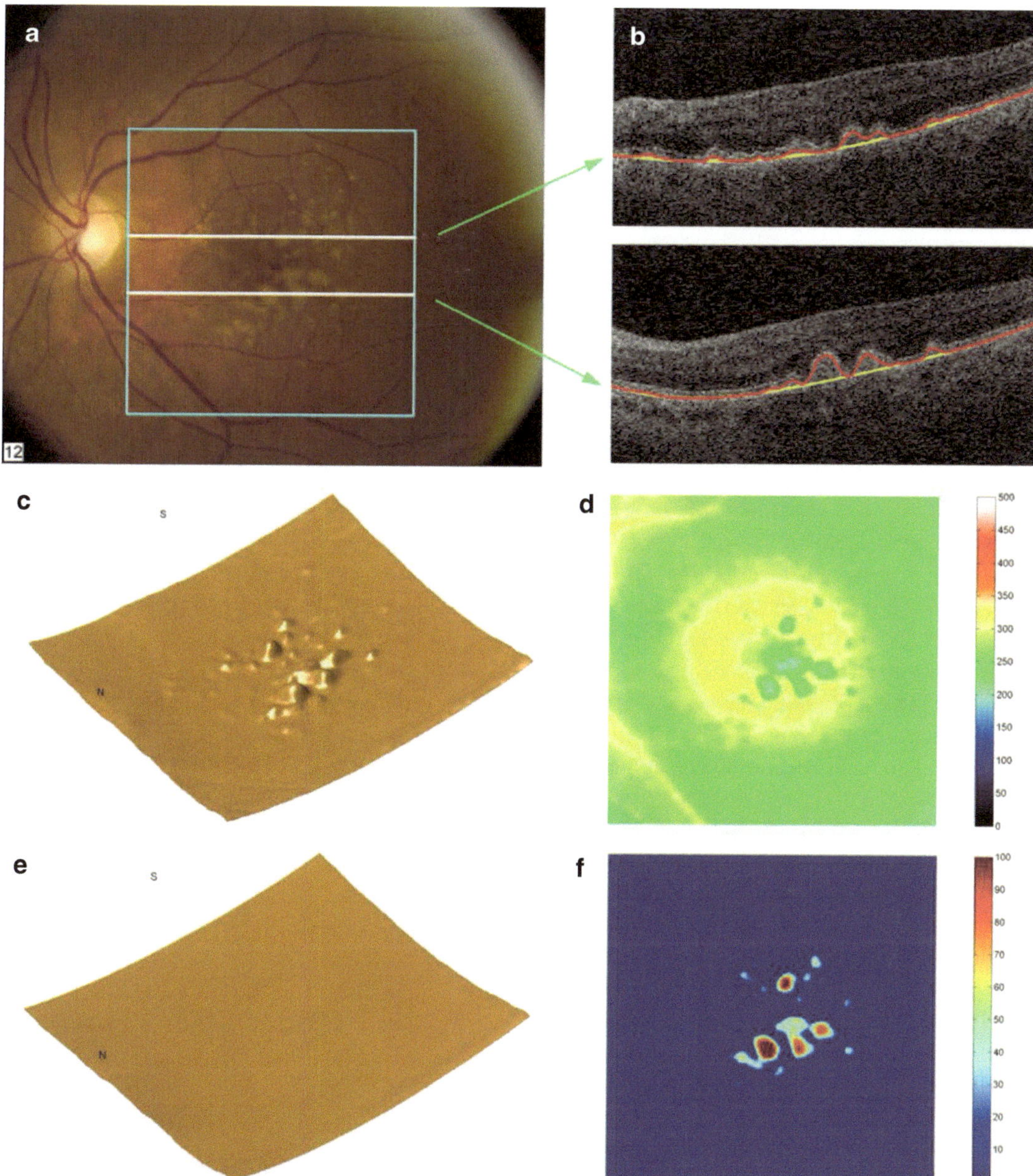

Fig. 13.2 SD-OCT imaging of small- to medium-sized drusen. (**a**) Color fundus photo with a superimposed SD-OCT dataset indicated by the blue square. (**b**) Two cross-sectional SD-OCT B-scans correspond to the retinal locations marked by white lines on the color fundus photo. The segmentation of the RPE is shown in red, and the RPE floor (RPE fit = free of any deformations) is shown in yellow. (**c**) Surface rendering of the RPE segmentation. (**d**) Retinal thickness map. (**e**) Surface rendering of the RPE floor. (**f**) Drusen thickness map (Figure, courtesy of Giovanni Gregori, Gregori G et al. 2011)

significantly fewer errors in drusen detection than the 3D OCT-1000 instrument ($p<0.001$). Due to the fact that the Spectralis instrument does not offer a true RPE segmentation, it performed poorly.

13.5 Following Drusen Growth with SD-OCT Imaging

Population-based trials studied the natural history of drusen to determine risk factors for disease progression (Chew et al. 2014; Cukras et al. 2010; Klein et al. 2007; Sparrow et al. 1997). Drusen size and number, extent of pigmentary abnormalities, and extent of involvement in one or both eyes are known risk factors for the development of late AMD (Ferris et al. 2013). Furthermore, the underlying genetics with the presence or absence of at-risk and/or protective alleles influences the phenotype of AMD, as well as its progression. For example, the COMPLETE study showed a significant association between the number of at-risk alleles in complement factor H (CFH; rs1061170) carried by a patient and the increase in drusen volume over 6 and 12 months ($p < 0.001$) (de Amorim Garcia Filho et al. 2014). In another study, a significant association was found between the area and volume of macular drusen in an Amish AMD population and the number of at-risk CFH alleles (CFH; rs12038333) carried by these patients (Chavali et al. 2015).

In addition to being able to measure drusen volume, SD-OCT imaging has revealed that drusen are not stable structures and far more dynamic than originally appreciated using color fundus imaging. Drusen undulate over time and undergo repeated cycles of growth and shrinkage, with growth more likely than shrinkage (Yehoshua et al. 2011b), and the risk of progression to either GA or MNV increases as drusen enlarge (Chew et al. 2014; Cukras et al. 2010; Ferris et al. 2013; Schlanitz et al. 2015; Yehoshua et al. 2011b). Drusen can also spontaneously regress without leaving any traces (Bressler et al. 1995; Klein et al. 2007; Sparrow et al. 1997), which would be the most desirable outcome in a clinical trial (Fig. 13.3).

Yehoshua et al. followed the natural course of drusen over 1 year, measuring drusen volume and area. For analyzing drusen volume, it was found that a cube root transformation of drusen volume has distinct advantages over using the traditional volume measurement, and these advantages were similar to the advantages of using the square root transformation strategy when measuring and following GA (Yehoshua et al. 2011a, b, 2014, 2015). By using the cube root volume of the drusen volume measurement, we found that a constant test-retest standard deviation was achieved regardless of the baseline drusen size, so measuring a defined increase or decrease in the drusen volume over time was independent of baseline drusen size and so it became easier to determine if drusen actually grew or decreased in size. If this strategy wasn't applied, then larger drusen volumes would appear to grow faster than smaller drusen volumes, which were not actually true, just as we observed for the growth rates of larger areas GA, which appeared to grow faster in the absence of the square root transformation strategy (Feuer et al. 2013).

An ideal baseline drusen volume to study in clinical trials was found to be a drusen volume of at least 0.03 mm^3 (cube root volume 0.31 mm) within a circular region with 3 mm in diameter centered on the fovea (de Amorim Garcia Filho et al. 2014; Yehoshua et al. 2011b). Natural history data on drusen showed that this drusen volume corresponded to a drusen area that included large drusen (125 μm), which were easily seen on color fundus photos, and this drusen volume could also be easily measured by SD-OCT. In addition, this drusen volume could decrease by more than 90 % and still be accurately measured using the SD-OCT algorithm for drusen volume measurements (Yehoshua et al. 2011b).

13.6 SD-OCT Drusen Volume as an Endpoint for Clinical Trials

Historically, drusen were manually graded in large clinical trials such as the AREDS and the laser to drusen trials (Parodi et al. 2009) and were quantified using digital high-quality color fundus images. The FDA-approved, commercially available, and fully automated SD-OCT drusen segmentation algorithm offers an accurate, reliable, and standardized method for following drusen morphology over time (Gregori et al. 2011, 2014; Yehoshua et al. 2010, 2011b, 2013) and does not require reading center involvement. The SD-OCT algorithm defines drusen as elevations of the overlying RPE above a minimal threshold and provides both area and volume measurements.

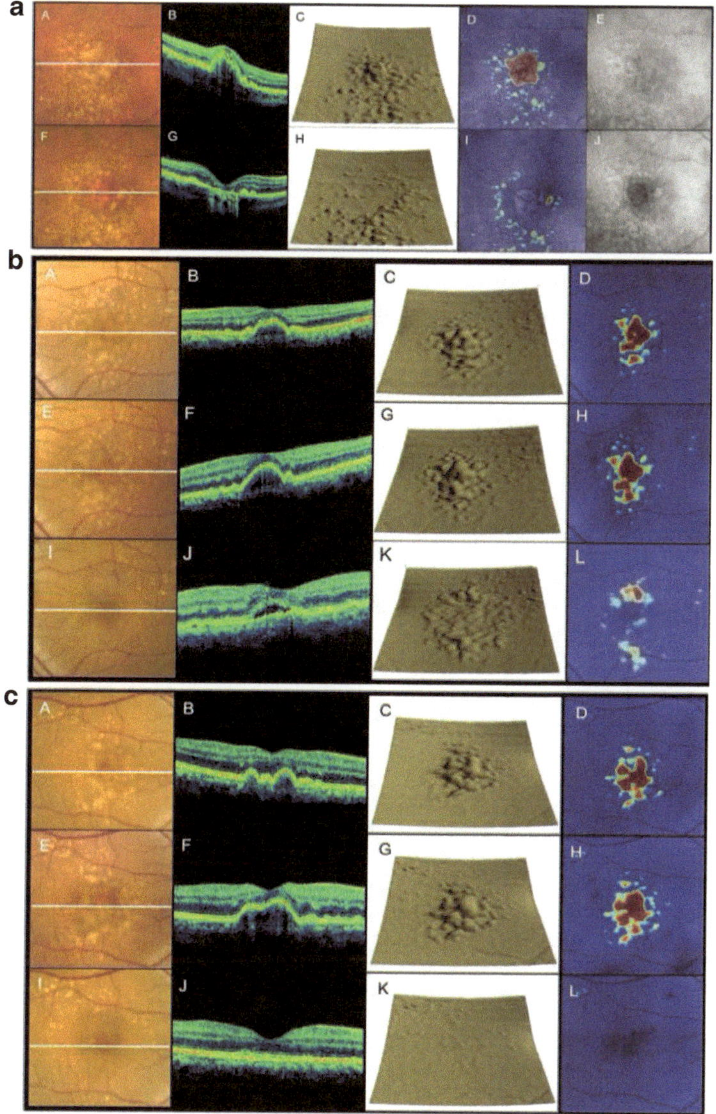

Fig. 13.3 Examples of how drusen can change over time with different outcomes such as GA, MNV, or regression without any sequelae. Panel (**a**) 76-year-old woman (*right eye*) with drusen at baseline and developed drusen associated atrophy over 12 months. Color fundus photos with a white line representing the location of the OCT B-scans (*A*, *F*), horizontal cross-sectional B-scans (*B*, *G*), RPE segmentation maps (*C*, *H*), hybrid map made of OCT fundus image and drusen thickness map (*D*, *I*), and fundus autofluorescence (*E*, *J*). At 12 months, GA appears with an area of 1.28 mm^2. Images are shown at baseline (*A–E*) and 12 months follow-up (*F–J*). Panel (**b**). A 64-year-old woman (*left eye*) with drusen at baseline and developed macular neovascularization (MNV) over 15 months. Drusen were found to increase in volume and then regress, eventually leading to MNV. Color fundus photos with a *white line* representing the location of the OCT B-scans (*A*, *E*, *I*), horizontal B-scans (*B*, *F*, *J*), RPE segmentation maps (*C*, *G*, *K*), hybrid map made of OCT fundus image, and drusen thickness map (*D*, *H*, *L*). Images are shown at baseline (*A–D*), at 6 months (*E–H*), and at 15 months of follow-up (*I–L*). Baseline drusen volume was 0.19 mm^3 (*D*) and 0.23 mm^3 at 6 months (*H*). Panel (**c**). A 64-year-old woman (*right eye*) with drusen at baseline and spontaneous drusen regression over 6 months without progressing to late AMD (MNV and/or GA). Color fundus photos with a *white line* representing the location of the OCT B-scans (*A*, *E*, *I*), horizontal B-scans (*B*, *F*, *J*), RPE segmentation maps (*C*, *G*, *K*), hybrid map made of OCT fundus image, and drusen thickness map (*D*, *H*, *L*). Images are shown at baseline (*A–D*), at 3 months (*E–H*), and 6 months follow-up (*I–L*). Baseline drusen volume was 0.21 mm^3 (*D*), 0.26 mm^3 at 3 months (*H*), and 0.001 mm^3 at 6 months follow-up (*L*). (Figure courtesy of Zohar Yehoshua, modified from Yehoshua Z et al. 2011b)

When testing new therapies for intermediate AMD (iAMD), we proposed the use of a composite endpoint in clinical trials rather than the use of the traditional visual acuity (VA) endpoint (Schaal et al. 2016). This allowed for the design of shorter proof-of-concept studies, with the goal of intervening earlier in the course of the disease before late AMD develops. In such a study targeting drusen, failure would be defined as drusen growth, formation of neovascularization, or conversion to GA, which are the three most likely outcomes when following iAMD patients. The advantage of using composite endpoints is the need of fewer patients, shorter study duration, and lower study costs. A drusen baseline volume of 0.03 mm^3 has been shown to be suitable to follow drusen growth and/or decrease (de Amorim Garcia Filho et al. 2014; Yehoshua et al. 2011b), and the cube root strategy should be used to evaluate drusen growth/shrinkage over time.

References

Age-Related Eye Disease Study Research G (2001) The Age-Related Eye Disease Study system for classifying age-related macular degeneration from stereoscopic color fundus photographs: the Age-Related Eye Disease Study Report Number 6. Am J Ophthalmol 132:668–681

Bartlett H, Eperjesi F (2007) Use of fundus imaging in quantification of age-related macular change. Surv Ophthalmol 52:655–671

Baumann B, Gotzinger E, Pircher M et al (2010) Segmentation and quantification of retinal lesions in age-related macular degeneration using polarization-sensitive optical coherence tomography. J Biomed Opt 15:061704

Bird AC, Bressler NM, Bressler SB et al (1995) An international classification and grading system for age-related maculopathy and age-related macular degeneration. The International ARM Epidemiological Study Group. Surv Ophthalmol 39:367–374

Bressler NM, Munoz B, Maguire MG et al (1995) Five-year incidence and disappearance of drusen and retinal pigment epithelial abnormalities. Waterman study. Arch Ophthalmol 113:301–308

Chavali VR, Diniz B, Huang J et al (2015) Association of OCT derived drusen measurements with AMD associated-genotypic SNPs in Amish population. J Clin Med 4:304–317

Chen Q, Leng T, Zheng LL et al (2014) An improved optical coherence tomography-derived fundus projection image for drusen visualization. Retina 34:996–1005

Chew EY, Clemons TE, Agron E et al (2014) Ten-year follow-up of age-related macular degeneration in the age-related eye disease study: AREDS report no. 36. JAMA Ophthalmol 132:272–277

Chiu SJ, Izatt JA, O'Connell RV et al (2012) Validated automatic segmentation of AMD pathology including drusen and geographic atrophy in SD-OCT images. Invest Ophthalmol Vis Sci 53:53–61

Cukras C, Agron E, Klein ML et al (2010) Natural history of drusenoid pigment epithelial detachment in age-related macular degeneration: Age-Related Eye Disease Study Report No. 28. Ophthalmology 117:489–499

Curcio CA, Messinger JD, Sloan KR et al (2013) Subretinal drusenoid deposits in non-neovascular age-related macular degeneration: morphology, prevalence, topography, and biogenesis model. Retina 33:265–276

Davis MD, Gangnon RE, Lee LY et al (2005) The Age-Related Eye Disease Study severity scale for age-related macular degeneration: AREDS Report No. 17. Arch Ophthalmol 123:1484–1498

de Amorim Garcia Filho CA, Yehoshua Z, Gregori G et al (2014) Change in drusen volume as a novel clinical trial endpoint for the study of complement inhibition in age-related macular degeneration. Ophthalmic Surg Lasers Imaging Retina. 45:18–31

Ferris FL 3rd, Wilkinson CP, Bird A et al (2013) Clinical classification of age-related macular degeneration. Ophthalmology 120:844–851

Feuer WJ, Yehoshua Z, Gregori G et al (2013) Square root transformation of geographic atrophy area measurements to eliminate dependence of growth rates on baseline lesion measurements: a reanalysis of age-related eye disease study report no. 26. JAMA Ophthalmol 131:110–111

Folgar FA, Yuan EL, Sevilla MB et al (2016) Drusen volume and retinal pigment epithelium abnormal thinning volume predict 2-year progression of age-related macular degeneration. Ophthalmology 123:39–50.e1

Friberg TR, Huang L, Palaiou M, Bremer R (2007) Computerized detection and measurement of drusen in age-related macular degeneration. Ophthalmic Surg Lasers Imaging 38:126–134

Gotzinger E, Pircher M, Geitzenauer W et al (2008) Retinal pigment epithelium segmentation by polarization sensitive optical coherence tomography. Opt Express 16:16410–16422

Gregori G, Wang F, Rosenfeld PJ et al (2011) Spectral domain optical coherence tomography imaging of drusen in nonexudative age-related macular degeneration. Ophthalmology 118:1373–1379

Gregori G, Yehoshua Z, Garcia Filho CA et al (2014) Change in drusen area over time compared using spectral-domain optical coherence tomography and color fundus imaging. Invest Ophthalmol Vis Sci 55:7662–7668

Jain N, Farsiu S, Khanifar AA et al (2010) Quantitative comparison of drusen segmented on SD-OCT versus drusen delineated on color fundus photographs. Invest Ophthalmol Vis Sci 51:4875–4883

Klein R, Davis MD, Magli YL et al (1991) The Wisconsin age-related maculopathy grading system. Ophthalmology 98:1128–1134

Klein R, Klein BE, Tomany SC et al (2002) Ten-year incidence and progression of age-related maculopathy: The Beaver Dam eye study. Ophthalmology 109:1767–1779

Klein R, Klein BE, Knudtson MD et al (2007) Fifteen-year cumulative incidence of age-related macular degeneration: the Beaver Dam Eye Study. Ophthalmology 114:253–262

Ouyang Y, Heussen FM, Hariri A et al (2013) Optical coherence tomography-based observation of the natural history of drusenoid lesion in eyes with dry age-related macular degeneration. Ophthalmology 120:2656–2665

Parodi MB, Virgili G, Evans JR (2009) Laser treatment of drusen to prevent progression to advanced age-related macular degeneration. Cochrane Database Syst Rev (3):CD006537

Sarks SH, Arnold JJ, Killingsworth MC, Sarks JP (1999) Early drusen formation in the normal and aging eye and their relation to age related maculopathy: a clinicopathological study. Br J Ophthalmol 83:358–368

Schaal KB, Rosenfeld PJ, Gregori G, et al (2016) Anatomic Clinical Trial Endpoints for Nonexudative Age-Related Macular Degeneration. Ophthalmology 123:1060–79.

Schlanitz FG, Ahlers C, Sacu S et al (2010) Performance of drusen detection by spectral-domain optical coherence tomography. Invest Ophthalmol Vis Sci 51:6715–6721

Schlanitz FG, Sacu S, Baumann B et al (2015) Identification of drusen characteristics in age-related macular degeneration by polarization-sensitive optical coherence tomography. Am J Ophthalmol 160:335–344.

Smith RT, Chan JK, Nagasaki T et al (2005) A method of drusen measurement based on reconstruction of fundus background reflectance. Br J Ophthalmol 89:87–91

Sparrow JM, Dickinson AJ, Duke AM et al (1997) Seven year follow-up of age-related maculopathy in an elderly British population. Eye (Lond) 11:315–324

Sugita M, Zotter S, Pircher M et al (2013) Motion artifact and speckle noise reduction in polarization sensitive optical coherence tomography by retinal tracking. Biomed Opt Express 5:106–122

Wang JJ, Foran S, Smith W, Mitchell P (2003) Risk of age-related macular degeneration in eyes with macular drusen or hyperpigmentation: the Blue Mountains Eye Study cohort. Arch Ophthalmol 121:658–663

Wu Z, Luu CD, Ayton LN et al (2014) Optical coherence tomography-defined changes preceding the development of drusen-associated atrophy in age-related macular degeneration. Ophthalmology 121:2415–2422

Yehoshua Z, Rosenfeld PJ, Gregori G, Penha F (2010) Spectral domain optical coherence tomography imaging of dry age-related macular degeneration. Ophthalmic Surg Lasers Imaging 41(Suppl):S6–S14

Yehoshua Z, Rosenfeld PJ, Gregori G et al (2011a) Progression of geographic atrophy in age-related macular degeneration imaged with spectral domain optical coherence tomography. Ophthalmology 118:679–686

Yehoshua Z, Wang F, Rosenfeld PJ et al (2011b) Natural history of drusen morphology in age-related macular degeneration using spectral domain optical coherence tomography. Ophthalmology 118:2434–2441

Yehoshua Z, Gregori G, Sadda SR et al (2013) Comparison of drusen area detected by spectral domain optical coherence tomography and color fundus imaging. Invest Ophthalmol Vis Sci 54:2429–2434

Yehoshua Z, de Amorim Garcia Filho CA, Nunes RP et al (2014) Systemic complement inhibition with eculizumab for geographic atrophy in age-related macular degeneration: the COMPLETE study. Ophthalmology 121:693–701

Yehoshua Z, de Amorim Garcia Filho CA, Nunes RP et al (2015) Comparison of geographic atrophy growth rates using different imaging modalities in the COMPLETE study. Ophthalmic Surg Lasers Imaging Retina 46:413–422

Zweifel SA, Spaide RF, Curcio CA et al (2010) Reticular pseudodrusen are subretinal drusenoid deposits. Ophthalmology 117:303–312.e1

14 Geographic Atrophy Secondary to Age-Related Macular Degeneration

Moritz Lindner, Monika Fleckenstein, Julia Steinberg, Steffen Schmitz-Valckenberg, and Frank G. Holz

Contents

14.1 Introduction

Atrophy of the retinal pigment epithelium (RPE) represents a common end stage of various retinal diseases including advanced age-related macular degeneration (AMD), where it is termed geographic atrophy (GA). While choroidal neovascularization (CNV) is the most common cause of acute severe visual loss in AMD, approximately 20 % of AMD patients who are legally blind have lost central vision due to GA (Friedman et al. 2004; Klaver et al. 1998; Klein et al. 2002; Mitchell et al. 1995; Sunness et al. 1999).

Histologically, areas of GA are characterized by loss of the RPE and of outer layers of the neurosensory retina and the choriocapillaris (Green and Key 1977; Sarks et al. 1988). While en face imaging methods, in particular fundus autofluorescence (FAF) confocal scanning laser ophthalmoscopy (cSLO), readily identify areas of geographic atrophy, spectral domain optical coherence tomography (SD-OCT) enables a detailed view on the cross-sectional morphology of the atrophic lesion, its boundaries, and its perilesional alterations (Fleckenstein et al. 2008). Recent findings indicate that distinct morphologic findings identified in SD-OCT scans may even predict atrophy progression (Fleckenstein et al. 2011; Hariri et al. 2014; Moussa et al. 2013; Stetson et al. 2014).

14.2 Atrophic Area

In the atrophic area, the loss of the outer retinal layers can be visualized by SD-OCT imaging in vivo. The typical SD-OCT characteristics of geographic atrophy include loss of the outer nuclear layer (ONL) and the outer hyperreflective bands (external limiting membrane [ELM],

M. Lindner, MD • M. Fleckenstein, MD
J. Steinberg, MD • S. Schmitz-Valckenberg, MD
F.G. Holz, MD (✉)
Department of Ophthalmology, University of Bonn, Bonn, Germany
e-mail: Frank.Holz@ukb.uni-bonn.de

C.H. Meyer et al. (eds.), *Spectral Domain Optical Coherence Tomography in Macular Diseases*, DOI 10.1007/978-81-322-3610-8_14

ellipsoid zone, interdigitation zone, inner part of the RPE-Bruch's membrane [BM] complex) resulting in direct apposition of the outer plexiform layer (OPL) and BM (Fig. 14.1a) (Ahlers et al. 2010; Fleckenstein et al. 2008; Michels et al. 2008; Wolf-Schnurrbusch et al. 2008). The band representing the RPE (inner portion of the RPE-BM complex) appears to be entirely lost, while the outer portion of the RPE-BM complex (assumed BM) continues through the atrophy (Figs. 14.1a and 14.3) (Fleckenstein et al. 2008). In the area of atrophy, SD-OCT imaging further reveals a choroidal signal enhancement that is explained by increased penetration of the light through the area of RPE atrophy (Figs. 14.2, 14.3, 14.4, 14.6, 14.7, and 14.9) (Fleckenstein et al. 2008; Wolf-Schnurrbusch et al. 2008). The margins of the area with increased choroidal reflectiveness have been shown to be the OCT parameter which correlates best with the borders of GA as monitored in fundus autofluorescence images (Schmitz-Valckenberg et al. 2011) (Fig. 14.2). Within the atrophic lesion, SD-OCT imaging may reveal various morphologic features including:

Plaques at the level of the former RPE-BM complex correlating with highly reflective lesions in the IR image (Fig. 14.1b) (Fleckenstein et al. 2008).

Clumps that rest on the thin remainder of RPE-BM, scattered throughout the atrophy. They may be noted also in other retinal layers (Fig. 14.1d) (Fleckenstein et al. 2008).

Irregular elevations in place of the inner portion of the RPE-BM band (Fig. 14.1c) (Fleckenstein et al. 2008; Ooto et al. 2014).

Elevations with crown-like appearance with presumed debris beneath these structures, also termed hyperreflective pyramidal structures (Fig. 14.1g) (Bonnet et al. 2014; Fleckenstein et al. 2008).

Larger accumulations of irregularly highly reflecting material (Fig. 14.1h) (Fleckenstein et al. 2008).

Branching, round, or ovoid hyporeflective structures with a hyperreflective border located in the outer nuclear layer (termed outer retinal tubulations – ORT) (Zweifel et al. 2009).

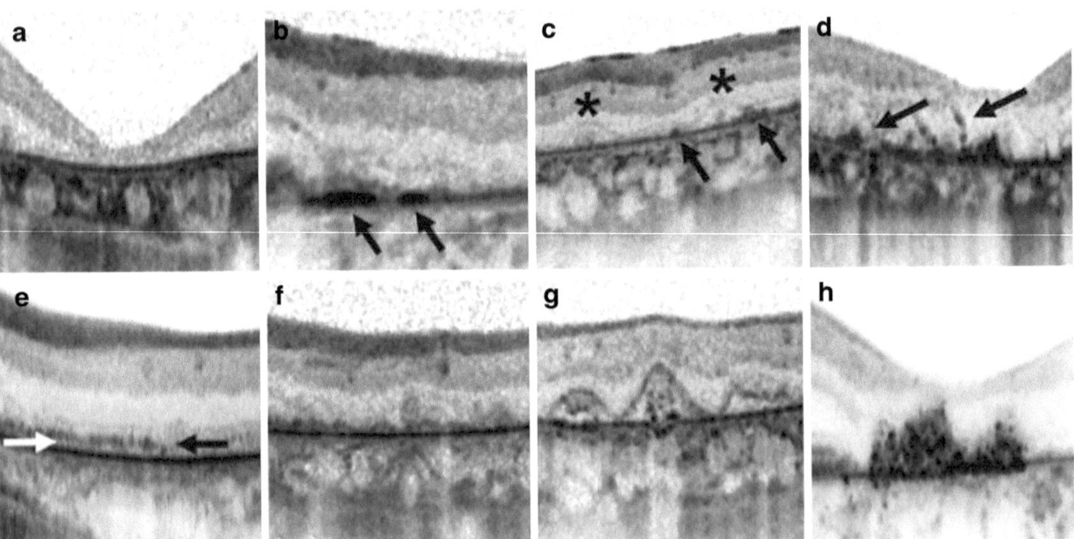

Fig. 14.1 Alterations within the area of geographic atrophy. (**a**) SD-OCT showing the absence of the outer retinal layers and remaining of a thin line on the outer margin of the original site of band 4, most likely representing Bruch's membrane. (**b–d**) SD-OCT showing plaques (**b**, *arrows*), elevations (**b**, *asterisks*), and clumps (**d**, *arrows*) based on the remaining of band 4. (**e**) SD-OCT showing a dotted line, seemingly continuing the elevated part of band 4 that splits at the atrophy margin that can be especially found in the "diffuse-trickling" FAF phenotype (Fleckenstein et al. 2011). (**f–h**) SD-OCT showing irregular elevations (**f**), crown-like elevations filled with hyperreflective "debris" (**g**), and irregular hyperreflective material (**h**) also based on band 4 that can be distinguished from the previous findings (Image obtained from Fleckenstein et al. 2008)

A thin, discontinuous hyperreflective band between the inner nuclear layer (INL) and the remaining outer part of RPE-BM band may be visible. This dotted band is most pronounced close to the atrophy border zone (Fig. 14.1e) (Fleckenstein et al. 2008, 2011).

The nature and the prognostic relevance of most of these structures are yet unknown. Elevations or

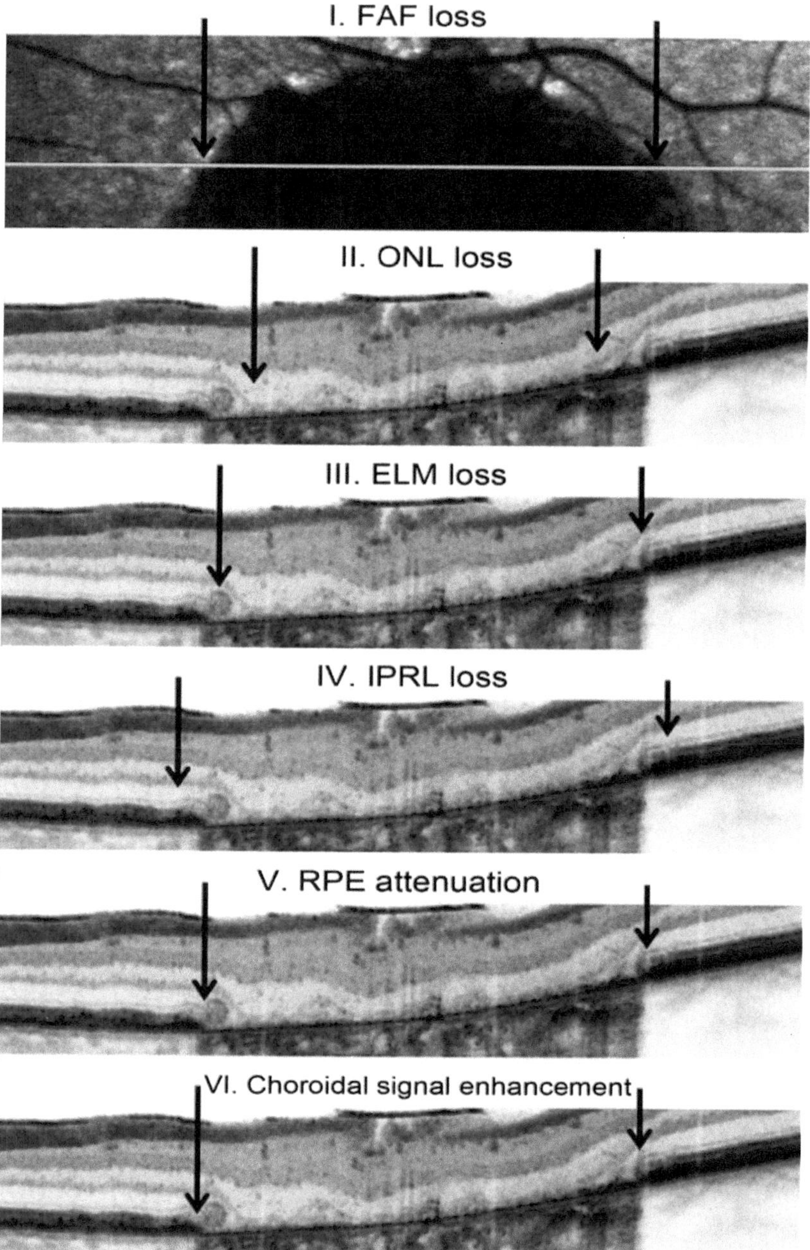

Fig. 14.2 Sequential loss of outer retinal bands. (*I*) Atrophy border in fundus autofluorescence image for comparison. (*II–VI*) SD-OCT showing loss of retinal bands ordered from the inner to outer retina. First, the ellipsoid zone (termed inner segment/outer segment photoreceptor layer [*IPRL*] here) is disrupted (*IV*). This is followed by choroidal signal enhancement (*VI*), visible RPE attenuations (*V*), external limiting membrane (*ELM*) loss (*III*), and the entire outer nuclear layer (*ONL*) loss (*II*) (Image obtained from Schmitz-Valckenberg et al. (2011), with permission)

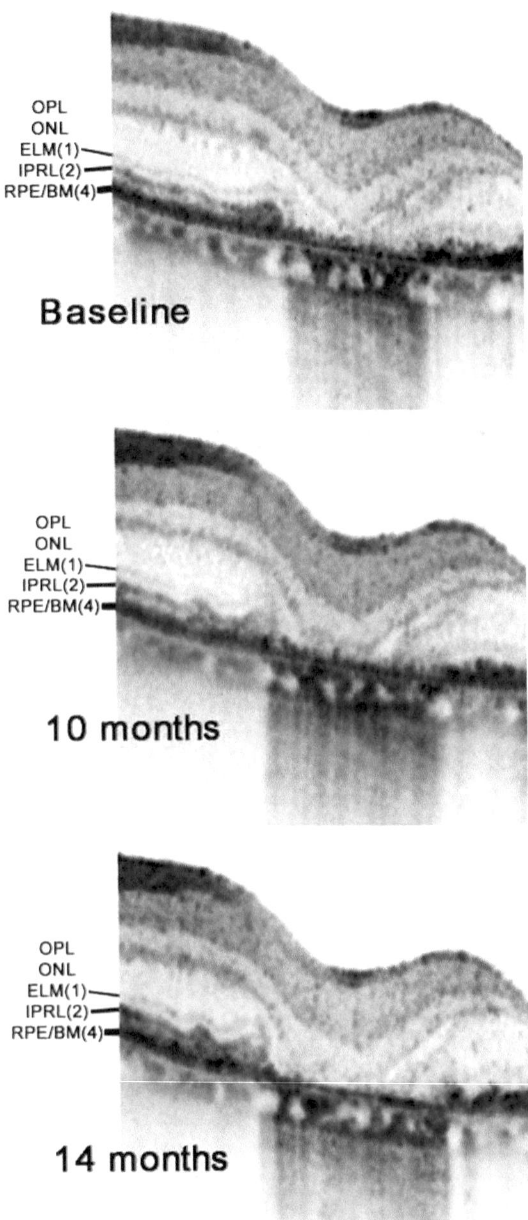

Fig. 14.3 Visualization of the progression of geographic atrophy. Serial SD-OCT imaging shows atrophy enlargement over time as progressive loss of the inner part of the RPE-BM complex, the ellipsoid zone, and the ELM, respectively, and thinning of hyporeflective band representing the ONL at the border of atrophy. Moving into the atrophic lesion, the ONL progressively thins, and the hyperreflective band above (*OPL*) approaches the remaining part of band 4 (assumed Bruch's membrane) (Image with permission from Fleckenstein et al. 2010)

accumulations of highly reflective material as well as plaques at the former RPE level might represent residual sub-RPE deposits and reflect various stages of regressing drusen, which may develop focal calcification and become increasingly irregular (Fleckenstein et al. 2008; Green and Key 1977; Sarks et al. 1988). The thin, discontinuous hyperreflective band between the INL and the remaining outer part of RPE-BM band is predominantly present in the "diffuse-trickling" GA phenotype, which is associated with rapid atrophy progression (Fleckenstein et al. 2011; Moussa et al. 2013). ORT are hypothesized to represent degenerating photoreceptors that rearrange in a tubular fashion. With respect to the prediction of atrophy progression rates, recent works have produced competing results showing that ORT predict significantly faster (Moussa et al. 2013) or slower progression rates (Hariri et al. 2014).

14.3 Atrophy Border Zone

Atrophic areas typically enlarge over time. During this process, not all outer retinal layers are lost at the same time. Loss of the ellipsoid zone may spatially precede the loss of the remainder OCT bands (Fleckenstein et al. 2008; Schmitz-Valckenberg et al. 2011). It is followed by attenuations in the RPE, first becoming more transparent to light reflecting from the choroid ("choroidal signal enhancement") and subsequently showing visible RPE alterations (Schmitz-Valckenberg et al. 2011). Complete ONL loss can usually be observed within the area of RPE loss (94 % of the cases) (Bearelly et al. 2009; Schmitz-Valckenberg et al. 2011). However, ONL loss does not occur abrupt. It rather thins gradually initiating on average 61 μm outside of the atrophy borders. Loss of ELM starts slightly inside the border of RPE atrophy (Fig. 14.2) (Bearelly et al. 2009). The inner retinal layers usually remain intact across the atrophic border (Wolf-Schnurrbusch et al. 2008). The morphologic alterations as described here are associated with remarkable functional impairments as shown by microperimetric examinations

(Sayegh et al. 2014). In a longitudinal study, it could be confirmed that expansion of GA patches was accompanied by advancing the loss of ELM, ellipsoid zone, the inner part of the RPE-BM complex, and a thinning of the ONL (Fig. 14.3) (Fleckenstein et al. 2010). In accordance with a progressive thinning of these layers, a decrease of retinal thickness over time (average – 14 μm/y) could be observed (Fleckenstein et al. 2010).

The exact shape of outer retinal layer loss at the atrophy border underlies interindividual differences. Three main types of atrophy border can be discriminated (Fig. 14.4). A first classification introduced by Brar et al. classified two distinct border types (Brar et al. 2009). Type 1 shows smooth margins and no alterations of the outer retina (Fig. 14.4a), while type 2 exhibits severe alterations in the outer retinal layers and irregular margins with or without increased optical reflectivity of the RPE (Fig. 14.4b). Subsequently, an additional border type termed "splitting" was described that is characterized by a splitting of the RPE-BM complex (Fig. 14.4c) (Fleckenstein et al. 2011). Of note, these atrophy border types are not patient or eye specific. Rather surrounding a single atrophic lesion, several of these types may occur. Little is known about the impact of border morphology on atrophy progression. A recent longitudinal study suggests that disruption of the ellipsoid zone predicts the direction of atrophy growth (Nunes et al. 2013). This observation suggests that photoreceptor damage occurs prior to RPE loss (Schmitz-Valckenberg et al. 2011). The "splitting" type atrophy border was shown to be predominant in the rapidly progressing "diffuse-trickling" type of GA (Fleckenstein et al. 2011). Consequently the "splitting" border type itself is also associated with rapid atrophy progression (Moussa et al. 2013). Using minimum intensity en face SD-OCT projections, a recent study found a tendency of GA progression to preferentially occur in areas of increased minimum intensity. The minimum intensity of an OCT A-scan is found in the ONL; these results thus suggest that alterations in this zone precede atrophy development (Stetson et al. 2014). To date it has not been investigated if these changes in minimum intensity are exactly correlated with the decrease in ONL thickness that has been observed to precede RPE loss (Bearelly et al. 2009).

14.4 Perilesional Zone

Heterogeneous changes can be noted in the perilesional zone of GA, which encompass retinal areas with visible abnormalities on the fundus photograph, SLO image, or SD-OCT outside the atrophic patches. In some sections, the retinal layers appear without noticeable alterations either of the inner or the outer retinal layers. Alterations of ellipsoid zone and RPE-BM complex may impede observation of the interdigitation zone (Fig. 14.5b–k), and changes can be so intense that the four outer hyperreflective OCT bands become indistinguishable (Fig. 14.5g). Thinning and thickening of the RPE-BM complex are common (Fig. 14.5b) and highly reflecting, segmented plaques may be observed in this band

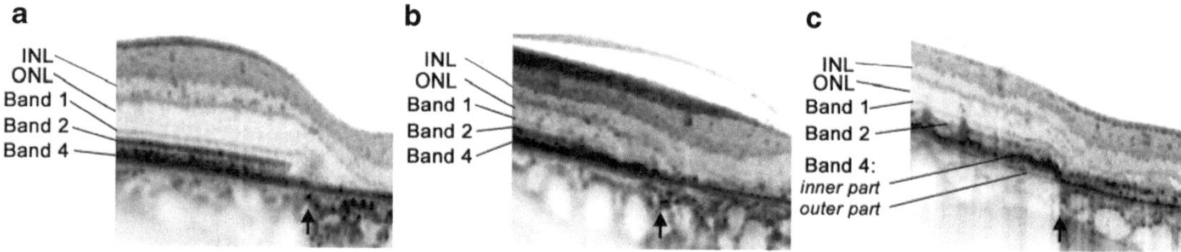

Fig. 14.4 Different types of borders as visualized by SD-OCT. (**a**, **b**) The assumed RPE-BM complex (*band 4*) narrows; and an outer layer remains throughout the atrophic area (assumed Bruch's membrane). According to Brar et al. (2009), the margin depicted in (**a**) represents a type 1 border with smooth margins and no alterations of the outer retina, and the margin in (**b**) represents a type 2 border with severe alterations in the outer retinal layers and irregular margins. (**c**) In contrast to (**a**) and (**b**), the "splitting" border is characterized by splitting of the RPE-BM complex in inner and outer regions (Image obtained from Fleckenstein et al. 2011)

(Fig. 14.5c). Elongated elevations (not correlated by funduscopically visible drusen) and dome-shaped elevations that correlate with drusen in fundus images (Fig. 14.5d–f) may occur (Fleckenstein et al. 2008). Beneath drusen, a thin line usually remains present on the former level of the RPE-BM complex (Fig. 14.5c–f). These dome-shaped elevations may precede atrophy development (Fleckenstein et al. 2010). A recent study identified pathological changes occurring before the development of drusen-associated atrophy using SD-OCT, which was defined as "nascent" GA (Wu et al. 2014). Unique features in these areas included subsidence of the OPL and INL and development of a hyporeflective wedge-shaped band within the limits of the OPL (Wu et al. 2014). There are several changes that can be observed on top of such a dome-shaped elevation, but may also occur independently (Fleckenstein et al. 2008). Apical extensions of the thickened RPE-BM complex can be observed with and without associated disruptions in the other outer retinal bands. These apical extensions may have clumps above the tips in different retinal layers (Fig. 14.5g–i). Such vertical extensions had spike-like appearances, beginning at the level of the RPE-BM complex, with extension through the overlying bands (Fig. 14.5h) (Fleckenstein et al. 2008). Longitudinal observations show that these findings may be considered as a continuum with clumps on the RPE-BM complex initially not disrupting the ellipsoid zone or ELM migrating toward the inner retinal layers and disrupting the retinal bands between. The clumps may either fade with time or precede atrophy development (Fleckenstein et al. 2010). Hyperreflective clumps may be found also independently of underlying spikelike lesions and can be noted at the level of the OPL. Underneath those clumps, outer retinal layers usually appear disrupted as if a piece of the RPE-BM complex had been torn out and broken through the layers above to finally localize at the assumed OPL level (Fig. 14.5j) (Fleckenstein et al. 2008). In the perilesional zone, a mottled irregular appearance of the RPE-BM complex accompanied by small elevations of the ellipsoid zone, commonly associated with a reticular drusen pattern in the FAF and IR images (Fig. 14.5k), may be present. Occasionally an increased distance between ellipsoid zone and RPE-BM complex can be found (Fig. 14.5l). In one eye of a patient, typically multiple such alterations can be detected.

14.5 Morphology of the Spared Fovea

Typically, atrophic patches initially occur in the parafoveal retina. Over time, several atrophic patches may coalesce, and new atrophic areas may occur. This can result in a horseshoe- and later ringlike configuration of atrophy surrounding the fovea. Thus, the fovea itself may remain uninvolved in the atrophic process until late in the course of the disease, a phenomenon referred to as "foveal sparing" (Sunness et al. 1995; Sarks et al. 1988). When the fovea finally becomes involved, a dramatic loss in visual acuity occurs, and less benefit would be expected from any future therapeutic intervention aiming to slow down or halt the natural course of the disease (Maguire and Vine 1986; Sunness et al. 1999). In SD-OCT scans of a healthy macula, the foveal depression (resulting in the physiological absence of the inner retinal layers in this area) is visualized (Fig. 14.6a). In patients with AMD and GA, the "spared fovea" may exhibit various alterations. Frequently an irregular and broad band of increased reflectivity at the site of the three outer hyperreflective bands can be found making details of these three bands invisible (Schmitz-Valckenberg et al. 2009). However the ELM usually remains visible. Interestingly when the atrophy does not entirely surround the fovea, outer retinal bands may be distinguishable (Wolf-Schnurrbusch et al. 2008). In the spared fovea, the ONL was found to be markedly swollen (Fig. 14.6b) (Schmitz-Valckenberg et al. 2009). Recent results suggest that not the entire ONL but rather the Henle's fiber layer was thickened. This implies that not a swelling of the photoreceptor nuclei themselves but rather their axons or of the Müller cells is responsible of the observed thickening (Mones et al. 2013). Surrounding atrophy of the outer

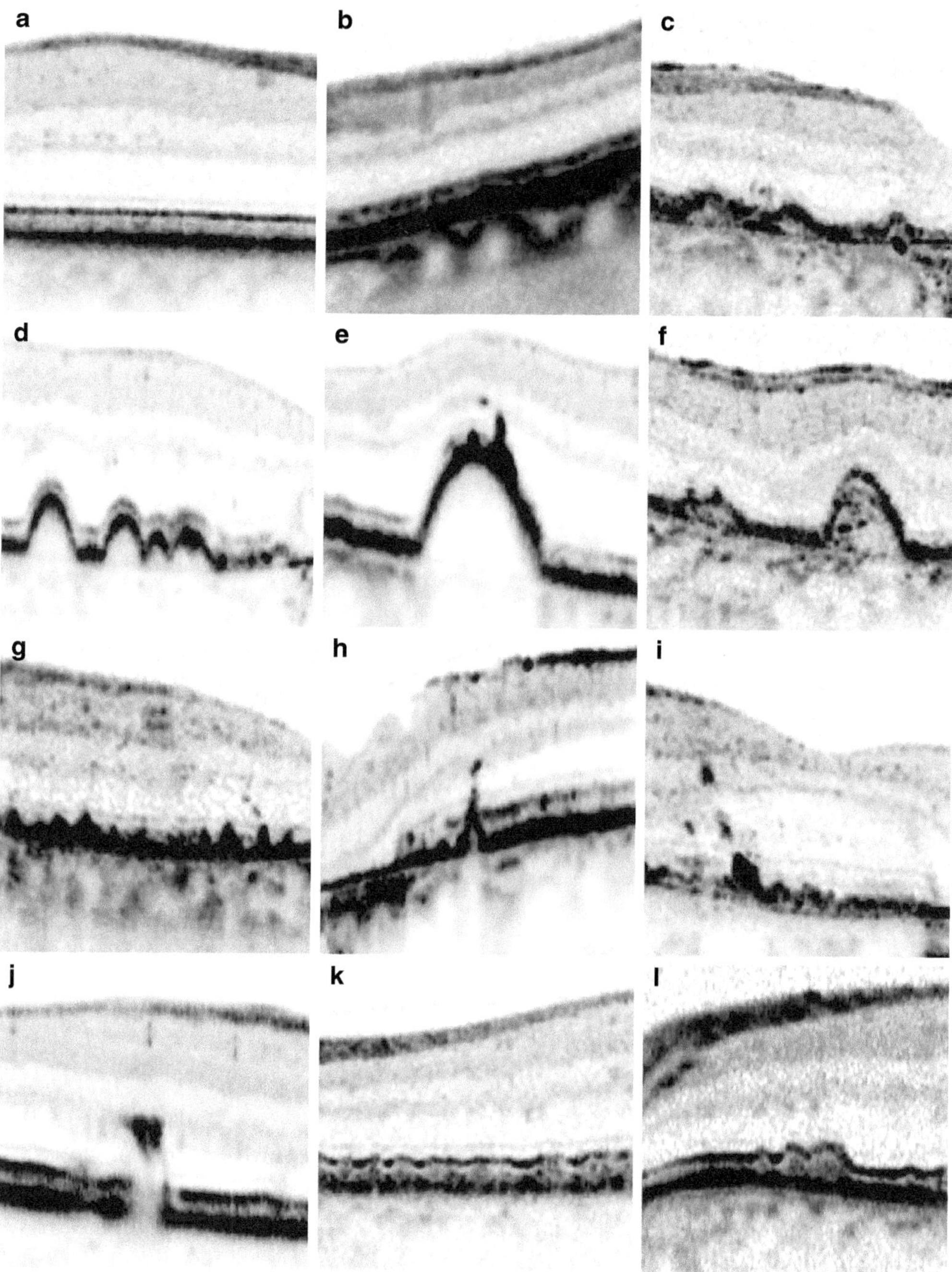

Fig. 14.5 Alterations of the perilesional zone. (**a**) SD-OCT scan obtained from a clinically normal appearing retina. (**b**) SD-OCT showing thickening of the RPE-BM complex. (**c**) SD-OCT showing elongation and elevation of the RPE-BM complex with plaques beneath. (**d**) SD-OCT showing dome-shaped elevations with preserved layers above. (**e**) SD-OCT showing dome-shaped elevation with clumps at the top. (**f**) SD-OCT showing dome-shaped elevation with backscattering material beneath. (**g**) SD-OCT showing apical extensions of the RPE-BM complex. (**h**) SD-OCT showing a spike with a clump at the tip. (**i**) SD-OCT showing clumps at different retinal levels. (**j**) SD-OCT showing a clump in the OPL with disrupted bands beneath. (**k**) SD-OCT showing small elevations of the ellipsoid zone and mottled RPE-BM complex. (**l**) SD-OCT showing increased distance between both bands (Figure copyright: Fleckenstein et al. 2008)

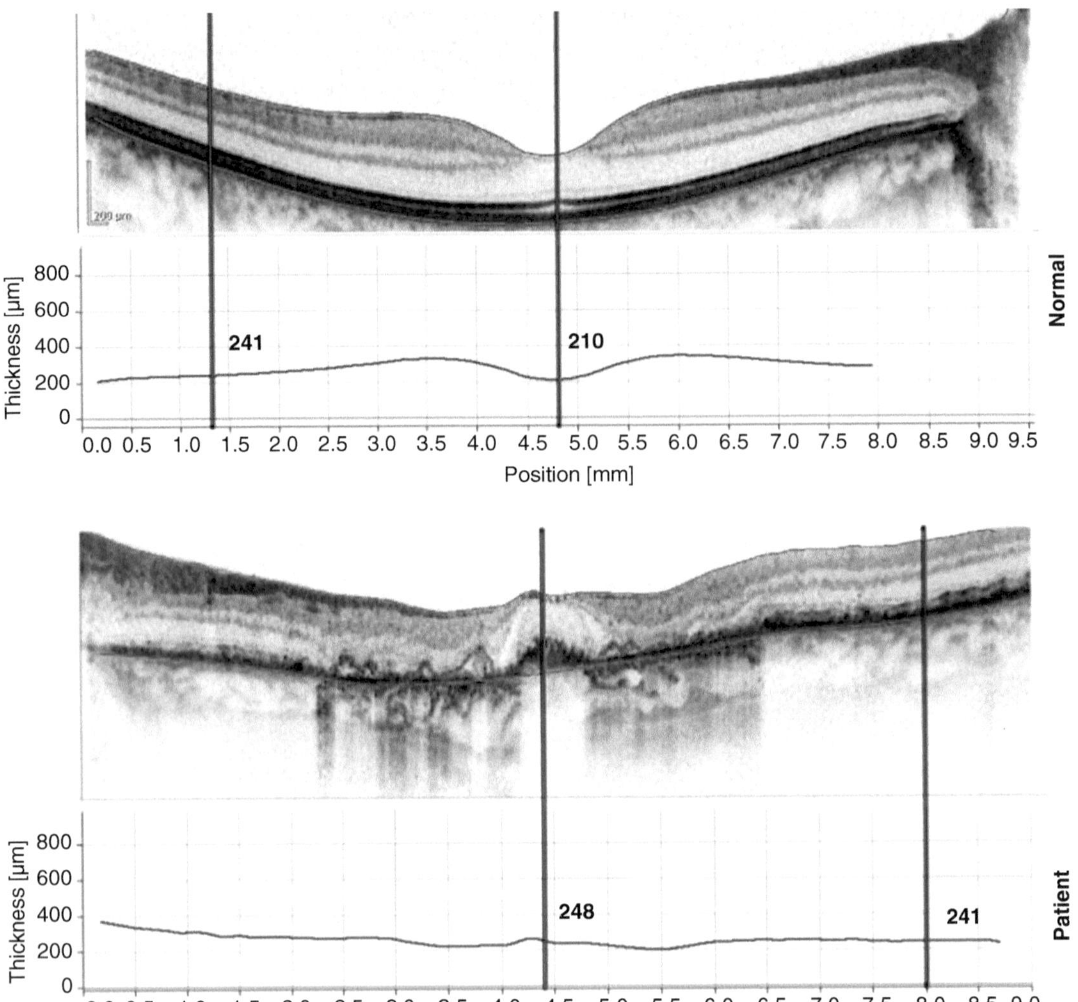

Fig. 14.6 Comparison of the foveal structure as observed in SD-OCT in a clinically healthy retina of a right eye (*upper panel*) and a left eye with GA and foveal sparing (*lower panel*). Underneath the SD-OCT images, retinal thickness curves are shown. In GA with foveal sparing, the subfoveal retinal thickness is increased as compared to the surrounding atrophic areas. The inner retinal layers appeared distorted and moved into the perifoveal atrophy (Image obtained from Schmitz-Valckenberg et al. (2009), with permission)

retinal layers together with this foveal swelling leads to a loss of the usual concave configuration of the foveal pit. Instead the inner retinal layers show a convex shape. The inner retinal layers appear to be distorted and to have a tendency toward perifoveal atrophy. At the site of atrophy, marked retinal thinning and the absence of the characteristic morphology of outer retinal layers are present (Schmitz-Valckenberg et al. 2009). At the edge between atrophy and spared fovea, so-called "wedge" hyperreflective structures ranging from the inner portion of the RPE-BM complex to the inner limit of the outer plexiform layer can be found in 70 % of the cases (Mones et al. 2012).

14.6 Evaluation of the Choroid in Geographic Atrophy

Choriocapillary atrophy is a well-described feature of GA in AMD (Green and Key 1977; Sarks et al. 1988), and a more general involvement of the choroid in the process of atrophy development has been hypothesized (Friedman 1997, 2004, 2008). Several recent studies made advantage of the newly developed enhanced depth imaging (EDI) modality in SD-OCT devices that enables the evaluation of structures beyond the Bruch's membrane, in particular the entire choroid and the choroido-scleral interface (Fig. 14.6a). Thereby reproducible measurement of choroidal thickness (CT) becomes possible (Margolis and Spaide 2009; Spaide et al. 2008). Works on early stages of AMD have revealed controversial results finding the CT decreased or unchanged in these patients (Adhi et al. 2014; Chung et al. 2011; Coscas et al. 2014; Jonas et al. 2014; Jirarattanasopa et al. 2012; Kang et al. 2014; Kim et al. 2011; Koizumi et al. 2011; Lee et al. 2013; Manjunath et al. 2011; Noori et al. 2012; Sigler and Randolph 2013; Wood et al. 2011). In contrast, three recent studies have assessed CT in GA in particular and consistently find that the choroid is thinned in eyes with this late-stage manifestation of AMD (Adhi et al. 2014; Lee et al. 2013; Lindner et al. 2015) (Fig. 14.6b). The extent of thinning exceeds the dimension that could be attributable to choriocapillary thinning alone; thus these findings suggest a more general role of the choroid in GA. Yet the extent of choroidal thinning seems to be different in distinct subtypes of GA (Lindner et al. 2015). Longitudinal data assessing whether GA development precedes choroidal thinning or vice versa are still missing.

Two recent developments may add to the understanding of choroidal changes in geographic atrophy in the future. Long-wavelength OCT devices provide an enhanced visibility of sub-RPE structures analogously to the EDI mode but with even higher contrast that could well enable automated segmentation of even very thick choroids (Kajic et al. 2012; Haas et al. 2014). In addition the phase variance OCT enables visualization of moving tissues, i.e., the blood circulating through the choroid including the choriocapillaris (Kim et al. 2013; Mahmud et al. 2013; Schwartz et al. 2013). By this method, individual visualization of Haller's layer, Sattler's layer, and the choriocapillaris appears to be achievable and has therefore the potential to give a more detailed view on the changes occurring in the choroid in GA (Kim et al. 2013). Besides studying the pathogenesis of GA, visualization of the choroid by SD-OCT becomes additionally relevant for tracking GA progression. The signal from the choroid is usually obscured by the RPE. In areas of GA, where the RPE is missing, an increased signal from the RPE can be detected, resulting in a sharp contrast between atrophic and non-atrophic retina (Chen et al. 2013; Hu et al. 2013; Schmitz-Valckenberg et al. 2011; Yehoshua et al. 2013).

14.7 Atrophy Area Quantification in SD-OCT Images

For studying natural history and to obtain a sensitive outcome measure for therapeutic trials in geographic atrophy, it is of particular importance to determine the size of the GA and its change over time. Today atrophy area as determined in blue FAF cSLO images is widely accepted to perform this task. GA area quantification in FAF images has additionally been accepted as an outcome measure for clinical trials by the Food and Drug Administration (FDA). However, the blue-light-excited autofluorescence wavelengths are obscured by the macula pigment; therefore, using this method alone might reach its limits when measuring atrophy borders in close proximity to the fovea. For this reason, several recent works aim to establish methods to quantify atrophic areas in high-density SD-OCT volume scans or reconstructed en face OCT images (Baumann et al. 2010; Chen et al. 2013; Diniz et al. 2015; Gotzinger et al. 2008; Hu et al. 2013; Lujan et al. 2009; Nunes et al. 2013; Schmitz-Valckenberg et al. 2011; Yehoshua et al. 2013) (Fig. 14.7).

Outer retinal atrophy leads to a remarkable decrease in retinal thickness; it was therefore tested if retinal thickness maps could serve for the measurement of GA areas (Schutze et al. 2011). Yet, Schutze et al. showed that this method is prone to errors and did not achieve good agreements with FAF measurements (Schutze et al. 2011). These observations highlight the need for refined atrophy segmentation strategies in SD-OCT scans.

A possible more precise approach is the analysis of a particular retinal layer in SD-OCT. The area of enhanced choroidal contrast revealed to exhibit a good correlation with the atrophy margins as visualized in FAF suggesting that the latter could be a helpful structure to determine GA size in SD-OCT scans (Sayegh et al. 2011; Schmitz-Valckenberg et al. 2011). Recent advances in the analysis of en face SD-OCT projections and so-called sub-RPE slabs (en face OCT images created of the portion of OCT signal arising from beneath the RPE) facilitate the delineation of the choroidal contrast-enriched area (i.e., the atrophy, Fig. 14.8)

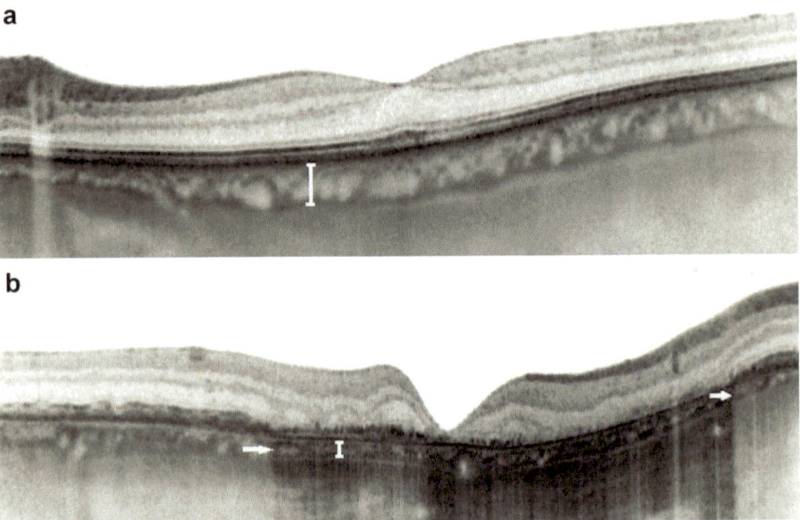

Fig. 14.7 SD-OCT scan obtained in EDI mode through the fovea of a clinically healthy macula (**a**) and a macula of an eye with GA (**b**). A notable thinning of the choroid as measured from the inner part of band 4 to the choroido-scleral margin (*white bars*) can be observed comparing (b) to (a). There is no apparent relationship between GA border (*arrow*) and thinning of the choroid

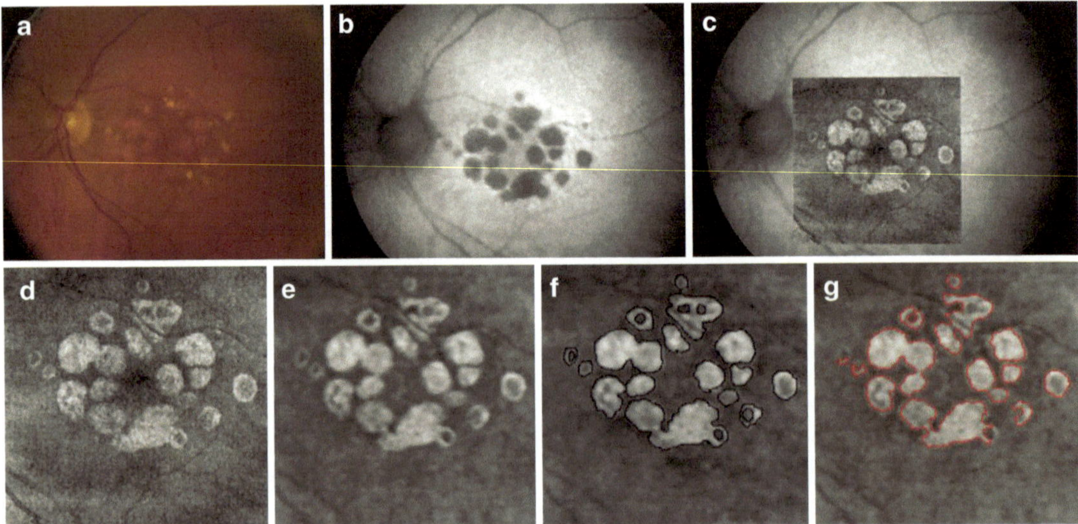

Fig. 14.8 Automated GA detection in an SD-OCT volume scan. Example of a geographic atrophy as imaged in color fundus photography (**a**), fundus autofluorescence (**b**), and en face SD-OCT reconstruction projected into an autofluorescence image (**c**). SD-OCT en face image as shown in (c) (**d**) and corresponding sub-RPE slab (**e**). Demarcation of the GA area (**f**) manually outlined and (**g**) outlined by automatic segmentation algorithm in a sub-RPE slab image (Image obtained from Yehoshua et al. (2013), with permission)

(Chen et al. 2013; Hu et al. 2013; Lujan et al. 2009; Schutze et al. 2011; Yehoshua et al. 2011; Yehoshua et al. 2013). Recent works additionally showed that good intergrader agreements can be obtained for deciding on foveal involvement into the atrophy and for atrophy width measurement (Forte et al. 2013; Moussa et al. 2015). Another new approach is based on the segmentation of the RPE in polarization-sensitive (PS)-OCT, based on that layer's depolarizing character (Gotzinger et al. 2008). On this basis, a novel segmentation algorithm was developed that allows automatic segmentation of atrophic zones (Fig. 14.9) (Baumann et al. 2010).

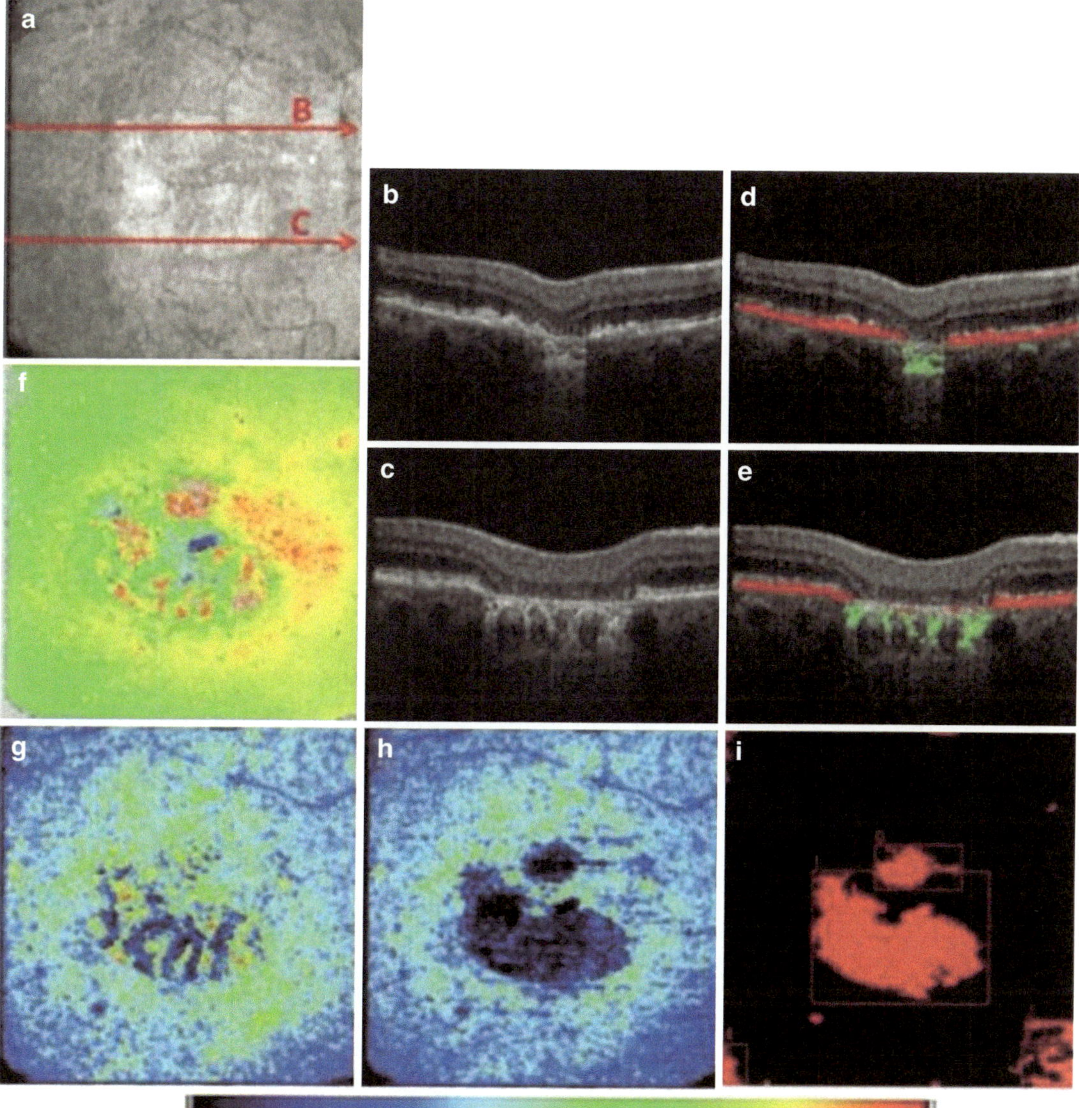

Fig. 14.9 Determination of geographic atrophy area using polarization-sensitive SD-OCT scans. (**a**) En face image reconstructed from an SD-OCT volume scan. (**b–e**) Single scans obtained as demarked in (a). (**d**, **e**) Overlay of the SD-OCT scans shown in (b) and (c), respectively, with depolarizing structures. An evaluation band is demarked to evaluate only depolarizing structures of interest (highlighted in red, mainly corresponding to the RPE). (**f**) Retinal thickness map. (**g**, **h**) Maps of depolarizing pixels throughout the whole imaging depth (**g**) and only within the evaluation band (**h**). (**i**) Binary map as calculated from (h). *Red areas* represent detected atrophy (Image obtained from Baumann et al. (2010), with permission)

References

Adhi M, Lau M, Liang MC, Waheed NK, Duker JS (2014) Analysis of the thickness and vascular layers of the choroid in eyes with geographic atrophy using spectral-domain optical coherence tomography. Retina 34:306–312

Ahlers C, Gotzinger E, Pircher M, Golbaz I, Prager F, Schutze C, Baumann B, Hitzenberger CK, Schmidt-Erfurth U (2010) Imaging of the retinal pigment epithelium in age-related macular degeneration using polarization-sensitive optical coherence tomography. Invest Ophthalmol Vis Sci 51: 2149–2157

Baumann B, Gotzinger E, Pircher M, Sattmann H, Schuutze C, Schlanitz F, Ahlers C, Schmidt-Erfurth U, Hitzenberger CK (2010) Segmentation and quantification of retinal lesions in age-related macular degeneration using polarization-sensitive optical coherence tomography. J Biomed Opt 15:061704

Bearelly S, Chau FY, Koreishi A, Stinnett SS, Izatt JA, Toth CA (2009) Spectral domain optical coherence tomography imaging of geographic atrophy margins. Ophthalmology 116:1762–1769

Bonnet C, Querques G, Zerbib J, Oubraham H, Garavito RB, Puche N, Souied EH (2014) Hyperreflective pyramidal structures on optical coherence tomography in geographic atrophy areas. Retina 34:1524–1530

Brar M, Kozak I, Cheng L, Bartsch DU, Yuson R, Nigam N, Oster SF, Mojana F, Freeman WR (2009) Correlation between spectral-domain optical coherence tomography and fundus autofluorescence at the margins of geographic atrophy. Am J Ophthalmol 148: 439–444

Chen Q, de Sisternes L, Leng T, Zheng L, Kutzscher L, Rubin DL (2013) Semi-automatic geographic atrophy segmentation for SD-OCT images. Biom Opt Express 4:2729–2750

Chung SE, Kang SW, Lee JH, Kim YT (2011) Choroidal thickness in polypoidal choroidal vasculopathy and exudative age-related macular degeneration. Ophthalmology 118:840–845

Coscas F, Puche N, Coscas G, Srour M, Francais C, Glacet-Bernard A, Querques G, Souied EH (2014) Comparison of macular choroidal thickness in adult onset foveomacular vitelliform dystrophy and age-related macular degeneration. Invest Ophthalmol Vis Sci 55:64–69

Diniz B, Rodger DC, Chavali V, MacKay T, Lee SY, Stambolian D, Sadda SV (2015) Drusen and RPE atrophy automated quantification by optical coherence tomography in an elderly population. Eye (Lond) 29:272–279

Fleckenstein M, CharbelIssa P, Helb HM, Schmitz-Valckenberg S, Finger RP, Scholl HP, Loeffler KU, Holz FG (2008) High-resolution spectral domain-OCT imaging in geographic atrophy associated with age-related macular degeneration. Invest Ophthalmol Vis Sci 49:4137–4144

Fleckenstein M, Schmitz-Valckenberg S, Adrion C, Kramer I, Eter N, Helb HM, Brinkmann CK, CharbelIssa P, Mansmann U, Holz FG (2010) Tracking progression with spectral-domain optical coherence tomography in geographic atrophy caused by age-related macular degeneration. Invest Ophthalmol Vis Sci 51:3846–3852

Fleckenstein M, Schmitz-Valckenberg S, Martens C, Kosanetzky S, Brinkmann CK, Hageman GS, Holz FG (2011) Fundus autofluorescence and spectral-domain optical coherence tomography characteristics in a rapidly progressing form of geographic atrophy. Invest Ophthalmol Vis Sci 52:3761–3766

Forte R, Querques G, Querques L, Leveziel N, Benhamou N, Souied EH (2013) Multimodal evaluation of foveal sparing in patients with geographical atrophy due to age-related macular degeneration. Retina 33: 482–489

Friedman E (1997) A hemodynamic model of the pathogenesis of age-related macular degeneration. Am J Ophthalmol 124:677–682

Friedman E (2004) Update of the vascular model of AMD. Br J Ohthalmol 88:161–163

Friedman E (2008) The pathogenesis of age-related macular degeneration. Am J Ophthalmol 146:348–349

Friedman DS, O'Colmain BJ, Munoz B, Tomany SC, McCarty C, de Jong PT, Nemesure B, Mitchell P, Kempen J (2004) Prevalence of age-related macular degeneration in the United States. Arch Ophthalmol 122:564–572

Gotzinger E, Pircher M, Geitzenauer W, Ahlers C, Baumann B, Michels S, Schmidt-Erfurth U, Hitzenberger CK (2008) Retinal pigment epithelium segmentation by polarization sensitive optical coherence tomography. Opt Express 16:16410–16422

Green WR, Key SN 3rd (1977) Senile macular degeneration: a histopathologic study. Trans Am Ophthalmol Soc 75:180–254

Haas P, Esmaeelpour M, Ansari-Shahrezaei S, Drexler W, Binder S (2014) Choroidal thickness in patients with reticular pseudodrusen using 3D-1060 nm OCT maps. Invest Ophthalmol Vis Sci 55:2674

Hariri A, Nittala MG, Sadda SR (2014) Outer retinal tubulation as a predictor of the enlargement amount of geographic atrophy in age-related macular degeneration. Ophthalmology 122:407–413

Hu Z, Medioni GG, Hernandez MT, Hariri A, Wu X, Sadda SR (2013) Segmentation of the geographic atrophy in spectral-domain optical coherence tomography and fundus autofluorescence images. Invest Ophthalmol Vis Sci 54:8375–8383

Jirarattanasopa P, Ooto S, Nakata I, Tsujikawa A, Yamashiro K, Oishi A, Yoshimura N (2012) Choroidal thickness, vascular hyperpermeability, and complement factor H in age-related macular degeneration and polypoidal choroidal vasculopathy. Invest Ophthalmol Vis Sci 53:3663–3672

Jonas JB, Forster TM, Steinmetz P, Schlichtenbrede FC, Harder BC (2014) Choroidal thickness in age-related macular degeneration. Retina 34:1149–1155

Kajic V, Esmaeelpour M, Povazay B, Marshall D, Rosin PL, Drexler W (2012) Automated choroidal segmentation of 1060 nm OCT in healthy and pathologic eyes using a statistical model. Biom Opt Express 3:86–103

Kang HM, Kwon HJ, Yi JH, Lee CS, Lee SC (2014) Subfoveal choroidal thickness as a potential predictor of visual outcome and treatment response after intravitreal ranibizumab injections for typical exudative age-related macular degeneration. Am J Ophthalmol 157:1013–1021

Kim SW, Oh J, Kwon SS, Yoo J, Huh K (2011) Comparison of choroidal thickness among patients with healthy eyes, early age-related maculopathy, neovascular age-related macular degeneration, central serous chorioretinopathy, and polypoidal choroidal vasculopathy. Retina 31:1904–1911

Kim DY, Fingler J, Zawadzki RJ, Park SS, Morse LS, Schwartz DM, Fraser SE, Werner JS (2013) Optical imaging of the chorioretinal vasculature in the living human eye. Proceedings of the National Academy of Sciences of the United States of America

Klaver CC, Wolfs RC, Vingerling JR, Hofman A, de Jong PT (1998) Age-specific prevalence and causes of blindness and visual impairment in an older population: the Rotterdam Study. Arch Ophthalmol 116: 653–658

Klein R, Klein BE, Tomany SC, Meuer SM, Huang GH (2002) Ten-year incidence and progression of age-related maculopathy: The Beaver Dam eye study. Ophthalmology 109:1767–1779

Koizumi H, Yamagishi T, Yamazaki T, Kawasaki R, Kinoshita S (2011) Subfoveal choroidal thickness in typical age-related macular degeneration and polypoidal choroidal vasculopathy. Graefe's Arch Clin Exp Ophthalmol 249:1123–1128

Lee JY, Lee DH, Yoon YH (2013) Correlation between subfoveal choroidal thickness and the severity or progression of nonexudative age-related macular degeneration. Invest Ophthalmol Vis Sci 54:7812–7818

Lindner M, Bezatis A, Czauderna J, Becker E, Brinkmann CK, Schmitz-Valckenberg S, Fimmers R, Holz FG, Fleckenstein M (2015) Choroidal thickness in geographic atrophy secondary to age-related macular degeneration. Invest Ophthalmol Vis Sci 56:875–882

Lujan BJ, Rosenfeld PJ, Gregori G, Wang F, Knighton RW, Feuer WJ, Puliafito CA (2009) Spectral domain optical coherence tomographic imaging of geographic atrophy. Ophthalmic Surg Lasers Imaging Off J Int Soc Imaging Eye. 40:96–101

Maguire P, Vine AK (1986) Geographic atrophy of the retinal pigment epithelium. Am J Ophthalmol 102:621–625

Mahmud MS, Cadotte DW, Vuong B, Sun C, Luk TW, Mariampillai A, Yang VX (2013) Review of speckle and phase variance optical coherence tomography to visualize microvascular networks. J Biomed Opt 18:50901

Manjunath V, Goren J, Fujimoto JG, Duker JS (2011) Analysis of choroidal thickness in age-related macular degeneration using spectral-domain optical coherence tomography. Am J Ophthalmol 152:663–668

Margolis R, Spaide RF (2009) A pilot study of enhanced depth imaging optical coherence tomography of the choroid in normal eyes. Am J Ophthalmol 147:811–815

Michels S, Pircher M, Geitzenauer W, Simader C, Gotzinger E, Findl O, Schmidt-Erfurth U, Hitzenberger CK (2008) Value of polarisation-sensitive optical coherence tomography in diseases affecting the retinal pigment epithelium. Br J Opthalmol 92:204–209

Mitchell P, Smith W, Attebo K, Wang JJ (1995) Prevalence of age-related maculopathy in Australia. The Blue Mountains Eye Study. Ophthalmology 102:1450–1460

Mones J, Biarnes M, Trindade F (2012) Hyporeflective wedge-shaped band in geographic atrophy secondary to age-related macular degeneration: an underreported finding. Ophthalmology 119:1412–1419

Mones J, Biarnes M, Trindade F, Arias L, Alonso J (2013) Optical coherence tomography assessment of apparent foveal swelling in patients with foveal sparing secondary to geographic atrophy. Ophthalmology 120:829–836

Moussa K, Lee JY, Stinnett SS, Jaffe GJ (2013) Spectral domain optical coherence tomography-determined morphologic predictors of age-related macular degeneration-associated geographic atrophy progression. Retina 33:1590–1599

Moussa NB, Georges A, Capuano V, Merle B, Souied EH, Querques G (2015) Multi Color imaging in the evaluation of geographic atrophy due to age-related macular degeneration. Br J Ohthalmol 99:842–847

Noori J, RiaziEsfahani M, Hajizadeh F, Zaferani MM (2012) Choroidal mapping; a novel approach for evaluating choroidal thickness and volume. J Ophthalmic Vis Res 7:180–185

Nunes RP, Gregori G, Yehoshua Z, Stetson PF, Feuer W, Moshfeghi AA, Rosenfeld PJ (2013) Predicting the progression of geographic atrophy in age-related macular degeneration with SD-OCT en face imaging of the outer retina. Ophthalmic Surg Lasers Imaging Retina 44:344–359

Ooto S, Vongkulsiri S, Sato T, Suzuki M, Curcio CA, Spaide RF (2014) Outer retinal corrugations in age-related macular degeneration. JAMA Ophthalmol 132:806–813

Sarks JP, Sarks SH, Killingsworth MC (1988) Evolution of geographic atrophy of the retinal pigment epithelium. Eye (Lond) 2:552–577

Sayegh RG, Simader C, Scheschy U, Montuoro A, Kiss C, Sacu S, Kreil DP, Prunte C, Schmidt-Erfurth U (2011) A systematic comparison of spectral-domain optical coherence tomography and fundus autofluorescence in patients with geographic atrophy. Ophthalmology 118:1844–1851

Sayegh RG, Kiss CG, Simader C, Kroisamer J, Montuoro A, Mittermuller TJ, Azhary M, Bolz M, Kreil DP, Schmidt-Erfurth U (2014) A systematic correlation of morphology and function using spectral domain optical coherence tomography and microperimetry in patients with geographic atrophy. Br J Ophthalmol 98:1050–1055

Schmitz-Valckenberg S, Fleckenstein M, Helb HM, CharbelIssa P, Scholl HP, Holz FG (2009) In vivo imaging of foveal sparing in geographic atrophy secondary to age-related macular degeneration. Invest Ophthalmol Vis Sci 50:3915–3921

Schmitz-Valckenberg S, Fleckenstein M, Gobel AP, Hohman TC, Holz FG (2011) Optical coherence tomography and autofluorescence findings in areas with geographic atrophy due to age-related macular degeneration. Invest Ophthalmol Vis Sci 52:1–6

Schutze C, Ahlers C, Sacu S, Mylonas G, Sayegh R, Golbaz I, Matt G, Stock G, Schmidt-Erfurth U (2011) Performance of OCT segmentation procedures to assess morphology and extension in geographic atrophy. Acta Ophthalmol 89:235–240

Schwartz DM, Fingler J, Kim DY, Zawadzki RJ, Morse LS, Park SS, Fraser SE, Werner JS (2013) Phase-variance optical coherence tomography: a new technique for non-invasive angiography. Ophthalmology 121:180–187

Sigler EJ, Randolph JC (2013) Comparison of macular choroidal thickness among patients older than age 65 with early atrophic age-related macular degeneration and normals. Invest Ophthalmol Vis Sci 54:6307–6313

Spaide RF, Koizumi H, Pozzoni MC (2008) Enhanced depth imaging spectral-domain optical coherence tomography. Am J Ophthalmol 146:496–500

Stetson PF, Yehoshua Z, Garcia Filho CA, PortellaNunes R, Gregori G, Rosenfeld PJ (2014) OCT minimum intensity as a predictor of geographic atrophy enlargement. Invest Ophthalmol Vis Sci 55:792–800

Sunness JS, Bressler NM, Maguire MG (1995) Scanning laser ophthalmoscopic analysis of the pattern of visual loss in age-related geographic atrophy of the macula. Am J Ophthalmol 119:143–151

Sunness JS, Gonzalez-Baron J, Applegate CA, Bressler NM, Tian Y, Hawkins B, Barron Y, Bergman A (1999) Enlargement of atrophy and visual acuity loss in the geographic atrophy form of age-related macular degeneration. Ophthalmology 106:1768–1779

Wolf-Schnurrbusch UE, Enzmann V, Brinkmann CK, Wolf S (2008) Morphologic changes in patients with geographic atrophy assessed with a novel spectral OCT-SLO combination. Invest Ophthalmol Vis Sci 49: 3095–3099

Wood A, Binns A, Margrain T, Drexler W, Povazay B, Esmaeelpour M, Sheen N (2011) Retinal and choroidal thickness in early age-related macular degeneration. Am J Ophthalmol 152:1030–1038.e1032

Wu Z, Luu CD, Ayton LN, Goh JK, Lucci LM, Hubbard WC, Hageman JL, Hageman GS, Guymer RH (2014) Optical coherence tomography-defined changes preceding the development of drusen-associated atrophy in age-related macular degeneration. Ophthalmology 121:2415–2422

Yehoshua Z, Rosenfeld PJ, Gregori G, Feuer WJ, Falcao M, Lujan BJ, Puliafito C (2011) Progression of geographic atrophy in age-related macular degeneration imaged with spectral domain optical coherence tomography. Ophthalmology 118:679–686

Yehoshua Z, Garcia Filho CA, Penha FM, Gregori G, Stetson PF, Feuer WJ, Rosenfeld PJ (2013) Comparison of geographic atrophy measurements from the OCT fundus image and the sub-RPE slab image. Ophthalmic Surg Lasers Imaging Retina 44:127–132

Zweifel SA, Engelbert M, Laud K, Margolis R, Spaide RF, Freund KB (2009) Outer retinal tubulation: a novel optical coherence tomography finding. Arch Ophthalmol 127:1596–1602

15 Neovascular Age-Related Macular Degeneration

Reinhard Told, Sebastian M. Waldstein, and Ursula Schmidt-Erfurth

Contents

R. Told, MD, PhD
Department of Ophthalmology, Medical University of Vienna, Vienna, Austria
e-mail: reinhard.told@meduniwien.ac.at

S.M. Waldstein, MD • U. Schmidt-Erfurth, MD (✉)
Department of Ophthalmology and Optometry, Medical University of Vienna, Vienna, Austria
e-mail: ursula.schmidt-erfurth@meduniwien.ac.at

15.1 Introduction

Since OCT's invention over 20 years ago (Fercher et al. 1993; Huang et al. 1991; Swanson et al. 1993), it has become important for visualizing static and, nowadays, dynamic retinal tissue properties. The invention of spectral domain OCT (SD-OCT) about 10 years later (de Boer et al. 2003; Wojtkowski et al. 2002) revolutionized ophthalmic imaging once more. Visualization of microstructural changes in the retina and surrounding tissues became possible with scan averaging (Sakamoto et al. 2008), active eye-tracking, raster scanning patterns, enhanced depth imaging (EDI) (Spaide et al. 2008), and 1050-nm light sources for

C.H. Meyer et al. (eds.), *Spectral Domain Optical Coherence Tomography in Macular Diseases*, DOI 10.1007/978-81-322-3610-8_15

deeper tissue penetration (Unterhuber et al. 2005). These techniques allowed ophthalmologists to assign specific anatomical compartments and retinal layers and accurately compare changes in the course of disease. Neovascular age-related macular degeneration (nAMD) is one of the diseases that has benefited most from advancements in OCT technology (Geitzenauer et al. 2011). Consequently, noninvasive SD-OCT imaging has become essential in nAMD diagnosis and follow-up in daily clinical routine.

15.2 Neovascular Age-Related Macular Degeneration (nAMD) Classification

Historically, nAMD was classified based on fluorescein angiography, which located the choroidal neovascularization (CNV) complex in relation to the retinal pigment epithelium (RPE) layer and laid the basis for our current OCT-based classification (Macular-Photocoagulation-Study-Group 1991). The first pattern was described as *occult CNV* lesions or "poorly defined forms of CNV with no directly identifiable neovascular vessels." In the occult pattern, the CNV lesion lies beneath the RPE, which makes it more difficult to angiographically distinguish it from unaffected regions. In the early phase, occult CNVs are characterized by fibrovascular pigment epithelial detachment (PED) appearing as stippled hyperfluorescence followed by persistent staining or leakage in the overlying subretinal space. Finally, late-stage leakage of indeterminate origin visible as "speckled hyperfluorescence" with blurry borders and pooling in the overlying retinal layers becomes apparent.

Classic CNV lesions are located between the RPE and the neurosensory retina and were defined as "an area of well-demarcated choroidal hyperfluorescence." During angiography, a marked leakage from the CNV becomes evident, and the spreading of the diffuse leakage blurs the margin of the membrane in the late phase (Freund et al. 1993).

The description of *occult CNV* lesions became more refined with the advent of indocyanine green (ICG) angiography as the near-infrared transmission of ICG allows a detailed look under the RPE and thus at the choroidal vasculature (Bischoff and Flower 1985). Occult CNV shows changing patterns during ICG angiography. Hot spots and ICG plaques are descriptions for well-defined changes in the mid to late phase and are located within the same area as the occult CNV lesion in fluorescein angiography (FA). Classic CNV lesions are hard to discriminate in ICG angiography because the surrounding vascular tissue emits an intense fluorescence signal (Gelisken et al. 1998).

As early as 1994, it was suggested that CNV classification should be based on structure and anatomical location (Gass 1994). This idea received little attention because of the lack of technology to adequately image CNV lesions. Regard for Gass' approach changed dramatically when OCT technology became available. However, the approach was not adopted until the use of SD-OCT systems became widespread as the resolution and speed of its predecessor, time domain (TD)-OCT, was inadequate for detailed analysis of CNV. In 2010, CNV classification was adapted using FA and OCT characteristics: CNV lesions were divided into type 1 (corresponding to occult CNV), type 2 (corresponding to classic CNV), and type 3 intraretinal neovascularization (retinal angiomatous proliferation, RAP) (Yannuzzi et al. 2001; Zacks and Johnson 2004). Polypoidal choroidal vasculopathy (PCV) was added as a fourth entity, categorized as a subtype of type 1 CNV (Freund et al. 2010). The simultaneous presence of characteristics of types 1, 2, or 3 is referred to as mixed forms of CNV.

Both OCT and FA are essential to reliably distinguish between CNV subtypes. Jung et al. compared the fluorescein angiography classification (Macular-Photocoagulation-Study-Group 1991) and the anatomic classification (FA and SD-OCT) (Freund et al. 2010). They found agreement between the two classification systems to be good; however, the combination of FA and OCT clearly identified more type 3 and mixed lesions, a result – according to Jung et al.– to be expected because of the difficulties in identifying type 3 and mixed neovascularization in fluorescein angiography (Jung et al. 2014).

The European Society of Retina Specialists (EURETINA) Schmidt-Erfurth et al. (2014a), the

American Academy of Ophthalmology (AAO) (AAO 2015), and the Royal College of Ophthalmologists (RCOphth) (Chakravarthy et al. 2013) state that FA and ICG are mandatory for the initial diagnosis of nAMD and provide the base for visualization of neovascular changes as well as dynamic criteria such as perfusion and exudation. The effect of anti-VEGF therapy can be effectively monitored by OCT imaging, preferably by SD-OCT.

15.3 Compartment-Based nAMD Features on Optical Coherence Tomography

Table 15.1 gives an overview of the most important morphologic characteristics occurring in the course of exudative AMD. They are explained in more detail in the following paragraphs.

15.3.1 Subretinal Pigment Epithelium Features

Advances in spectral domain OCT, particularly the EDI mode and swept-source (SS)-OCT using longer wavelengths, allow a closer look at the structures present under the RPE in nAMD. Growth of choroidal neovascularization beneath the RPE causes pigment epithelial detachment (PED), separating Bruch's membrane and the RPE. The appearance of PEDs varies greatly in size and content. PEDs are categorized as serous or fibrovascular based on the PED content on OCT scans (Zayit-Soudry et al. 2007). Serous PEDs are caused by fluid accumulation between the RPE and Bruch's membrane and appear as hyporeflective, dome-shaped lesions on SD-OCT (Fig. 15.1a). Fibrovascular PEDs are often irregularly shaped and filled with moderately hyperreflective content (Fig. 15.1b). However, most lesions are of a mixed configuration, and both serous and fibrovascular components are frequently present in the same eye in the course of nAMD. Various OCT signs associated with PED were reported, yet none became a valid OCT biomarker (prechoroidal cleft, triple-layer sign, hyperreflective line) for CNV activity or RPE tear (Khan et al. 2012; Mukai et al. 2014; Nagiel et al. 2013; Spaide 2009). The results of the VIEW 2 trial, the largest study ever in nAMD therapy with over 1200 patients, show that PED is the primary indi-

Table 15.1 Common nAMD features that can be appreciated on OCT images

OCT feature	Description
PED (pigment epithelial detachment)	Areas of detached pigment epithelium. The lesion is filled with serous fluid and/or fibrovascular tissue
SHRM (subretinal hyperreflective material)	Thickening of the outer reflective band, mostly in association with fibrosis
SRF (subretinal fluid)	Area of low reflectivity between the outer retina and the RPE
IRC (intraretinal cysts)	Intraretinal cystoid areas of low reflectivity
ORT (outer retinal tubulation)	Branching hyporeflective lesion in the outer retina with hyperreflective border
IRF (intraretinal fluid)	Increased retinal thickness with reduced retinal reflectivity; frequently in association with IRC

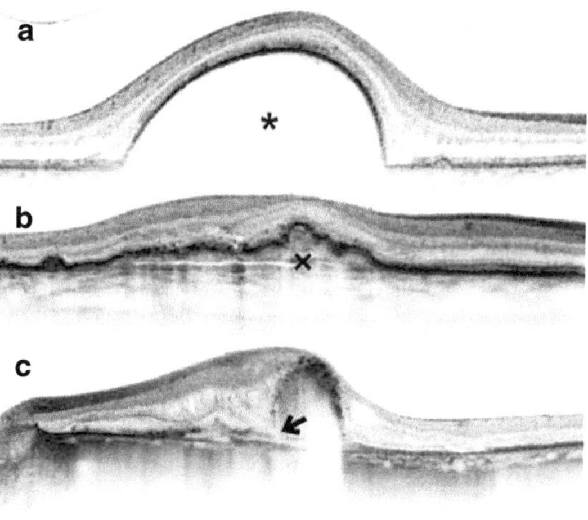

Fig. 15.1 Pigment epithelial detachment (PED). (**a**) Serous PED: SD-OCT showing dome-shaped PED swelling (*) with serous content. (**b**) Fibrovascular PED: SD-OCT showing hyperreflective content (*x*) and irregular contour. (**c**) RPE tear: SD-OCT showing RPE discontinuity (*black arrow*) adjacent to PED after anti-VEGF treatment

cator for progressive nAMD activity and the underlying event for visual loss under PRN (pro re nata, treatment as needed) treatment (Schmidt-Erfurth et al. 2015). PEDs can collapse in response to anti-VEGF therapy due to fibrosis of the fibrovascular content and reduced fluid exudation (Fig. 15.1b).

RPE tears may result during the course of the disease and after anti-VEGF treatment. Eyes with fibrovascular PEDs, where the CNV is attached to the RPE, are especially prone to RPE tears. SD-OCT showed that RPE tears usually occur after the first anti-VEGF treatment, as contraction of the CNV induces tension on bare RPE areas, leading to adjacent tears if the RPE is not stabilized by CNV or attached to Bruch's membrane (Nagiel et al. 2013). Post-tear OCT images reveal a discontinuous RPE layer (Fig. 15.1c).

15.3.2 Subretinal Features

The subretinal compartment is located between the neurosensory retina and the RPE. SD-OCT can visualize type 2 and also type 3 neovascularization at the subretinal site. Neovascularizations appear as hyperreflective, inhomogeneous convolutes (Sulzbacher et al. 2011). Follow-up of patients receiving anti-VEGF therapy shows a shrinking and flattening of the CNV lesion in association with fibrosis, which becomes visible on SD-OCT as a hyperreflective subretinal area (You et al. 2012). However, although the total lesion size does not change significantly under anti-VEGF therapy (Framme et al. 2010; Kiss et al. 2009), the retinal morphology starts reorganizing and CNV stabilizes (You et al. 2012) or regresses with subsequent geographic atrophy development (Channa et al. 2015).

Because the neovascular process takes place in the subretinal space, exudation leads to focal detachments of the neurosensory retina and subretinal fluid (SRF) accumulation. In VIEW 2, SRF was the most frequent OCT finding (84 %) in newly diagnosed nAMD patients (Schmidt-Erfurth et al. 2015). *Subretinal fluid* can be easily detected on OCT as a hyporeflective space under the neurosensory retina (Fig. 15.2a). If subretinal fluid is present in combination with a PED, fluid typically pools on both sides of the PED leading to a triangular configuration of the hyporeflective areas (Fig. 15.2b). Contrary to earlier literature, where SRF was considered a strong sign for CNV activity with the need of immediate treatment (Bolz et al. 2010), there is recent evidence that SRF that is refractory to anti-VEGF treatment still allows the visual improvement to be maintained. Jang et al. suggest that monthly injections should be questioned when refractory SRF is present (Jang et al. 2014).

The optical density ratio of SRF in SD-OCT may help in distinguishing CNV from other entities associated with CNV and fluid exudation such as central serous chorioretinopathy (CSC). It characterizes the optical density of fluids accumulating in the retina in comparison with the optical densities of the vitreous body. Optical densities were reported to be statistically significantly higher in CNV than in other diseases. The component-laden SRF in nAMD is therefore thought to comprise elements potentially toxic to the blood-retinal barrier, resulting in blood-retinal barrier dysfunction. This has been shown to be disadvantageous for visual outcome (Ahlers et al. 2008, 2009).

Subretinal hyperreflective material (SRHM) is mainly associated with type 2 and 3 CNV lesions (Liakopoulos et al. 2008), where neoangiogenetic vessels intrude into the subretinal space (Grossniklaus and Green 2004). With anti-VEGF

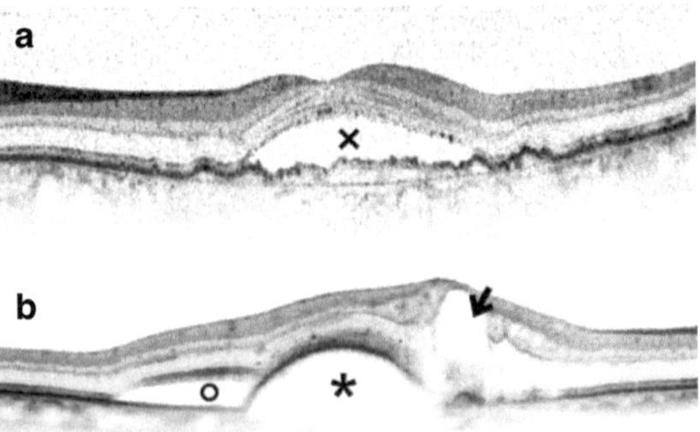

Fig. 15.2 Subretinal fluid. (**a**) SD-OCT showing subretinal fluid (*x*) in neovascular age-related macular degeneration. (**b**) SD-OCT shows serous pigment epithelial detachment (PED, *) with triangular-shaped subretinal fluid (SRF, °) on the left side and cystic changes (IRC) on the right side (*black arrow*)

therapy, these neovascular convolutes reorganize and the fibrous component increases, which leads to the formation of a well-demarcated scar (Fig. 15.3) (Keane et al. 2012). SRHM appears as a subretinal hyperreflective area on OCT images. The functional impact of SRHM was investigated in the CATT study population. Baseline SRHM was found to lead to an increased likelihood of scar formation (Daniel et al. 2014) as well as a continuing loss of visual function (Ying et al. 2014).

15.3.3 Intraretinal Features

The intraretinal compartment is severely affected in nAMD, firstly by neovascularizations type 2 and 3 and secondly by fluid exudations from these lesions. Moreover, late-stage type 1 lesions are frequently associated with intraretinal changes. These morphological changes translate into diffuse retinal swelling/edema and intraretinal cystoid fluid on OCT.

Intraretinal cystoid fluid (IRC) appears as round hyporeflective spaces of various size, predominantly in the inner and outer nuclear layers. IRC usually indicates exudative activity of the underlying CNV. In a recent study, about 40 % of patients developed IRC at least once during the first year after treatment was initiated. In 80 % of patients presenting with exudative cystoid fluid, cystoid fluid reoccurred less than three times during the first year of treatment. Cystoid fluid resolving during the loading interval (first 3 months of anti-VEGF treatment) is referred to as exudative (Fig. 15.4a); cystoid fluid persistent after the first 3 months is considered degenerative cystoid fluid (Fig. 15.4c) (Schmidt-Erfurth et al. 2015). The presence of exudative cystoid fluid is an important finding on OCT as cysts are associated with a higher risk for visual loss associated with fibrosis and atrophy (Gianniou et al. 2015). Therefore, intraretinal cystoid fluid is considered the most relevant prognostic biomarker in nAMD (Ritter et al. 2014). In end-stage AMD, intraretinal cystoid fluid may be present above the atrophic scar, which appears as a hyperreflective and thickened RPE on OCT. A sharp demarcation indicates the borderline between scar with cystoid changes and healthy retina. The presence of degenerative cystoid fluid and an underlying fibrotic scar are thought to be irreversible, and patients may not benefit from further anti-VEGF therapy.

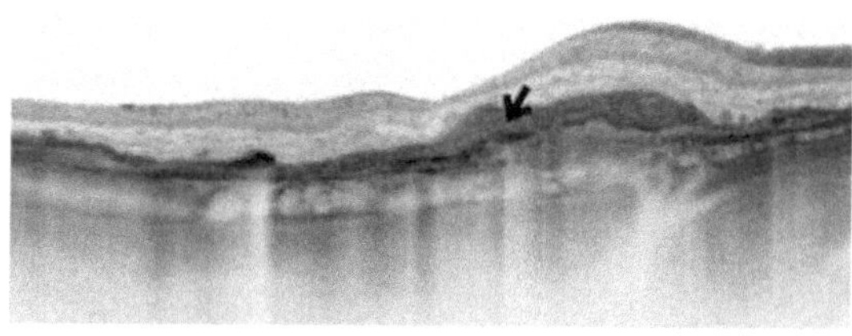

Fig. 15.3 Subretinal hyperreflective material (SHRM). SS-OCT showing subretinal hyperreflective material (*black arrow*) after multiple anti-VEGF injections

15.3.3.1 Outer Retinal Tubulation

Zweifel et al. characterized outer retinal tubulation (ORT) based on OCT. ORTs are branching tubular structures found in the outer nuclear layer (Fig. 15.5); however, ORT are not pathognomonic for nAMD (Zweifel et al. 2009). ORTs are

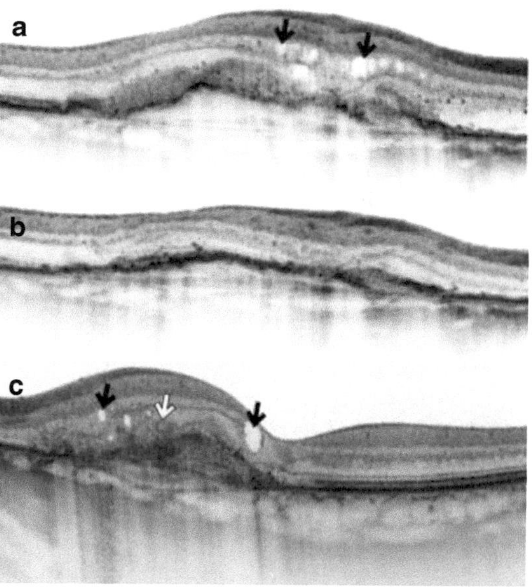

Fig. 15.4 Intraretinal cystoid fluid (IRC). (**a**) SD-OCT showing exudative IRC (*black arrow*) with underlying pigment epithelial detachment before treatment. (**b**) SD-OCT showing resolved IRC one month after antiangiogenetic treatment. (**c**) SS-OCT showing subretinal hyperreflective material (SHRM) with overlying degenerative IRC (*black arrow*) and outer retinal tubulation (ORT, *white arrow*)

present in other eye diseases as well, such as retinitis pigmentosa or in association with angioid streaks (Ellabban et al. 2012; Tulvatana et al. 1999). Histopathological analysis shows that ORTs largely consist of cones in various phases of degeneration lacking outer segments and inner segments, morphologically altered mitochondria, and external limiting membrane delineating the luminal wall (Schaal et al. 2015). On SD-OCT, ORT has a tubelike appearance with hyporeflective centers and hyperreflective borders. En face images reveal branching networks emanating from neovascular lesions (Wolff et al. 2012). When reviewing OCT scans, care must be taken to distinguish ORT from intraretinal cysts or subretinal fluid without a hyperreflective border. ORTs are commonly present outside the foveal central 1-mm area, but progress centrally in the course of the disease (Lee et al. 2014). A recent study based on the CATT (comparison of anti-VEGF treatment trails) population suggests that ORTs are an important finding on OCT as eyes with ORT have significantly worse visual acuity (VA) at baseline and after 2 years than eyes without ORT change (Lee et al. 2014). VA outcomes were consistent with previous findings in which ORT had been associated with significantly worse VA; however, under anti-VEGF treatment, an increase in VA was still recorded (Faria-Correia et al. 2013).

15.3.4 Vitreo-macular Interface

The vitreo-macular interface has gained scientific interest with the availability of high-resolution imaging techniques and raster scanning options. The age group of AMD patients, which is elderly, usually presents with a complete posterior vitreous detachment. This is the antelocation and liquification of the vitreous body and the separation of the vitreous cortex from the retina (Kakehashi et al. 1994). Vitreous adhesions have been found to be more common in the eyes with CNV than in the healthy control eyes (Mojana et al. 2008). A firm adherence of the vitreous is seen at the natural adhesion sites in nAMD (Fig. 15.6). Local inflammatory processes are thought to lead to the vitreous adhesion at the site of CNV (Mayr-Sponer et al. 2013). However, there is currently no evidence that the adhesive vitreous promotes or causes the development of CNV (Waldstein et al. 2012, 2014).

With SD, and more so with SS-OCT (Liu and Zhang 2014), it is possible to visualize and characterize the vitreous attachment. Complete detachment, focal adhesion, and detachment from the macula with adhesion at the optic disc or vessel arcades as well as complete attachment have been described. A retinal angiomatous proliferation (RAP) was present in 88 % of patients with juxtafoveally localized vitreo-macular adhesion, and the adhesion area was colocalized with the area of the RAP. In general, the area of adhesion corresponded directly to the area of CNV (Krebs et al. 2011). A recent study including 255 treatment-naïve patients with nAMD found that the vitreo-macular adhesions resolved in about 40 % after several months of anti-VEGF therapy (Waldstein et al. 2014). The configuration of the vitreo-macular interface has been shown to have an important influence on the visual outcome. Eyes with vitreo-macular adhesion might benefit

Fig. 15.5 Outer retinal tubulation (ORT). SD-OCT showing hyperreflective borders (*white arrow*) as well as SRHM and overlying neurosensory atrophy after multiple anti-VEGF treatments

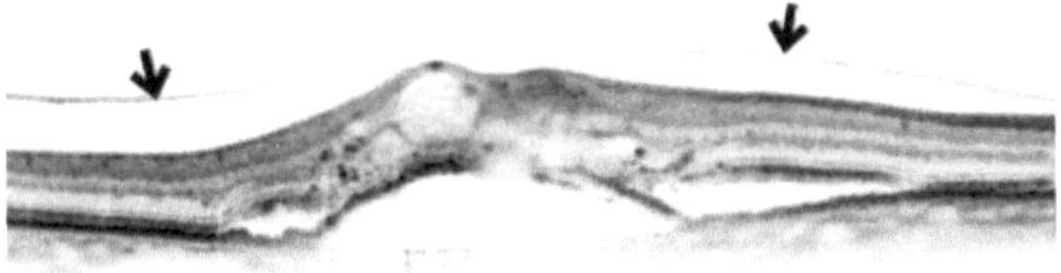

Fig. 15.6 Vitreo-macular adhesion. SD-OCT showing partial posterior vitreous detachment (*black arrow*) in nAMD with serous pigment epithelial detachment (*PED*), subretinal fluid (*SRF*), and intraretinal cystoid fluid (*IRC*)

from a fixed therapy regime with intensive retreatment, whereas eyes with posterior vitreous detachment may achieve adequate disease control with a PRN regime and lower retreatment frequency (Mayr-Sponer et al. 2013).

Besides vitreo-macular adhesion, *vitreo-macular traction* is an important finding in nAMD as it leads to severe disorganization of retinal architecture (Green-Simms and Bakri 2011; Schulze et al. 2008). Vitreo-macular tractions are easily visualized with SD and SS-OCT. The retinal contour and the angle of insertion give information on the nature of the traction and the need for surgery (Duker et al. 2013).

15.4 Neovascular Age-Related Macular Degeneration Subtype Characteristics on SD-OCT

Accurate identification of exudative AMD subtypes and characteristics is a prerequisite when aiming for individualized therapy whereby physicians can predict which patients will respond well in, e.g., a strict monthly or PRN regime. In the following paragraphs, the anatomic classification of CNV based on FA and OCT (Freund et al. 2010) is used to introduce OCT characteristics of the different CNV lesions, which are defined as type 1 (sub-RPE), type 2 (subretinal), type 3 (intraretinal), or mixed. PCV is categorized as a form of type 1 CNV. Types 1, 2, and 3 correspond to occult, classic, and RAP (retinal angiomatous proliferation) lesions in FA angiography.

Jung et al. assessed the frequency of newly diagnosed exudative AMD subtypes with SD-OCT. Type 1 (sub-RPE) was most frequent with 40 %, followed by type 3 (intraretinal) with 34 %, mixed neovascularization because of AMD with 17 %, and type 2 (subretinal) CNV with 9 % (Jung et al. 2014). These findings are in good agreement with other studies, yet the incidence of type 3/RAP was higher, which might be explained firstly by the fact that the current SD-OCT resolution is beneficial for RAP identification (Mathew et al. 2014) and secondly by the large differences in incidence among ethnic groups. RAP incidence has been reported as 0.8–4.5 % in a Japanese cohort (Hirami et al. 2009; Maruko et al. 2007) and 4.5 % in a Chinese cohort (Liu et al. 2007) and is overall rare in African-American AMD patients (Yannuzzi et al. 2008). Type 3 incidence in white patients varies from 10 to 22 % (Gross et al. 2005; Slakter et al. 2000; Yannuzzi et al. 2001).

Various studies have investigated the correlation between fundus fluorescein angiography and SD-OCT. Mathew et al. reported high sensitivity (86–98 %) and specificity (84–100 %) of SD-OCT in identification of nAMD subtypes. Weighted kappa statistics assessing the agreement between fundus (F) FA and SD-OCT showed an almost perfect agreement (0.85) (Mathew et al. 2014). However, a recent meta-analysis that compared the accuracy of OCT with alternative tests, most importantly FA, in monitoring and detecting disease activity, found substantial disagreement between OCT and FA in nAMD follow-up. Although OCT (TD and SD) was highly sensitive, it was moderately specific in determining nAMD activity. Consequently, Castillo and coauthors do not recommend the sole use of OCT for detection of AMD reactivation (Castillo et al. 2015), which is in agreement with current guidelines (AAO 2015; Chakravarthy et al. 2013; Schmidt-Erfurth et al. 2014a, b).

15.4.1 Type 1 Lesion

Type 1 neovascularization corresponds mainly to the occult form of CNV and is defined as hyperreflective areas posterior of the RPE in SD-OCT, which is frequently associated with PED. The 3D en face map of the RPE layer reveals a dome-shaped area with an area of fibrovascular material (Malamos et al. 2009). Enhanced depth imaging (EDI) helps to visualize and localize the content of the whole fibrovascular PED. The en face projection of the hyperreflective material perfectly matches the hyper-fluorescent neovascularization in ICG angiography (Coscas et al. 2012).

Often type 1 CNV lesions are clinically silent for a long time because the overlaying neurosensory retina remains dry and the retinal architecture is maintained. Clinically manifest type 1 CNV lesions are characterized by exudative features on OCT, where mostly subretinal fluid can be seen. Subretinal fluid on OCT is a clear sign to initiate anti-VEGF therapy. With disease progression, disruption of the blood-retinal barrier and alterations of the RPE layer occur, and consequently intraretinal cystoid spaces appear on OCT.

15.4.2 Polypoidal Choroidal Vasculopathy

Today, there is widespread consensus that polypoidal choroidal vasculopathy is a subtype of type 1 nAMD. But whether or not it could be a distinct entity of the choroidal vasculature is still discussed. It has a high prevalence in Asian patients and is more frequent in Asian male than female patients as opposed to Caucasian people where it occurs more often in female than in male patients (Imamura et al. 2010). Clinical signs of polypoidal lesions are very diverse, which is why initial diagnosis is confirmed by ICG angiography, which identifies polypoidal dilatations and branching networks of choroidal vessels.

On SD-OCT, PCV neovascularizations appear as sub-RPE lesions, with multiple large and small PEDs attaching to the outer surface of the RPE, as well as branching communications. With SS-OCT, polypoidal structures were identified between the RPE and Bruch's membrane. Branching vascular networks above and below Bruch's membrane as well as choroidal vascular abnormalities were found. En face OCT maps located under the RPE visualize the entire topography of polypoidal lesions best. This has been shown in SD and SS-OCT systems (Alasil et al. 2015; Imamura et al. 2010; Saito et al. 2008; Sayanagi et al. 2015), the latter systems being superior. En face view may also reveal the "hematocrit sign," describing a lesion where blood is presumed to be separated into corpuscular and serous components (Imamura et al. 2010).

15.4.3 Type 2 Lesion

In type 2 CNV, the RPE layer is penetrated by the neovascular tissue, which grows within the subretinal space. As the origin of the subretinal neovascular complex lies within the choroid, type 2 CNV is connected to a type 1 choroidal lesion. Type 2 neovascular membranes are identified as hyperreflective and thickened areas anterior to the RPE in SD-OCT. Because of the vessel leakage, intraretinal fluid in the form of cysts is one of the first signs visible on OCT. SD-OCT has been shown to be the method of choice in type 2 CNV: FA and ICG angiography underestimate the size of the neovascular complex as the area of the associated edema cannot be delineated in FA and ICG angiography (Sulzbacher et al. 2011). Type 2 lesions usually improve in tissue morphology with anti-VEGF therapy by regress in retinal thickness, RPE regrowth, and ellipsoid zone/interdigitation zone rearrangement, indicating improved tissue function. CNV diameters, however, remained stable, which is particularly true for the occult components of the CNV lesion (Framme et al. 2010; You et al. 2012).

15.4.4 Type 3/Retinal Angiomatous Proliferation

The type 3 AMD subtype is also known as retinal angiomatous proliferation (RAP) and is characterized by neovascularization, presumed to originate from the retina (Sayanagi et al. 2014). Type 3 was first described in 1996 as a deep retinal anomalous complex with advanced Bruch's membrane changes and severe visual loss (Hartnett et al. 1996) and is considered the second most frequent form of AMD (Jung et al. 2014) with varying numbers reported.

Today we know that depending on the stage of the disease, intraretinal neovascularizations are not limited anterior of the RPE, as a retinochoroidal anastomosis is present on SD-OCT in the late stage of the disease (Yannuzzi et al. 2001). Also IRC in combination with PED are a common characteristic (Rouvas et al. 2010; Schmidt-Erfurth et al. 2014). Outer retinal layer disorganization becomes evident on OCT with progression of the disease (Querques et al. 2013).

15.5 Optical Coherence Tomography Biomarkers and Clinical Implications

OCT is currently the most frequently used device in exudative AMD management. Ever since OCT became available, a huge effort has been made to identify OCT biomarkers that facilitate nAMD management and provide solid surrogate variables for treatment response and functional prognosis. In the first approach of defining OCT-guided retreatment criteria for anti-VEGF therapy, Fung et al. were able to show that the number of retreatments could be reduced in the OCT-guided group compared with a fixed treatment regime. The visual acuity outcome of the OCT-based retreatment group was comparable to the fixed regimen used in phase III clinical trials (Fung et al. 2007). However, these favorable initial results could never be replicated on a large scale. Thus, it is essential to understand the precise relation between morphologic retina changes over time and functional outcomes and to establish guidelines for nAMD treatment. The following paragraphs introduce established and promising future OCT criteria.

15.5.1 Central Retinal Thickness (CRT)

CRT was first used in the ANCHOR and MARINA trials and served as a secondary outcome measure (Brown et al. 2006; Rosenfeld et al. 2006). Both studies employed a fixed treatment regimen with monthly intravitreal injections. CRT change became the most frequent criteria for retreatment decisions when nAMD treatment was individualized applying PRN (pro re nata, treatment as needed) treatment based on predefined retreatment criteria (Fung et al. 2007; Holz et al. 2011; Schmidt-Erfurth et al. 2011). The Comparison of Age-Related Macular Degeneration Trials (CATT) later suggested that retreatment should be based on a zero-tolerance strategy of fluid seen on OCT by eradication as early as possible (Martin et al. 2012). Switching from low-resolution TD-OCT to high-resolution SD-OCT by eradication led to more retreatment numbers being reported (Busbee et al. 2013) because the high resolution and large number of scans possible with SD-OCT revealed small occurrences of fluid. Major et al. affirmed the superiority of SD-OCT over TD-OCT as it revealed more exudative disease activity (Major et al. 2014).

Today CRT-based PRN treatment is still the most commonly used regimen in Europe (Schmidt-Erfurth et al. 2014). Therefore, it is not surprising that all recent OCT devices provide false-color-coded retinal thickness maps that give a first impression of macular topography (Fig. 15.7). The maps are usually divided into nine subfields (Early-Treatment-Diabetic-Retinopathy-Study-Group 1985); the center field equates to the CRT, which is defined as the average retinal thickness within a 1-mm circular area centered on the fovea. Great attention should be paid to OCT B scans as increases in retinal thickness comprise a multitude of pathological retinal changes.

Despite its popularity, treatment based solely on CRT is already outdated. CRT only correlates with visual function in treatment-naïve patients and during the loading phase (first 3 months with monthly intravitreal anti-VEGF injections) (Bolz et al. 2010). Simader et al. were able to show that the change in CRT from baseline does not correlate with best-corrected visual acuity (BCVA) after a 3-month loading interval (Simader et al. 2014).

Various pharmaceutical trials have considered the reduction in CRT a therapeutic success, although it is known that CRT is not necessarily associated with improved retinal function (Chakravarthy et al. 2012; Cohen et al. 2013; Martin et al. 2011; Roberts et al. 2014). The mismatch between CRT and BCVA emphasizes the need for OCT biomarkers that better indicate a functional benefit from nAMD therapy.

15.5.1.1 Value for Clinical Routine

As functional outcomes correlate poorly with CRT and subtle changes are inadequately mir-

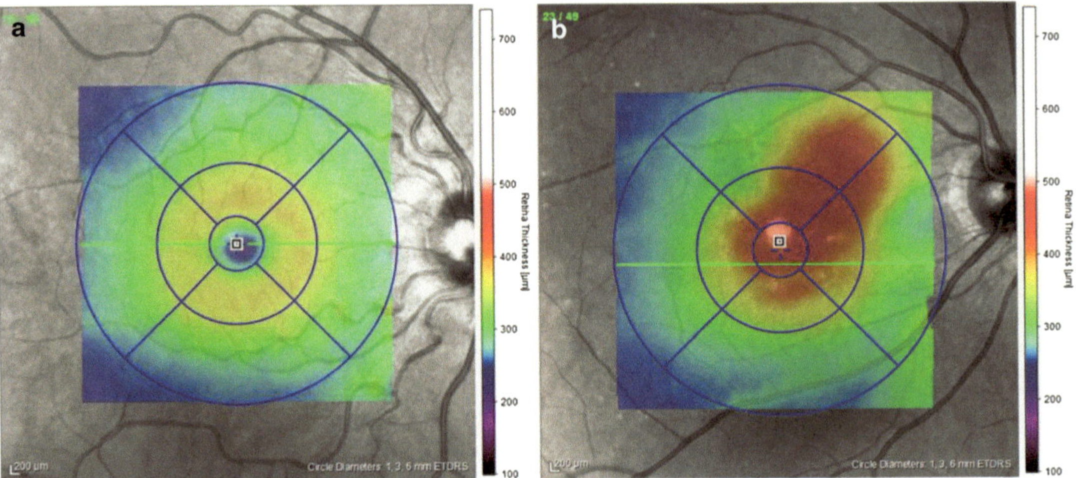

Fig. 15.7 False color-coded retinal thickness maps. (**a**) Healthy eye. (**b**) Neovascular age-related macular degeneration with intra retinal cystoid fluid

rored in CRT, solely relying on CRT to make clinical decisions or using CRT as retreatment criteria in clinical trials is not recommended. However, CRT gives a first impression of retinal topography.

15.5.2 External Limiting Membrane (ELM) and Ellipsoid Zone

The integrity of the external limiting membrane (ELM) and the ellipsoid zone as assessed by OCT correlates well with visual acuity in patients with nAMD. Müller cells and photoreceptors are assumed to connect at the ELM layer. Thus, ELM together with ellipsoid zone is considered a criterion that directly reflects photoreceptor function. However, ELM is no predictor for individual loss or recovery in BCVA, but rather mirrors the current functional state of the retina (Roberts et al. 2014). It has to be kept in mind that ELM integrity is not pathognomonic for nAMD. A correlation with visual acuity has also been found in retinal detachment, retinal vein occlusion, and macular hole (Chhablani et al. 2013; Landa et al. 2012; Wakabayashi et al. 2009; Wolf-Schnurrbusch et al. 2011). A small body of evidence suggests that the ellipsoid zone status in nAMD is a good indicator for BCVA after anti-VEGF injections (Sayanagi et al. 2009; Ueda-Arakawa et al. 2012). However, adjacent lesions make it very difficult to delineate the state of the photoreceptor layers in OCT, for example, shadowing or signal transmission occurs due to the changed retinal architecture in disease.

15.5.2.1 Value for Clinical Routine

The biggest challenge for using outer retinal bands/layers as biomarkers in nAMD is accurately quantifying subtle changes in these contours. Also, the predictive value for visual acuity is questionable, as so far there is no reliable data which indicates that assessing changes in outer retinal layers has the power to predict visual acuity in the course of the disease. The huge effort being made to automatically process OCT data might allow changes in the outer retinal layers to be accurately assessed in the future.

15.5.3 Optical Density Ratio

The optical density ratio (ODR) might be a valuable biomarker in nAMD as it correlates well with BCVA under anti-VEGF therapy and may be useful for differentiation as well as prognosis (Ahlers et al. 2009). As described previously, the ODR compares the optical density of fluid accumulation in or under the retina to the optical density of the vitreous body. Optical density ratios change in the course of the disease because the blood-retinal barrier regains function under anti-VEGF therapy and prevents the CNV from leaking. A high optical density signal indicates increased reflectivity of the fluid accumulation, which is assumed to be caused by the protein concentration in the SRF (Baek and Park 2015) and is therefore thought to be a direct indicator for the blood-retinal barrier function (Ahlers et al. 2009; Baek and Park 2015; Neudorfer et al. 2012). Further, Ahlers et al. showed that ODR changes correlate well with BCVA changes under anti-VEGF therapy (Ahlers et al. 2009).

15.5.3.1 Value for Clinical Routine

A small body of evidence suggests that the optical density ratio might become a biomarker in future to help distinguish between diseases associated with fluid accumulation. Studies with larger sample sizes and longer follow-up are however needed to determine sensitivity and specificity for clinical use.

15.5.4 Outer Retinal Tubulation (ORT)

We have mentioned outer retinal tabulation previously as findings of the intraretinal space, containing degenerated photoreceptors, almost exclusively cones, and Müller cells (Schaal et al. 2015). ORT may be misdiagnosed as new fluid in the retina which lacks the hyperreflective border. The prevalence of ORT in the first year of anti-VEGF treatment is around 17 % and increases to over 40 % after 4 years (Dirani et al. 2015). ORT may be considered a valuable OCT biomarker for future clinical trials as BCVA and retinal sensitivity (microperimetry) were shown to be significantly worse in nAMD eyes with ORT than ORT-free eyes, both at baseline and after 1–2 years' follow-up (Faria-Correia et al. 2013; Lee et al. 2014; Dirani et al. 2015; Iaculli et al. 2015).

15.5.4.1 Value for Clinical Routine

ORT is known to be associated with a reduced visual prognosis in nAMD, yet not to be pathognomonic. Therefore, further research is needed to establish ORT as an OCT biomarker for future treatment decisions.

15.5.5 Intraretinal Cysts (IRC), Subretinal Fluid (SRF), Pigment Epithelial Detachment (PED)

So far, most clinical trials investigating flexible PRN treatment have shown that PRN is inferior to strict monthly injections. The first clinical anti-VEGF trials using various treatment regimen have given insight into detailed morphologic changes in sub-/intraretinal fluid compartments and their correlation with functional outcomes such as BCVA.

Three pathologic changes affecting central retinal morphology have been described in nAMD patients; intraretinal cystoid fluid (IRC, Fig. 15.4), subretinal fluid (SRF, Fig. 15.2a), and pigment epithelial detachment (PED, Fig. 15.1) (Jaffe et al. 2013; Schmidt-Erfurth et al. 2015; Simader et al. 2014). A comprehensive subgroup analysis of the VIEW II data (Schmidt-Erfurth et al. 2014) showed a clear association between the PRN regime and visual acuity loss in patients presenting with primary PED at baseline (Schmidt-Erfurth et al. 2015). A significant drop in BCVA was found in this subgroup contrasting with the loss of one or two letters after gross averaging of the whole study population. After stratification for retinal morphologies, it became evident that all patients other than those with initial PED have constant BCVA readings. This finding exemplifies the need for solid OCT biomarkers to provide the best individualized disease management.

Under anti-VEGF therapy, IRC and SRF were resorbed in 70–80 % of patients, whereas PED vanished in only 50 %. Patients with SRF only had good BCVA at baseline followed by improvement under therapy. Patients with IRC with or without PED had poor BCVA at baseline and did not gain as many letters as the first group under anti-VEGF therapy. However, PED did regress under continuous therapy, but switching from fixed to flexible PRN treatment led to a reactivation of this subretinal lesion. We suggest that the elevation of the retinal pigment epithelium (RPE) is the morphologic correlate for nAMD activity, and the associated loss in visual acuity caused by secondary degenerative intraretinal cystoid fluid formation is the functional manifestation. This is in good agreement with the finding that the occurrence of IRC is correlated with a loss in BCVA in the eyes with PED (Schmidt-Erfurth et al. 2015). The eyes with subretinal fluid (SRF) had the best visual prognosis. IRC and fibrovascular PED at baseline influenced BCVA prognosis negatively (Ritter et al. 2014; Schmidt-Erfurth et al. 2015).

These results clearly contrast with the current convention that PRN is inferior to a fix OCT-based therapy regimen, highlighting the need to consider morphologic OCT variables in the future. However, final conclusions regarding retinal morphologic retreatment criteria are still lacking, and further studies are needed to identify or confirm OCT biomarkers. As for now, expert guidelines recommend that IRC, SRF, and PED should be incorporated into treatment protocols (Schmidt-Erfurth et al. 2014). Monthly monitoring is advised using SD-OCT because of its ability to visualize even small morphologic changes, which is essential when monitoring a disease with the potential to progress rapidly leading to irreversible loss of vision if treatment is deferred.

15.5.5.1 Value for Clinical Routine

Current data suggests that patients with nAMD and intraretinal cystoid fluid should be diagnosed early and treatment should be initiated as soon as possible because accumulation of intraretinal fluid may lead to irreversible neurosensory damage. A physician deciding whether to retreat patients who have cystic degeneration with underlying RPE atrophy should bear in mind that degenerative IRC have a low potential for responding to anti-VEGF therapy.

Usually, SRF is easily managed with anti-VEGF therapy. SRF is known to be linked to a benign course of the disease and in most cases responds to treatment at extended intervals (treat-and-extend regimen). Recent data shows that PED should be included in retreatment decisions (PED growth in SD-OCT), especially in flexible anti-VEGF treatment plans. The risk for RPE tear in large PEDs also has to be kept in mind and discussed with the patient.

15.6 Functional Extensions and Future Developments

With advanced OCT systems commercially available, the great challenge is to find ways to enhance tissue contrast or add functional tools to obtain more information in addition to the recording of morphological structures and thus extend the clinical applicability of OCT. Functional approaches are of great interest as early diagnosis of retinal changes is known to be of vital importance because structural pathologies might be linked to irreversible damage and visual loss. Future therapeutic strategies will most likely aim for disease-modifying interventions and individualized treatment regimes to protect the functional abilities and morphologic integrity of the retina. Doppler OCT and polarization-sensitive OCT are currently most commonly used in retinal studies. These systems measure functional variables such as blood flow and velocity, as well as enhanced tissue contrast.

15.6.1 Doppler OCT

Doppler OCT obtains high-resolution OCT images and information about functional blood flow and velocity (Wang et al. 1995; Werkmeister et al. 2008). Wang et al. were the first to report total retinal blood flow (Wang et al. 2007), and other groups followed (Baumann et al. 2011; Blatter et al. 2013; Dai et al. 2013; Doblhoff-Dier et al. 2014). Various eye diseases such as age-related macular degeneration (Ehrlich et al. 2009; Pemp and Schmetterer 2008), diabetic retinopathy (Clermont and Bursell 2007; Pemp and Schmetterer 2008; Wang et al. 2011b), and glaucoma (Costa et al. 2014; Schmidl et al. 2011) were shown to be linked to early changes in blood flow. Early changes in blood flow regulation can be detected by using flicker light stimulation. The response to flicker light was altered in nAMD and normalized after anti-VEGF treatment (Lanzl et al. 2011). Today, flickering light stimulation is incorporated into Doppler OCT setups (Clermont and Bursell 2007; Leitgeb 2007; Pemp and Schmetterer 2008; Wang et al. 2011a, b), with the aim of early diagnosing ocular diseases such as nAMD.

15.6.2 OCT Angiography

From a clinical point of view, visualization of the retinal and choroidal vasculature is the most advanced application of Doppler OCT. The optical Doppler effect creates motion-related image contrast in vessels, which can be extracted by software-based post-processing (Schwartz et al. 2014). This is why this technique is also called optical coherence angiography or OCTA (Makita et al. 2006). OCTA has already been commercialized based on an SD-OCT system (e.g. Angiovue, Optovue, Fremont, CA, USA), allowing fast and detailed visualization of the retinal and choroidal microcirculation (Fig. 15.8). With improvements in the technology, it has become possible to distinguish CNV from the surrounding retinal or choroidal vasculature in en face (coronal) projections as well as to quantify the CNV area (Flores-Moreno et al. 2015; Jia et al. 2012; Moult et al. 2014) and visualize CNV vessel architecture in the course of anti-VEGF treatment. This treatment results in abnormal vessel configurations, which can possibly be explained by treatment-related pruning of vessel sprouts (Spaide 2015). So far studies using OCTA have mostly had a descriptive character, but lately obtaining quantitative information such as vessel density, flow index, and areas of nonperfusion (Jia et al. 2015) has also become possible, adding valuable information, for example, in nAMD follow-up. Also, a recent study investigating CNV of various origins concluded that OCTA is ideal for identifying neovascularization and adjacent fluid noninvasively and without the use of contrast agents (de Carlo et al. 2015). The same conclusions were drawn in a study investigating the value of OCTA for early identification and treatment response of type 3 neovascularization (RAP) (Dansingani et al. 2015). The main advantage of OCTA is that it is label-free, given the risks associated with the dye fluorescein (López-Sáez et al. 1998), the current gold standard for nAMD diagnosis (Schmidt-Erfurth et al. 2014a, b; AAO 2015; Chakravarthy et al. 2013). Future nAMD treatment will probably be guided by the presence or absence of flow-related contrast or areas of non- or hyperperfusion on OCTA, which could indicate CNV activity.

Currently, the main shortcoming of OCTA is that it is only sensitive to blood flow and not to static leakage sites. This is because it is motion that creates image contrast. Scientists are already searching for contrast enhancing agents to over-

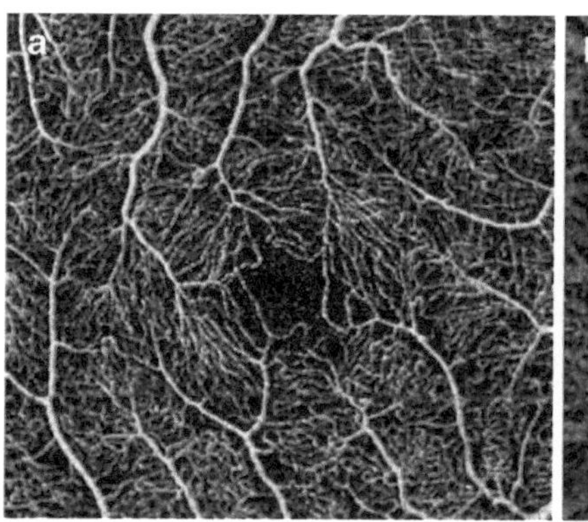

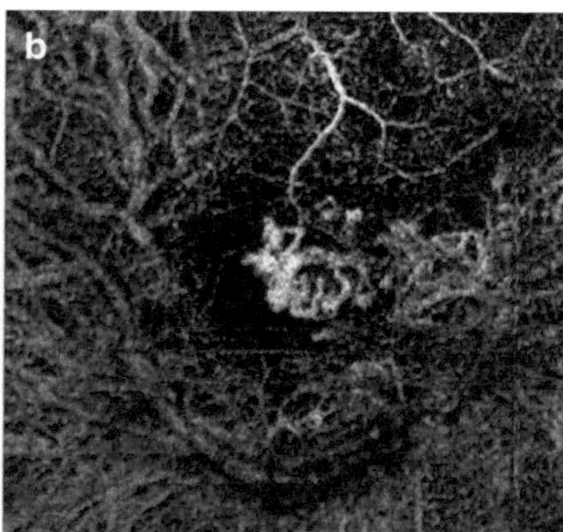

Fig. 15.8 Neovascular age-related macular degeneration in OCTA. (**a**) OCTA (Angiovue, Optovue, CA, USA) showing superficial, parafoveal microcirculation of a healthy eye. (**b**) OCTA showing hyperreflective vessels representing flow in a subfoveal CNV lesion

come this problem. Biocompatible gold nanoparticles, for example, might have the potential to increase tissue contrast and highlight static leakage sites in nAMD (Gordon and Jayagopal 2014; Lee et al. 2003).

OCT angiography has several compelling characteristics such as acquisition times of a few seconds and the possibility of visualizing abnormalities in a three-dimensional manner, making it promising for extended future clinical use.

15.6.3 Polarization-Sensitive Optical Coherence Tomography

Polarization-sensitive OCT (*PS-OCT*) was one of the first OCT advances. It is sensitive to depth-resolved tissue properties (de Boer et al. 1999; de Boer et al. 1997) and is based on the principle that light has additional properties to those used in intensity-based OCT setups. Light properties assessed with PS-OCT are for example reflectivity, retardation, optic axis orientation, and the degree of polarization uniformity, all of which can be altered by tissue-light interactions. PS-OCT is of special interest in nAMD as it allows distinct documentation of the RPE condition during the course of the disease (Ahlers et al. 2010), with RPE migration and atrophy being two variables of CNV activity, or changes in the course of anti-VEGF treatment (Fig. 15.9) (Schütze et al. 2015). PS-OCT is also used to automatically quantify drusen dynamics (Schlanitz et al. 2011), a vital sign for the progression of AMD regardless of its endpoint (geographic atrophy (Baumann et al. 2010)/CNV (Schütze et al. 2015)). Therefore, PS-OCT is promising for upcoming nAMD treatment regimens and follow-up.

15.6.4 Adaptive Optics Optical Coherence Tomography (AO-OCT)

The aim of better resolution reached the cellular level with an approach called adaptive optics OCT. AO-OCT systems are similar to wave front analyzers, which are able to compensate for ocular aberrations by means of a deformable mirror.

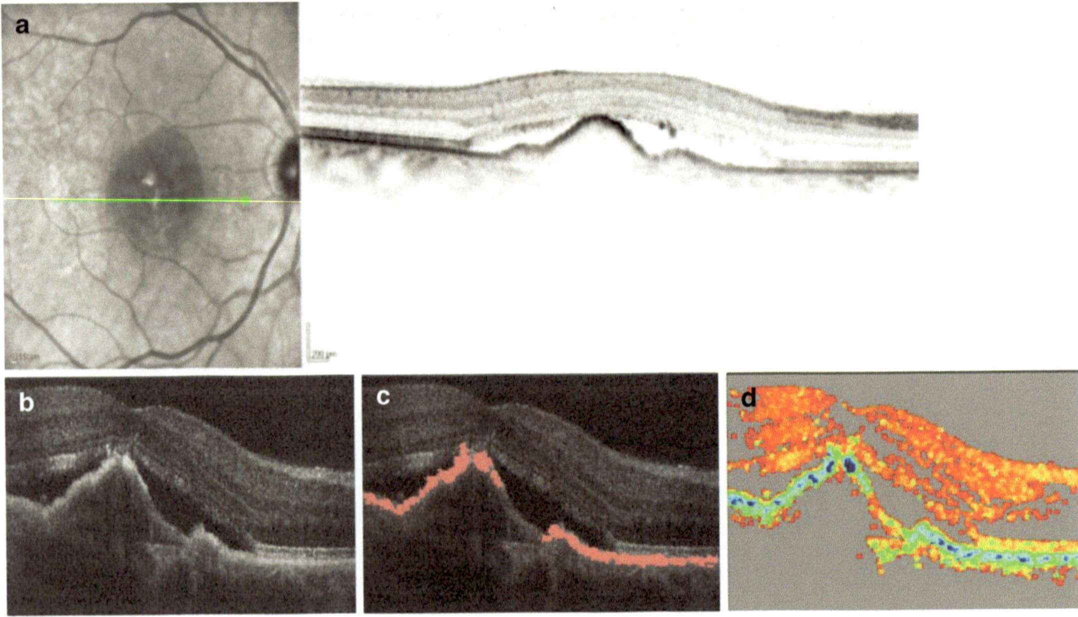

Fig. 15.9 Neovascular age-related macular degeneration in polarization sensitive OCT. (**a**) SD-OCT showing nAMD lesion. (**b**) PS-OCT intensity image. (**c**) PS-OCT intensity image + RPE segmentation (*red*). (**d**) DOPU map (degree of polarization uniformity)

This technique originated from astronomy and allows unprecedented resolution (Drexler and Fujimoto 2008). Today, single photoreceptor imaging is possible, as recently demonstrated by Felberer et al. (Felberer et al. 2014). Preliminary data in AMD suggest AO-OCT images show morphological changes similar to postmortem histological studies in RPE areas that appear normal on fundus autofluorescence (FAF) (Rossi et al. 2013). However, further studies are needed to explore the potential of this new approach in AMD.

15.7 Proof of Concepts

Despite reaching the cellular level of resolution, further innovation is still expected in the coming years. Exciting and promising proofs of concepts which could herald our diagnostic tools for tomorrow's nAMD management have already been published. A few which make use of the OCT principle are pointed out in the following paragraphs.

Spectroscopic OCT is a functional extension of OCT, allowing, for example, oxygen measurements in combination with OCT measurements (Lu et al. 2008; Liu and Kang 2010). As changes in oxygen consumption are associated with changes in various diseases, including AMD (Geirsdottir et al. 2014), it could facilitate future oxygen measurements and help diagnose retinal diseases earlier.

Photoacoustic tomography (PAT) is based on acoustic detection of optical absorption (Xia et al. 2014). This technology is expected to provide high image resolution at the molecular level as ultrasound scatters less than light in tissue. In ophthalmology, PAT could enable oxygen saturation mapping and high-resolution visualization of retinal and choroidal vascularization (Liu and Zhang 2014; Song et al. 2013).

The current gold standard when it comes to functional measurements of the retina is electrophysiology. It is time consuming and has limited depth resolution. *Optophysiology* is an OCT-based, contact-free technique that allows optical imaging of retinal responses to stimuli such as light flickering. Additionally, is possible to obtain depth information with optophysiology. It is based on the principle that light exposure on dark-adapted retinas leads to a change in local tissue reflectivity, which represents functional changes and can be measured and visualized on morphologic OCT images (Bizheva et al. 2006; Drexler and Fujimoto 2008).

References

AAO (2015) Age-related macular degeneration PPP – updated 2015. http://www.aao.org/ppp. Accessed 21 Apr 2015

Ahlers C, Golbaz I, Stock G, Fous A, Kolar S, Pruente C, Schmidt-Erfurth U (2008) Time course of morphologic effects on different retinal compartments after ranibizumab therapy in age-related macular degeneration. Ophthalmology 115:46. doi:10.1016/j.ophtha.2008.05.017

Ahlers C, Golbaz I, Einwallner E, Dunavölgyi R, Malamos P, Stock G, Pruente C, Schmidt-Erfurth U (2009) Identification of optical density ratios in subretinal fluid as a clinically relevant biomarker in exudative macular disease. Invest Ophthalmol Vis Sci 50:3417–3424. doi:10.1167/iovs.08-2759

Ahlers C, Götzinger E, Pircher M, Golbaz I, Prager F, Schütze C, Baumann B, Hitzenberger CK, Schmidt-Erfurth U (2010) Imaging of the retinal pigment epithelium in age-related macular degeneration using polarization-sensitive optical coherence tomography. Invest Ophthalmol Vis Sci 51:2149–2157. doi:10.1167/iovs.09-3817

Alasil T, Ferrara D, Adhi M, Brewer E, Kraus MF, Baumal CR, Hornegger J, Fujimoto JG, Witkin AJ, Reichel E, Duker JS, Waheed NK (2015) En face imaging of the choroid in polypoidal choroidal vasculopathy using swept-source optical coherence tomography. Am J Ophthalmol 159:634–64300. doi:10.1016/j.ajo.2014.12.012

Baek J, Park Y-HH (2015) Optical density ratio in the subretinal fluid: differentiating chronic central serous chorioretinopathy and polypodial choroidal vasculopathy. Am J Ophthalmol 159:386–392. doi:10.1016/j.ajo.2014.11.011

Baumann B, Gotzinger E, Pircher M, Sattmann H, Schuutze C, Schlanitz F, Ahlers C, Schmidt-Erfurth U, Hitzenberger CK (2010) Segmentation and quantification of retinal lesions in age-related macular degeneration using polarization-sensitive optical coherence tomography. J Biomed Opt 15:61704. doi:10.1117/1.3499420

Baumann B, Potsaid B, Kraus MF, Liu JJ, Huang D, Hornegger J, Cable AE, Duker JS, Fujimoto JG (2011) Total retinal blood flow measurement with ultrahigh speed swept source/Fourier domain OCT. Biomed Opt Express 2:1539–1552. doi:10.1364/BOE.2.001539

Bischoff PM, Flower RW (1985) Ten years experience with choroidal angiography using indocyanine green dye: a new routine examination or an epilogue? Doc Ophthalmol Adv Ophthalmol 60:235–291

Bizheva K, Pflug R, Hermann B, Povazay B, Sattmann H, Qiu P, Anger E, Reitsamer H, Popov S, Taylor JR, Unterhuber A, Ahnelt P, Drexler W (2006) Optophysiology: depth-resolved probing of retinal physiology with functional ultrahigh-resolution optical coherence tomography. Proc Natl Acad Sci U S A 103:5066–5071. doi:10.1073/pnas.0506997103

Blatter C, Coquoz S, Grajciar B, Singh AS, Bonesi M, Werkmeister RM, Schmetterer L, Leitgeb RA (2013) Dove prism based rotating dual beam bidirectional Doppler OCT. Biomed Opt Express 4:1188–1203. doi:10.1364/BOE.4.001188

Bolz M, Simader C, Ritter M, Ahlers C, Benesch T, Prünte C, Schmidt-Erfurth U (2010) Morphological and functional analysis of the loading regimen with intravitreal ranibizumab in neovascular age-related macular degeneration. Br J Ophthalmol 94:185–189. doi:10.1136/bjo.2008.143974

Brown DM, Kaiser PK, Michels M, Soubrane G, Heier JS, Kim RY, Sy JP, Schneider S, Group AS (2006) Ranibizumab versus verteporfin for neovascular age-related macular degeneration. N Engl J Med 355:1432–1444. doi:10.1056/NEJMoa062655

Busbee BG, Ho AC, Brown DM, Heier JS, Suñer IJ, Li Z, Rubio RG, Lai P, Group HS (2013) Twelve-month efficacy and safety of 0.5 mg or 2.0 mg ranibizumab in patients with subfoveal neovascular age-related macular degeneration. Ophthalmology 120:1046–1056. doi:10.1016/j.ophtha.2012.10.014

Castillo MM, Mowatt G, Elders A, Lois N, Fraser C, Hernández R, Amoaku W, Burr JM, Lotery A, Ramsay CR, Azuara-Blanco A (2015) Optical coherence tomography for the monitoring of neovascular age-related macular degeneration: a systematic review. Ophthalmology 122:399–406. doi:10.1016/j.ophtha.2014.07.055

Chakravarthy U, Harding SP, Rogers CA, Downes SM, Lotery AJ, Wordsworth S, Reeves BC, Investigators IS (2012) Ranibizumab versus bevacizumab to treat neovascular age-related macular degeneration: one-year findings from the IVAN randomized trial. Ophthalmology 119:1399–1411. doi:10.1016/j.ophtha.2012.04.015

Chakravarthy U, Williams M, Group AMDG (2013) The Royal College of Ophthalmologists Guidelines on AMD: Executive Summary. Eye (London) 27:1429–1431. doi:10.1038/eye.2013.233

Channa R, Sophie R, Bagheri S, Shah SM, Wang J, Adeyemo O, Sodhi A, Wenick A, Ying HS, Campochiaro PA (2015) Regression of choroidal neovascularization results in macular atrophy in anti-vascular endothelial growth factor-treated eyes. Am J Ophthalmol 159(9–19):e11–e12. doi:10.1016/j.ajo.2014.09.012

Chhablani J, Kim JS, Freeman WR, Kozak I, Wang H-YY, Cheng L (2013) Predictors of visual outcome in eyes with choroidal neovascularization secondary to age related macular degeneration treated with intravitreal bevacizumab monotherapy. Int J Ophthalmol 6:62–66. doi:10.3980/j.issn.2222-3959.2013.01.13

Clermont AC, Bursell S-EE (2007) Retinal blood flow in diabetes. Microcirculation (New York) 14:49–61. doi:10.1080/10739680601072164

Cohen SY, Mimoun G, Oubraham H, Zourdani A, Malbrel C, Queré S, Schneider V, Group LS (2013) Changes in visual acuity in patients with wet age-related macular degeneration treated with intravitreal ranibizumab in daily clinical practice: the LUMIERE study. Retina (Philadelphia) 33:474–481. doi:10.1097/IAE.0b013e31827b6324

Coscas F, Coscas G, Querques G, Massamba N, Querques L, Bandello F, Souied EH (2012) En face enhanced depth imaging optical coherence tomography of fibrovascular pigment epithelium detachment. Invest Ophthalmol Vis Sci 53:4147–4151. doi:10.1167/iovs.12-9878

Costa VP, Harris A, Anderson D, Stodtmeister R, Cremasco F, Kergoat H, Lovasik J, Stalmans I, Zeitz O, Lanzl I, Gugleta K, Schmetterer L (2014) Ocular perfusion pressure in glaucoma. Acta Ophthalmol 92:66. doi:10.1111/aos.12298

Dai C, Liu X, Zhang HF, Puliafito CA, Jiao S (2013) Absolute retinal blood flow measurement with a dual-beam Doppler optical coherence tomography. Invest Ophthalmol Vis Sci 54:7998–8003. doi:10.1167/iovs.13-12318

Daniel E, Toth CA, Grunwald JE, Jaffe GJ, Martin DF, Fine SL, Huang J, Ying GS, Hagstrom SA, Winter K, Maguire MG, Comparison of Age-related Macular Degeneration Treatments Trials Research G (2014) Risk of scar in the comparison of age-related macular degeneration treatments trials. Ophthalmology 121:656–666. doi:10.1016/j.ophtha.2013.10.019

Dansingani KK, Naysan J, Freund KB (2015) En face OCT angiography demonstrates flow in early type 3 neovascularization (retinal angiomatous proliferation). Eye 29:703–706. doi:10.1038/eye.2015.27

de Boer JF, Milner TE, van Gemert MJ, Nelson JS (1997) Two-dimensional birefringence imaging in biological tissue by polarization-sensitive optical coherence tomography. Opt Lett 22:934–936

de Boer JF, Milner TE, Nelson JS (1999) Determination of the depth-resolved stokes parameters of light backscattered from turbid media by use of polarization-sensitive optical coherence tomography. Opt Lett 24:300–302

de Boer JF, Cense B, Park BH, Pierce MC, Tearney GJ, Bouma BE (2003) Improved signal-to-noise ratio in spectral-domain compared with time-domain optical coherence tomography. Opt Lett 28:2067–2069

de Carlo TE, Bonini Filho MA, Chin AT, Adhi M, Ferrara D, Baumal CR, Witkin AJ, Reichel E, Duker JS, Waheed NK (2015) Spectral-domain optical coherence tomography angiography of choroidal neovascularization. Ophthalmology 122:1228–1238. doi:10.1016/j.ophtha.2015.01.029

Dirani A, Gianniou C, Marchionno L, Decugis D, Mantel I (2015) Incidence of outer retinal tubulation in ranibizumab-treated Age-related macular degeneration. Retina 35:1166–1172. doi:10.1097/IAE.0000000000000439

Doblhoff-Dier V, Schmetterer L, Vilser W, Garhöfer G, Gröschl M, Leitgeb RA, Werkmeister RM (2014) Measurement of the total retinal blood flow using dual beam fourier-domain doppler optical coherence tomography with orthogonal detection planes. Biomed Opt Express 5:630–642. doi:10.1364/BOE.5.000630

Drexler W, Fujimoto JG (2008) State-of-the-art retinal optical coherence tomography. Prog Retin Eye Res 27:45–88. doi:10.1016/j.preteyeres.2007.07.005

Duker JS, Kaiser PK, Binder S, de Smet MD, Gaudric A, Reichel E, Sadda SR, Sebag J, Spaide RF, Stalmans P (2013) The international vitreomacular traction study group classification of vitreomacular adhesion, traction, and macular hole. Ophthalmology 120:2611–2619. doi:10.1016/j.ophtha.2013.07.042

Early-Treatment-Diabetic-Retinopathy-Study-Group (1985) Photocoagulation for diabetic macular edema. Early treatment diabetic retinopathy study report number 1. Early treatment diabetic retinopathy study research group. Arch Ophthalmol 103:1796–1806

Ehrlich R, Kheradiya NS, Winston DM, Moore DB, Wirostko B, Harris A (2009) Age-related ocular vascular changes. Graefes Arch Clin Exp Ophthalmol 247:583–591. doi:10.1007/s00417-008-1018-x

Ellabban AA, Hangai M, Yamashiro K, Nakagawa S, Tsujikawa A, Yoshimura N (2012) Tomographic fundus features in pseudoxanthoma elasticum: comparison with neovascular age-related macular degeneration in Japanese patients. Eye (London) 26:1086–1094. doi:10.1038/eye.2012.101

Faria-Correia F, Barros-Pereira R, Queirós-Mendanha L, Fonseca S, Mendonça L, Falcão MS, Brandão E, Falcão-Reis F, Carneiro AM (2013) Characterization of neovascular age-related macular degeneration patients with outer retinal tubulations. Ophthalmol J Int d'ophtalmol Int J Ophthalmol Zeitschrift für Augenheilkunde 229:147–151. doi:10.1159/000346854

Felberer F, Kroisamer J-SS, Baumann B, Zotter S, Schmidt-Erfurth U, Hitzenberger CK, Pircher M (2014) Adaptive optics SLO/OCT for 3D imaging of human photoreceptors in vivo. Biomed Opt Express 5:439–456. doi:10.1364/BOE.5.000439

Fercher AF, Hitzenberger CK, Drexler W, Kamp G, Sattmann H (1993) In vivo optical coherence tomography. Am J Ophthalmol 116:113–114

Flores-Moreno I, Arias-Barquet L, Rubio-Caso MJ, Ruiz-Moreno JM, Duker JS, Caminal JM (2015) En face swept-source optical coherence tomography in neovascular age-related macular degeneration. Br J Ophthalmol 99:1260–1267. doi:10.1136/bjophthalmol-2014-306422

Framme C, Panagakis G, Birngruber R (2010) Effects on choroidal neovascularization after anti-VEGF upload using intravitreal ranibizumab, as determined by spectral domain-optical coherence tomography. Invest Ophthalmol Vis Sci 51:1671–1676. doi:10.1167/iovs.09-4496

Freund KB, Yannuzzi LA, Sorenson JA (1993) Age-related macular degeneration and choroidal neovascularization. Am J Ophthalmol 115:786–791

Freund KB, Zweifel SA, Engelbert M (2010) Do we need a new classification for choroidal neovascularization in age-related macular degeneration? Retina (Philadelphia) 30:1333–1349. doi:10.1097/IAE.0b013e3181e7976b

Fung AE, Lalwani GA, Rosenfeld PJ, Dubovy SR, Michels S, Feuer WJ, Puliafito CA, Davis JL, Flynn HW, Esquiabro M (2007) An optical coherence tomography-guided, variable dosing regimen with intravitreal ranibizumab (Lucentis) for neovascular age-related macular degeneration. Am J Ophthalmol 143:566–583. doi:10.1016/j.ajo.2007.01.028

Gass JD (1994) Biomicroscopic and histopathologic considerations regarding the feasibility of surgical excision of subfoveal neovascular membranes. Trans Am Ophthalmol Soc 92:91

Geirsdottir A, Hardarson SH, Olafsdottir OB, Stefánsson E (2014) Retinal oxygen metabolism in exudative age-related macular degeneration. Acta Ophthalmol 92:27–33. doi:10.1111/aos.12294

Geitzenauer W, Hitzenberger CK, Schmidt-Erfurth UM (2011) Retinal optical coherence tomography: past, present and future perspectives. Br J Ophthalmol 95:171–177. doi:10.1136/bjo.2010.182170

Gelisken F, Inhoffen W, Schneider U, Stroman G, Kreissig I (1998) Indocyanine green angiography in classic choroidal neovascularization. Jpn J Ophthalmol 42:300–303

Gianniou C, Dirani A, Jang L, Mantel I (2015) Refractory intraretinal or subretinal fluid in neovascular age-related macular degeneration treated with intravitreal ranizubimab: Functional and Structural Outcome. Retina (Philadelphia) 35:1195–1201. doi:10.1097/IAE.0000000000000465

Gordon AY, Jayagopal A (2014) Engineering of nanoscale contrast agents for optical coherence tomography. J Nanomedicine Nanotechnol Suppl 5:4. doi:10.4172/2157-7439.S5-004

Green-Simms AE, Bakri SJ (2011) Vitreomacular traction and age-related macular degeneration. Semin Ophthalmol 26:137–138. doi:10.3109/08820538.2011.559512

Gross NE, Aizman A, Brucker A, Klancnik JM, Yannuzzi LA (2005) Nature and risk of neovascularization in the fellow eye of patients with unilateral retinal angiomatous proliferation. Retina (Philadelphia) 25:713–718

Grossniklaus HE, Green WR (2004) Choroidal neovascularization. Am J Ophthalmol 137:496–503. doi:10.1016/j.ajo.2003.09.042

Hartnett ME, Weiter JJ, Staurenghi G, Elsner AE (1996) Deep retinal vascular anomalous complexes in advanced age-related macular degeneration. Ophthalmology 103:2042–2053

Hirami Y, Mandai M, Takahashi M, Teramukai S, Tada H, Yoshimura N (2009) Association of clinical characteristics with disease subtypes, initial visual acuity, and visual prognosis in neovascular age-related macular degeneration. Jpn J Ophthalmol 53:396–407. doi:10.1007/s10384-009-0669-4

Holz FG, Amoaku W, Donate J, Guymer RH, Kellner U, Schlingemann RO, Weichselberger A, Staurenghi G, Group SS (2011) Safety and efficacy of a flexible dosing regimen of ranibizumab in neovascular age-related macular degeneration: the SUSTAIN study. Ophthalmology 118:663–671. doi:10.1016/j.ophtha.2010.12.019

Huang D, Swanson EA, Lin CP, Schuman JS, Stinson WG, Chang W, Hee MR, Flotte T, Gregory K, Puliafito CA et al (1991) Optical coherence tomography. Science 254:1178–1181

Iaculli C, Barone A, Scudieri M, Giovanna Palumbo M, Delle Noci N (2015) OUTER RETINAL TUBULATION: characteristics in patients with neovascular age-related macular degeneration. Retina 35:1979–1984. doi:10.1097/IAE.0000000000000609

Imamura Y, Engelbert M, Iida T, Freund KB, Yannuzzi LA (2010) Polypoidal choroidal vasculopathy: a review. Surv Ophthalmol 55:501–515. doi:10.1016/j.survophthal.2010.03.004

Jaffe GJ, Martin DF, Toth CA, Daniel E, Maguire MG (2013) Macular morphology and visual acuity in the comparison of age-related macular degeneration treatments trials. Ophthalmology 120:1860–1870

Jang L, Gianniou C, Ambresin A, Mantel I (2014) Refractory subretinal fluid in patients with neovascular age-related macular degeneration treated with intravitreal ranibizumab: visual acuity outcome. Graefes Arch Clin Exp Ophthalmol 253:1211–1216. doi:10.1007/s00417-014-2789-x

Jia Y, Morrison JC, Tokayer J, Tan O, Lombardi L, Baumann B, Lu CD, Choi W, Fujimoto JG, Huang D (2012) Quantitative OCT angiography of optic nerve head blood flow. Biomed Opt Express 3:3127–3137. doi:10.1364/BOE.3.003127

Jia Y, Bailey ST, Hwang TS, McClintic SM, Gao SS, Pennesi ME, Flaxel CJ, Lauer AK, Wilson DJ, Hornegger J, Fujimoto JG, Huang D (2015) Quantitative optical coherence tomography angiography of vascular abnormalities in the living human eye. Proc Natl Acad Sci U S A 112:E2395–E2402. doi:10.1073/pnas.1500185112

Jung JJ, Chen CY, Mrejen S, Gallego-Pinazo R, Xu L, Marsiglia M, Boddu S, Freund KB (2014) The incidence of neovascular subtypes in newly diagnosed neovascular age-related macular degeneration. Am J Ophthalmol 158:769–77900. doi:10.1016/j.ajo.2014.07.006

Kakehashi A, Schepens CL, Trempe CL (1994) Vitreomacular observations. I Vitreomacular adhesion and hole in the premacular hyaloid. Ophthalmology 101:1515–1521

Keane PA, Patel PJ, Liakopoulos S, Heussen FM, Sadda SR, Tufail A (2012) Evaluation of age-related macular degeneration with optical coherence tomography. Surv Ophthalmol 57:389–414. doi:10.1016/j.survophthal.2012.01.006

Khan S, Engelbert M, Imamura Y, Freund KB (2012) Polypoidal choroidal vasculopathy: simultaneous indocyanine green angiography and eye-tracked spectral domain optical coherence tomography findings. Retina (Philadelphia) 32:1057–1068. doi:10.1097/IAE.0b013e31823beb14

Kiss CG, Geitzenauer W, Simader C, Gregori G, Schmidt-Erfurth U (2009) Evaluation of ranibizumab-induced changes in high-resolution optical coherence tomographic retinal morphology and their impact on visual function. Invest Ophthalmol Vis Sci 50:2376–2383. doi:10.1167/iovs.08-2017

Krebs I, Glittenberg C, Zeiler F, Binder S (2011) Spectral domain optical coherence tomography for higher precision in the evaluation of vitreoretinal adhesions in exudative age-related macular degeneration. Br J Ophthalmol 95:1415–1418. doi:10.1136/bjo.2010.192385

Landa G, Gentile RC, Garcia PM, Muldoon TO, Rosen RB (2012) External limiting membrane and visual outcome in macular hole repair: spectral domain OCT analysis. Eye (London) 26:61–69. doi:10.1038/eye.2011.237

Lanzl IM, Seidova S-FF, Maier M, Lohmann C, Schmidt-Trucksäss A, Halle M, Kotliar KE (2011) Dynamic retinal vessel response to flicker in age-related macular degeneration patients before and after vascular endothelial growth factor inhibitor injection. Acta Ophthalmol 89:472–479. doi:10.1111/j.1755-3768.2009.01718.x

Lee TM, Oldenburg AL, Sitafalwalla S, Marks DL, Luo W, Toublan FJ, Suslick KS, Boppart SA (2003) Engineered microsphere contrast agents for optical coherence tomography. Opt Lett 28:1546–1548

Lee JY, Folgar FA, Maguire MG, Ying G-sS, Toth CA, Martin DF, Jaffe GJ, Group CR (2014) Outer retinal tubulation in the comparison of age-related macular degeneration treatments trials (CATT). Ophthalmology 121:2423–2431. doi:10.1016/j.ophtha.2014.06.013

Leitgeb RA (2007) Optical coherence tomography-high resolution imaging of structure and function. Eng Med Biol Soc 2007:530–532. doi:10.1109/IEMBS.2007.4352344

Liakopoulos S, Ongchin S, Bansal A, Msutta S, Walsh AC, Updike PG, Sadda SR (2008) Quantitative optical coherence tomography findings in various subtypes of neovascular age-related macular degeneration. Invest Ophthalmol Vis Sci 49:5048–5054. doi:10.1167/iovs.08-1877

Liu X, Kang JU (2010) Depth-resolved blood oxygen saturation assessment using spectroscopic common-path Fourier domain optical coherence tomography. IEEE Trans Biomed Eng 57:2572–2575. doi:10.1109/TBME.2010.2058109

Liu W, Zhang HF (2014) Noninvasive in vivo imaging of oxygen metabolic rate in the retina. Conf Proc Annu Int Conference IEEE Eng Med Biol Soc IEEE Eng Med Biol Soc Annu Conf 2014:3865–3868. doi:10.1109/EMBC.2014.6944467

Liu Y, Wen F, Huang S, Luo G, Yan H, Sun Z, Wu D (2007) Subtype lesions of neovascular age-related macular degeneration in Chinese patients. Graefes Arch Clin Exp Ophthalmol 245:1441–1445. doi:10.1007/s00417-007-0575-8

López-Sáez MP, Ordoqui E, Tornero P, Baeza A, Sainza T, Zubeldia JM, Baeza ML (1998) Fluorescein-induced allergic reaction. Ann Allergy Asthma Immunol Off Publ Am Coll Allergy Asthma Immunol 81(5 Pt 1):428–430. doi:10.1016/S1081-1206(10)63140-7

Lu CW, Lee CK, Tsai MT, Wang YM, Yang CC (2008) Measurement of the hemoglobin oxygen saturation level with spectroscopic spectral-domain optical coherence tomography. Opt Lett 33:416–418

Macular-Photocoagulation-Study-Group (1991) Subfoveal neovascular lesions in age-related macular degeneration. Guidelines for evaluation and treatment in the macular photocoagulation study. Macular Photocoagulation Study Group. Arch Ophthalmol 109:1242–1257

Major JC, Wykoff CC, Mariani AF, Chen E, Croft DE, Brown DM (2014) Comparison of spectral-domain and time-domain optical coherence tomography in the detection of neovascular age-related macular degeneration activity. Retina (Philadelphia) 34:48–54. doi:10.1097/IAE.0b013e3182965743

Makita S, Hong Y, Yamanari M, Yatagai T, Yasuno Y (2006) Optical coherence angiography. Opt Express 14:7821–7840

Malamos P, Sacu S, Georgopoulos M, Kiss C, Pruente C, Schmidt-Erfurth U (2009) Correlation of high-definition optical coherence tomography and fluorescein angiography imaging in neovascular macular degeneration. Invest Ophthalmol Vis Sci 50:4926–4933. doi:10.1167/iovs.09-3610

Martin DF, Maguire MG, Ying GS, Grunwald JE, Fine SL, Jaffe GJ, Group CR (2011) Ranibizumab and bevacizumab for neovascular age-related macular degeneration. N Engl J Med 364:1897–1908. doi:10.1056/NEJMoa1102673

Martin DF, Maguire MG, Fine SL, Ying GS, Jaffe GJ, Grunwald JE, Toth C, Redford M, Ferris FL 3rd, Comparison of Age-Related Macular Degeneration Treatments Trials Research G (2012) Ranibizumab and bevacizumab for treatment of neovascular age-related macular degeneration: two-year results. Ophthalmology 119:1388–1398. doi:10.1016/j.ophtha.2012.03.053

Maruko I, Iida T, Saito M, Nagayama D, Saito K (2007) Clinical characteristics of exudative age-related macular degeneration in Japanese patients. Am J Ophthalmol 144:15–22. doi:10.1016/j.ajo.2007.03.047

Mathew R, Pefkianaki M, Kopsachilis N, Brar M, Richardson M, Sivaprasad S (2014) Correlation of fundus fluorescein angiography and spectral-domain optical coherence tomography in identification of membrane subtypes in neovascular age-related macular degeneration. Ophthalmol J Int d'ophtalmol Int J Ophthalmol Zeitschrift für Augenheilkunde 231:153–159. doi:10.1159/000355091

Mayr-Sponer U, Waldstein SM, Kundi M, Ritter M, Golbaz I, Heiling U, Papp A, Simader C, Schmidt-Erfurth U (2013) Influence of the vitreomacular interface on outcomes of ranibizumab therapy in neovascular age-related macular degeneration. Ophthalmology 120:2620–2629. doi:10.1016/j.ophtha.2013.05.032

Mojana F, Cheng L, Bartsch DU, Silva GA, Kozak I, Nigam N, Freeman WR (2008) The role of abnormal vitreomacular adhesion in age-related macular degeneration: spectral optical coherence tomography and surgical results. Am J Ophthalmol 146(2):218–227. doi:10.1016/j.ajo.2008.04.027

Moult E, Choi W, Waheed NK, Adhi M, Lee B, Lu CD, Jayaraman V, Potsaid B, Rosenfeld PJ, Duker JS, Fujimoto JG (2014) Ultrahigh-speed swept-source OCT angiography in exudative AMD. Ophthalmic Surg Lasers Imaging Retina 45:496–505. doi:10.3928/23258160-20141118-03

Mukai R, Sato T, Kishi S (2014) A hyporeflective space between hyperreflective materials in pigment epithelial detachment and Bruch's membrane in neovascular age-related macular degeneration. BMC Ophthalmol 14:159. doi:10.1186/1471-2415-14-159

Nagiel A, Freund KB, Spaide RF, Munch IC, Larsen M, Sarraf D (2013) Mechanism of retinal pigment epithelium tear formation following intravitreal anti-vascular endothelial growth factor therapy revealed by spectral-domain optical coherence tomography. Am J Ophthalmol 156:981–98800. doi:10.1016/j.ajo.2013.06.024

Neudorfer M, Weinberg A, Loewenstein A, Barak A (2012) Differential optical density of subretinal spaces. Invest Ophthalmol Vis Sci 53:3104–3110. doi:10.1167/iovs.11-8700

Pemp B, Schmetterer L (2008) Ocular blood flow in diabetes and age-related macular degeneration. Can J Ophthalmol J Can d'ophtalmol 43:295–301. doi:10.3129/i08-049

Querques G, Souied EH, Freund KB (2013) Multimodal imaging of early stage 1 type 3 neovascularization with simultaneous eye-tracked spectral-domain optical coherence tomography and high-speed real-time angiography. Retina (Philadelphia) 33:1881–1887. doi:10.1097/IAE.0b013e3182923448

Ritter M, Simader C, Bolz M, Deák GG, Mayr-Sponer U, Sayegh R, Kundi M, Schmidt-Erfurth UM (2014) Intraretinal cysts are the most relevant prognostic biomarker in neovascular age-related macular degeneration independent of the therapeutic strategy. Br J Ophthalmol 98:1629–1635. doi:10.1136/bjophthalmol-2014-305186

Roberts P, Mittermueller TJ, Montuoro A, Sulzbacher F, Munk M, Sacu S, Schmidt-Erfurth U (2014) A quantitative approach to identify morphological features relevant for visual function in ranibizumab therapy of neovascular AMD. Invest Ophthalmol Vis Sci 55:6623–6630. doi:10.1167/iovs.14-14293

Rosenfeld PJ, Brown DM, Heier JS, Boyer DS, Kaiser PK, Chung CY, Kim RY, Group MS (2006) Ranibizumab for neovascular age-related macular degeneration. N Engl J Med 355:1419–1431. doi:10.1056/NEJMoa054481

Rossi EA, Rangel-Fonseca P, Parkins K, Fischer W, Latchney LR, Folwell MA, Williams DR, Dubra A, Chung MM (2013) In vivo imaging of retinal pigment epithelium cells in age related macular degeneration. Biomed Opt Express 4:2527–2539. doi:10.1364/BOE.4.002527

Rouvas AA, Papakostas TD, Ntouraki A, Douvali M, Vergados I, Ladas ID (2010) Angiographic and OCT features of retinal angiomatous proliferation. Eye (Lond) 24:1633. doi:10.1038/eye.2010.134

Saito M, Iida T, Nagayama D (2008) Cross-sectional and en face optical coherence tomographic features of polypoidal choroidal vasculopathy. Retina (Philadelphia) 28:459–464. doi:10.1097/IAE.0b013e318156db60

Sakamoto A, Hangai M, Yoshimura N (2008) Spectral-domain optical coherence tomography with multiple B-scan averaging for enhanced imaging of retinal diseases. Ophthalmology 115:1071. doi:10.1016/j.ophtha.2007.09.001

Sayanagi K, Sharma S, Kaiser PK (2009) Photoreceptor status after antivascular endothelial growth factor therapy in exudative age-related macular degeneration. Br J Ophthalmol 93:622–626. doi:10.1136/bjo.2008.151977

Sayanagi K, Gomi F, Ikuno Y, Akiba M, Nishida K (2014) Comparison of spectral-domain and high-penetration OCT for observing morphologic changes in age-related macular degeneration and polypoidal choroidal vasculopathy. Graefes Arch Clin Exp Ophthalmol 252:3–9. doi:10.1007/s00417-013-2474-5

Sayanagi K, Gomi F, Akiba M, Sawa M, Hara C, Nishida K (2015) En-face high-penetration optical coherence tomography imaging in polypoidal choroidal vasculopathy. Br J Ophthalmol 99:29–35. doi:10.1136/bjophthalmol-2013-304658

Schaal KB, Freund KB, Litts KM, Zhang Y, Messinger JD, Curcio CA (2015) OUTER RETINAL TUBULATION IN ADVANCED AGE-RELATED MACULAR DEGENERATION: optical coherence tomographic findings correspond to histology. Retina 35:1339–1350. doi:10.1097/IAE.0000000000000471

Schlanitz FG, Baumann B, Spalek T, Schütze C, Ahlers C, Pircher M, Götzinger E, Hitzenberger CK, Schmidt-Erfurth U (2011) Performance of automated drusen detection by polarization-sensitive optical coherence tomography. Invest Ophthalmol Vis Sci 52:4571–4579. doi:10.1167/iovs.10-6846

Schmidl D, Garhofer G, Schmetterer L (2011) The complex interaction between ocular perfusion pressure and ocular blood flow - relevance for glaucoma. Exp Eye Res 93:141–155. doi:10.1016/j.exer.2010.09.002

Schmidt-Erfurth U, Eldem B, Guymer R, Korobelnik J-FF, Schlingemann RO, Axer-Siegel R, Wiedemann P, Simader C, Gekkieva M, Weichselberger A, Group ES (2011) Efficacy and safety of monthly versus quarterly ranibizumab treatment in neovascular age-related macular degeneration: the EXCITE study. Ophthalmology 118:831–839. doi:10.1016/j.ophtha.2010.09.004

Schmidt-Erfurth U, Chong V, Loewenstein A, Larsen M, Souied E, Schlingemann R, Eldem B, Monés J, Richard G, Bandello F, European Society of Retina S (2014a) Guidelines for the management of neovascular age-related macular degeneration by the European Society of Retina Specialists (EURETINA). Br J Ophthalmol 98:1144–1167. doi:10.1136/bjophthalmol-2014-305702

Schmidt-Erfurth U, Kaiser PK, Korobelnik J-FF, Brown DM, Chong V, Nguyen QD, Ho AC, Ogura Y, Simader C, Jaffe GJ, Slakter JS, Yancopoulos GD, Stahl N, Vitti R, Berliner AJ, Soo Y, Anderesi M, Sowade O, Zeitz O, Norenberg C, Sandbrink R, Heier JS (2014b) Intravitreal aflibercept injection for neovascular age-related macular degeneration: ninety-six-week results of the VIEW studies. Ophthalmology 121:193–201. doi:10.1016/j.ophtha.2013.08.011

Schmidt-Erfurth U, Waldstein SM, Deak G-GG, Kundi M, Simader C (2015) Pigment epithelial detachment followed by retinal cystoid degeneration leads to vision loss in treatment of neovascular age-related macular degeneration. Ophthalmology 122:822–832. doi:10.1016/j.ophtha.2014.11.017

Schulze S, Hoerle S, Mennel S, Kroll P (2008) Vitreomacular traction and exudative age-related macular degeneration. Acta Ophthalmol 86:470–481. doi:10.1111/j.1755-3768.2008.01210.x

Schütze C, Wedl M, Baumann B, Pircher M, Hitzenberger CK, Schmidt-Erfurth U (2015) Progression of retinal pigment epithelial atrophy in antiangiogenic therapy of neovascular age-related macular degeneration. Am J Ophthalmol 159:1100–1114.e1. doi:10.1016/j.ajo.2015.02.020

Schwartz DM, Fingler J, Kim DY, Zawadzki RJ, Morse LS, Park SS, Fraser SE, Werner JS (2014) Phase-variance optical coherence tomography: a technique for noninvasive angiography. Ophthalmology 121:180–187. doi:10.1016/j.ophtha.2013.09.002

Simader C, Ritter M, Bolz M, Deák GG, Mayr-Sponer U, Golbaz I, Kundi M, Schmidt-Erfurth UM (2014) Morphologic parameters relevant for visual outcome during anti-angiogenic therapy of neovascular age-related macular degeneration. Ophthalmology 121:1237–1245. doi:10.1016/j.ophtha.2013.12.029

Slakter JS, Yannuzzi LA, Schneider U, Sorenson JA, Ciardella A, Guyer DR, Spaide RF, Freund KB, Orlock DA (2000) Retinal choroidal anastomoses and occult choroidal neovascularization in age-related macular degeneration. Ophthalmology 107:742. doi:10.1016/S0161-6420(00)00009-9

Song W, Wei Q, Jiao S, Zhang HF (2013) Integrated photoacoustic ophthalmoscopy and spectral-domain optical coherence tomography. J Vis Exp JoVE 71:e4390. doi:10.3791/4390

Spaide RF (2009) Enhanced depth imaging optical coherence tomography of retinal pigment epithelial detachment in age-related macular degeneration. Am J Ophthalmol 147:644–652. doi:10.1016/j.ajo.2008.10.005

Spaide RF (2015) Optical coherence tomography angiography signs of vascular abnormalization with antiangiogenic therapy for choroidal neovascularization. Am J Ophthalmol 160:6–16. doi:10.1016/j.ajo.2015.04.012

Spaide RF, Koizumi H, Pozzoni MC, Pozonni MC (2008) Enhanced depth imaging spectral-domain optical coherence tomography. Am J Ophthalmol 146(4):496–500. doi:10.1016/j.ajo.2008.05.032

Sulzbacher F, Kiss C, Munk M, Deak G, Sacu S, Schmidt-Erfurth U (2011) Diagnostic evaluation of type 2 (classic) choroidal neovascularization: optical coherence tomography, indocyanine green angiography, and fluorescein angiography. Am J Ophthalmol 152:799–8060. doi:10.1016/j.ajo.2011.04.011

Swanson EA, Izatt JA, Hee MR, Huang D, Lin CP, Schuman JS, Puliafito CA, Fujimoto JG (1993) In vivo retinal imaging by optical coherence tomography. Opt Lett 18:1864–1866

Tulvatana W, Adamian M, Berson EL, Dryja TP (1999) Photoreceptor rosettes in autosomal dominant retinitis pigmentosa with reduced penetrance. Arch Ophthalmol 117:399–402

Ueda-Arakawa N, Tsujikawa A, Yamashiro K, Ooto S, Tamura H, Yoshimura N (2012) Visual prognosis of eyes with submacular hemorrhage associated with exudative age-related macular degeneration. Jpn J Ophthalmol 56:589–598. doi:10.1007/s10384-012-0191-y

Unterhuber A, Povazay B, Hermann B, Sattmann H, Chavez-Pirson A, Drexler W (2005) In vivo retinal optical coherence tomography at 1040 nm-enhanced penetration into the choroid. Optics express 13(9): 3252–3258

Wakabayashi T, Oshima Y, Fujimoto H, Murakami Y, Sakaguchi H, Kusaka S, Tano Y (2009) Foveal microstructure and visual acuity after retinal detachment repair: imaging analysis by Fourier-domain optical coherence tomography. Ophthalmology 116:519–528. doi:10.1016/j.ophtha.2008.10.001

Waldstein SM, Sponer U, Simader C, Sacu S, Schmidt-Erfurth U (2012) Influence of vitreomacular adhesion on the development of exudative age-related macular degeneration: 4-year results of a longitudinal study. Retina (Philadelphia, Pa) 32:424–433. doi:10.1097/IAE.0b013e3182278b80

Waldstein SM, Ritter M, Simader C, Mayr-Sponer U, Kundi M, Schmidt-Erfurth U (2014) Impact of vitreomacular adhesion on ranibizumab mono- and combination therapy for neovascular age-related macular degeneration. Am J Ophthalmol 158:328–3360. doi:10.1016/j.ajo.2014.04.028

Wang XJ, Milner TE, Nelson JS (1995) Characterization of fluid flow velocity by optical Doppler tomography. Opt Lett 20:1337–1339

Wang Y, Bower BA, Izatt JA, Tan O, Huang D (2007) In vivo total retinal blood flow measurement by Fourier domain Doppler optical coherence tomography. J Biomed Opt 12:41215. doi:10.1117/1.2772871

Wang Y, Fawzi AA, Tan O, Zhang X, Huang D (2011a) Flicker-induced changes in retinal blood flow assessed by Doppler optical coherence tomography. Biomed Opt Express 2:1852–1860. doi:10.1364/BOE.001852

Wang Y, Fawzi AA, Varma R, Sadun AA, Zhang X (2011b) Pilot study of optical coherence tomography measurement of retinal blood flow in retinal and optic nerve diseases. Invest Ophthalmol Vis Sci 52:840–845. doi:10.1167/iovs.10-5985

Werkmeister RM, Dragostinoff N, Pircher M, Götzinger E, Hitzenberger CK, Leitgeb RA, Schmetterer L (2008) Bidirectional Doppler Fourier-domain optical coherence tomography for measurement of absolute flow velocities in human retinal vessels. Opt Lett 33:2967–2969

Wojtkowski M, Leitgeb R, Kowalczyk A, Bajraszewski T, Fercher AF (2002) In vivo human retinal imaging by Fourier domain optical coherence tomography. J Biomed Opt 7:457–463. doi:10.1117/1.1482379

Wolff B, Matet A, Vasseur V, Sahel J-AA, Mauget-Faÿsse M (2012) En face OCT imaging for the diagnosis of outer retinal tubulations in age-related macular degeneration. J Ophthalmol 2012:542417. doi:10.1155/2012/542417

Wolf-Schnurrbusch UE, Ghanem R, Rothenbuehler SP, Enzmann V, Framme C, Wolf S (2011) Predictors of short-term visual outcome after anti-VEGF therapy of macular edema due to central retinal vein occlusion. Invest Ophthalmol Vis Sci 52:3334–3337. doi:10.1167/iovs.10-6097

Xia J, Yao J, Wang LV (2014) Photoacoustic tomography: principles and advances. Electromagn waves (Cambridge, Mass) 147:1–22

Yannuzzi LA, Negrão S, Iida T, Carvalho C, Rodriguez-Coleman H, Slakter J, Freund KB, Sorenson J, Orlock D, Borodoker N (2001) Retinal angiomatous proliferation in age-related macular degeneration. Retina (Philadelphia, Pa) 21:416–434

Yannuzzi LA, Freund KB, Takahashi BS (2008) Review of retinal angiomatous proliferation or type 3 neovascularization. Retina (Philadelphia, Pa) 28:375–384. doi:10.1097/IAE.0b013e3181619c55

Ying GS, Kim BJ, Maguire MG, Huang J, Daniel E, Jaffe GJ, Grunwald JE, Blinder KJ, Flaxel CJ, Rahhal F, Regillo C, Martin DF, Group CR (2014) Sustained visual acuity loss in the comparison of age-related macular degeneration treatments trials. JAMA Ophthalmol 132:915–921. doi:10.1001/jamaophthalmol.2014.1019

You JY, Chung H, Kim HC (2012) Evaluation of changes in choroidal neovascularization secondary to age-related macular degeneration after anti-VEGF therapy using spectral domain optical coherence tomography. Curr Eye Res 37:438–445. doi:10.3109/02713683.2011.647227

Zacks DN, Johnson MW (2004) Retinal angiomatous proliferation: optical coherence tomographic confirmation of an intraretinal lesion. Arch Ophthalmol (Chicago, Ill : 1960) 122:932–933. doi:10.1001/archopht.122.6.932

Zayit-Soudry S, Moroz I, Loewenstein A (2007) Retinal pigment epithelial detachment. Surv Ophthalmol 52:227–243. doi:10.1016/j.survophthal.2007.02.008

Zweifel SA, Engelbert M, Laud K, Margolis R, Spaide RF, Freund KB (2009) Outer retinal tubulation: a novel optical coherence tomography finding. Arch Ophthalmol 127:1596–1602. doi:10.1001/archophthalmol.2009.326

16 Polypoidal Choroidal Vasculopathy

Ichiro Maruko and Tomohiro Iida

Contents

16.1 Introduction

Polypoidal choroidal vasculopathy (PCV) is a disease reported by Yannuzzi et al. (1990) in 1990 and is now considered one of phenotypes of age-related macular degeneration (AMD). While exudative AMD is seen in approximately 5–10 % of western populations, various previous reports have confirmed that its prevalence is high in Asian countries including Japan (Ahuja et al. 2000; Byeon et al. 2008; Kwok et al. 2002; Maruko et al. 2007; Sho et al. 2003; Wen et al. 2004; Yannuzzi et al. 1999). According to our research, in which classification of AMD subtypes using fluorescein and indocyanine green angiography was conducted to 289 cases of patients with exudative AMD newly found in 2 years from 2003 to 2005, PCV, typical AMD, and retinal angiomatous proliferation (RAP) were seen in 158 (54.7 %), 102 (35.3 %), and 13 (4.5 %) cases, respectively (Maruko et al. 2007). While our report is a hospital-based study, when considered in connection with other reports, it shows that approximately half of cases suspected of exudative AMD are most likely to be diagnosed as PCV; therefore, PCV can be considered as one of the most major subtypes rather than a special type of exudative AMD in Japan. Meanwhile, there are some combined cases in which patients have PCV in one eye and typical AMD in the other in our report, so they are figured as disease groups with clinical overlap even though they have different phenotypes (Maruko et al. 2007, 2010). Also, it is shown that there is no large difference of genetic background in development of PCV and exudative AMD (Kondo et al. 2007; Gotoh et al. 2009).

I. Maruko, MD • T. Iida, MD (✉)
Department of Ophthalmology, Tokyo Women's Medical University School of Medicine, Tokyo, Japan
e-mail: iida@oph.twmu.ac.jp

C.H. Meyer et al. (eds.), *Spectral Domain Optical Coherence Tomography in Macular Diseases*,
DOI 10.1007/978-81-322-3610-8_16

PCV is definitionally structured with branch vascular network vessels and polypoidal formation around the tip. While these can be observed only as weak hyperfluorescence (occult type) with fluorescein angiography, indocyanine green angiography definitely shows these structures. Hence, the frequency of PCV might be underestimated at hospitals where indocyanine green angiography is not operated routinely. A certain example of diagnostic criteria for PCV by Japanese study group of PCV (2005) is defined as one which meets one of the following conditions: (1) Orange-red raised lesion is seen with funduscopy. (2) Typical polypoidal structure is seen with indocyanine green angiography. Also, an uncertain example is defined as one which meets one of the following conditions: (1) Only abnormal blood vessel networks are seen with indocyanine green angiography. (2) Only recurrent hemorrhagic serous retinal pigment epithelial detachment (PED) is seen. The typical polypoidal structure is torose or botryoid on indocyanine green angiography. The abnormal blood vessel networks are the ones which can be differentiated with normal choroid blood vessels by their running path and calibers of blood vessels at choroid membrane in the early phase of imaging with indocyanine green angiography, and it is said that they often show planate hyperfluorescence at the late phase. While those diagnostic criteria are Japanese ones, accurate diagnosis is needed for PCV since it can cause severe subretinal or retinal pigment epithelial bleeding followed by poor visual acuity or even type 2 CNV followed by bad prognosis of visual acuity. The criteria can be useful for doctors who diagnose such diseases. Some examples of differential diseases include typical AMD and central serous chorioretinopathy (CSC). Typical AMD especially type 1 is difficult to be identified. In addition, when only abnormal blood vessel networks are seen as an uncertain example of PCV, there are some cases impossible to be identified even using indocyanine green angiography. CSC, a disease which starts in middle age and causes serous retinal detachment (SRD) in a macula area, is sometimes difficult to be identified since it is sometimes seen in elderly people at the age of 50 or older and can be followed by atrophy of retinal pigment epithelium (RPE) (Spaide et al. 1996).

On the other hand, optical coherence tomography (OCT) can be a useful remark in diagnosis of PCV. Polypoidal structure is observed as a steep protrusion of retinal pigment epithelium (RPE). This is thought that a protrusion of RPE caused by polypoidal structure is observed secondarily (Saito et al. 2008a). Still, it can last even after treatment and regression of polypoidal structure, and the same remark can be observed in hemorrhagic PED or some other diseases. Therefore, it is difficult to diagnose only with this protrusion, and an angiographic examination is still needed for definite diagnosis.

With respect to treatment, research was conducted to 469 cases of 471 eyes with 1 year progress on verteporfin photodynamic therapy (PDT) in 13 facilities in Japan (Japanese Age-Related Macular Degeneration Tial (JAT) Study Group 2003) in accordance with new PDT guideline in 2008 (Tano 2008); it reported that the average visual acuity of the 146 eyes with PCV significantly improved from 0.15 to 0.19. Furthermore, reports regarding long-term progress showed it was possible to maintain the improved visual acuity for more than 2 years (Akaza et al. 2011; Saito et al. 2008b). These results insist that PDT is effective for PCV treatment. In the meantime, opportunities to choose therapy with anti-vascular epithelial growth factor (VEGF) agent have increased recently since it has only a few chances of complications and since a percentage of subretinal hemorrhage after PDT is relatively high (about 10%). On the other hand, some reports say that therapy with anti-VEGF agent for PCV makes exudation reduced but does not result in resolution of polypoidal lesion in many cases (Gomi et al. 2008; Hikichi et al. 2010; Kokame et al. 2009). EVEREST study (Koh et al. 2012) also reports that therapy with anti-VEGF agent alone is harder to obtain regression of polypoidal structure than that with PDT, so combined therapy with PDT and anti-VEGF agent has been attempted. Aflibercept has recently received attention because of a report showing it has the same function to resolve polypoidal lesion with anti-VEGF agent alone as PDT (Koizumi et al. 2015a).

Meanwhile, a large amount of recent reports regarding choroidal thickness of AMD using OCT indicates that PCV is thicker than typical AMD, and RAP is even thinner than typical AMD. Chung et al. (Chung et al. 2011) and Koizumi et al. (2011) reported that choroidal thickening in eyes with PCV was comparable to choroidal thinning in eyes with typical AMD. These findings might indicate that there are some differences in choroidal abnormalities between PCV and typical AMD. Sasahara et al. (Sasahara et al. 2006) reported that indocyanine green angiography showed much more choroidal vascular hyperpermeability similar to CSC in eyes with PCV than in eyes with typical AMD (Yannuzzi et al. 2000). Choroidal thickening in eyes with PCV might result from choroidal vascular hyperpermeability, and choroidal changes by various therapies have received attention recently (Koizumi et al. 2015b; Maruko et al. 2011, 2013; Yamazaki et al. 2012).

16.2 Typical Polypoidal Choroidal Vasculopathy

With OCT, polypoidal structure is observed as a steep, dome-shaped protrusion of RPE. Moderate reflection at some parts inside of this RPE protrusion is considered as polyp blood vessels themselves (Iijima et al. 1999, 2000; Otsuji et al. 2000). Areas of branch vascular network vessels are observed as two hyperreflective lines (double-layer sign) (Khan et al. 2012; Ojima et al. 2009; Sato et al. 2007; Tsujikawa et al. 2007). These lines are RPE and the Bruch membrane, and the network vessels are thought to be located between those two layers.

There are some cases of PCV associated with serous pigment epithelium detachment (PED). Polypoidal structure is sometimes located in a marginal edge of the PED (notch sign), and it is also observed as a dome-shaped protrusion of RPE besides the edge of PED on OCT.

16.3 Polypoidal Choroidal Vasculopathy Associated with Serous Retinal Detachment

Some cases of PCV show SRD without hemorrhage. In such cases, it can be hard to differentiate it with CSC using only foveal cross-hair OCT. Since steep, dome-shaped protrusions of RPE can be observed in areas of polypoidal structure as mentioned before, it is necessary to scan the whole part of SRD. Radial scan can be useful as well. Branch vascular network vessels are observed as double-layer sign connected to polypoidal structure. In many cases, PCV associated with SRD has thick choroid, which makes it easy to be mistaken for CSC.

16.4 Polypoidal Choroidal Vasculopathy with Macular Hematoma

PCV is sometimes accompanied with a large amount of macular hemorrhage. In such a case, the backward of the macular hematoma may not be visualized clearly even using swept source OCT or EDI-OCT. Subretinal hemorrhage is the major lesion of PCV with hematoma, and it is rare to result in preretinal hemorrhage or sub-internal limiting membrane hemorrhage. It is the important point to differentiate it with a case of macular hemorrhage caused by rupture of retinal arteriolar macroaneurysm. In addition, whereas choroid in PCV is thick, it tends to be thin in the case of rupture of retinal arteriolar macroaneurysm since it is seen in elderly people; this fact is used in diagnosis as well.

16.5 Optic Disc Type of Polypoidal Choroidal Vasculopathy

Early reports of PCV introduced some cases in which polypoidal structure and branch vascular network vessels were located around optic discs. Now, it is known that most lesions are seen in macular areas (Yannuzzi et al. 1997). Although it can be completely normal with OCT if there is no lesion in macular areas, SRD sometimes reaches to central fovea. Polypoidal structure is observed as a steep, dome-shaped protrusion of RPE like other types of PCV.

16.6 Choroidal Changes in Polypoidal Choroidal Vasculopathy After Treatment

Choroidal thickness in PCV is relatively thicker than other subtypes of AMD as mentioned above. In addition, the choroidal thickness seems to change after PDT and/or intravitreal injection of anti-VEGF. Maruko et al. (2011) described the choroidal thickness decreased after PDT for PCV. On the other hand, Yamazaki et al. (2012) reported 1-year results of the choroidal thinning after intravitreal ranibizumab as needed, and Koizumi et al. (2015a, b) mentioned the choroidal thickness reduction after intravitreal aflibercept in their short-term results.

Moreover, the choroidal thickness changes in PCV might be associated with the activity of PCV according to the latest researches. Maruko et al. (2013) reported the choroidal thickness at PCV recurrence returned to the baseline level after choroidal thinning as a result of combination therapy with intravitreal ranibizumab and PDT. The choroidal thickness in this case was maintained thinner than that in nonrecurrent cases even at 1 year.

16.7 Case Report

Case 1: Typical Polypoidal Choroidal Vasculopathy

76 year-old male; 0.2 corrected vision in the left eye:

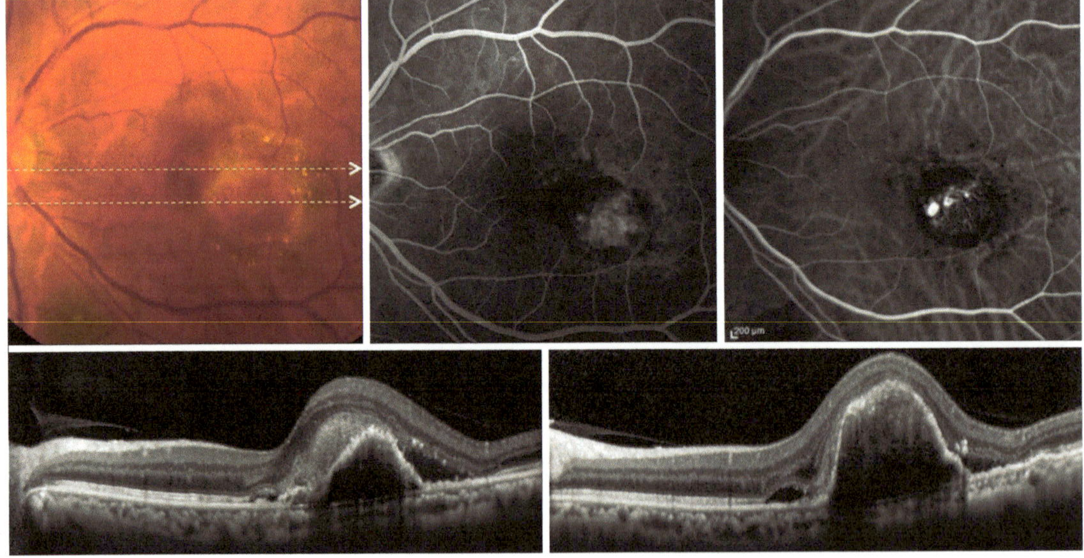

1. Color image

   Orange-red raised lesion with hard exudate is seen in the temporal to foveal.
2. Fluorescein angiography

   The orange lesion is observed as weak hyperfluorescence-like occult type of AMD.
3. Indocyanine green angiography

   Polypoidal structure and surrounding branch vascular network vessels can be observed.
4. OCT horizontal scan at the fovea

   Polypoidal structure can be observed as a steep, dome-shaped protrusion of RPE, and branch vascular network vessels connected to polypoidal structure are observed as double-layer sign. Moderate reflection, which presumably is fibrin, above the polypoidal lesion is observed at the subfovea. SRD is also observed in the area adjacent to RPE protrusion. The choroid is not thickened in this case. Subfoveal choroidal thickness is 203 μm.
5. OCT horizontal scan at the center of polypoidal lesion

   OCT image shows RPE protrusion at the center of the polypoidal lesion, and the inside of this protrusion is observed as the moderate reflection.

Case 2: PCV with Large PED

74 year-old male; 0.1 corrected vision in the left eye:

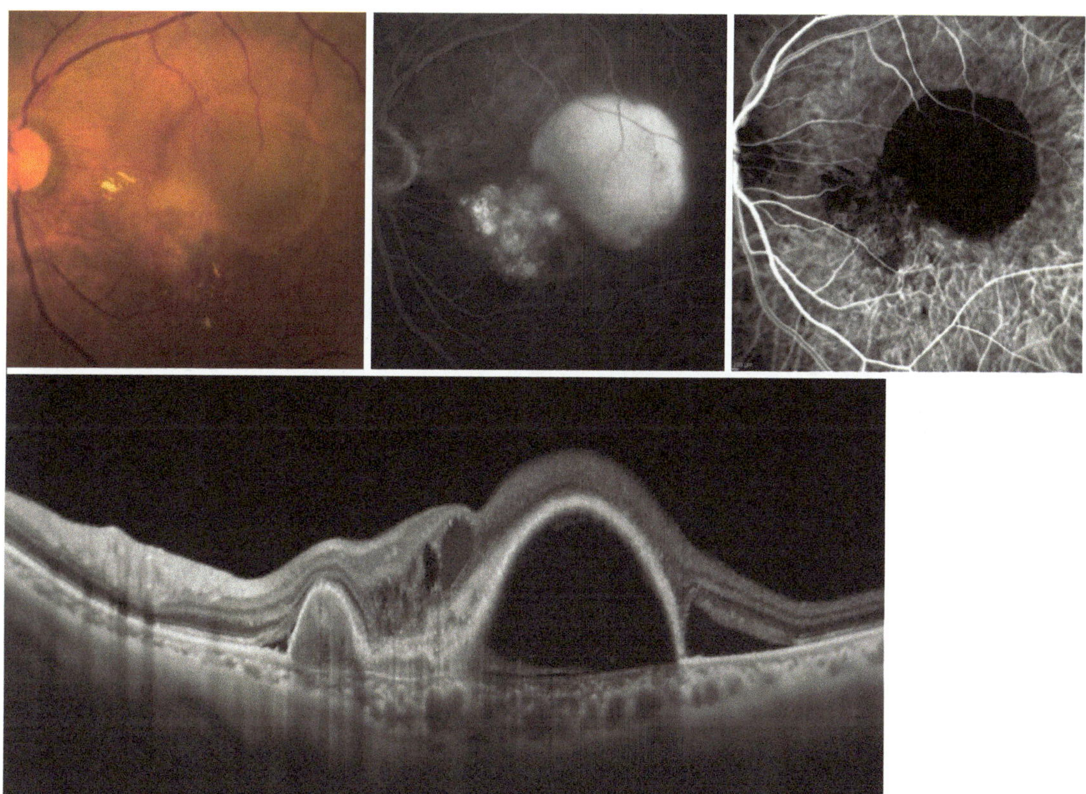

1. Color image

   Large circular serous PED is seen in central fovea. Orange lesion with hard exudate is observed in the nasal side of the large PED.
2. Fluorescein angiography

   Weak hyperfluorescence can be observed in the nasal side of PED.
3. Indocyanine green angiography

   PED is observed as hypofluorescence since it is blocked, and polypoidal structure can be observed in its nasal side (notch sign).
4. OCT (horizontal section)

   Large PED is observed at the subfovea to temporal macula. Polypoidal structure can be observed as a steep, dome-shaped protrusion of RPE in the nasal side of the fovea, and branch vascular network vessels connected to polypoidal structure and large PED are observed as double-layer sign. Inside of the polypoidal structure is seen as the moderate reflection.

Case 3: PCV Associated with Serous Retinal Detachment 75 year-old male; 0.6 corrected vision in the right eye:

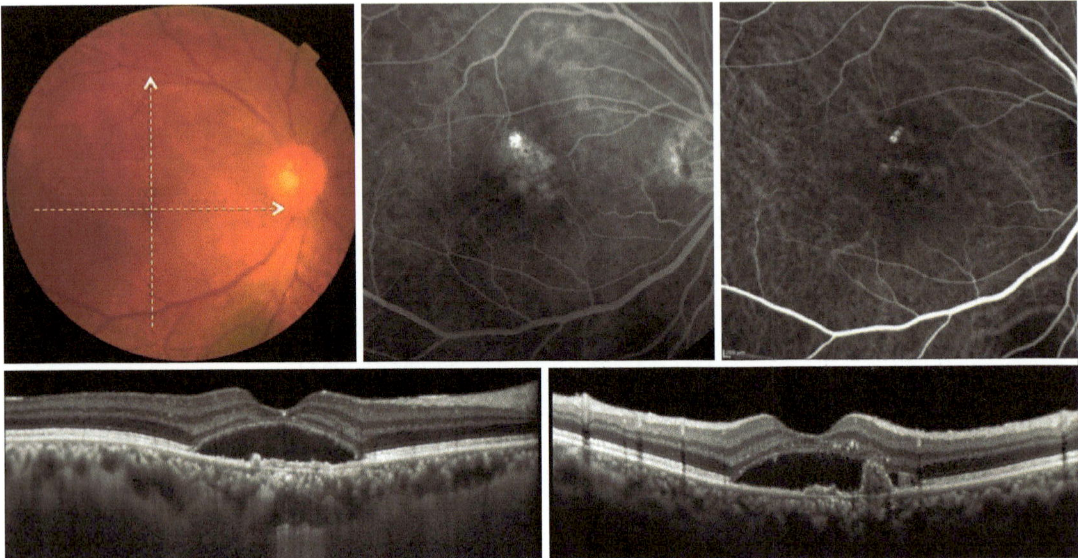

1. Color image

   SRD is seen at the fovea.
2. Fluorescein angiography

   Weak hyperfluorescence is observed in the upper part of macula.
3. Indocyanine green angiography

   Polypoidal structure is found in the area within hyperfluorescence seen on fluorescein angiography.
4. OCT (horizontal section)

   SRD can be observed. There are some small, irregular protrusions of RPE. The choroid is relatively thickened in this case. Subfoveal choroidal thickness is 337 μm.
5. OCT (vertical section)

   Steep protrusions of RPE can be observed in the upper area of the fovea, consistent with the polypoidal structure seen on indocyanine green angiography. Branch vascular network vessels are observed as double-layer sign connected to RPE protrusion.

Case 4: PCV with Macular Hematoma
87 year-old male; 0.1 corrected vision in the right eye:

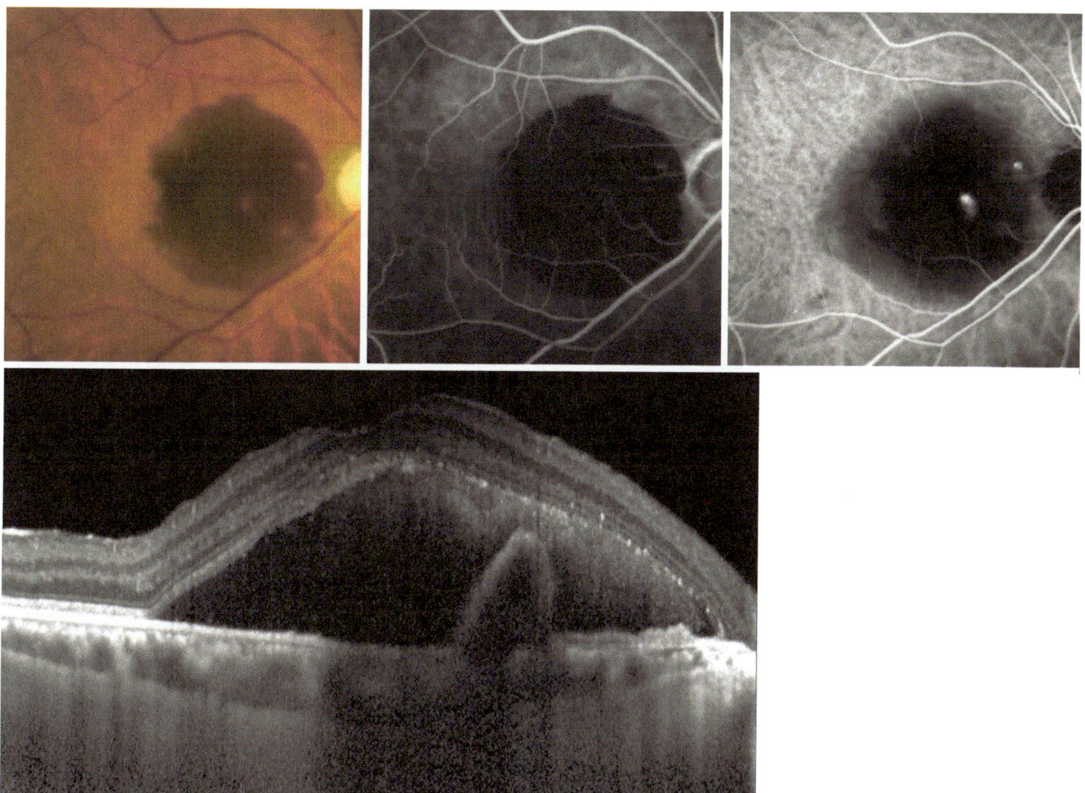

1. Color image
   Subretinal hematoma is seen at the macular area.
2. Fluorescein angiography
   Macular hemorrhage is observed as hypofluorescence since it is blocked.
3. Indocyanine green angiography
   Polypoidal structure can be observed in the nasal side of the fovea and temporal side of the disc.
4. OCT horizontal scan using EDI technique
   Polypoidal structure can be observed as steep, dome-shaped protrusions of RPE within the subretinal space. Inside of the subretinal space is observed as the moderate reflection, consistent with macular hematoma. Although it is unclear because of the hematoma, subfoveal choroidal thickness is 271 μm.

Case 5: Optic Disc Type of PCV

71 year-old male; 0.5 corrected vision in the right eye:

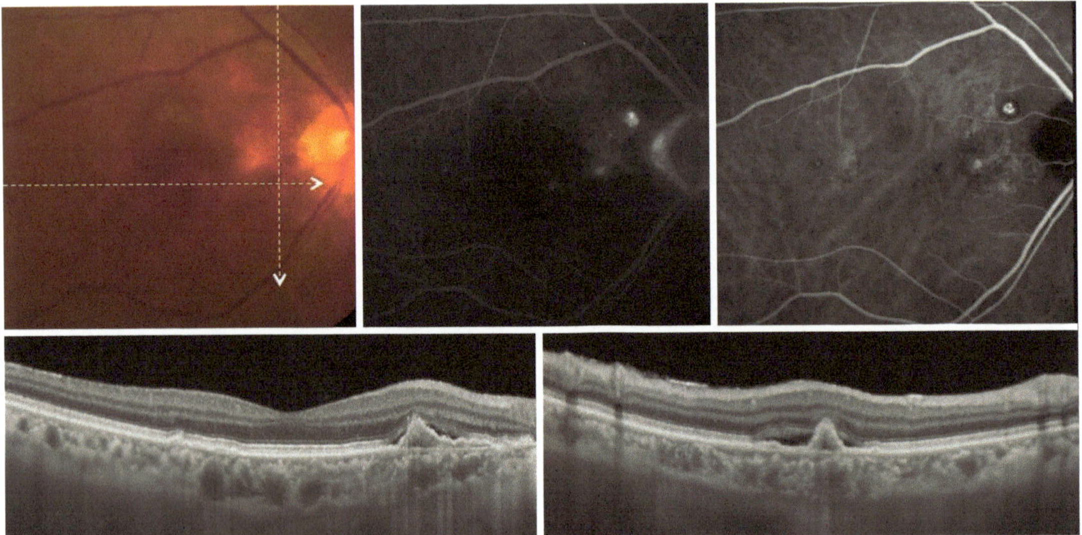

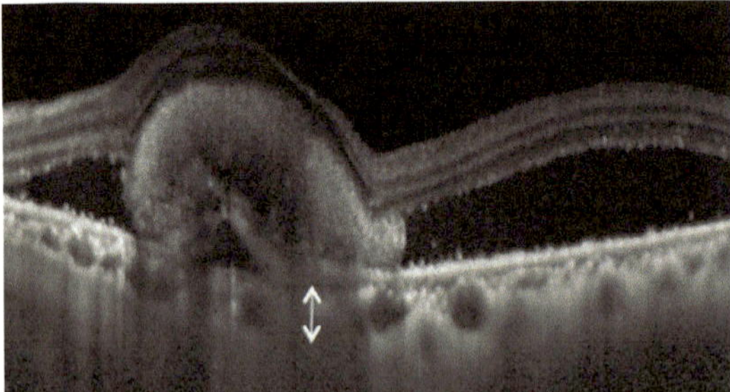

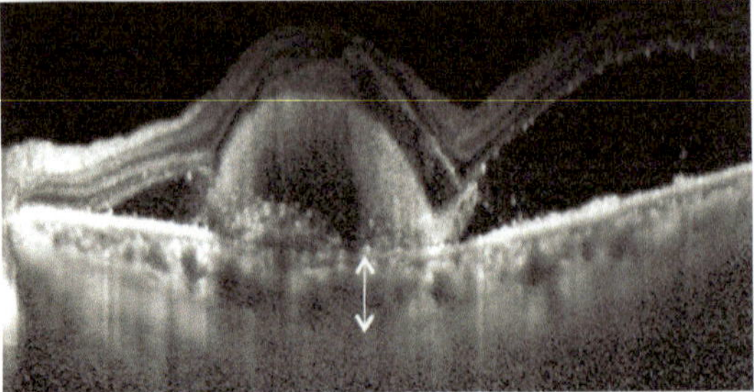

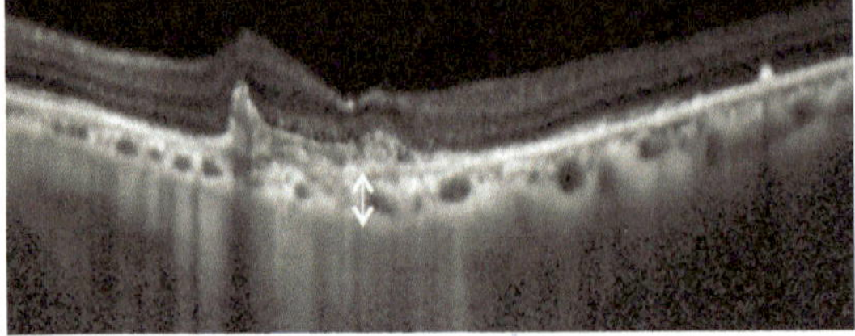

1. Color image

   There is no SRD in the fovea, and orange-red raised lesion is seen in the temporal to the optic disc.
2. Fluorescein angiography

   Weak hyperfluorescence can be observed from the temporal to the optic disc.
3. Indocyanine green angiography

   Polypoidal structure can be observed in the temporal to the optic disc, and branch vascular network vessels are surrounded on the temporal side of the optic disc.
4. OCT (horizontal section)

   OCT image shows almost normal at the fovea, and RPE irregularity is observed in the nasal side of the fovea.
5. OCT (vertical section near the optic disc)

   Polypoidal structure can be observed as steep, dome-shaped protrusions of RPE just in the temporal side of the disc.

Case 6: Choroidal Change After PDT

78 year-old male; 0.1 corrected vision in the left eye:

1. OCT at baseline
   SRD can be observed. There is an irregular RPE protrusion with hyperreflection considered as fibrin. Subfoveal choroidal thickness is 235 μm.
2. OCT 2 days after PDT
   Subfoveal choroidal thickness is thickened at 280 μm. At the same time, SRD gets tall, and retinal edema is also seen.
3. OCT 3 months after PDT
   Subfoveal choroidal thickness has reduced to 142 μm. SRD and retinal edema have been resolved. On the other hand, protrusions of RPE have been still observed although the size becomes smaller.

Case 7: Choroidal Thinning After Intravitreal Injection of Anti-VEGF

81 year-old male; 0.3 corrected vision in the right eye:

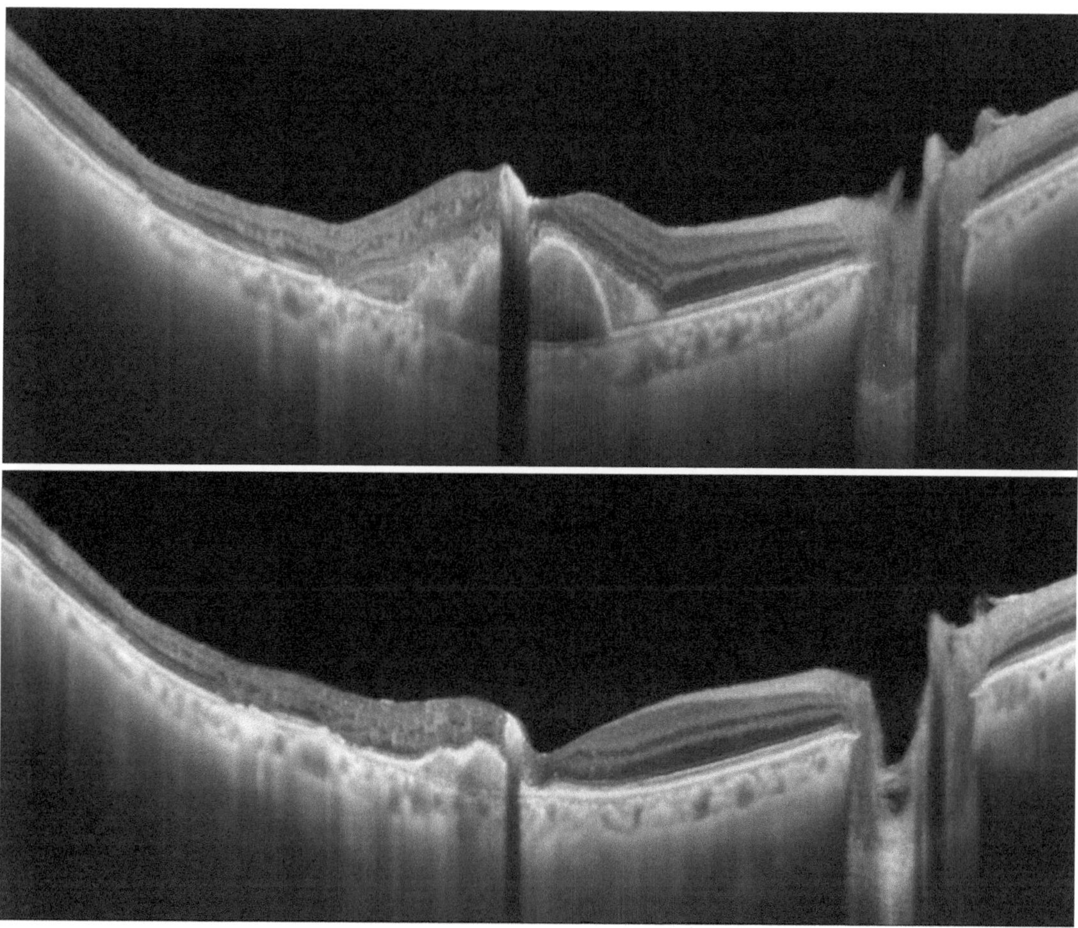

1. OCT at baseline
   There are some irregular RPE protrusions and SRD. Subfoveal choroidal thickness is 200 μm.
2. OCT after three monthly intravitreal injections of anti-VEGF
   Subfoveal choroidal thickness has decreased to 158 μm. While SRD and retinal edema have no longer been observed, protrusions of RPE have remained.

References

Ahuja RM, Stanga PE, Vingerling JR et al (2000) Polypoidal choroidal vasculopathy in exudative and hemorrhagic pigment epithelial detachments. Br J Ophthalmol 84:479–484

Akaza E, Yuzawa M, Mori R (2011) Three-year follow-up results of photodynamic therapy forpolypoidal choroidal vasculopathy. Jpn J Ophthalmol 55:39–44

Byeon SH, Lee SC, Oh HS (2008) Incidence and clinical patterns of polypoidal choroidal vasculopathy in Korean patients. Jpn J Ophthalmol 52:57–62

Chung SE, Kang SW, Lee JH et al (2011) Choroidal thickness in polypoidal choroidal vasculopathy and exudative age-related macular degeneration. Ophthalmology 118:840–845

Gomi F, Sawa M, Sakaguchi H et al (2008) Efficacy of intravitrealbevacizumab for polypoidal choroidal vasculopathy. Br J Ophthalmol 92:70–73

Gotoh N, Nakanishi H, Hayashi H et al (2009) ARMS2 (LOC387715) variants in Japanese patients with exudative age-related macular degeneration and polypoidal choroidalvasculopathy. Am J Ophthalmol 147:1037–1041

Hikichi T, Ohtsuka H, Higuchi M et al (2010) Improvement of angiographic findings of polypoidal choroidal vasculopathy after intravitreal injection of ranibizumab monthly for 3 months. Am J Ophthalmol 150:674–682

Iijima H, Imai M, Gohdo T et al (1999) Optical coherence tomography of idiopathic polypoidal choroidal vasculopathy. Am J Ophthalmol 127:301–305

Iijima H, Iida T, Imai M et al (2000) Optical coherence tomography of orange-red subretinallesions in eyes with idiopathic polypoidal choroidal vasculopathy. Am J Ophthalmol 129:21–26

Japanese Age-Related Macular Degeneration Tial (JAT) Study Group:Japanese age-relatedmacular degeneration trial (2003) 1-year results of photodynamic therapy with verteporfin in Japanese patients with subfoveal choroidal neovascularization secondary to age-related macular degeneration. Am J Ophthalmol 136:1049–1061

Japanese study group of polypoidal choroidal vasculopathy (2005) Criteria for diagnosis of polypoidal choroidal vasculopathy. Nihon Ganka Gakkai Zasshi 109:417–427

Khan S, Engelbert M, Imamura Y et al (2012) Polypoidal choroidal vasculopathy: simultaneous indocyanine green angiography and eye-tracked spectral domain optical coherencetomography findings. Retina 32:1057–1068

Koh A, Lee WK, Chen LJ et al (2012) EVEREST study: efficacy and safety of verteporfin photodynamic therapy in combination with ranibizumab or alone versus ranibizumabmonotherapy in patients with symptomatic macular polypoidal choroidal vasculopathy. Retina 32:1453–1464

Koizumi H, Yamagishi T, Yamazaki T et al (2011) Subfoveal choroidal thickness in typical age-related macular degeneration and polypoidal choroidal vasculopathy. Graefes Arch Clin Exp Ophthalmol 249:1123–1128

Koizumi H, Kano M, Yamamoto A et al (2015a) Aflibercept therapy for polypoidal choroidalvasculopathy: short-term results of a multicentre study. Br J Ophthalmol 99:1284–1288. doi:10.1136/bjophthalmol-2014-306432

Koizumi H, Kano M, Yamamoto A et al (2015b) Short-term changes in choroidal thickness after aflibercept therapy for neovascular age-related macular degeneration. Am J Ophthalmol 159:627–633

Kokame GT, Yeung L, Lai JC (2009) Continuous anti-VEGF treatment with ranibizumabforpolypoidal choroidal vasculopathy: 6-month results. Br J Ophthalmol 94:297–301

Kondo N, Honda S, Ishibashi K et al (2007) LOC387715/HTRA1 variants in polypoidal choroidal vasculopathy and age-related macular degeneration in a Japanese population. Am J Ophthalmol 144:608–612

Kwok AK, Lai TY, Chan CW et al (2002) Polypoidal choroidal vasculopathy in Chinese patients. Br J Ophthalmol 86:892–897

Maruko I, Iida T, Saito M et al (2007) Clinical characteristics of exudative age-related macular degeneration in Japanese patients. Am J Ophthalmol 144:15–22

Maruko I, Iida T, Saito M et al (2010) Combined cases of polypoidal choroidal vasculopathy and typical age-related macular degeneration. Graefes Arch Clin Exp Ophthalmol 248:361–368

Maruko I, Iida T, Sugano Y et al (2011) Subfoveal retinal and choroidal thickness after verteporfin photodynamic therapy for polypoidal choroidal vasculopathy. Am J Ophthalmol 151:594–603

Maruko I, Iida T, Oyamada H et al (2013) Choroidal thickness changes after intravitreal ranibizumab and photodynamic therapy in recurrent polypoidal choroidal vasculopathy. Am J Ophthalmol 156:548–556

Ojima Y, Hangai M, Sakamoto A et al (2009) Improved visualization of polypoidal choroidal vasculopathy lesions using spectral-domain optical coherence tomography. Retina 29:52–59

Otsuji T, Takahashi K, Fukushima I et al (2000) Optical coherence tomographic findings of idiopathic polypoidal choroidal vasculopathy. Ophthalmic Surg Lasers 31:210–214

Saito M, Iida T, Nagayama D (2008a) Cross-sectional and en face optical coherence tomographic features of polypoidal choroidal vasculopathy. Retina 28:459–469

Saito M, Iida T, Nagayama D (2008b) Photodynamic therapy with verteporfin for age-related macular degeneration or polypoidal choroidal vasculopathy: comparison of the presence of serous retinal pigment epithelial detachment. Br J Ophthalmol 92:1642–1647

Sasahara M, Tsujikawa A, Musashi K et al (2006) Polypoidal choroidal vasculopathy with choroidal vascular hyperpermeability. Am J Ophthalmol 142:601–607

Sato T, Kishi S, Watanabe G et al (2007) Tomographic features of branching vascular networks in polypoidal choroidal vasculopathy. Retina 27:589–594

Sho K, Takahashi K, Yamada H et al (2003) Polypoidal choroidal vasculopathy: incidence, demographic features, and clinical characteristics. Arch Ophthalmol 121:1392–1396

Spaide RF, Campeas L, Haas A et al (1996) Central serous chorioretinopathy in younger and older adults. Ophthalmology 103:2070–2080

Tano Y, Ophthalmic PDT Study Group (2008) Guidelines for PDT in Japan. Ophthalmology 115:585–585

Tsujikawa A, Sasahara M, Otani A et al (2007) Pigment epithelial detachment in polypoidal choroidal vasculopathy. Am J Ophthalmol 143:102–111

Wen F, Chen C, Wu D et al (2004) Polypoidal choroidal vasculopathy in elderly Chinese patients. Graefes Arch Clin Exp Ophthalmol 242:625–629

Yamazaki T, Koizumi H, Yamagishi T et al (2012) Subfoveal choroidal thickness after ranibizumab therapy for neovascular age-related macular degeneration: 12-month results. Ophthalmology 119:1621–1627

Yannuzzi LA, Sorenson J, Spaide RF et al (1990) Idiopathic polypoidal choroidal vasculopathy (IPCV). Retina 10:1–8

Yannuzzi LA, Ciardella A, Spaide RF et al (1997) The expanding clinical spectrum of idiopathic polypoidal choroidal vasculopathy. Arch Ophthalmol 115:478–485

Yannuzzi LA, Wong DW, Sforzolini BS et al (1999) Polypoidal choroidal vasculopathy and neovascularized age-related macular degeneration. Arch Ophthalmol 117:1503–1510

Yannuzzi LA, Freund KB, Goldbaum M et al (2000) Polypoidal choroidal vasculopathy masquerading as central serous chorioretinopathy. Ophthalmology 107:767–777

17 Macular Telangiectasia

Peter Charbel Issa, Simone Müller,
Tjebo F.C. Heeren, and Frank G. Holz

Contents

17.1 Introduction

This chapter contains excerpts, reprinted from Charbel Issa et al. (2013) with permission from Elsevier.

Macular telangiectasia type 2 (MacTel type 2) is a retinal disease with characteristic degenerative changes within the macular area (Charbel Issa et al. 2013). Concurrent alterations of the macular vascular network and the unknown cause of the disease have led to a variety of different descriptive terms, including idiopathic juxtafoveolar telangiectasia type 2, perifoveal telangiectasia, and others. Although funduscopy may reveal characteristic changes, the diagnosis based on clinical examination may sometimes be challenging. Fluorescein angiography has long been the gold standard to diagnose the disease. However, it has recently emerged that noninvasive optical coherence tomography (OCT) may also be particularly helpful in making the diagnosis. Herein, we provide a summary on the clinical phenotype of MacTel type 2 and describe the variety of presentations on OCT imaging.

17.2 Clinical Findings

Disease manifestations of MacTel type 2 are largely confined to an oval central retinal area that is slightly larger horizontally than vertically, while the peripheral retina appears unaffected. Five stages of the disease have been proposed by Gass and Blodi (Gass and Blodi 1993) based on funduscopy and fluorescein angiography (FA). Stage 1 (Fig. 17.1a) is ophthalmoscopically inconspicuous but shows hyperfluorescence in late phase FA. Stage 2 (Fig. 17.1b) is defined by a reduced parafoveolar retinal transparency seen as a peculiar graying. Stage 3 (Fig. 17.1c) is characterized by the presence of so-called right-angled vessels that end with a blunted tip and

P. Charbel Issa, MD (✉) • S. Müller, MD
T.F.C. Heeren, MD • F.G. Holz, MD
Department of Ophthalmology, University of Bonn, Bonn, Germany
e-mail: Peter.Issa@ukb.uni-bonn.de

C.H. Meyer et al. (eds.), *Spectral Domain Optical Coherence Tomography in Macular Diseases*, DOI 10.1007/978-81-322-3610-8_17

seem to bend into deeper retinal layers. Stage 4 (Fig. 17.1d) is defined by ophthalmoscopically visible retinal pigment plaques, probably due to proliferation of pigment epithelial cells within areas of photoreceptor loss. Stage 5 is defined by the presence of a secondary neovascular complex. These neovascular lesions usually originate from the retinal vasculature and are thus different from choroidal neovascularization as mostly observed in patients with age-related macular degeneration. It should be noted that a neovascular complex may develop at any time point in the disease process. Thus, it rather represents a complication of the disease and not the natural end point (Charbel Issa et al. 2013). Retinal crystalline deposits can be found in 40–70 % of eyes with MacTel type 2 and are also a characteristic finding in this disease. Eventually, visual function is determined by a localized atrophy of the photoreceptor layer which is the common finding in late disease stages (Charbel Issa et al. 2013).

In patients with MacTel type 2, all disease manifestations are usually most pronounced and most obvious temporal to the foveal center. Within the same area, retinal function is most affected (paracentral scotoma).

MacTel type 2 shows a unique depletion of the macular pigment in the central retina (Charbel Issa et al. 2008c, 2009b; Helb et al. 2008), resulting in increased reflectivity on confocal blue reflectance imaging and an increased fundus autofluorescence signal due to reduced absorption of the excitation light (Charbel Issa et al. 2008c, 2013).

17.3 Optical Coherence Tomography

High-resolution optical coherence tomography (OCT) has been proven very useful for the diagnosis of MacTel type 2 and for the follow-up of affected patients. Even patients without any obvious funduscopic changes can be identified using OCT. In recent years, several features have been identified that characterize MacTel type 2 and rarely occur in other diseases (Charbel Issa et al. 2012; Gaudric et al. 2006).

The characteristic findings on OCT imaging may be present in various combinations. The changes are usually most prominent temporal to the foveal center. Larger longitudinal studies exploring the natural history on OCT imaging are still lacking. However, based on exemplary case studies, clinical experience, and the correlation with other imaging techniques and functional parameters, a time course of alterations may be suggested (Fig. 17.2).

The earliest subtle changes on OCT imaging may include temporal enlargement of the foveal pit (Fig. 17.2b), which then appears asymmetric with its thinnest sector temporal to the anatomic foveal center (Gillies et al. 2009; Charbel Issa 2016). This minor structural alteration appears to be due to changes in the outer nuclear/Henle's fiber layer thickness. However, if capillary leakage occurs within the same area, this asymmetric thinning may disappear due to a slight thickening mainly within the inner retinal layers (Fig. 17.2c). Such vascular leakage may be associated with a slightly increased reflectivity of inner neurosensory layers.

Within the inner retina, hyporeflective cavities (Fig. 17.2d–f) may develop which are usually located in the foveal pit with a predilection for the temporal slope. These atrophic hyporeflective spaces may have the appearance on funduscopy of a lamellar macular hole ("pseudo-lamellar macular hole"). In contrast to other diseases such as diabetic maculopathy or Irvine-Gass syndrome, there is no angiographic

Fig. 17.1 Stages of macular telangiectasia type 2. (**a**) Stage 1. No or only subtle changes on funduscopy (*left*). Leakage in fluorescein angiography, late phase (*middle* picture: early phase, *right* picture: late phase). The SD-OCT shows an interruption of the ellipsoid zone (*arrows*) and intraretinal cystoid spaces (*asterisk*). (**b**) Stage 2. There is a peculiar graying of the retina seen on funduscopy. (**c**) Stage 3. The *arrow* indicates a "right-angled venule." OCT shows slight thickening of the inner retina, which is not always seen. (**d**) Stage 4 is characterized by pigment plaques. In this case, crystalline deposits are also seen. The pigment plaques are seen as hyperreflective changes in SD-OCT and are related to outer retinal atrophy (*arrows*)

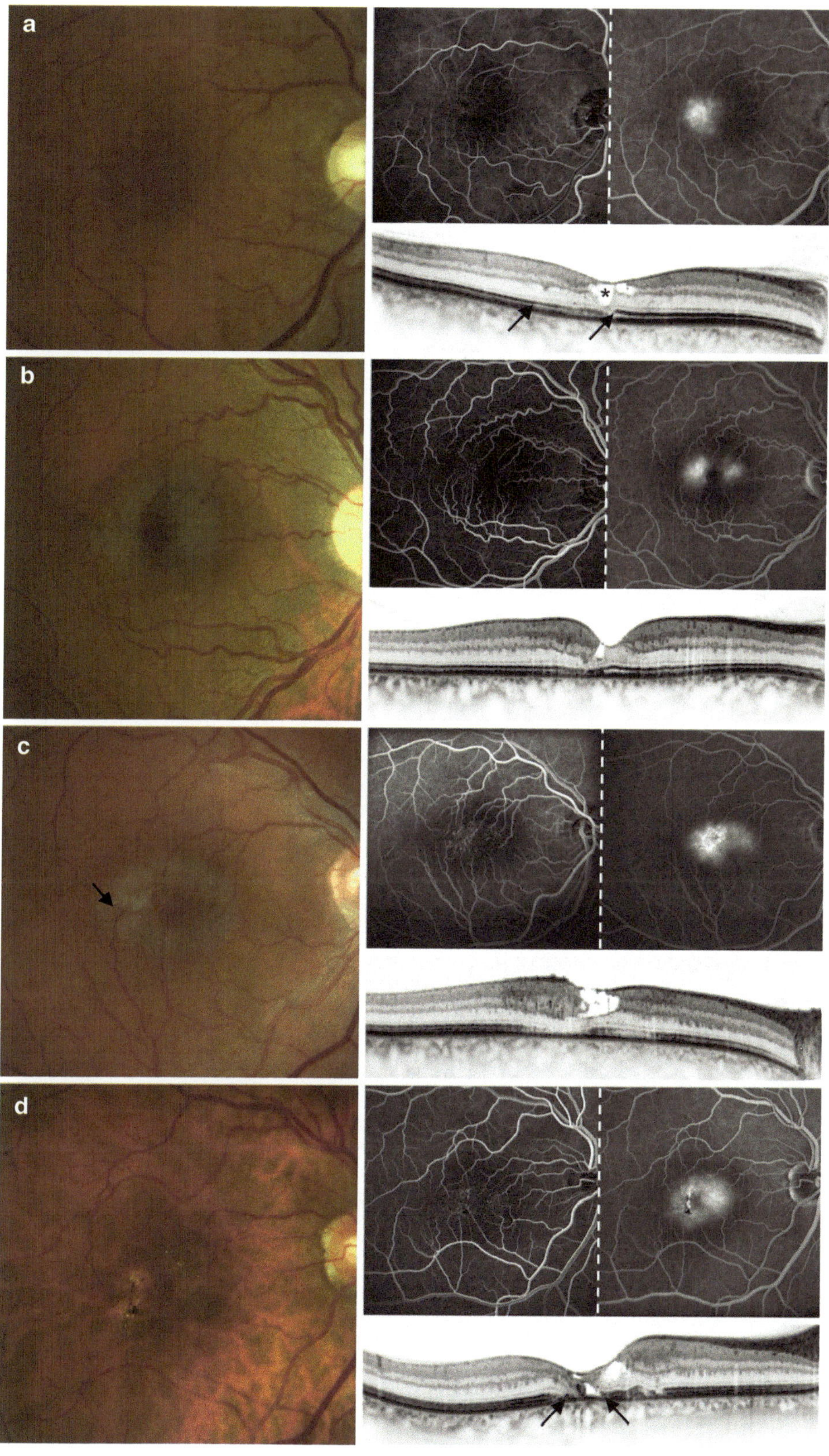
a
b
c
d
*

leakage and pooling of fluorescein dye into the hyporeflective cavities in MacTel type 2 (Koizumi et al. 2006), and there is no similar neurosensory thickening. The hyporeflective cavities in MacTel type 2 were shown to have a reflectivity different from exudative macular cysts (Barthelmes et al. 2008). These differences suggest that atrophy, as may be found in retinal

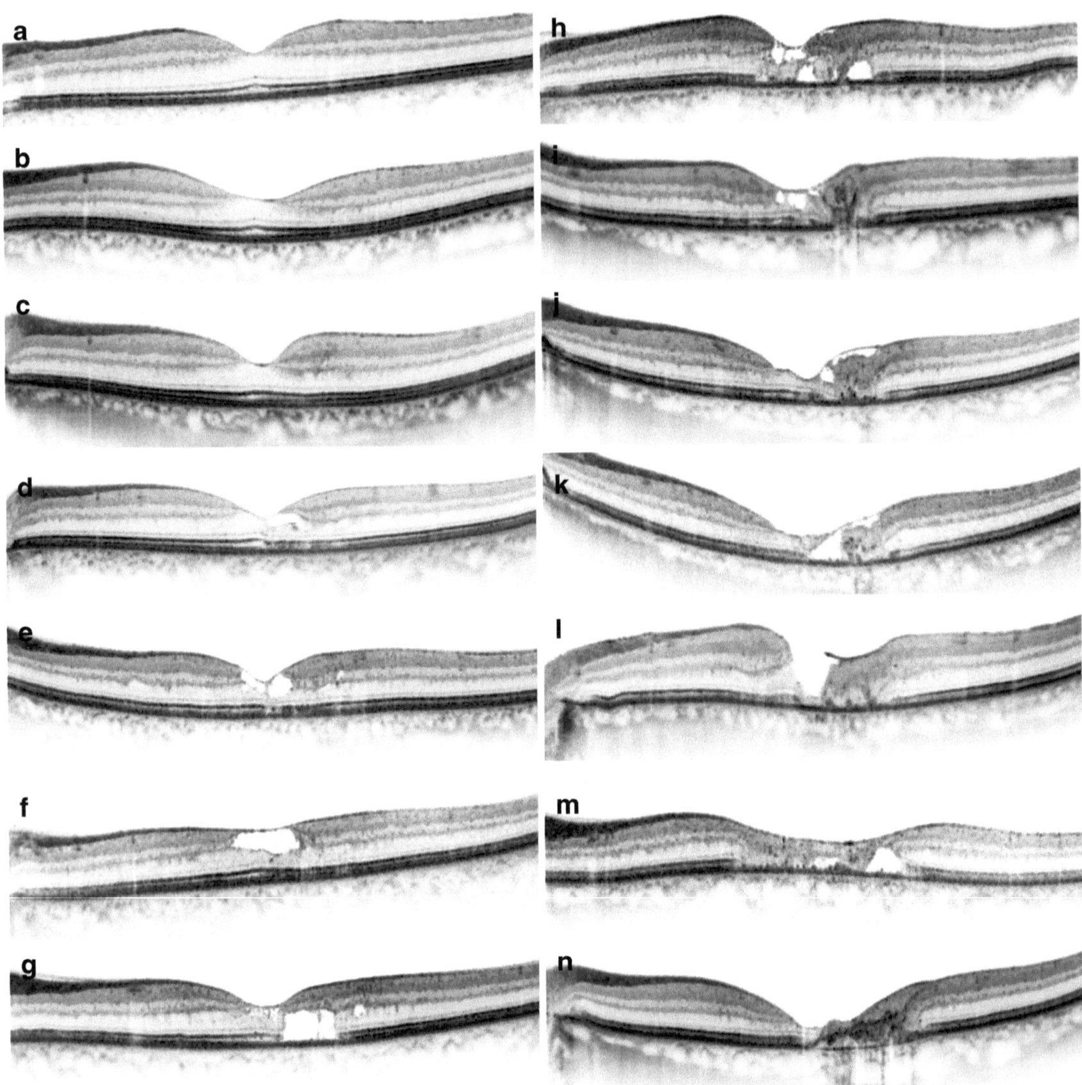

Fig. 17.2 Spectral domain OCT findings in patients with MacTel type 2. The optic nerve head is always to the *left side* in each of these horizontal scans through the foveal center. (**a**) Normal retina. (**b**) An asymmetric foveal contour may occur very early in the disease. (**c**) Hyperreflectivity within the inner retinal layers due to capillary leakage may also be an early finding. (**d–f**) Hyporeflective cavities within the inner foveal layers may remain without marked functional loss. There is some discontinuity of the highly reflective line above the retinal pigment epithelium and thinning of the outer nuclear layer mainly centrally and temporal to the foveal center. (**g**) Hyporeflective cavities within the outer retina. (**h**) Collapse of such outer retinal cavities. (**i, j**) Atrophic outer retina with hyperreflective pigment plaques. (**k**) The inner retinal layers appear to detach from the inner limiting membrane. (**l**) A lamellar macular hole may develop after disruption of the inner limiting membrane. (**m, n**) Localized complete atrophy of the outer retina with reactive pigment epithelial proliferation (Reprinted from Charbel Issa et al. (2013) with permission from Elsevier)

dystrophies, rather than exudation leads to the formation of these cavities in MacTel type 2. While outer retinal cavities appear to be due to tissue loss in the photoreceptor layer (see below), inner hyporeflective cavities might also result from loss of structural integrity with a pathophysiology similar to that seen in X-linked retinoschisis or retinitis pigmentosa. As well, detachment of the foveolar neurosensory retina from the inner limiting membrane may result in a foveal hyporeflective cavity and an apparent flattening of the foveal pit, especially in presence of additional thinning of the paracentral retina (Fig. 17.2f). Inner hyporeflective cavities may decrease with disease progression, possibly due to loss of supporting structures, surrounding atrophy and sometimes decreasing leakage.

Another sign that is considered characteristic of the disease is the disruption of the line now attributed to the ellipsoid zone. This sign may occur relatively early but is also observed in later disease stages. Discontinuity of this highly reflective line usually starts temporal to the foveola and is one of the most frequent findings in MacTel type 2 on OCT imaging. Modeling of 2-dimensional en face views (Fig. 17.3) at the level of the inner segment-outer segment border from densely recorded B-scans has been shown to reveal the extent of loss of this structural alteration (Sallo et al. 2012a, b). In a recent follow-up study, reappearance of a previously disrupted ellipsoid zone was shown in areas with preserved external limiting membrane. It was concluded that the latter might be a good prognostic factor (Wang et al. 2015).

In few eyes, accumulation of subretinal debris appears evident within the foveal area. The histopathological correlate was suggested to be degenerated photoreceptor elements that have lipofuscin-like autofluorescent properties, possibly explaining increased foveal autofluorescence and the funduscopic appearance of a yellowish foveal spot that is

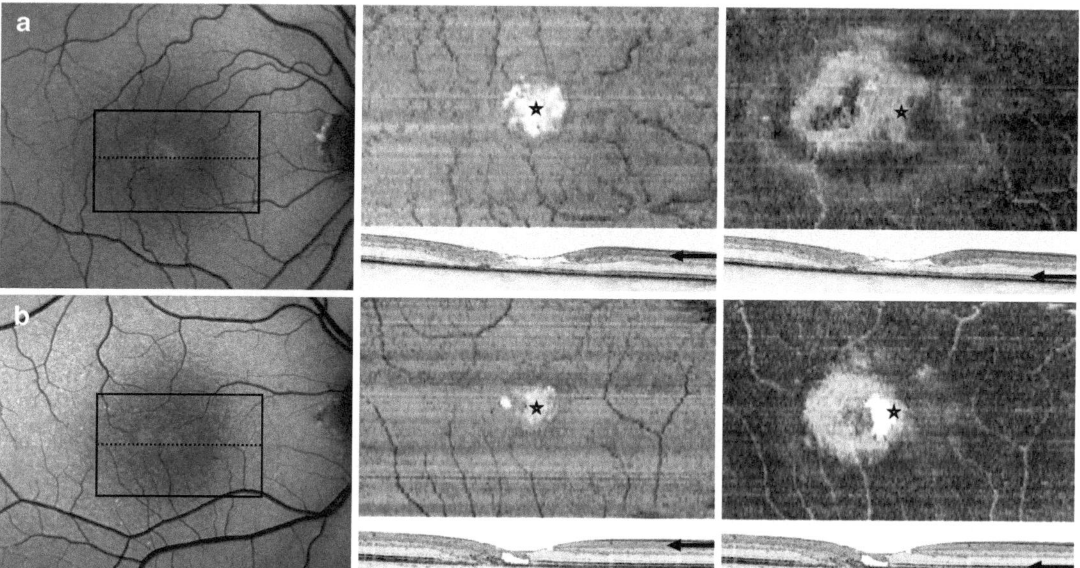

Fig. 17.3 "En face" view of OCT volume scans. The *left* image shows the correspondent fundus autofluorescence, the *black box* marks the position of the volume scan. The *dotted line* indicates the position of the B-scan shown in the *middle* and *right* image. The *asterisk* marks the foveal center. The *arrow* marks the retinal plane the position of the en-face image. The *middle* images are aligned parallel to the inner limiting membrane to show the inner retinal layers. There is a *round hole* centered on the foveola. The *right* images are aligned parallel the RPE band and show the topographic distribution of the disruption of the line representing the ellipsoid zone of the photoreceptors. In patient (**a**), the area of altered reflectivity within the ellipsoid zone corresponds to the entire retinal area affected by disease, whereas in patient (**b**), this area is more confined to an area centered temporal to the foveola (Reprinted from Charbel Issa et al. (2013) with permission from Elsevier)

apparent in a small subset of eyes (Cherepanoff et al. 2012).

With disease progression, atrophy of the outer neurosensory retina, i.e., the photoreceptor layer, becomes increasingly prevalent (Fig. 17.2g–n). Possibly depending on the integrity of supporting structures, outer hyporeflective cavities may develop (Fig. 17.2g–h) and increase within the photoreceptor layer, then subsequently collapse leading to apposition of inner retinal layers onto the pigment epithelium (Fig. 17.2j–n). Such apposition often occurs without the intermediate stage of cavitation within the photoreceptor layer.

Hyperreflective intraretinal lesions (Fig. 17.2i) are usually associated with pigment plaques. They may first appear as slightly prominent hyperreflective elevation within areas of photoreceptor atrophy, progressing into the retinal tissue. Larger lesions may present as a flat hyperreflective structure in the inner retinal layer, masking features of the underlying tissue. Secondary neovascular complexes may present as a hyperreflective lesion on OCT images. In these cases the lesion typically is located in or external to the outer neurosensory retinal layers.

Quantitative analysis of OCT data showed decreased thickness of the central neurosensory retina in most studies, likely due to thinning mainly within the photoreceptor layer (Krivosic et al. 2009). Characteristic retinal thickness maps are shown in Fig. 17.4 that highlight asymmetry of the foveal depression, loss of retinal contour, and a general thinning of the macular area secondary to outer retinal atrophy. It has been pointed out that apparent normal or slightly increased macular thickness may occur due to the low-grade macular edema superimposed on the atrophic neurosensory retina (Charbel Issa et al. 2008a, b). Increased macular thickness measurements may be found in MacTel type 2 eyes with marked capillary leakage and only little atrophy, in eyes with foveal detachment, pronounced pigment proliferation (Gaudric et al. 2006) or neovascular membranes.

Choroidal thickness was also assessed in patients with MacTel type 2 using enhanced depth OCT imaging and is still controversial. Chhablani et al. found no different subfoveal choroidal thickness than in healthy controls (Chhablani et al. 2014), whereas a Nunes et al. (Nunes et al. 2015) suggested a thicker subfoveal choroid in patients with MacTel type 2.

17.4 Optical Coherence Tomography Angiography

So far, data is sparse about visible changes in OCT angiography (Spaide et al. 2015; Thorell et al. 2014). Using this technique, the observation was confirmed that the structural vascular changes are concentrated in the deeper capillary plexus between the inner nuclear layer (INL) and the outer plexiform layer (OPL). This observation has already been described by Gass on stereoscopic fluorescein angiography before OCT had been clinically available (Gass and Blodi 1993). Additionally, there seems to be a rarification of the outer capillary plexus within the juxtafoveal region. This rarification is visible as thinner and less densely packed capillary plexus (Spaide et al. 2015). However, since OCT angiography is only able to detect vessels with flow, it may be that for instance occluded vessels would not be visible.

17.5 Functional Impairment and Structure-Function Correlation

In early stages, functional impairment may be mild with no or only slight reduction in best corrected visual acuity (BCVA). Epidemiologic studies revealed a mean BCVA of 20/40 in over 500 eyes (Clemons et al. 2010). Approximately half of the eyes had a BCVA of 20/32 or better and 16 % of 20/20 or better. A BCVA worse than 20/200 is rarely observed in MacTel type 2. However, reduced visual abilities such as reading difficulties disproportional to the level of BCVA are frequently reported and may affect the patient's quality of life significantly (Finger et al. 2009). Patients may also report perception of metamorphopsia (Charbel Issa et al. 2009a)

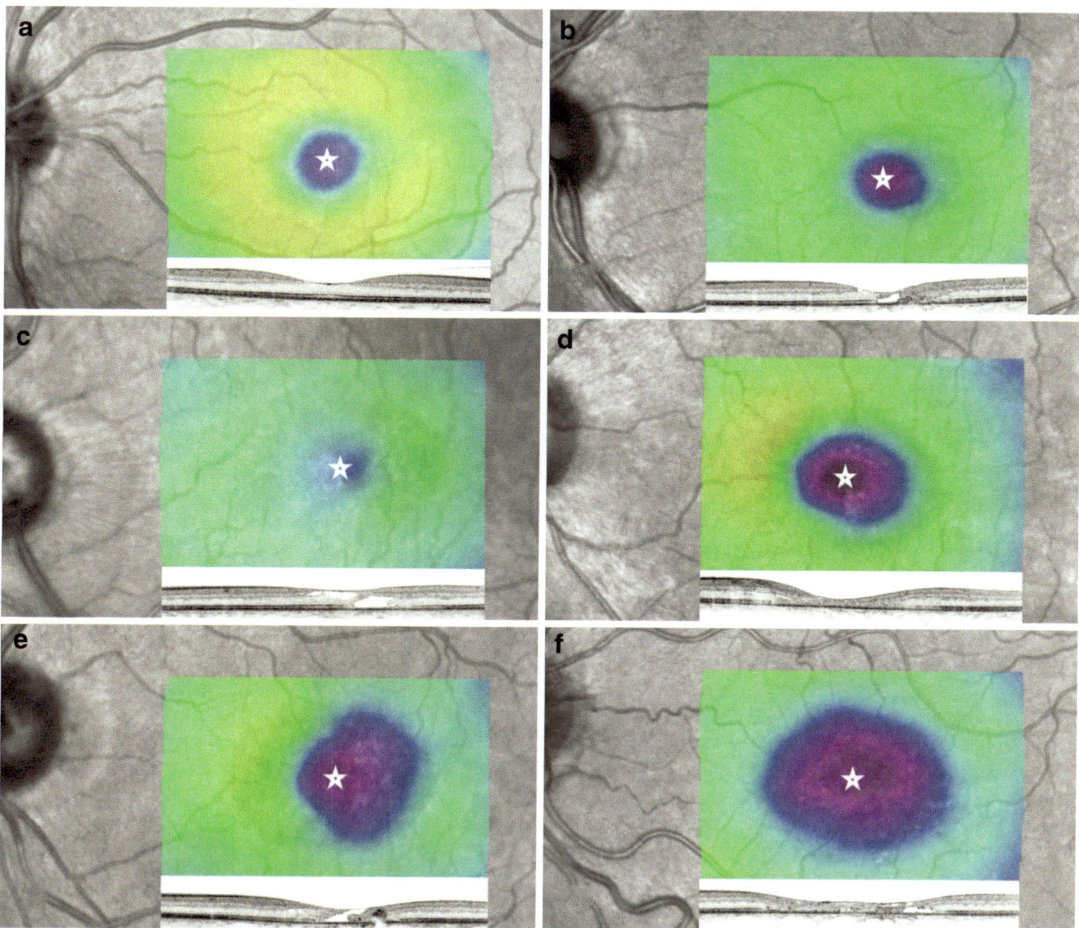

Fig. 17.4 Retinal thickness maps in an age-matched normal control (**a**) and patients with MacTel type 2 (**b–f**), representing the phenotypic variability. The B-scan underneath each thickness map was recorded through the foveal center (marked by an *asterisk*). Overall, there is an asymmetry of the foveal depression, a loss of retinal contour, and a general thinning of the macular area. In later disease stages, there is pronounced retinal thinning due to outer retinal atrophy (Reprinted from Charbel Issa et al. (2013) with permission from Elsevier)

and/or a positive scotoma that can be best detected and followed by microperimetry (Heeren et al. 2015).

Paracentral scotomata in patients with MacTel type 2 usually are small and well defined. Only in much progressed disease stages, they may enlarge to cover a central area of up to about 8–10° horizontally and less vertically. The epicenter of function loss in MacTel type 2 was shown to be located about 2° temporal/temporal inferior to the foveal center (Charbel Issa et al. 2007; Heeren et al. 2015).

By the use of microperimetry for mapping functional changes, deep paracentral scotomata have been identified as a characteristic functional consequence of the disease process. Structure-function correlation revealed well-defined progressive focal photoreceptor loss to be the underlying cause for functional loss in MacTel type 2 (Fig. 17.5).

In various diseases, such as diabetic macular edema or central serous chorioretinopathy, there appears to be an association of retinal function with retinal thickness measures. However, in MacTel type 2, conclusions on retinal function based on total retinal thickness measurements may be less valid due to low-grade retinal edema over a partial atrophic retina (Charbel Issa et al. 2008a). Therefore, it is more

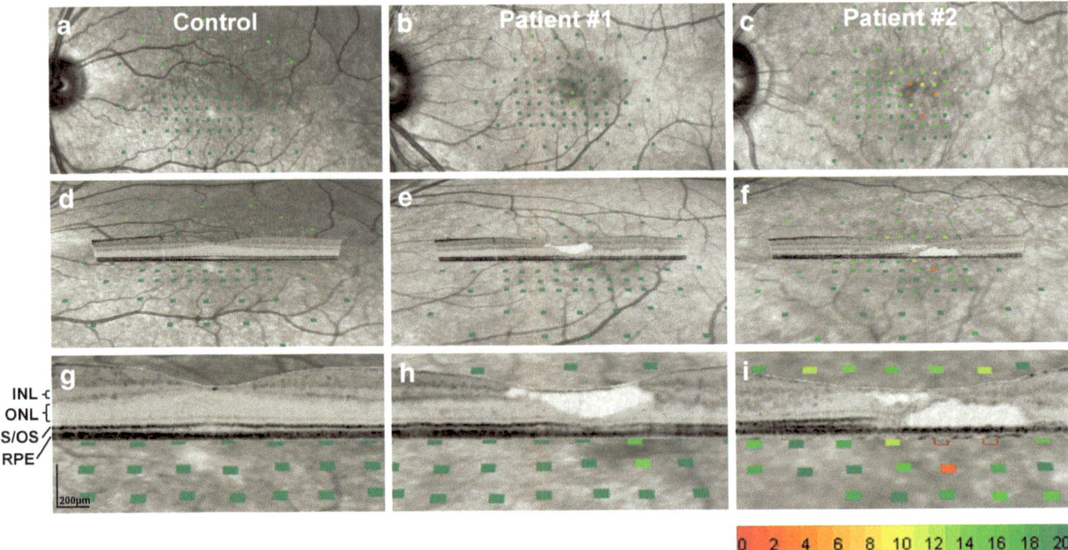

Fig. 17.5 Correlation of topographic and tomographic retinal imaging with functional mapping. Retinal sensitivity data derived from microperimetry (**a–c**) are presented according to the scale below (**i**). Open rectangles demonstrate absolute defects. The first column illustrates findings in a normal subject, the middle and right column in two patients with macular telangiectasia type 2. The first row shows functional maps superimposed on near-infrared confocal scanning laser ophthalmoscopy (cSLO) images of the central retina. The second and third row (**d–i**) show the functional maps superimposed on the back-tilted cSLO images and a high-resolution spectral-domain optical coherence tomography (SD-OCT) scan. The lower panels (**g–i**) show enlarged cutouts of the middle row (**d–f**). For the normal subject, selected anatomical layers of the retina are indicated for orientation on the left-hand side of panel g (*INL* inner nuclear layer, *ONL* outer nuclear layer, *IS/OS* junction of the inner and outer photoreceptor segment or "ellipsoid zone," *RPE* retinal pigment epithelium). The tissue defect within the inner retina (**e**, **h**) is associated with a normal or slightly decreased retinal light sensitivity (*green squares*), whereas damage to the outer retina (the photoreceptor layers) was accompanied by a strong loss of retinal sensitivity (*red* filled and *red open squares*; **f**, **i**) (Reprinted from Charbel Issa et al. (2010))

appropriate to qualitatively analyze the retinal morphology for identifying structural associations with functional deficits in MacTel type 2.

An example for such an approach is provided in Fig. 17.5; functional preservation on microperimetry testing can be found if degeneration spares the photoreceptors but causes quite extensive disruption of the inner retina. However, degenerative alterations of the photoreceptor layer result in an absolute and well-demarcated paracentral scotoma.

It was noted previously that an absolute scotoma is always present in MacTel type 2 stages 4 and 5 (see above). However, we have observed a substantial number of patients presenting with an absolute scotoma in stage 3 disease (Heeren et al. 2015). Probably photoreceptor atrophy as the underlying structural correlate appears earlier in the course of the disease than the ophthalmoscopically visible signs of stage 4 and 5. This emphasizes the importance of high-resolution SD-OCT and microperimetry testing in this disease entity to fully understand individual disease manifestations and their functional relevance.

References

Barthelmes D, Gillies MC, Sutter FKP (2008) Quantitative OCT analysis of idiopathic perifoveal telangiectasia. Invest Ophthalmol Vis Sci 49:2156–2162. doi:10.1167/iovs.07-0478

Charbel Issa P, Helb H-M, Rohrschneider K, Holz FG, Scholl HPN (2007) Microperimetric assessment of patients with type 2 idiopathic macular telangiectasia. Invest Ophthalmol Vis Sci 48:3788–3795. doi:10.1167/iovs.06-1272

Charbel Issa P, Helb H-M, Holz FG, Scholl HPN, MacTel Study Group (2008a) Correlation of macular function with retinal thickness in nonproliferative type 2 idiopathic macular telangiectasia. Am J Ophthalmol 145:169–175. doi:10.1016/j.ajo.2007.08.028

Charbel Issa P, Finger RP, Holz FG, Scholl HPN (2008b) Eighteen-month follow-up of intravitreal bevacizumab in type 2 idiopathic macular telangiectasia. Br J Ophthalmol 92:941–945. doi:10.1136/bjo.2007.129627

Charbel Issa P, Berendschot TT, Staurenghi G, Holz FG, Scholl HPN (2008c) Confocal blue reflectance imaging in type 2 idiopathic macular telangiectasia. Invest Ophthalmol Vis Sci 49:1172–1177. doi:10.1167/iovs.07-0636

Charbel Issa P, Holz FG, Scholl HPN (2009a) Metamorphopsia in patients with macular telangiectasia type 2. Doc Ophthalmol 119:133–140. doi:10.1007/s10633-009-9190-9

Charbel Issa P, van der Veen RLP, Stijfs A, Holz FG, Scholl HPN, Berendschot TT (2009b) Quantification of reduced macular pigment optical density in the central retina in macular telangiectasia type 2. Exp Eye Res 89:25–31. doi:10.1016/j.exer.2009.02.006

Charbel Issa P, Troeger E, Finger R, Holz FG, Wilke R, Scholl HPN (2010) Structure-function correlation of the human central retina. PLoS One 5:e12864. doi:10.1371/journal.pone.0012864

Clemons TE, Gillies MC, Chew EY, Bird AC, Peto T, Figueroa MJ, Harrington MW, MacTel Research Group (2010) Baseline characteristics of participants in the natural history study of macular telangiectasia (MacTel) MacTel Project Report No. 2. Ophthalmic Epidemiol 17:66–73. doi:10.3109/09286580903450361

Charbel Issa P, Gillies MC, Chew EY, Bird AC, Heeren T, Peto T, Holz FG, Scholl HPN (2013) Macular telangiectasia type 2. Prog Retin Eye Res 34:49–77. doi:10.1016/j.preteyeres.2012.11.002

Charbel Issa P, Heeren TF, Kupitz EH, Holz FG, Berendschot TT (2016) Very early disease manifestations of macular telangiectasia type 2. Retina 36: 524–534. doi:10.1097/IAE.0000000000000863

Cherepanoff S, Killingsworth MC, Zhu M, Nolan T, Hunyor AP, Young SH, Hageman GS, Gillies MC (2012) Ultrastructural and clinical evidence of subretinal debris accumulation in type 2 macular telangiectasia. Br J Ophthalmol 96:1404–1409. doi:10.1136/bjophthalmol-2011-301009

Chhablani J, Kozak I, Jonnadula GB, Venkata A, Narayanan R, Pappuru RR, Rao PS (2014) Choroidal thickness in macular telangiectasia type 2. Retina 34:1819–1823. doi:10.1097/IAE.0000000000000180

Finger RP, Charbel Issa P, Fimmers R, Holz FG, Rubin GS, Scholl HPN (2009) Reading performance is reduced by parafoveal scotomas in patients with macular telangiectasia type 2. Invest Ophthalmol Vis Sci 50:1366–1370. doi:10.1167/iovs.08-2032

Gass JD, Blodi BA (1993) Idiopathic juxtafoveolar retinal telangiectasis. Update of classification and follow-up study. Ophthalmology 100:1536–154

Gaudric A, Ducos de Lahitte G, Cohen SY, Massin P, Haouchine B (2006) Optical coherence tomography in group 2A idiopathic juxtafoveolar retinal telangiectasis. Arch Ophthalmol 124:1410–1419. doi:10.1001/archopht.124.10.1410

Gillies MC, Zhu M, Chew E, Barthelmes D, Hughes E, Ali H, Holz FG, Scholl HPN, Charbel Issa P (2009) Familial asymptomatic macular telangiectasia type 2. Ophthalmology 116:2422–2429. doi:10.1016/j.ophtha.2009.05.010

Helb H-M, Charbel Issa P, van der Veen RLP, Berendschot TTJM, Scholl HPN, Holz FG (2008) Abnormal macular pigment distribution in type 2 idiopathic macular telangiectasia. Retina 28:808–816. doi:10.1097/IAE.0b013e31816d81aa

Heeren TFC, Clemons T, Scholl HPN, Bird AC, Holz FG, Charbel Issa P (2015) Progression of vision loss in macular telangiectasia type 2. Invest Ophthalmol Vis Sci 56:3905–3912. doi:10.1167/iovs.15-16915

Koizumi H, Iida T, Maruko I (2006) Morphologic features of group 2A idiopathic juxtafoveolar retinal telangiectasis in three-dimensional optical coherence tomography. Am J Ophthalmol 142:340–343. doi:10.1016/j.ajo.2006.03.021

Krivosic V, Tadayoni R, Massin P, Erginay A, Gaudric A (2009) Spectral domain optical coherence tomography in type 2 idiopathic perifoveal telangiectasia. Ophthalmic Surg Lasers Imaging 40:379–384

Nunes RP, Goldhardt R, de Amorim Garcia Filho CA, Thorell MR, Abbey AM, Kuriyan AE, Modi YS, Shah M, Yehoshua Z, Gregori G, Feuer W, Rosenfeld PJ (2015) Spectral-domain optical coherence tomography measurements of choroidal thickness and outer retinal disruption in macular telangiectasia type 2. Ophthalmic Surg Lasers Imaging Retina 46:162–170. doi:10.3928/23258160-20150213-17

Sallo FB, Peto T, Egan C, Wolf-Schnurrbusch UEK, Clemons TE, Gillies MC, Pauleikhoff D, Rubin GS, Chew EY, Bird AC (2012a) The IS/OS junction layer in the natural history of type 2 idiopathic macular telangiectasia. Invest Ophthalmol Vis Sci 53:7889–7895. doi:10.1167/iovs.12-10765

Sallo FB, Peto T, Egan C, Wolf-Schnurrbusch UEK, Clemons TE, Gillies MC, Pauleikhoff D, Rubin GS, Chew EY, Bird AC (2012b) "En face" OCT imaging of the IS/OS junction line in type 2 idiopathic macular telangiectasia. Invest Ophthalmol Vis Sci 53:6145–6152. doi:10.1167/iovs.12-10580

Spaide RF, Klancnik JM, Cooney MJ (2015) Retinal vascular layers in macular telangiectasia type 2 imaged by optical coherence tomographic angiography. JAMA Ophthalmol 133:66–73. doi:10.1001/jamaophthalmol.2014.3950

Thorell MR, Zhang Q, Huang Y, An L, Durbin MK, Laron M, Sharma U, Stetson PF, Gregori G, Wang RK, Rosenfeld PJ (2014) Swept-source OCT angiography of macular telangiectasia type 2. Ophthalmic Surg Lasers Imaging Retina 45:369–380. doi:10.3928/23258160-20140909-06

Wang Q, Tuten WS, Lujan BJ, Holland J, Bernstein PS, Schwartz SD, Duncan JL, Roorda A (2015) Adaptive optics microperimetry and OCT images show preserved function and recovery of cone visibility in macular telangiectasia type 2 retinal lesions. Invest Ophthalmol Vis Sci 56:778–786. doi:10.1167/iovs.14-15576

18 Central Serous Chorioretinopathy

Angie H.C. Fong and Timothy Y.Y. Lai

Contents

A.H.C. Fong, FRCS • T.Y.Y. Lai, FRCS, FRCOphth (✉)
Department of Ophthalmology and Visual Sciences, The Chinese University of Hong Kong, Hong Kong, China
e-mail: tyylai@cuhk.edu.hk

18.1 Introduction

18.1.1 Definition and Pathogenesis

Central serous chorioretinopathy (CSC) was originally described by Albrecht von Graefe in

C.H. Meyer et al. (eds.), *Spectral Domain Optical Coherence Tomography in Macular Diseases*, DOI 10.1007/978-81-322-3610-8_18

1866 as "central recurrent retinitis" (Von Graefe 1866). Since then our understanding of CSC has progressed considerably. Gass in 1967 named the disease as central serous chorioretinopathy and proposed choriocapillaris hyperpermeability as the cause of CSC (Gass 1967). This hypothesis was later supported by studies using indocyanine green angiography (ICGA) which showed multifocal areas of choroidal vascular hyperpermeability in eyes with CSC.

CSC is characterized by serous retinal detachment of the neurosensory retina at the posterior pole, sometimes associated with serous detachment of the retinal pigment epithelium (RPE). It is thought that the pathogenic mechanism for CSC is associated with a hyperdynamic choroidal circulation. The resulting elevated hydrostatic pressure of choroid causes elevation of the RPE, which in turn causes serous pigment epithelial detachments (PEDs). RPE might subsequently undergo tiny rips, which causes leakage into the subretinal space leading to neurosensory retinal detachment (Nicholson et al. 2013; Ross et al. 2011). Factors such as elevated serum glucocorticoid, *Helicobacter pylori* infection, and gene polymorphisms (eg, complement factor H) have been suggested to contribute to the pathogenesis of CSC (Miki et al. 2014).

18.1.2 Epidemiology

CSC develops more frequently in men, with a male to female ratio of approximately six to one. The mean age of onset is around 41 years of age, but CSC can be found in young patients or in patients over 60 years old. The disease occurs most frequently in Asians and Whites and less frequently in the African-American populations, although the disease appeared to behave more aggressively in blacks (Ross et al. 2011). CSC is usually unilateral at initial presentation; however, bilateral cases have been reported to occur in up to 40 %. Chronic cases of CSC tend to have bilateral involvement (Gäckle et al. 1998a, b).

18.1.3 Natural History

Traditionally, CSC was thought to be a benign and self-limiting condition (Gass 1967). However, we now classify CSC broadly into acute (or classic) and chronic forms. Only the acute form carries a favorable prognosis of being a self-limiting condition, in which the serous macular detachment usually resolves after 3 months. Although these cases with acute CSC are usually not associated with loss of visual acuity, subtle changes in retinal sensitivity and contrast may occur (Bajarboura 2001). The chronic cases can be divided into chronic CSC following a single episode, recurrent resolving CSC, and recurrent chronic CSC. The proportion of eyes with recurrent CSC has been estimated to be around 30 % (Castro-Correia et al. 1992). The chronic form of CSC is sometimes characterized by diffuse RPE change, indicating widespread decompensation of the RPE, and has been referred to as diffuse retinal pigment epitheliopathy (DRPE) (Polak et al. 1995). The chronic subretinal fluid could be absorbed by the RPE due to diffuse dysfunction and loss of RPE, and the presence of fluid causes progressive photoreceptor death and may result in permanent visual loss (Nicholson et al. 2013).

Another rare form of CSC is the bullous variant, characterized by inferiorly gravitating fluid causing bullous exudative retinal detachment. It can be primary or associated with the use of systemic corticosteroid, organ transplant, and pregnancy (Gass 1973). Favorable outcome has been described for these cases which tend to be self-limiting. Otsuka and colleagues described a series of 25 cases of bullous CSC in which 52 % achieved a visual acuity of 20/20 or better and 80 % achieved 20/40 (Otsuka et al. 2002).

18.1.4 Why Spectral-Domain Optical Coherence Tomography (SD-OCT) Is Useful in Central Serous Chorioretinopathy?

OCT is one of the primary imaging techniques used in the diagnosis and management of

CSC. Compared with time-domain OCT (TD-OCT), spectral-domain OCT (SD-OCT) has a 43–100 times higher image acquisition speed. It has a higher signal-to-noise ratio and can capture high-quality images of retinal microstructures up to 1 μm axial resolution (Wojtkowski et al. 2005). SD-OCT provides a convenient, noninvasive way to evaluate the presence and resolution of subretinal fluid and other pathology in CSC. Changes in the photoreceptor layers, outer nuclear layer (ONL), or the external limiting membrane (ELM) can be clearly visualized. Visualization of these structures is useful because the ELM, ONL thickness, and the continuity of the photoreceptor inner and outer segment (IS/OS) junction are positively correlated with visual function and carries important prognostic significance. Also, using eye-tracking device, the same cross-sectional area can be scanned at each visit, so that the morphological changes at the same location can be accurately evaluated longitudinally. Early macular changes in CSC such as shallow subretinal fluid or serous PED might be subtle and missed on fundus examination, but these changes will be clearly visualized in SD-OCT examination.

As the main pathology of CSC lies in the choroid, imaging of the choroid is important in the evaluation of CSC. Enhanced depth imaging OCT (EDI-OCT) is such an imaging technique that is now commercially available with various SD-OCT machines. In EDI-OCT, the choroid is placed closer to the zero-delay plane compared with the retina, thus placing the most focused portion of the OCT scan on the choroid. An enhanced image of the choroid, from the Bruch's membrane to the suprachoroidal space, can then be obtained. This is a useful tool to provide in vivo cross-sectional histological information of choroidal vessels, as well as choroidal thickness, in normal and disease states.

Another new development using the SD-OCT is the coronal imaging or en face OCT imaging. Using three-dimensional reconstruction of transverse images of SD-OCT, a virtual "macula block" can be imaged, and coronal sections recreated from these scans, otherwise known as the C-scan or en face OCT. Using this technology, coronal sections of the retina, subretinal space, and choroid can be visualized, allowing collection of new information that complements other investigations. For example, choroidal venous dilatation under the abnormal RPE can be visualized on en face EDI-OCT whereby it will only appear as a hyperdynamic circulation on ICGA.

18.2 SD-OCT Changes and Findings in Central Serous Chorioretinopathy

18.2.1 Subretinal Fluid in Central Serous Chorioretinopathy

The hallmark of CSC is the accumulation of subretinal fluid (SRF) under the neurosensory retina causing a serous retinal detachment (SRD) (Fig. 18.1). Three-dimensional analysis of the SRF configuration in CSC using SD-OCT shows that the morphology of SRF in CSC changes over time (Ahn et al. 2013). The height of the SRD is higher in acute CSC compared with chronic CSC (Song et al. 2012). Ahn and colleagues evaluated the ratio of peak height to the greatest basal diameter of the SRD and found that the ratio was higher in acute than chronic CSC (Ahn et al. 2013) (Fig. 18.1). Early dynamic changes in SRF are more often observed in acute than chronic CSC, and the changing pattern differs according to prognosis. Eyes with spontaneous resolution often show symmetrical shrinking of SRF, while eyes with persistent fluid showed flattening and elongation of the SRF, turning the basal area into an oval shape. It is possible that the inferior shifting of SRF as observed in OCT is a result of the gravitational effect on the SRF, which is greater with persistent SRF in chronic CSC. Fluorescein angiography (FA) has demonstrated inferior gravitational tracts often described as hourglass configuration which can be seen extending from the macula to the inferior retina in chronic CSC eyes, where the SRF dissects its way down through

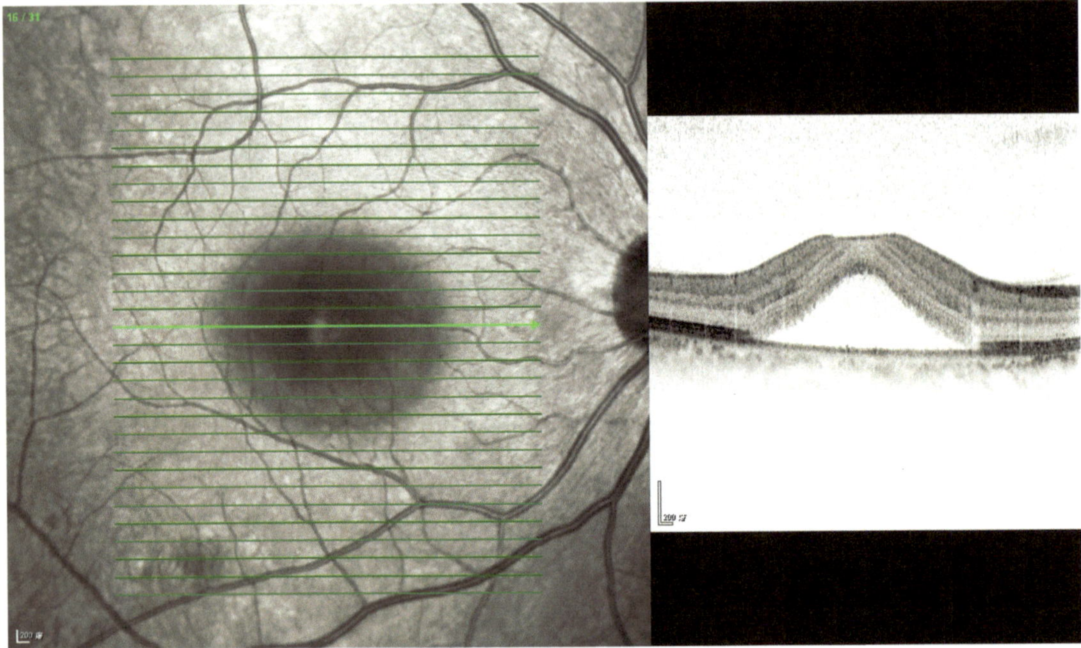

Fig. 18.1 Acute central serous chorioretinopathy. SD-OCT showing high height of subretinal fluid relative to the basal diameter of the fluid

the subretinal space due to a high specific gravity (Yannuzzi et al. 1984).

18.2.2 Fibrin in Central Serous Chorioretinopathy

As early as 1967, Gass reported the presence of cloudy white exudate surrounding PED in patients with CSC with accompanying evidence of angiographic leakage (Gass 1967). Subsequent studies found that fibrin is present from 19 to 62 % of eyes with CSC (Ooto et al. 2010; Shinojima et al. 2010; Kim et al. 2012; Nair et al. 2012). The presence of fibrin indicates serous exudate, rich in protein, pigment granules, or homogeneous hyaline-like masses (Gass 1967). Fibrin appears as a hyper-reflective lump in the subretinal space on SD-OCT (Fig. 18.2), often overlying small PED, corresponding to leakage sites on FA (Kim et al. 2012). En face OCT scanning often shows a break in the PED associated with fibrin indicating active leakage from these PEDs. Shinjojima and colleagues visualized fibrin-like substance beneath the RPE in 62 % of eyes and suggested that plasma components, including fibrinogen, might be released from choriocapillaris and form fibrin beneath RPE, which leak into the subretinal space through defects in the RPE (Shinojima et al. 2010). Smooth protrusions of the RPE are also associated with fibrin in eyes with CSC.

In eyes with acute CSC, characteristic focal dipping or sagging of the posterior retina (Fujimoto et al. 2008; Song et al. 2012; Nair et al. 2012; Kim et al. 2012) could be seen accompanying fibrin over the leakage site in up to 38 % of eyes at a mean of 8 days after disease onset (Song et al. 2012) (Fig. 18.3). Song et al. suggested that this might be a result of a focal residual attachment of the retina with reactive exudation that persisted until the detachment of neurosensory retina from the RPE was complete. Therefore, focal dipping or sagging of the posterior retina associated with fibrin may be an early indicator of acute CSC. Subretinal fibrinous exudates were observed in around 24 % of eyes with early chronic CSC in their study that persisted into the late chronic stage.

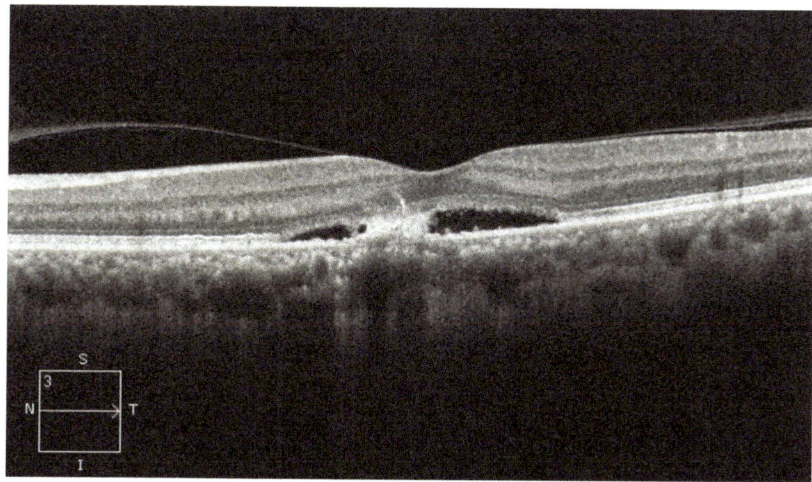

Fig. 18.2 Fibrin in central serous chorioretinopathy. SD-OCT scan showing subretinal fluid with hyper-reflective material due to fibrin in acute central serous chorioretinopathy

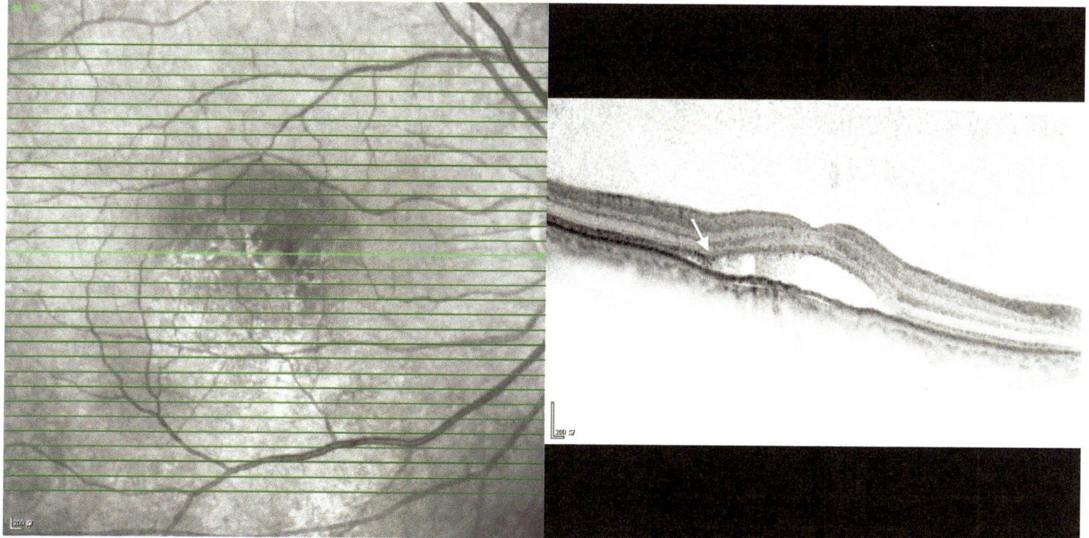

Fig. 18.3 SD-OCT showing fibrin in the subretinal fluid with focal dipping (*arrow*) of the posterior retina in acute central serous chorioretinopathy

18.2.3 Central Serous Chorioretinopathy with Bullous Serous Retinal Detachment

Gass in 1973 first described a series of five cases of bullous exudative retinal detachment as an unusual manifestation of CSC (Gass 1973). This rare presentation is thought to be an exaggerated form of typical CSC. Clinically, there is bullous retinal detachment with shifting subretinal fluid. There are large, single, or multiple-leaking PEDs which are often hidden under cloudy subretinal exudation (Sahu et al. 2000). FA reveals multiple foci of intense RPE leakage communicating with the detached subretinal space (Fig. 18.4). It is thought that proteins and fibrinogen escape into the subretinal space through these intensive leakage sites leading to the presence of a thick subretinal exudate which subsequently seals the leakage site (Fig. 18.5). Fibrin may also stimulate the fibrosis leading to formation of subretinal fibrotic membrane (Hooymans 1998; Schatz et al. 1995).

On SD-OCT scans, bullous neurosensory retinal detachments and large PEDs could be visualized. Spontaneous RPE rip appearing as a defect in the RPE with a rolled edge has also been reported (Lee et al. 2013) (Fig. 18.6). Due to the bullous appearance, bullous CSC might be mistaken with other diseases such as rhegmatogenous retinal detachment, idiopathic uveal effusion syndrome, multifocal choroiditis, Vogt-Koyanagi-Harada disease, choroidal metastasis, or lymphoma (Gass and Little 1995). Bullous CSC can be idiopathic in healthy individuals or can occur following high-dose corticosteroid therapy, organ transplantation, and hemodialysis or in pregnant women. Although most cases of bullous retinal detachment in CSC resolve either spontaneously, with discontinuation of steroid, following delivery or after laser photocoagulation, the visual outcome is usually variable. One series reported visual deterioration in all bullous CSC patients with 50% having a final vision of 20/200 or worse, while others reported a good outcome with 80 to 100% achieving vision of 20/40 or better (Fawzi et al. 2006; Gass 1973, 1991, 1992; Gass and Little 1995; Sahuet al. 2000).

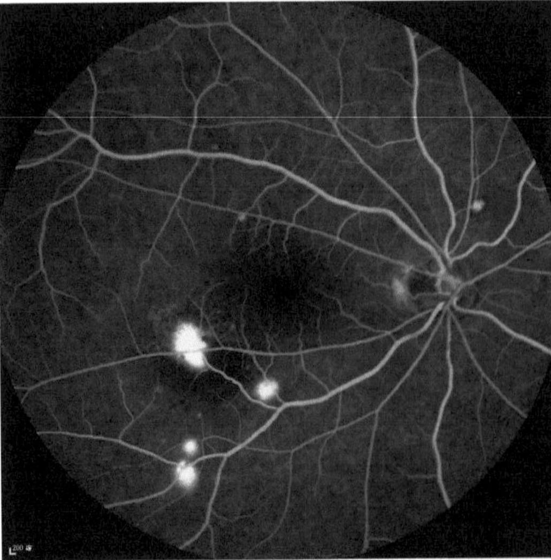

Fig. 18.4 Bullous central serous chorioretinopathy. Mid-phase fluorescein angiography of an eye showing multiple leakage sites

18.2.4 Degeneration of Photoreceptors and Outer Retinal Changes in Central Serous Chorioretinopathy

The inner segment/outer segment (IS/OS) junction of the photoreceptors, also known as the ellipsoid zone (EZ), shows up as a hyper-reflective line on OCT scans and has been found to be closely related to visual acuity. In normal individuals, the IS/OS line is continuous at the macula, while the IS/OS line is disrupted in various disease states. In CSC, the IS/OS line is usually not visible in eyes with serous retinal detachment but becomes visible again in the majority of eyes after resolution of the subretinal fluid (Kim et al. 2012). This indicates a disruption of the normal photoreceptor assembly during the serous macular detachment, which normalizes with phagocytosis of photoreceptor shed discs by the RPE upon reattachment.

During the acute phase of CSC, there is elongation of the photoreceptor OS, which is seen on SD-OCT as a thickened and smooth posterior surface of the detached retina (Ooto et al. 2011; Song et al. 2012). After several months, the posterior surface of the detached retina takes on a granulated or partially thinned appearance, and hyper-reflective dots begin to appear intraretinal or on the posterior retinal surface, reflecting accumulation of shed OS (Fujimoto et al. 2008; Kim et al. 2012; Ojima et al. 2007) (Fig. 18.7). In the late phase of CSC, the posterior surface of the retina is usually thinned due to long-standing shedding and disintegration of the photoreceptors. A chronic sustained serous retinal detachment results in the disruption of the outer photoreceptor layer, and atrophy of the RPE ensues.

SD-OCT findings of IS/OS line discontinuity, longer length of IS/OS disruption, thinning of the outer nuclear layer, disruption in external limiting membrane integrity, presence of hyper-

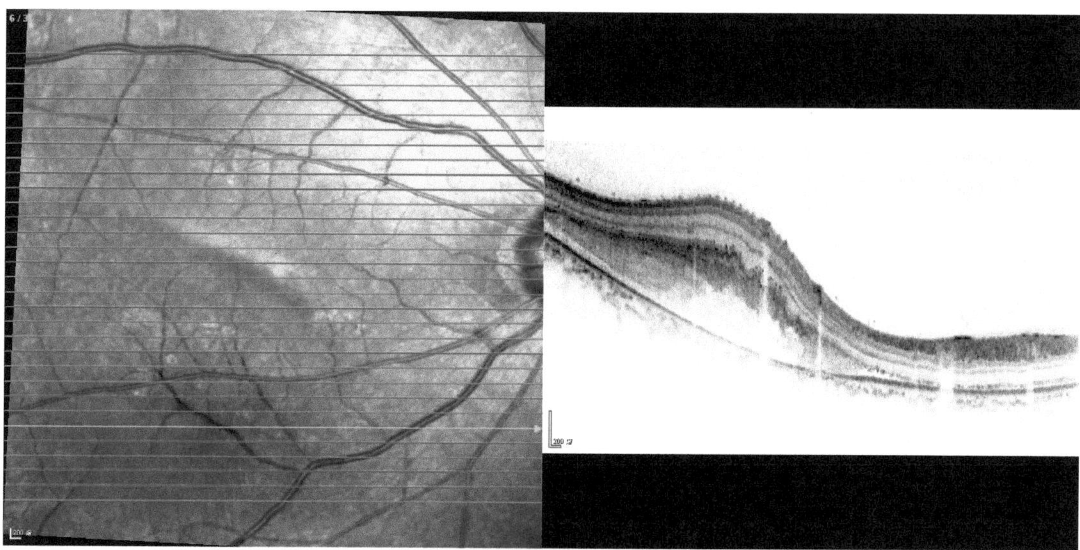

Fig. 18.5 SD-OCT of the same eye with bullous central serous chorioretinopathy showing large amount of subretinal fluid with exudate showing as hyper-reflective material beneath the neurosensory retina

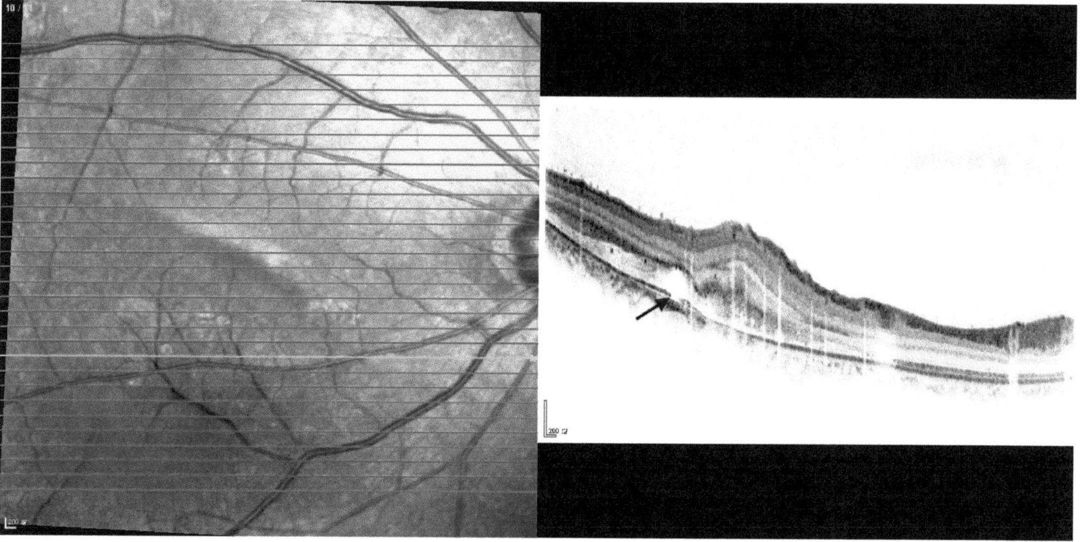

Fig. 18.6 SD-OCT in an eye with bullous central serous chorioretinopathy showing RPE rip appearing as a defect in the RPE with a rolled edge

reflective dots, and RPE hypertrophy have all been shown to be associated with poor final visual acuity in eyes with resolved CSC (Matsumoto et al. 2009; Ozdemir and Erol 2013; Yalcinbayir et al. 2014) (Fig. 18.8). Therefore, periodic imaging with SD-OCT in eyes with CSC is useful in assessing the visual prognosis of these patients.

18.2.5 Subretinal Deposits in Central Serous Chorioretinopathy

Yellowish deposits forming a reticulated leopard spot pattern have been reported in eyes with chronic neurosensory detachment caused by CSC (Iida et al. 2002). These deposits can be found within the areas of neurosensory detachment and

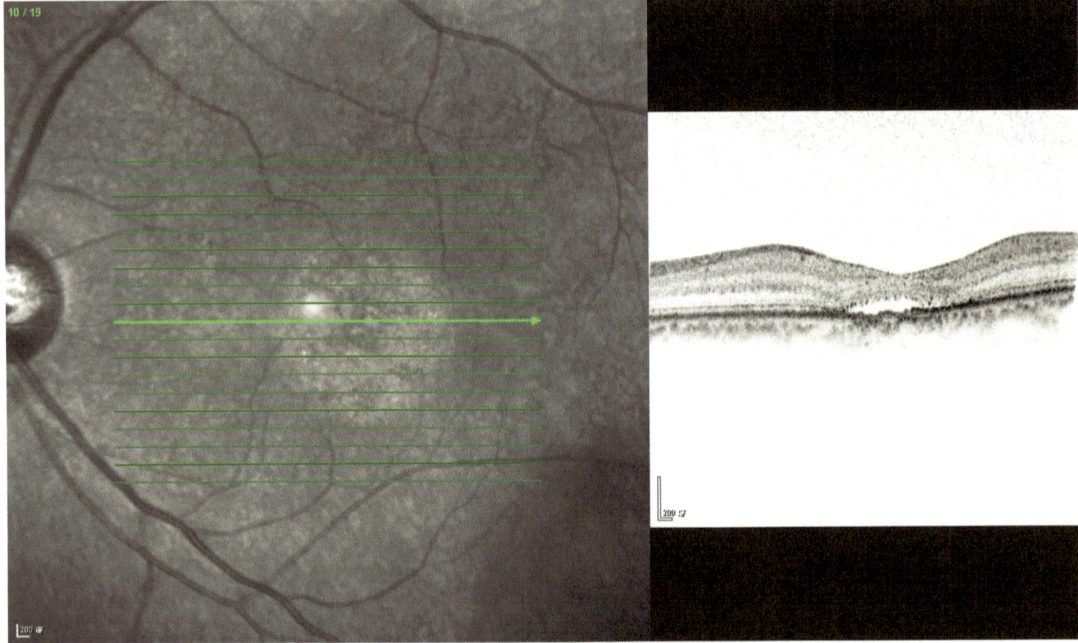

Fig. 18.7 SD-OCT showing shallow subretinal fluid with subretinal hyper-reflective dots and granulated and partially thinned retina

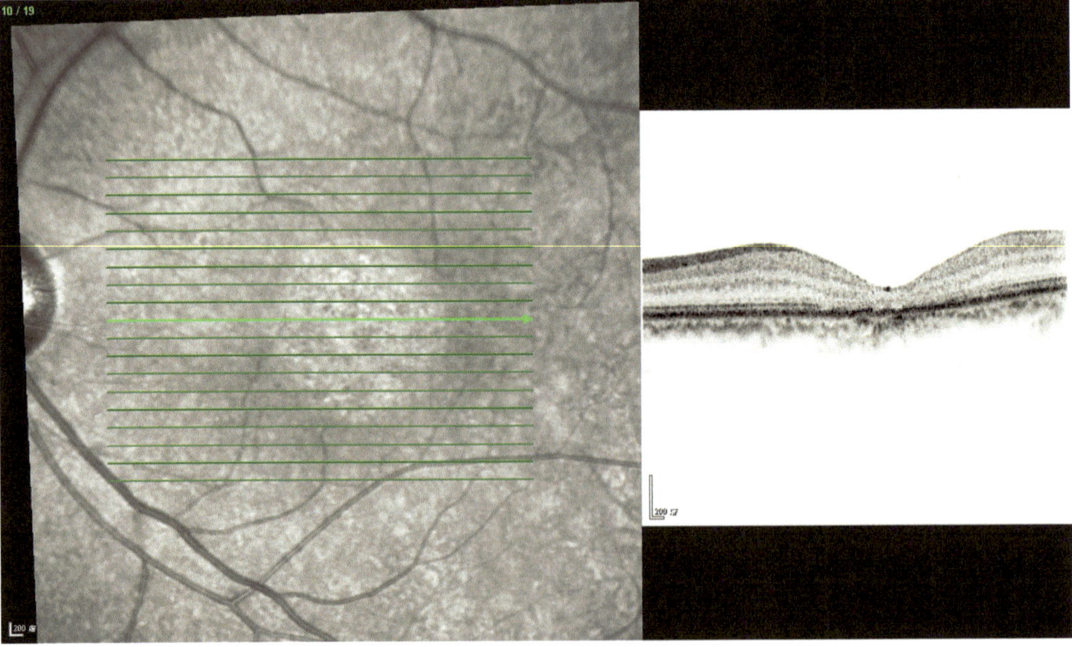

Fig. 18.8 SD-OCT showing disruption of ellipsoid zone after complete resolution of subretinal fluid in chronic CSC

increase in size and amount with increasing duration of symptoms (Wang et al. 2005). SD-OCT imaging of these yellowish drusen-like granular deposits correlated well with the hyper-reflective deposits found on the posterior surface of the neurosensory retina as well as in the sub-retinal cavity (Fig. 18.9). It has been suggested that these deposits are composed of fragments of photoreceptor OS that accumulate when they were unable to be phagocytosed by RPE due to presence of neurosensory detachment, especially when the detachment is prolonged for over 4 months (Pryds and Larsen 2013). Other possible explanations for these deposits include plasma proteins extruded from the choriocapillaris, inflammatory debris, and lipid exudate originating from occult choroidal neovascularization secondary to CSC (Wang et al. 2005). Eyes with foveal subretinal deposit on presentation usually do not recover to the full functional and structural status compared with the asymptomatic fellow eyes even after complete resolution of the neurosensory retinal detachment following treatment with photodynamic therapy. This seems to indicate that the subretinal deposits are associated with irreversible foveal damage in CSC (Pryds and Larsen 2013).

18.2.6 Decrease in Outer Nuclear Layer (ONL) Thickness in Central Serous Chorioretinopathy

While the time-domain OCT allows visualization of the IS/OS junction with a resolution of up to 10 μm, the SD-OCT has an axial resolution of up to 1 μm, which enables visualization the external limiting membrane (ELM), in addition to showing the IS/OS line more clearly. The outer nuclear layer (ONL) represents the cell bodies of the cone photoreceptors. The outer limit of the ONL is the ELM, while at the central fovea, the inner boundary of the ONL almost abuts the internal limiting membrane (ILM). Matsumoto and colleagues defined the distance between the ILM and ELM at the fovea as the ONL thickness and evaluated this in patients with CSC (Matsumoto et al. 2009). Eyes were classified into two groups according to

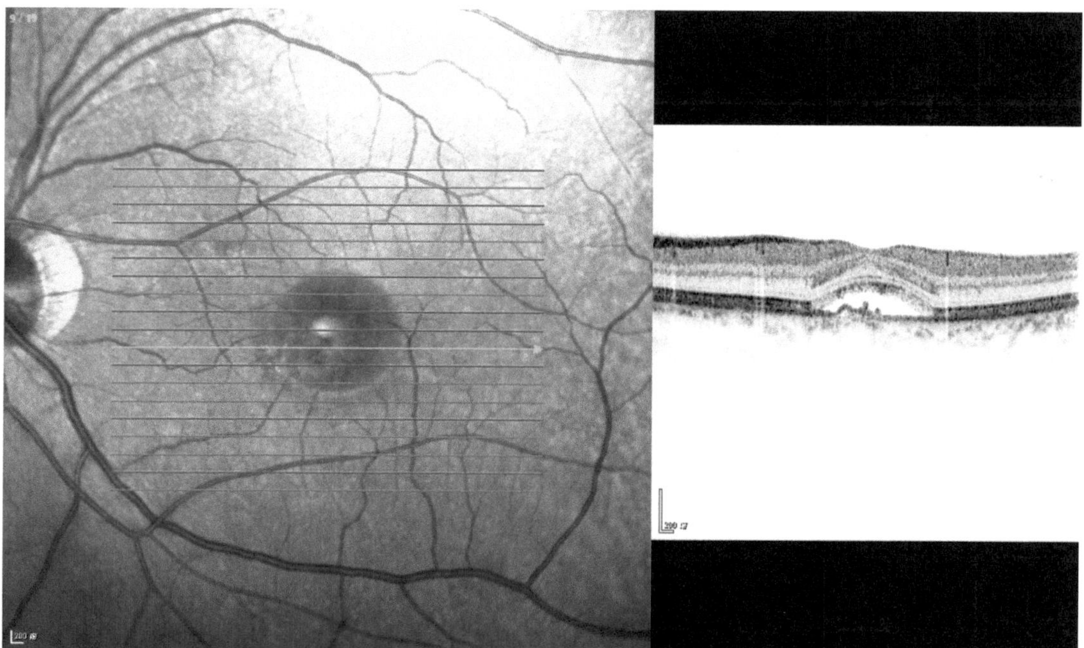

Fig. 18.9 SD-OCT in an eye with chronic CSC showing subretinal fluid with hyper-reflective deposits on the posterior surface of the neurosensory retina and in the subretinal space

BCVA. Eyes with BCVA poorer than 20/20 were found to have significantly thinner ONL compared with those with BCVA better than 20/20, which in turn was significantly thinner than the ONL of normal controls. It was hypothesized that in serous retinal detachment, the retinal insults begin in the photoreceptor OS, where the disruption of the physiological phagocytosis of the OS by RPE cells leads to elongation of the OS, which eventually leads to apoptosis of photoreceptor cell bodies and thinning of the ONL. The thinning of central foveal thickness has been replicated in other studies (Kim et al. 2012; Ooto et al. 2010). The ONL reflects photoreceptor volume and was found to be a more sensitive indicator of visual outcome than IS/OS junction disruption (Ooto et al. 2010).

18.2.7 Retinal Pigment Epithelial Layer Changes and Pigment Epithelial Defect in Central Serous Chorioretinopathy

Morphological alterations of the RPE invariably occur at the point of angiographic leakage on FA in CSC. They can be shown on both cross-sectional and en face SD-OCT scans as PED, RPE irregularities, RPE bulge or protrusions (defined as an absence of an optically clear space within the lesion in contrast with PED), RPE hyperplasia, and RPE micro-rip (Gupta et al. 2010a; Kim et al. 2012; Lehmann et al. 2013; Shinojima et al. 2010).

PEDs are found in nearly all eyes with acute CSC. They are shown to persist in chronic CSC and in quiescent eyes even after resolution of SRF (Fujimoto et al. 2008; Song et al. 2012). Serous PEDs in SD-OCT are characterized by separation of the RPE (shown as a hyper-reflective line) from the underlying Bruch's membrane with an optically empty space in between. PEDs in acute CSC tend to be semicircular in shape with a smooth surface (Fig. 18.10), while those in chronic CSCs are usually low or flat with a dimpled or irregular surface (Song et al. 2012) (Fig. 18.11). It has been postulated that in CSC, the RPE overlying the hyperpermeable choroidal circulation is damaged from the exudation and becomes dysfunctional. The increased hydrostatic pressure from the choroidal circulation pushes the RPE forward and thereby creating a PED. A "micro-rip" or blowout of the RPE can occur if the damage is severe, resulting in a focal leak which shows up as a leakage spot on fluorescein angiography (Fujimoto et al. 2008). These RPE micro-rips could be seen morphologically on SD-OCT scans (Kim et al. 2012). Once the fluid egresses from the sub-RPE space to the subretinal space, the pressure equalizes which causes the collapse of the PED. As the walls of the PED collapse, the RPE micro-rip may seal or bundle up appearing as RPE irregularities or hyperplasia on OCT (Gupta et al. 2010a, b; Shinojima et al. 2010). Once the RPE seals, the subretinal fluid will usually absorb leading to spontaneous CSC resolution.

Abnormalities in the RPE can be seen not only in eyes with active CSC but also in asymptomatic fellow eyes. Gupta and colleagues demonstrated that RPE bumps and PED could be seen in 94 % and 12 % of asymptomatic fellow eyes of CSC patients, respectively (Gupta et al. 2010b). The study provided evidence that CSC is a bilateral disease with asymmetrical clinical features. The RPE bumps may be related to underlying hyperpermeable choroid together with impaired RPE function leading to pooling of fluid in the sub-RPE space and might represent a preclinical or subclinical state of the disease. Yalcinbayir and colleagues noted that RPE bumps and hypertrophy were correlated with poor visual acuity, and the presence of these abnormalities on OCT may provide an indirect evidence of earlier photoreceptor damage and worse visual outcome (Yalcinbayir et al. 2014).

PED in CSC can also be visualized using en face OCT. They appear as circular with smooth inner silhouette on coronal section and are characterized by a hypo-reflective area surrounded by a well-defined hyper-reflective margin. PEDs tend to be located within or at the edge of serous retinal detachment (Lehmann et al. 2013). With the en face SD-OCT, RPE hyperplasia can be seen as a hyper-reflective area overlying the RPE

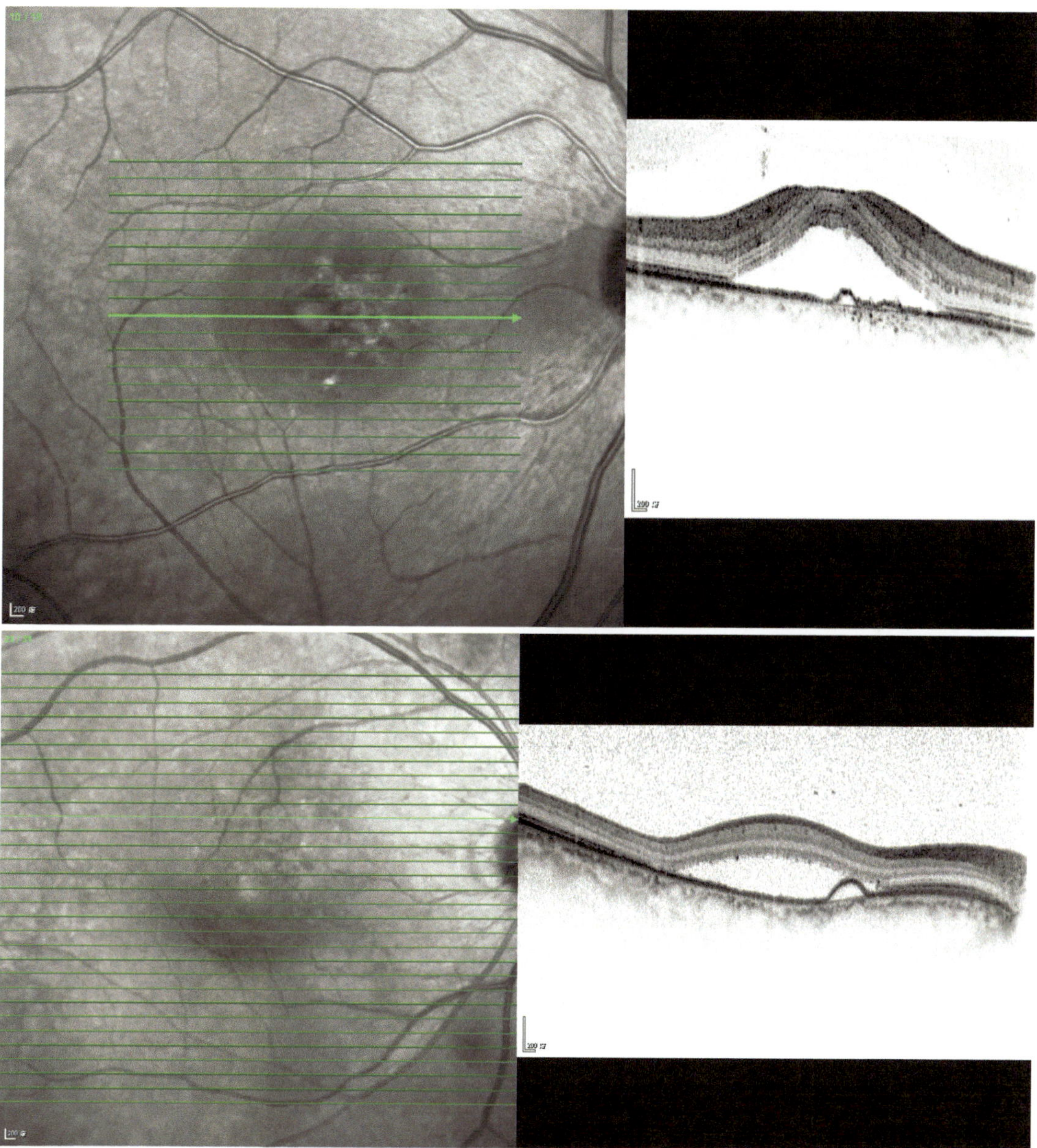

Fig. 18.10 SD-OCT of an eye with acute CSC showing subretinal fluid with semicircular-shaped PED with smooth surface

in 31 % of eyes with CSC (Lehmann et al. 2013). These areas of RPE hyperplasia are often located with small PEDs over the leakage points on FA. Under the RPE abnormalities, they noted choroidal cavitations, shown as multiple black hypo-reflective cystic lesions corresponding to abnormal choroidal dilatations on transverse EDI-OCT scans.

18.2.8 Secondary Choroidal Neovascularization in Central Serous Chorioretinopathy

Choroidal neovascularization (CNV) can arise as a complication of CSC, as with any other lesions of the RPE or the Bruch's membrane. It occurs more frequently in chronic retinal

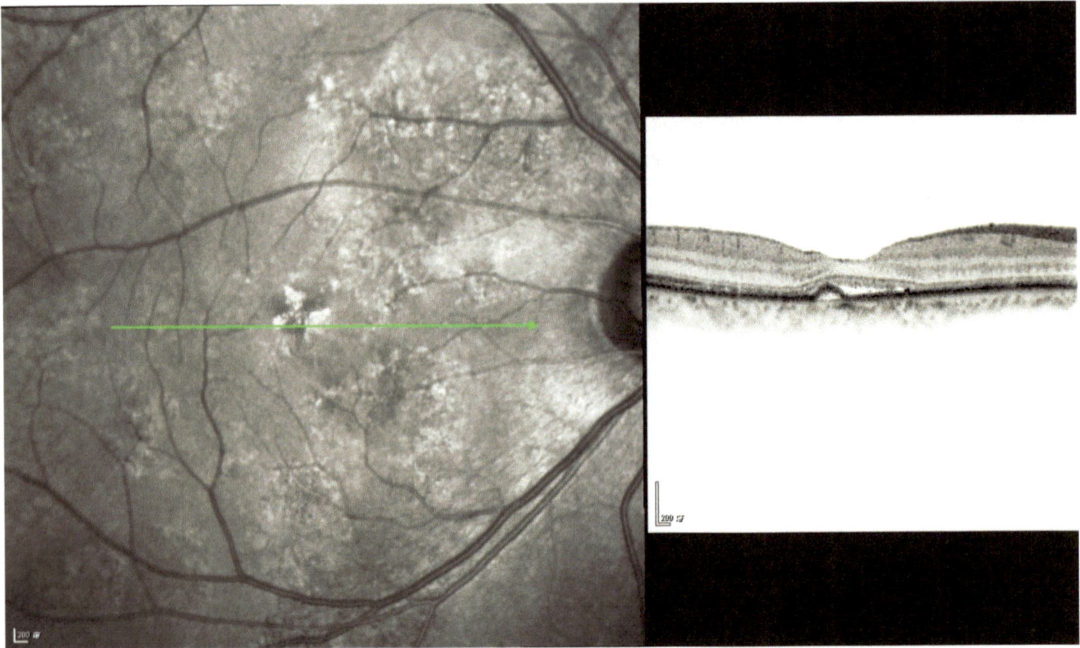

Fig. 18.11 SD-OCT of an eye with chronic CSC showing subretinal fluid with semicircular-shaped PED with dimpled surface

pigment epitheliopathy and has a reported incidence of 4 % (Chan et al. 2003). CNV may occur after a long period after resolution of the acute disease and might be confused with CNV associated with age-related macular degeneration (AMD) in older patients (Wang et al. 2005). CNV in long-standing CSC are more likely to be type 2 membranes (Chan et al. 2003), but associations with type 1 CNV and polypoidal choroidal vasculopathy (PCV) have also been reported (Fung et al. 2012). Patients who have received laser photocoagulation for CSC can also develop laser-induced CNV, with a reported incidence from 0.6 to 5 % (Matsunaga et al. 1995).

The exact hypothesis of secondary CNV in CSC is unclear. It is hypothesized that in normal eyes, the Bruch's membrane acts as a barrier against CNV formation (Fung et al. 2012). In cases of CSC, chronic RPE decompensation or splitting of the RPE/Bruch's membrane complex in serous PEDs together with ischemic changes of the choriocapillaris may be factors leading to CNV development (Chan et al. 2003; Levine et al. 1989).

CNV in CSC typically has classic features of a well-delineated membrane in the early phase with intense leakage in the late phase on FA (Cooper and Thomas 2000). OCT shows a subretinal membrane associated with subretinal fluid (Fig. 18.12). Intravitreal anti-vascular endothelial growth factor (anti-VEGF) therapy such as bevacizumab and ranibizumab has been investigated and appeared to be a useful treatment modality, with OCT resolution or reduction of the subretinal fluid and shrinkage of the CNV membrane (Konstantinidis et al. 2010; Montero et al. 2011; Nomura et al. 2012) (Fig. 18.13).

18.2.9 Enhanced Depth Imaging for Choroidal Changes in Central Serous Chorioretinopathy

Choroidal Thickness Imamura and colleagues (Imamura et al. 2009) demonstrated using EDI-OCT imaging that the subfoveal choroidal thickness was increased in both acute and chronic cases of CSC (Fig. 18.14). In the study, the mean

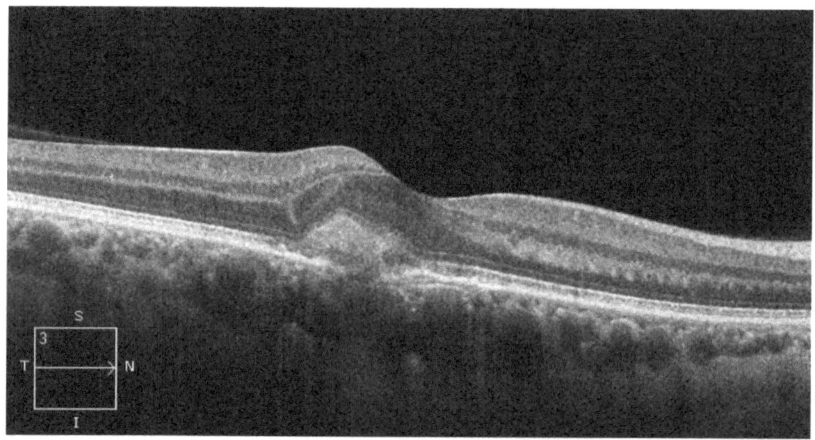

Fig. 18.12 SD-OCT of an eye with a history of CSC showing hyper-reflective lesion at the RPE level due to CNV formation

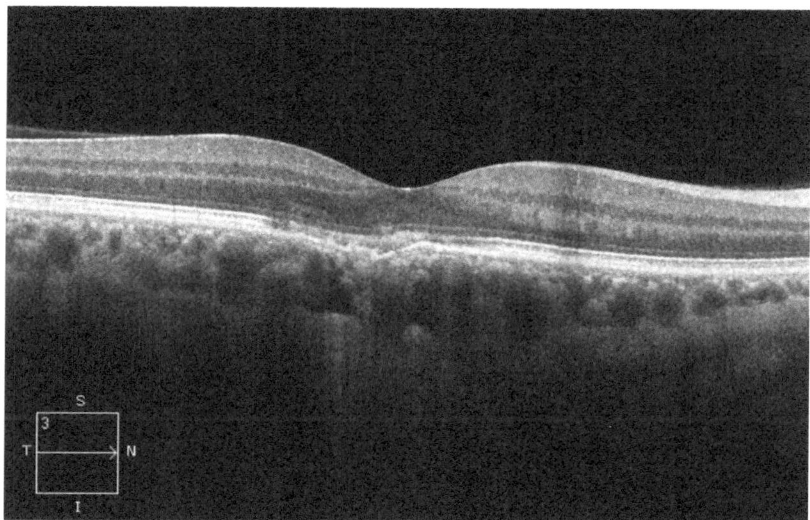

Fig. 18.13 SD-OCT after intravitreal anti-VEGF therapy for CNV secondary to CSC showing complete resolution of fluid and regression of the CNV

choroidal thickness was greater in eyes with CSC compared with normal eyes by a mean of 214 μm. The results provided evidence that there is expansion of the choroid as a result of the venous dilatation and increased hydrostatic pressure in the choroid in eyes with CSC.

Choroidal Vessels EDI-OCT imaging can be performed simultaneously with ICGA. Yang and colleagues showed that in the ICGA hyperfluorescent areas, there was reduction in hyperreflectivity beneath Bruch's membrane on EDI-OCT, suggesting thinning of the small to medium vessel layers of the choroid (Yang et al. 2013). Underneath this thinned layer, enlarged, hypo-reflective (similar to subretinal fluid) lumina were identified, suggesting dilatation of the large choroidal vessels. The diameters of the hypo-reflective choroidal lumina in hyperfluorescent ICGA areas were significantly associated with increased subfoveal choroidal thickness. They suggested interstitial edema may play a role in addition to choroidal dilatation.

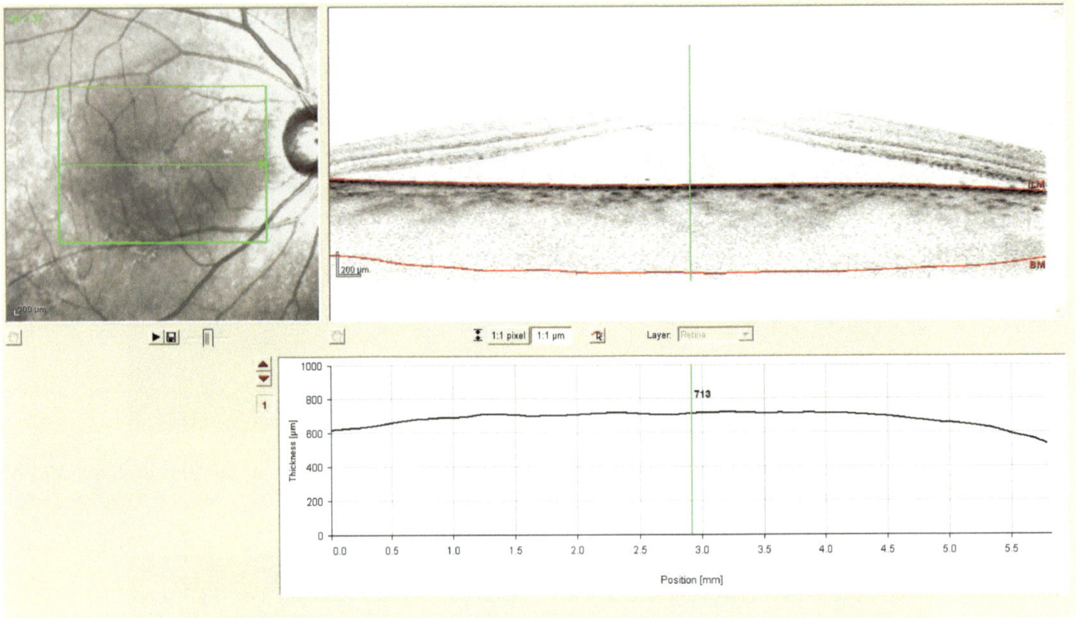

Fig. 18.14 EDI-OCT showing subretinal fluid with increased choroidal thickness in acute CSC

RPE Layer Changes A "double-layer sign" can be seen on EDI-OCT scans, most often in chronic CSC eyes where the RPE layer has an undulated non-dome-shaped appearance, while the underlying intact Bruch's membrane appears as a straight line. The space in between the double layer could either be hyper- or hypo-reflective, but hypo-reflectivity is seen in the majority of CSC eyes. This feature can also be found in eyes with PCV, where the space is hyper-reflective in most eyes with PCV. This can be used as one of the distinguishing features between the two diseases. It has been postulated that the difference in the reflectivity between eyes with PCV and CSC may be due to differences in the hyperpermeability of the choroidal vessels between the two diseases (Yang et al. 2013).

In both acute and chronic CSC, RPE hyperplasia that corresponds to focal leak on FA could be seen and can act as a guide to localize treatment area. Choroidal cavitation, defined as multiple, black hypo-reflective cystic lesions, could be seen in en face OCT at a layer just beneath the choriocapillaris, situated in areas of abnormal RPE. This could represent ischemic choroidal areas around focal hyper-fluorescent spot observed on FA (Lehmann et al. 2013).

18.2.10 Focal Choroidal Excavation in Central Serous Chorioretinopathy

Focal choroidal excavation (FCE) is a localized trough within the submacular choroid, along the RPE/Bruch's membrane complex line seen on SD-OCT scans. On fundus examination, FCE appears as mild pigmentary mottling or a small yellowish spot, which can only be confirmed with OCT imaging. It can be classified as conforming, if the photoreceptor tips are attached to the apical surface of the RPE (Fig. 18.15), or nonconforming if the photoreceptor tips and the RPE are separated (Fig. 18.16). Eyes with nonconforming type are generally more visually symptomatic as patients may develop metamorphopsia or blurred vision. FCE can also be classified in terms of its location: foveal if the foveal center is within the choroidal excavation or extrafoveal if the foveal center is not within the excavation.

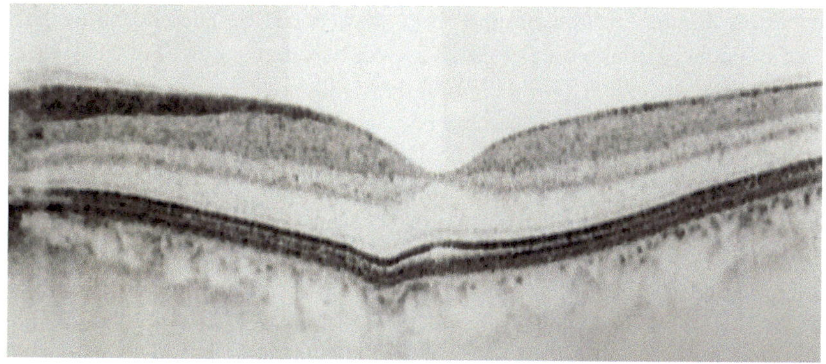

Fig. 18.15 SD-OCT of an eye with focal choroidal excavation showing photoreceptor layer is attached to the apical surface of the RPE in the excavation

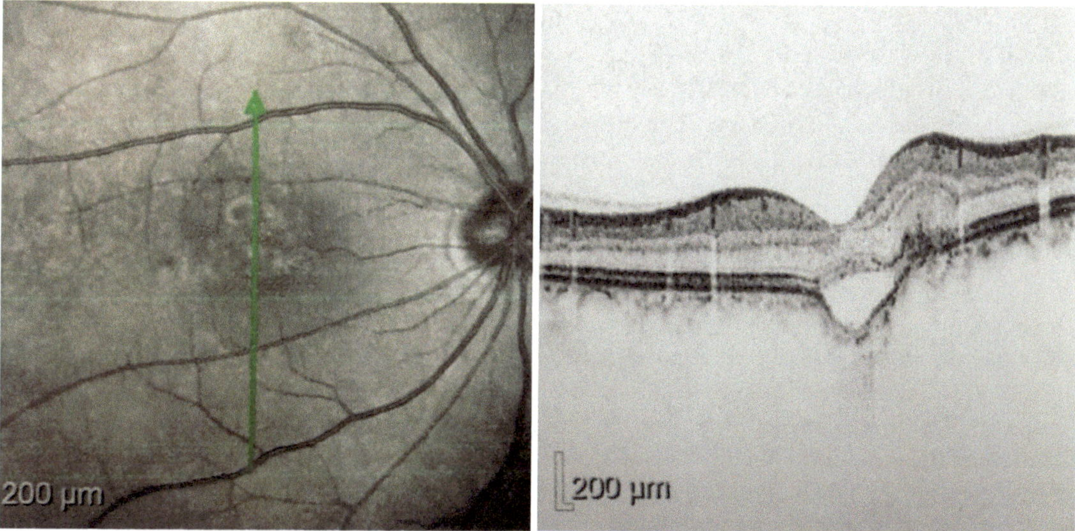

Fig. 18.16 SD-OCT of an eye with focal choroidal excavation showing photoreceptor layer is separated from the apical surface of the RPE in the excavation

While FCE was first reported in normal eyes, it is more commonly found in association with other macular diseases such as PCV and CNV (Lee and Lee 2014). In a small case series, FCE was found to be present in around 8 % of eyes with CSC, especially in myopic eyes (Ellabban et al. 2013). It is unclear whether FCE is a congenital or acquired condition, but FCE tends to remain unchanged over time. There are close topographic associations between FCE and CNV/PCV. It has been suggested that anatomic alterations or relative choroidal ischemia at the excavation site due to focal thinning could predispose FCE eyes to develop CNV at the excavated area (Lee and Lee 2014). FCE is often found to be within or next to leakage points seen in FA (Ellabban et al. 2013; Suzuki et al. 2014). Choroidal vascular hyperpermeability was found in nearly all eyes around the FCE or in a wide area outside the FCE (Luk et al. 2015). It remains unknown whether FCE plays a pathogenic role in the development of CSC.

En face SD-OCT imaging at the level beneath the FCE has shown unusual choroidal tissue devoid of normal large choroidal vessels bridging between the bottom of the excavation and the outer choroidal boundary (Ellabban et al. 2013). In some eyes, the outer boundary of the choroid seemed to be pulled inward, showing the underlying suprachoroidal space. This suggests a focal scarring process might be involved resulting in focal retraction of the RPE with FCE formation. This finding is supported by later studies where this hyper-reflective band was found in 54 % of eyes with FCE (Lee et al. 2014). This hyper-reflective layer was found to be associated with decreased choroidal thickness which further supports the theory that there is scarring and contraction of choroidal tissue in the development of FCE.

18.3 Correlation of SD-OCT Findings with Other Imaging Modalities

18.3.1 Fundus Autofluorescence

Fundus autofluorescence (FAF) is an imaging technique that reflects the intensity and spatial distribution of autofluorophores in the retina. The main autofluorophore is pyridinium bis-retinoid (AE2), contained in lipofuscin which is a breakdown product of phagocytosed photoreceptor OS. When stimulated by light of specific wavelengths, autofluorophore emits light which can be captured by imaging systems focusing on the RPE.

In acute CSC, there may be no abnormal FAF findings until after several months, when diffuse hyper-autofluorescence develops along the inferior border of the retinal detachment. This is due to buildup of autofluorescent materials in the subretinal space caused by impaired phagocytosis of the photoreceptor OS. There may also be small punctate hyper-autofluorescence, resulting in a granular appearance. These precipitates are common and can appear in up to 65 % of eyes with CSC (Maruko et al. 2011a). They correspond to hyper-reflective lesions in the outer retina or subretinal space in SD-OCT scans. It has been hypothesized that the precipitates could be accumulations of shed photoreceptor outer segments or engorged macrophages that have phagocytosed them (Nicholson et al. 2013).

In chronic CSC, there are often FAF changes that reflect large areas of RPE atrophy or damage. Gravity-driven descending tracts of subretinal fluid can be seen. These tracts appear hyper-autofluorescent when the fluid first occurs, then becoming increasingly hypo-autofluorescent as the underlying RPE is damaged in the path of the fluid. Imamura and colleagues classified hypo-autofluorescence in CSC into granular or confluent types (Imamura et al. 2011). They noted the granular type seemed to signify incomplete loss of RPE cells and therefore appeared as intermixed dots of normal autofluorescence and hypo-autofluorescence in between, while confluent type appears as a uniform hypo-autofluorescence, indicating confluent cell loss. This could be correlated with OCT scans where areas of hypo-autofluorescence on FAF are associated with atrophy of the RPE and the outer retina, as well as photoreceptor damage seen as IS/OS disruption on OCT scans (Spaide et al. 2008; Kim et al. 2013). The presence of granular or confluent hypo-autofluorescence at the macula or peripapillary area or descending tract from the macula has been shown to be a significant predictor for poor visual acuity.

Recent developments in autofluorescence imaging have used infrared (IR) or near-IR autofluorescence as the stimulating light source instead of the traditional short wavelength (SWL) autofluorescence. In these FAF images, melanin is the main autofluorophore, in contrast to lipofuscins in SWL autofluorescence. Granular hyper-IR autofluorescence was noted in CSC that changed to hypo-autofluorescence later in the disease course and is hypothesized to be due to modification of melanin in the RPE. Also, areas of simultaneous punctate hyper-IR autofluorescence and hyper-SWL autofluorescence could be seen. These areas correspond to RPE hyperplastic areas on OCT scans and are speculated to be hyperplastic RPE clumps (Sekiryu et al. 2010; Kim et al. 2013).

18.3.2 Fluorescein Angiography

Fluorescein angiography (FA) is widely used in the diagnosis and treatment of CSC. In acute CSC, the most characteristic feature is one or more expanding dots of fluorescein that pools in the serous retinal detachment. The classic "smokestack" appearance, where the dye rises from the leakage point to the top of the neurosensory detachment then spreads laterally due to osmotic gradient between old and new fluid within the detachment, is less commonly seen than the inkblot or mushroom-shaped dye pattern. The pinpoint leak on FA represents leakage of dye from the choroid through a focal RPE defect which is present in about 95 % of CSC cases. The leak is usually within 1500 μm of the fovea, most commonly in the supero-nasal quadrant as gravity pulls the fluid inferiorly (Ross et al. 2011).

Correlation of FA leakage points with cross-sectional SD-OCT scans shows RPE abnormalities in nearly all eyes. PEDs are present in 61–71 % of eyes, while a protruding or irregular RPE layer is seen in 32–100 % (Fujimoto et al. 2008; Kim et al. 2012; Shinojima et al. 2010). SD-OCT enables the detection of small or shallow PEDs which cannot be detected on FA alone. RPE micro-rips or defects within these PEDs or RPE irregularities have been matched precisely to leakage points on FA and provide further evidence that RPE abnormalities are involved in the pathogenesis of CSC (Kim et al. 2012). On follow-up assessment, these RPE rips undergo spontaneous closure, replaced by RPE hypertrophy (Gupta et al. 2010a).

In multifocal or chronic CSC, multiple areas of pinpoint leakage and neurosensory detachment filling could be seen. As the RPE is damaged from repeated neurosensory detachment and SRF, hyper-fluorescent window defects could be seen, often along gravitational tracts corresponding to areas of RPE atrophy. SD-OCT imaging of these window defects shows different degree of damage to the RPE or the outer retina including the IS/OS junction and the external limiting membrane (Kim et al. 2013).

18.3.3 Indocyanine Green Angiography

The use of indocyanine green angiography (ICGA) has shed much light on the pathophysiology of CSC. It is also used to guide treatment with verteporfin photodynamic therapy (PDT). Characteristically, ICGA shows initial hypofluorescence with delayed choroidal arterial filling, followed by mid-phase hyperfluorescence due to vascular hyperpermeability and late-phase washout of indocyanine green dye (Ross et al. 2011; Quin et al. 2013). It is suggested that the initial delayed arterial filling is due to choroidal capillary and venous congestion, as leakage from RPE on FA only occurs in areas where ICGA showed delayed arterial filling (Kitaya et al. 2003). Localized hyperfluorescence suggests areas of underlying choroidal hyperpermeability and dilatation.

With the use of en face EDI-OCT, it was demonstrated that areas of dilation of choroidal vascular network corresponded exactly with the choroidal abnormalities in ICGA. In contrast to hyperfluorescence on ICGA, dilated choroidal vessels show up as large hypo-reflective tubes in an interconnected network on en face EDI-OCT (Lehmann et al. 2013). Ferrara and colleagues further characterized these dilatations as focal or diffuse choroidal dilation (Ferrara et al. 2014). Dilatations are considered as focal if some vascular branches have larger caliber than the surrounding branches and as diffuse if the dilatations are relatively homogeneous. The areas of dilatation corresponded to areas of choroidal hyperperfusion on ICGA and are invariably found in eyes with overlying PED or RPE changes. En face EDI-OCT may be more advantageous than ICGA in assessing choroidal vessel dilatation as it can provide cross-sectional information about the choroidal vasculature in individual layers (choriocapillaris, Sattler's and Haller's layer could be separately analyzed), whereas in ICGA, all the layers are compressed into a two-dimensional image. In addition, en face OCT is noninvasive and can provide the same information on the choroidal vasculature using ICGA (Ferrara et al. 2014).

Table 18.1 Comparisons of OCT findings of macular disorders which might resemble CSC

OCT feature	Central serous chorioretinopathy	Polypoidal choroidal vasculopathy	Serous PED in AMD	Vogt-Koyanagi-Harada disease
Intraretinal fluid	Usually mild or minimal	Present	Present	Mild intraretinal cyst in acute phase
Subretinal fluid	Marked in acute phase	Mild	Mild	Marked in acute phase Can occur in multiple pockets
RPE level	Double-layer sign with hypo-reflective space. Circular PED	Double-layer sign with hyper-reflective space due to branching vascular network Sharp protrusion of RPE layer due to polyp	Irregular due to drusen or RPE atrophy	Undulations due to infiltration of inflammatory cells
EDI-OCT choroidal layer	Increased choroidal thickness Small- and medium-sized vessel thinning	Increased choroidal thickness	Reduced choroidal thickness	Increased choroidal thickness in acute phase Small- and medium-sized vessel thinning Dilation of large choroidal vessels
En face OCT	PED with smooth inner silhouette, uniform borders, and clear content	Branching vascular network	PED has irregular borders	N/A

18.4 Use of SD-OCT to Differentiate Other Conditions Mimicking Central Serous Chorioretinopathy (Table 18.1)

18.4.1 Polypoidal Choroidal Vasculopathy

Polypoidal choroidal vasculopathy (PCV) was first described by Yannuzzi in 1982. It is now considered a subtype of neovascular AMD which is characterized by aneurysmal or polyp-like abnormalities with a branching vascular network (BVN) of neovascularization in the inner choroidal vessels seen on ICGA. It typically shows multiple, recurrent serosanguineous detachment of the retina and RPE with leakage and bleeding from the polypoidal lesions or BVN (Ciardella et al. 2004). There are some similarities between PCV and chronic CSC which might lead to misdiagnosis of chronic CSC patients as having PCV and vice versa. Both diseases tend to occur in patients with younger age than typical AMD, and both conditions are associated with multifocal choroidal vascular hyperpermeability on ICGA, increased choroidal thickness, and dilated thin-walled choroidal vessels histologically (Mrejen and Spaide 2013; Sasahara et al. 2006). It has been suggested that chronic CSC may predispose to formation of polypoidal lesions and maybe an ocular risk factor for PCV (Koizumi et al. 2013; Sasahara et al. 2006). However, PCV is more commonly associated with subretinal exudation, fibrin deposition, and hemorrhages which generally leads to a poorer visual outcome.

OCT studies of eyes with PCV show sharp protrusions of the RPE correlating to orange red nodules seen clinically (Fig. 18.17). A characteristic "double-layer sign" consisting of a two lines at the RPE level with hyper-reflective material in between could be seen in PCV, and this is considered to correspond to the BVN (Sato et al. 2007). In CSC, although a similar double-layer sign could be seen, the space between the two layers is usually hypo-reflective (Yang et al. 2013).

Cystoid macula edema, lipid deposits, subretinal hemorrhage, and hemorrhagic PED are more commonly seen in PCV but not CSC (Ooto et al. 2011). In the retina, the thickness of the outer nuclear layer as well as the inner segment of the photoreceptor is decreased in both PCV and CSC, which correlates with poor visual acuity. However, in PCV, the thickness of the photoreceptor OS is thinner than normal individuals, while in CSC, the OS is similar or thicker than normal individuals (Ooto et al. 2010). Elongation of OS could be seen in CSC, but it is rare in PCV. This suggests that photoreceptors may be more severely damaged by the subretinal fluid in PCV than CSC, which often contains fibrin or hemorrhage. This leads to poorer visual outcome in PCV than CSC (Kim et al. 2012; Matsumoto et al. 2009; Ooto et al. 2010).

18.4.2 Serous Pigment Epithelial Detachment in Age-Related Macular Degeneration

The diagnosis of CSC can sometimes be confused with AMD, especially in cases of chronic CSC among older patients. Overlapping features of the two conditions include chronicity, RPE hyperplasia or atrophy, PED, subretinal fluid, cystoid macular degeneration, retinal atrophy, and hyperfluorescence on FA or ICGA (Fung et al. 2012). There are several ways to differentiate the two diseases using SD-OCT imaging. In CSC, the PED tends to be smaller and more circular and have a clear content (Cho et al. 2010). Subretinal fluid and hypertrophic outer retinal changes are more common in CSC than in AMD, but there is less intraretinal fluid in CSC compared with AMD (Lumbroso et al. 2011). On EDI-OCT imaging, choroidal thickness is usually increased in CSC, whereas the choroidal thickness is typically reduced in AMD. With en face OCT imaging, PEDs in CSC are circular with smooth inner silhouette, clear contents, and uniform borders, where the borders are often irregular in AMD. The OCT findings, combined with medical history (eg, steroid use), demographics (eg, younger patient), other clinical features (eg, absence of drusen), and features of other investigations (eg, bilateral vascular hyperpermeability on mid-phase ICGA), often enable clinicians to differentiate among these two disease entities.

18.4.3 Vogt-Koyanagi-Harada Disease

Vogt-Koyanagi-Harada (VKH) disease is an idiopathic granulomatous inflammatory disorder that affects the eyes, meninges, and skin. The main site of the intraocular inflammation is the choroid. The clinical course of VKH disease is divided into acute, chronic, and convalescent stages. Eyes during acute VKH disease stage are characterized by bilateral multifocal serous neurosensory detachments. In the convalescent stage, the retinal detachment resolves and develops late manifestations such as ocular depigmentation, peripheral nummular scars, pigmentary changes of the RPE, or recurrent chronic anterior uveitis.

VKH can sometimes be confused with CSC, especially in the acute stage where both conditions present with neurosensory retinal detachment. Differentiating between the two disease entities is important as VKH is treated with high-dose steroids while CSC is aggravated by steroid therapy. Characteristic FA findings for VKH disease include disseminated spotted choroidal hyperfluorescence and multifocal pockets of SRF with pooling of dye and with disc leakage, while CSC typically present with inkblot or smokestack leakage patterns, and the SRF is mainly limited to the posterior pole with no disc leakage.

Using SD-OCT, differentiating features for VKH from CSC include large wavy undulations of the RPE, presence of subretinal septa, and intraretinal cystic space (Vasconcelos-Santos et al. 2010). In acute VKH disease, intraretinal cystic spaces corresponded to areas of dye pooling on FA. The retina is split just above the IS/OS junction in these cystic structures, and a membranous structure, represented by a highly reflective line, is seen at the floor of these cysts and is continuous with the IS/OS line (Ishihara

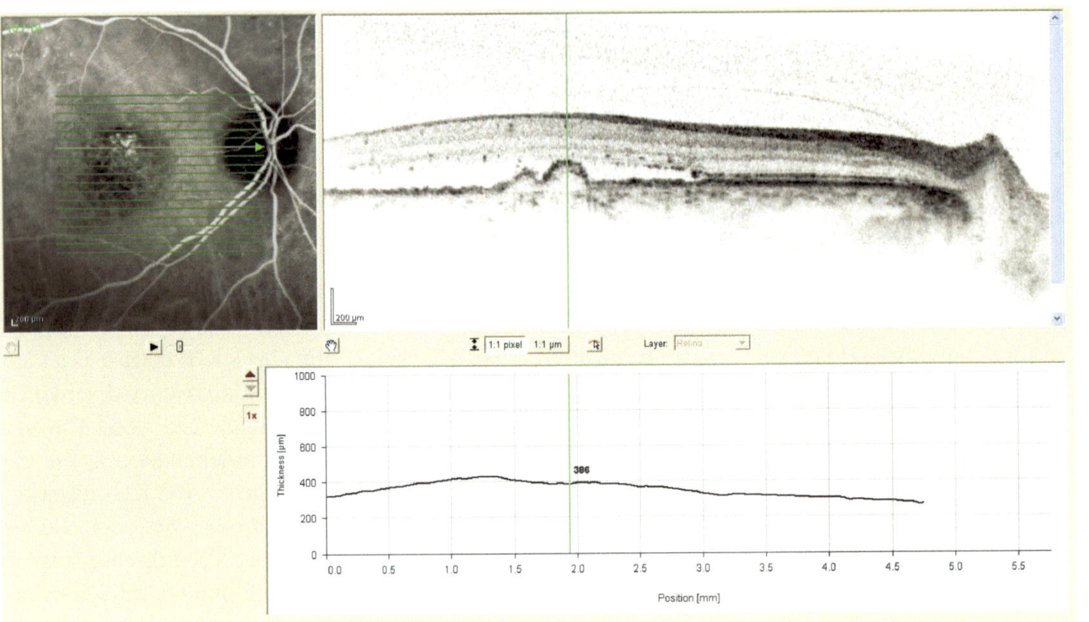

Fig. 18.17 SD-OCT showing subretinal fluid with nodular protrusions at the RPE level due to polypoidal choroidal vasculopathy corresponding to the nodular hyperfluorescence as seen in ICGA

et al. 2009). Ishihara and colleagues hypothesized that inflammatory products such as fibrin binds to a portion of the OS layer and is split from the IS in these cystoid spaces (Ishihara et al. 2009). In areas of serous retinal detachment, irregularity of the IS/OS junction could be seen. Characteristic wavy undulations of the RPE can often be found in areas adjacent to the serous retinal detachment, probably representing areas of infiltration of inflammatory cells in the choroid and choroidal folds (Gupta et al. 2009).

In the chronic or convalescent phase of VKH disease, SD-OCT imaging of the hypopigmented atrophic lesions in sunset glow fundi shows RPE loss with variable involvement of the outer retinal layers. RPE thickening suggesting RPE hypertrophy could be seen in areas with pigmented or disciform scars.

EDI-OCT imaging of eyes with acute VKH disease shows diffuse choroidal thickening compared with convalescent phase VKH (Fong et al. 2011; Montero et al. 2011). Localized thickening of the choroidal compartment with subsequent bulging of the RPE/Bruch's reflective complex anteriorly ("choroidal bulging") has been observed in convalescent VKH, and this might suggest ongoing subclinical inflammation (Sakata et al. 2014).

Fong and colleagues demonstrated a loss of inner choroidal hyper-reflective foci in VKH patients in both acute and convalescent stages using EDI-OCT imaging (Fong et al. 2011). It was hypothesized that these hyper-reflective foci represent pericapillary arterioles and venules, which were damaged by inflammation and caused stromal shrinking and small vessel dropout as shown on EDI-OCT. This hypothesis was later supported by further SD-OCT studies which showed loss of choriocapillaris layer in convalescent phase VKH, represented as a break in the hypo-reflective band just below the RPE/BM layer (Nazari et al. 2014). Eyes with CSC also showed a relative thinning of the inner choroidal layer of small- and medium-sized vessels. However, underneath the thinned inner choroidal layer, there is a relative dilation of the large choroidal vessels, shown as hypo-reflective lumina beneath the thinned inner choroidal layer, which contrasts with eyes with VKH disease (Yang et al. 2013).

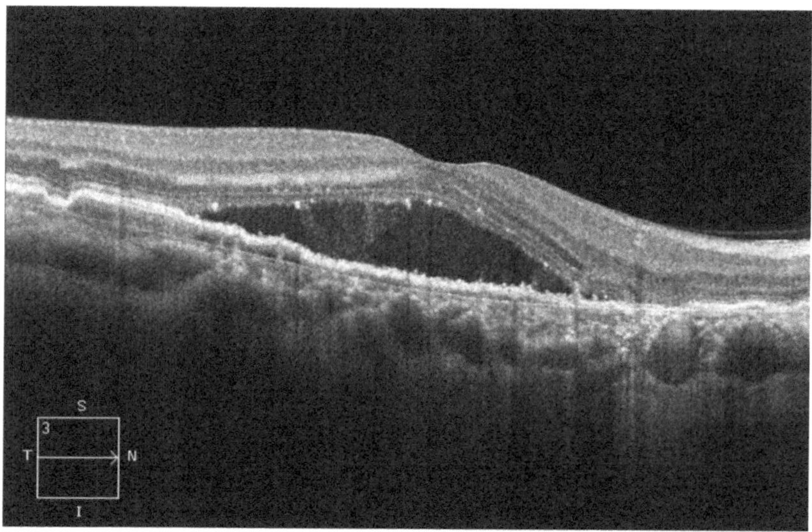

Fig. 18.18 SD-OCT showing subretinal fluid in CSC prior to photodynamic therapy with half-dose verteporfin

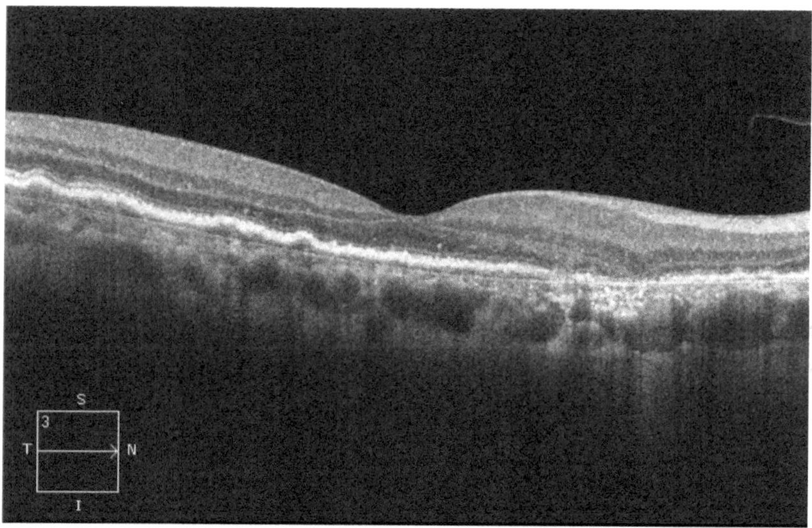

Fig. 18.19 SD-OCT 1 month after photodynamic therapy with half-dose verteporfin showing complete resolution of subretinal fluid

18.5 Use of SD-OCT for Treatment Monitoring in Central Serous Chorioretinopathy

18.5.1 Photodynamic Therapy

Verteporfin PDT is useful in promoting resolution of acute and chronic CSC as well as to prevent recurrences. It causes remodeling of the choroidal vasculature and reduces choroidal hyperpermeability and congestion thereby addressing the root cause of the disease. Early reports using standard protocol PDT for CSC reported 60–100 % success rates with improvement of visual outcome in both acute and chronic cases (Yannuzzi et al. 2012). However, potential problems including foveal RPE atrophy, choroidal ischemia, and secondary CNV were reported to occur with standard PDT. More recently safety enhanced PDT, either with reduced dose or fluence PDT, has been investigated with good results.

Chan and colleagues (Chan et al. 2008) performed a randomized control trial with half-dose verteporfin PDT for acute CSC eyes and found 95 % resolution of SRF in patients in the treatment group compared with 58 % in the placebo group. Reduced fluence, either by decreasing treatment time or energy output, was also found to be efficacious in speeding up subretinal fluid resolution with reduced complications such as CNV and choriocapillaris nonperfusion (Reibaldi et al. 2010).

SD-OCT imaging is useful in monitoring CSC following PDT in two ways. Firstly, it can monitor the height of serous retinal detachment following PDT and can detect any residual fluid that is not obvious on clinical examination (Figs. 18.18 and 18.19). Some eyes show a transient increase in exudation immediately following PDT, similar to eyes with CNV treated with PDT, with subsequent resolution of the subretinal fluid (Rogers et al. 2002). Secondly, by using EDI-OCT, subfoveal choroidal thickness can be assessed following PDT. Maruko and colleagues reported reduction of mean choroidal thickness from a baseline of 462 μm to 360 μm in PDT-treated eyes after 1 month, and ICGA showed decreased hyperpermeability (Maruko et al. 2010). This reduction was not seen in eyes treated with thermal laser photocoagulation.

18.5.2 Thermal Laser Photocoagulation

Conventional laser treatment for CSC is performed in CSC to obtain a confluent coagulation of moderate intensity covering the leakage point on FA. It is used to expedite the absorption of SRF in acute and chronic CSC, but it does not prevent recurrence (Nicholson et al. 2013). The exact mechanism of action for thermal laser in CSC is unclear, but it may cause direct sealing of the RPE leaking sites or by promoting RPE pumping function. Possible side effects include scotoma and late development of CNV, and therefore it is mainly used in chronic or refractory cases. However, it does not have a role in bullous variant of CSC (Liegl and Ulbig. 2014). Using SD-OCT to evaluate the photoreceptors before and after laser treatment in acute and chronic CSC, Odrobina and colleagues found that permanent damage to the photoreceptor layer and external limiting membrane occurred in 93 % of chronic CSC eyes but not in acute CSC eyes up to 12 months post-laser treatment and absorption of subretinal fluid (Odrobina et al. 2013). Changes include disruption of the foveal photoreceptor layer and external limiting membrane, persistent hyper-reflective subretinal deposits, and a noticeable RPE bulge, reflecting outer segment apoptosis and phagocytosis by RPE. This seems to indicate that early laser treatment of CSC results in quicker resolution of SRF and might reduce long-term photoreceptor damage and visual acuity loss.

While traditional laser is useful to shorten duration of serous detachment in CSC, it is not appropriate for juxtafoveal or subfoveal leakage points (leakage sites should be more than 375 μm from the fovea). A modified laser therapy with micropulse diode laser has been recently investigated, which involves applying a sub-threshold laser burn using a 810 nm diode laser to the leakage site, which leads to early resolution of serous retinal detachment in chronic CSC without leaving any visible scars on fundoscopy or on FA (Lanzetta et al. 2008; Roisman et al. 2013).

References

Ahn SE, Oh J, Oh JH et al (2013) Three-dimensional configuration of subretinal fluid in central serous chorioretinopathy. Invest Ophthalmol Vis Sci 54:5944–5952

Bajarborua D (2001) Long-term follow-up of idiopathic central serous chorioretinopathy without laser. Acta Ophthalmol Scand 79:417–421

Castro-Correia J, Coutinho MF, Rosas V et al (1992) Long term follow up of central serous retinopathy in 150 patients. Doc Ophthalmol 81:379–386

Chan WM, Lam DS, Lai TY et al (2003) Treatment of choroidal neovascularization in central serous chorioretinopathy by photodynamic therapy with verteporfin. Am J Ophthalmol 136:836–845

Chan WM, Lai TY, Lai RY et al (2008) Half-dose verteporfin photodynamic therapy for acute central serous chorioretinopathy: one-year results of a randomized controlled trial. Ophthalmology 115:1756–1765

Cho M, Athanikar A, Paccione J et al (2010) Optical coherence tomography features of acute central serous chorioretinopathy versus neovascular age-related macular degeneration. Br J Ophthalmol 94:597–599

Ciardella AP, Donsoff IM, Huang SJ et al (2004) Polypoidal choroidal vasculopathy. Surv Ophthalmol 49:25–37

Cooper BA, Thomas MA (2000) Submacular surgery to remove choroidal neovascularization associated with central serous chorioretinopathy. Am J Ophthalmol 130:187–191

Ellabban AA, Tsujikawa A, Ooto S et al (2013) Focal choroidal excavation in eyes with central serous chorioretinopathy. Am J Ophthalmol 56:673–683

Fawzi AA, Holland GN, Kreiger AE et al (2006) Central serous chorioretinopathy after solid organ transplantation. Ophthalmology 113:805–813

Ferrara D, Mohler KJ, Waheed N et al (2014) En-face enhanced-depth swept-source optical coherence tomography features of chronic central serous chorioretinopathy. Ophthalmology 121:719–726

Fong AH, Li KK, Wong D (2011) Choroidal evaluation using enhanced depth imaging spectral-domain optical coherence tomography in Vogt-Koyanagi-Harada disease. Retina 31:502–509

Fujimoto H, Gomi F, Wakabayashi T et al (2008) Morphologic changes in acute central serous chorioretinopathy evaluated by Fourier-domain optical coherence tomography. Ophthalmology 115: 1494–1500

Fung AT, Yannuzzi LA, Freund KB (2012) Type 1 (sub-retinal pigment epithelial) neovascularization in central serous chorioretinopathy masquerading as neovascular age-related macular degeneration. Retina 32:1829–1837

Gäckle HC, Lang GE, Freissler KA et al (1998a) Central serous chorioretinopathy. Clinical, fluorescein angiography and demographic aspects. Ophthalmologe 95:529–533

Gäckle HC, Lang GE, Freidler KA et al (1998b) Clinical fluorescein angiographic and demographic aspects in central serous chorioretinopathy. Ophthalmologe 95:529–533

Gass JDM (1967) Pathogenesis of disciform detachment of the neuroepithelium: II. Idiopathic central serous choroidopathy. Am J Ophthalmol 63:587–615

Gass JDM (1973) Bullous retinal detachment. An unusual manifestation of idiopathic central serous choroidopathy. Am J Ophthalmol 75:810–882

Gass JDM (1991) Central serous chorioretinopathy and white subretinal exudation during pregnancy. Arch Ophthalmol 109:677–681

Gass JDM (1992) Bullous retinal detachment and multiple retinal pigment epithelium detachments in patients receiving haemodialysis. Graefes Arch ClinExpOphthalmol 230:454–458

Gass JDM, Little H (1995) Bilateral bullous exudative retinal detachment complicating idiopathic central serous chorioretinopathy during systemic corticosteroid therapy. Ophthalmology 102:737–747

Gupta V, Gupta A, Gupta P et al (2009) Spectral-domain cirrus optical coherence tomography of choroidal striations seen in the acute stage of Vogt-Koyanagi-Harada disease. Am J Ophthalmol 147:148–153

Gupta V, Gupta P, Dogra MR et al (2010a) Spontaneous closure of retinal pigment epithelium microrip in the natural course of central serous chorioretinopathy. Eye (Lond) 24:595–599

Gupta P, Gupta V, Dogra MR et al (2010b) Morphological changes in the retinal pigment epithelium on spectral-domain OCT in the unaffected eyes with idiopathic central serous chorioretinopathy. Int Ophthalmol 30:175–181

Hooymans JM (1998) Fibrotic scar formation in central serous chorioretinopathy developed during systemic treatment with corticosteroids. Graefes Arch Clin Exp Ophthalmol 236:876–879

Iida T, Spaide RF, Haas A et al (2002) Leopard-spot pattern of yellowish subretinal deposits in central serous chorioretinopathy. Arch Ophthalmol 120:37–42

Imamura Y, Fujiwara T, Margolis R et al (2009) Enhanced depth imaging optical coherence tomography of the choroid in central serous chorioretinopathy. Retina 29:1469–1473

Imamura Y, Fujiwara T, Spaide RF (2011) Fundus autofluorescence and visual acuity in central serous chorioretinopathy. Ophthalmology 118:700–705

Ishihara K, Hangai M, Kita M et al (2009) Acute Vogt-Koyanagi-Harada disease in enhanced spectral-domain optical coherence tomography. Ophthalmology 116:1799–1807

Kim HC, Cho WB, Chung H (2012) Morphologic changes in acute central serous chorioretinopathy using spectral domain optical coherence tomography. Korean J Ophthalmol 26:347–354

Kim SK, Kim SW, Oh J et al (2013) Near-infrared and short-wavelength autofluorescence in resolved central serous chorioretinopathy: association with outer retinal layer abnormalities. Am J Ophthalmol 156:157–164

Kitaya N, Nagaoka T, Hikichi T et al (2003) Features of abnormal choroidal circulation in central serous chorioretinopathy. Br J Ophthalmol 87:709–712

Koizumi H, Yamagishi T, Yamazaki T et al (2013) Relationship between clinical characteristics of polypoidal choroidal vasculopathy and choroidal vascular hyperpermeability. Am J Ophthalmol 155:305–313

Konstantinidis L, Mantel I, Zografos L et al (2010) Intravitreal ranibizumab in the treatment of choroidal neovascularization associated with idiopathic central serous chorioretinopathy. Eur J Ophthalmol 20: 955–958

Lanzetta P, Furlan F, Morgante L et al (2008) Nonvisible subthreshold micropulse diode laser (810 nm) treatment of central serous chorioretinopathy. A pilot study. Eur J Ophthalmol 18:934–940

Lee JH, Lee WK (2014) Choroidal neovascularization associated with focal choroidal excavation. Am J Ophthalmol 157:710–718

Lee SB, Kim JY, Kim WJ et al (2013) Bilateral central serous chorioretinopathy with retinal pigment

epithelium tears following epidural steroid injection. In J Ophthalmol 61:514–515
Lee CS, Woo SJ, Kim YK et al (2014) Clinical and spectral-domain optical coherence tomography findings in patients with focal choroidal excavation. Ophthalmology 121:1029–1035
Lehmann M, Wolff B, Vasseur V et al (2013) Retinal and choroidal changes observed with 'En-face' enhanced-depth imaging OCT in central serous chorioretinopathy. Br J Ophthalmol 97:1181–1186
Levine R, Brucker AJ, Robinson F (1989) Long-term follow-up of idiopathic central serous chorioretinopathy by fluorescein angiography. Ophthalmology 96:854–859
Liegl R, Ulbig MW (2014) Central serous chorioretinopathy. Ophthalmologica 232:65–76, Epub ahead of print
Lumbroso B, Savastano MC, Rispoli M et al (2011) Morphologic differences, according to etiology, in pigment epithelial detachments by means of en-face optical coherence tomography. Retina 31:553–558
Luk FO, Fok AC, Lee A et al (2015) Focal choroidal excavation in patients with central serous chorioretinopathy. Eye (Lond) 29:453–459
Maruko I, Iida T, Sugano Y et al (2010) Subfoveal choroidal thickness after treatment of central serous chorioretinopathy. Ophthalmology 117:1792–1799
Maruko I, Iida T, Ojima A et al (2011a) Subretinal dot-like precipitates and yellow material in central serous chorioretinopathy. Retina 31:759–765
Maruko I, Tomohiro I, Sugano Y et al (2011b) Subfoveal choroidal thickness after treatment of Vogt-Koyanagi-Harada disease. Retina 31:510–517
Matsumoto H, Sato T, Kishi S (2009) Outer nuclear layer thickness at the fovea determines visual outcomes in resolved central serous chorioretinopathy. Am J Ophthalmol 148:105–110
Matsunaga H, Nangoh K, Uyama M et al (1995) Occurrence of choroidal neovascularization following photocoagulation treatment for central serous retinopathy. Nippon GankaGakkaiZasshi 99:460–468
Miki A, Kondo N, Yanagisawa S et al (2014) Common variants in the complement factor h gene confer genetic susceptibility to central serous chorioretinopathy. Ophthalmology 121:1067–1072
Montero JA, Ruiz-Moreno JM, Fernandez-Muñoz M (2011) Intravitreal bevacizumab to treat choroidal neovascularization following photodynamic therapy in central serous choroidopathy. Eur J Ophthalmol 21:503–505
Mrejen S, Spaide RF (2013) Optical coherence tomography: imaging of the choroid and beyond. Surv Ophthalmol 58:387–429
Nair U, Ganekal S, Soman M et al (2012) Correlation of spectral domain optical coherence tomography findings in acute central serous chorioretinopathy with visual acuity. Clin Ophthalmol 6:1949–1954
Nazari H, Hariri A, Hu Z et al (2014) Choroidal atrophy and loss of choriocapillaris in convalescent stage of Vogt-Koyanagi-Harada disease: in vivo documentation. J Ophthalmic Inflamm Infect 4:9
Nicholson B, Noble J, Forooghian F et al (2013) Central serous chorioretinopathy: update on pathophysiology and treatment. Surv Ophthalmol 58:103–126
Nomura Y, Obata R, Yanagi Y (2012) Intravitreal bevacizumab for iatrogenic choroidal neovascularization due to laser photocoagulation in central serous chorioretinopathy. Jpn J Ophthalmol 56:245–249
Odrobina D, Laudańska-Olszewska I, Gozdek P et al (2013) Morphologic changes in the foveal photoreceptor layer before and after laser treatment in acute and chronic central serous chorioretinopathy documented in spectral-domain optical coherence tomography. J Ophthalmol 2013:361513
Ojima Y, Hangai M, Sasahara M et al (2007) Three-dimensional imaging of the foveal photoreceptor layer in central serous chorioretinopathy using high-speed optical coherence tomography. Ophthalmology 114:2197–2207
Ooto S, Tsujikawa A, Mori S et al (2010) Thickness of photoreceptor layers in polypoidal choroidal vasculopathy and central serous chorioretinopathy. Graefes Arch Clin Exp Ophthalmol 248:1077–1086
Ooto S, Tsujikawa A, Mori S et al (2011) Retinal microstructural abnormalities in central serous chorioretinopathy and polypoidal choroidal vasculopathy. Retina 31:527–534
Otsuka S, Ohnba N, Nakao K (2002) A long-term follow-up study of severe variant of central serous chorioretinopathy. Retina 22:25–32
Ozdemir O, Erol MK (2014) Morphologic changes and visual outcomes in resolved central serous chorioretinopathy treated with ranibizumab. Cutan Ocul Toxicol 33(2):122–126, Epub ahead of print
Polak BCP, Baarsma GS, Snyers B (1995) Diffuse retinal pigment epitheliopathy complicating systemic corticosteroid treatment. Br J Ophthalmol 79:922–925
Pryds A, Larsen M (2013) Foveal function and thickness after verteporfin photodynamic therapy in central serous chorioretinopathy with hyperautofluorescent subretinal deposits. Retina 33:128–135
Quin G, Liew G, Ho IV et al (2013) Diagnosis and interventions for central serous chorioretinopathy: review and update. Clin Exp Ophthalmol 41:187–200
Reibaldi M, Cardascia N, Longo A et al (2010) Standard-fluence versus low-fluence photodynamic therapy in chronic central serous chorioretinopathy: a nonrandomized clinical trial. Am J Ophthalmol 149: 307–315
Rogers AH, Martidis A, Greenberg PB et al (2002) Optical coherence tomography findings following photodynamic therapy of choroidal neovascularization. Am J Ophthalmol 134:566–576
Roisman L, Magalhães FP, Lavinsky D et al (2013) Micropulse diode laser treatment for chronic central serous chorioretinopathy: a randomized pilot trial. Ophthalmic Surg Lasers Imaging Retina 44:465–470
Ross A, Ross AH, Mohamed Q (2011) Review and update of central serous chorioretinopathy. Curr Opin Ophthalmol 22:166–173

Sahu DK, Namperumalsamy P, Hilton GF et al (2000) Bullous variant of idiopathic central serous chorioretinopathy. Br J Ophthalmol 84:485–492

Sakata VM, da Silva FT, Hirata CE et al (2014) Choroidal bulging in patients with Vogt-Koyanagi-Harada disease in the non-acute uveitic stage. J Ophthalmic Inflamm Infect 4:6

Sasahara M, Tsujikawa A, Musashi K et al (2006) Polypoidal choroidal vasculopathy with choroidal vascular hyperpermeability. Am J Ophthalmol 142:601–607

Sato T, Kishi S, Watanabe G, Matsumoto H, Mukai R (2007) Tomographic features of branching vascular networks in polypoidal choroidal vasculopathy. Retina 27:589–594

Schatz H, McDonald HR, Johnson RN et al (1995) Subretinal fibrosis in central serous chorioretinopathy. Ophthalmology 102:1077–1088

Sekiryu T, Iida T, Maruko I et al (2010) Infrared fundus autofluorescence and central serous chorioretinopathy. Invest Ophthalmol Vis Sci 51:4956–4962

Shinojima A, Hirose T, Mori R et al (2010) Morphologic findings in acute central serous chorioretinopathy using spectral domain-optical coherence tomography with simultaneous angiography. Retina 30:193–202

Song IS, Shin YU, Lee BR (2012) Time-periodic characteristics in the morphology of idiopathic central serous chorioretinopathy evaluated by volume scan using spectral-domain optical coherence tomography. Am J Ophthalmol 154:366–375

Spaide RF, Koizumi H, Pozzoni MC (2008) Enhanced depth imaging spectral-domain optical coherence tomography. Am J Ophthalmol 146:496–500

Suzuki M, Gomi F, Hara C et al (2014) Characteristics of central serous chorioretinopathy complicated by focal choroidal excavation. Retina 4(6):1216–1222 [Epub ahead of print]

Vasconcelos-Santos DV, Sohn EH, Sadda S et al (2010) Retinal pigment epithelial changes in chronic Vogt-Koyanagi-Harada disease: fundus autofluorescence and spectral domain-optical coherence tomography findings. Retina 30:33–41

Von Graefe A (1866) Ueber central recidivierende retinitis. Graefes Arch Clin Exp Ophthalmol 12:211–215

Wang M, Sander B, la Cour M et al (2005) Clinical characteristics of subretinal deposits in central serous chorioretinopathy. Acta Ophthalmol Scand 83:691–696

Wojtkowski M, Srinivasan V, Fujimoto JG et al (2005) Three-dimensional retinal imaging with high speed ultrahigh resolution optical coherence tomography. Ophthalmology 112:1734–1746

Yalcinbayir O, Gelisken O, Akova-Budak B et al (2014) Correlation of spectral domain optical coherence tomography findings and visual acuity in central serous chorioretinopathy. Retina 34:705–712

Yang L, Jonas JB, Wei W et al (2013) Optical coherence tomography assisted enhanced depth imaging of central serous chorioretinopathy. Invest Ophthalmol Vis Sci 54:4659–4665

Yannuzzi LA, Shakin JL, Fisher YL et al (1984) Peripheral retinal detachments and retinal pigment epithelial atrophic tracts secondary to central serous pigment epitheliopathy. Ophthalmology 91:1554–1572

Yannuzzi LA, Slakter JS, Gross NE et al (2012) Indocyanine green angiography-guided photodynamic therapy for treatment of chronic central serous chorioretinopathy: a pilot study. Retina 32(Suppl 1): 288–298

Part III
Surgical Retina

19 Vitreomacular Traction and Epiretinal Membranes

Michael D. Tibbetts and Jay S. Duker

Contents

M.D. Tibbetts • J.S. Duker (✉)
New England Eye Center, Tufts Medical Center and Tufts Unviersity School of Medicine, Boston, MA, USA
e-mail: jduker@tuftsmedicalcenter.org

19.1 Introduction

Optical coherence tomography (OCT) has transformed the understanding of the anatomy of the vitreomacular interface (VMI) and pathologic processes that occur there. Since the first description of macular diseases with OCT in 1995, progressive advances in technology have made OCT the gold standard for the diagnosis and management of VMI diseases (Puliafito et al. 1995; Stalmans et al. 2013). Clinical biomicroscopic examination and other imaging modalities are limited in their capabilities to fully diagnose and document diseases of the VMI as vitreous membranes are often clinically invisible. Spectral domain OCT (SD-OCT) provides high-resolution images of the VMI with noninvasive capture and fast acquisition. SD-OCT enables the clinician to more accurately diagnose diseases of the VMI, informs treatment, and guides postoperative care (Folgar et al. 2012). The approval of ocriplasmin (Jetrea, ThromboGenics, Iselin, New Jersey) for pharmacologic vitreolysis of "symptomatic vitreomacular adhesion" has further stimulated interest in understanding the pathophysiology of the VMI (FDA 2012). These developments led to the formation of the International Vitreomacular Traction Study (IVTS) Group to create a strictly anatomic OCT-based classification system for the VMI and more specifically the vitreomacular interface (VMI) (Duker et al. 2013). The panel of vitreoretinal disease experts provided anatomic

C.H. Meyer et al. (eds.), *Spectral Domain Optical Coherence Tomography in Macular Diseases*,
DOI 10.1007/978-81-322-3610-8_19

definitions and classification of vitreomacular adhesion (VMA), vitreomacular traction (VMT), and full-thickness macular hole (FTMH). This classification system and the science upon which it is based inform the current diagnosis and management of diseases of the VMI.

19.2 Posterior Vitreous Detachment

The vitreous gel is attached to the internal limiting membrane (ILM) of the retina and all other contiguous structures of the inner eye (Bishop 2000; Sebag and Balazs 1989). The posterior vitreous cortex and ILM are attached by a glue-like matrix of macromolecules including fibronectin and laminin. Posterior vitreous detachment (PVD) is the result of gel liquefaction and weakening of the vitreoretinal adhesion. OCT reveals that PVD usually begins in the perifoveal macula (Johnson 2010; Uchino et al. 2001). The normal vitreous contains a posterior precortical vitreous pocket that was first described by anatomical studies but can be visualized on swept source OCT as a boat-shaped lacunae over the macula with the thinnest posterior vitreous cortex at the fovea (Itakura et al. 2013; Worst 1977). The concurrent liquefaction of the gel and progressive posterior vitreous cortex separation lead to nonpathologic PVD in half of the eyes by age 50 years and in almost all subjects age 80 years and older (Sebag 1987). In most eyes, concurrent vitreoretinal separation occurs at multiple sites and proceeds for decades before coalescing into a final separation from the macula and optic nerve. The vitreopapillary separation is signaled by the appearance of the Weiss ring, often with acute symptoms to signal the completion of a yearlong process. Symptoms of the completion of a PVD include light flashes caused by vitreous traction and floaters which may be due to blood, condensations of vitreous collagen, or glial tissue torn from the optic nerve (Steel and Lotery 2013). However, a subset of patients will have pathologic consequences of PVD known as an anomalous PVD (Sebag 2004). This most commonly occurs at sites of strong vitreous adherence including the vitreous base, optic disk, and macula. The pathologic consequences include retinal tears from traction at the vitreous base, vitreopapillary adhesion from traction on the optic nerve, and focal VMT of the macula (Stalmans et al. 2013).

In the IVTS classification, an anomalous PVD is defined as "a partial vitreous detachment with persistent attachment in the macular region featuring an anomalous strength of adhesion to one or more structures in the posterior pole, resulting in transactional deformation of retinal tissue" (Duker et al. 2013). The consensus panel utilized OCT-derived findings to define the pathologic progression of anomalous PVD at the VMI including vitreomacular traction (VMT) and full-thickness macular holes (FTMH). SD-OCT is clinically useful to determine if a PVD is complete, which may inform the management of VMI diseases.

19.3 Vitreomacular Adhesion

Vitreoretinal adhesion is a normal state as most eyes have complete adhesion between the vitreous and retina at birth. For the purposes of the IVTS-OCT classification, VMA is defined as "a specific stage of vitreous separation wherein partial detachment of the vitreous in the perifoveal area has occurred without retinal abnormalities" (Duker et al. 2013) (Fig. 19.1). In prior classification systems, VMA is the equivalent of a stage 1 PVD (Gaudric et al. 1999; Johnson 2010; Uchino et al. 2001). On OCT, VMA can be visualized as elevation of the cortical vitreous above the retinal surface. The remaining vitreous remains attached within a 3-mm radius of the fovea with an acute angle between the vitreous and inner retinal surface. The retina does not demonstrate any change in contour or morphologic features because of vitreous adhesion, and therefore, there is no expected visual impairment or symptoms. The eyes with VMA may be subclassified by the size of the adhesion as FOCAL $\leq$ 1500 μm or BROAD > 1500 μm. The 1500-μm cutoff is a known area of increased vitreous adhesion in the fovea and has been used in prior classification systems and reading center protocols (DeCroos et al. 2012; Koizumi et al. 2008). However, it is unclear whether the distinction between focal and broad VMA has prognostic

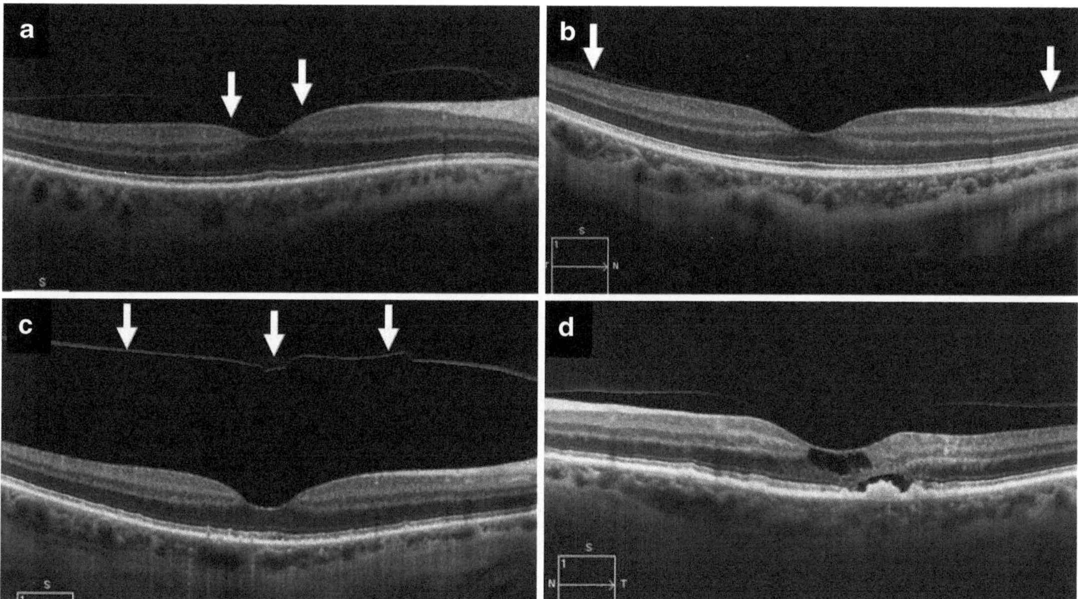

Fig. 19.1 Nonpathologic posterior vitreous detachment and vitreomacular adhesion. (**a**) Focal VMA (*arrows*) with normal foveal contour. (**b**) Broad VMA (*arrows*) with normal foveal contour. (**c**) Nonpathologic complete PVD. (**d**) Focal VMA with concurrent cystoid macular edema (CME), subretinal fluid, and drusen in a patient with CME post-cataract extraction and a history of age-related macular degeneration (Unless stated otherwise all SD-OCT images acquired with by Cirrus SD-OCT, Carl Zeiss Meditec, Inc., Dublin, CA)

significance for the development of VMT or FTMH. In most patients with VMA, the vitreous will separate spontaneously without pathological sequelae. VMA can also be classified as CONCURRENT if the OCT findings are associated with other macular abnormalities such as age-related macular degeneration or diabetic macular edema, and ISOLATED if no ocular disease is present (Duker et al. 2013). SD-OCT provides high-resolution images to judge whether VMA is isolated or concurrent (Fig. 19.1). For example, in the eyes with diabetic macular edema (DME), the angle of insertion of the vitreous adhesion may indicate whether the vitreous is causing traction and resultant distortion in the retinal architecture or is simply concurrent with the DME.

19.4 Vitreomacular Traction

Traction on the macula from the progression of a PVD can result in anatomic changes in the retina. These changes can include distortion in the contour of the foveal surface, intraretinal pseudocyst formation, elevation of the fovea from the RPE, or some combination that may result in reduced vision (Duker et al. 2013; Johnson 2010).

The IVTS defined vitreomacular traction (VMT) as the concurrence of detectable retinal anatomic changes on OCT with perifoveolar PVD (Duker et al. 2013) (Fig. 19.2). The criteria to define VMT include:

1. Evidence of perifoveal vitreous cortex detachment from the retinal surface
2. Macular attachment of the vitreous cortex within a 3-mm radius of the fovea
3. Association of attachment with distortion of the foveal surface, intraretinal structural changes, elevation of the fovea above the RPE, or a combination thereof, but no full-thickness interruption of all retinal layers

VMT can also be subclassified as FOCAL (≤1500 μm) or BROAD (>1500 μm) and ISOLATED or CONCURRENT similar to VMA (Koizumi et al. 2008). The surface area of VMT affects the anatomical distortion of the retina and the patient's symptomatology (Fig. 19.2) (Spaide et al. 2002; Yamada and Kishi 2005). For exam-

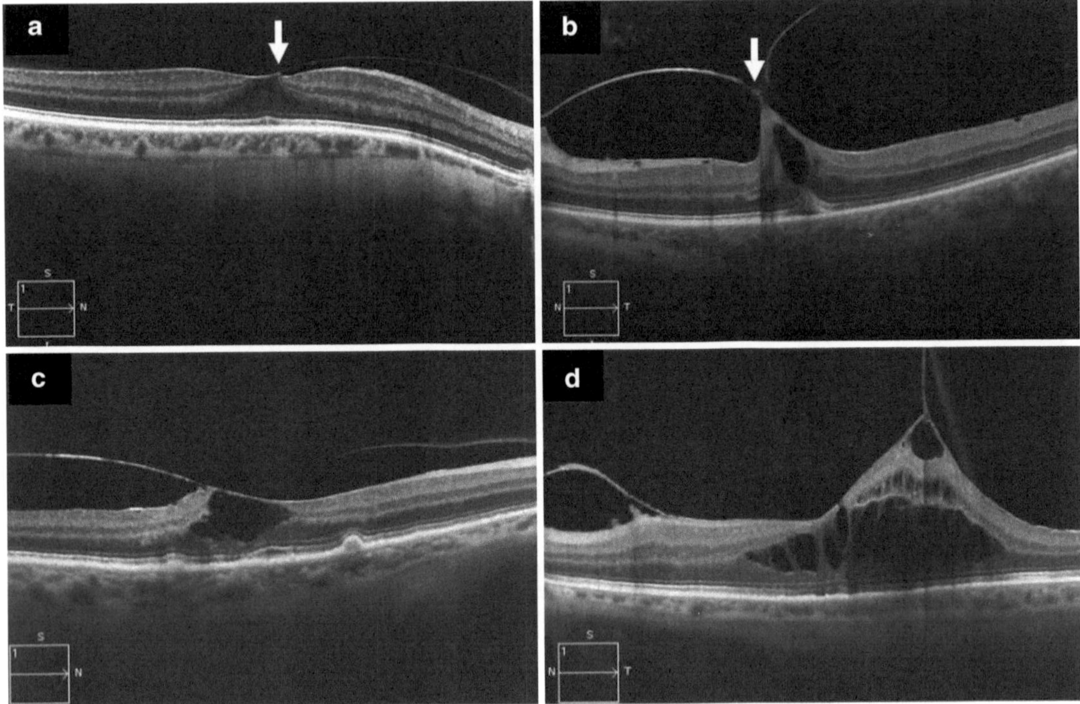

Fig. 19.2 Range of pathology of vitreomacular traction. (**a**) Focal VMT (*arrow*) with minimal distortion of the foveal architecture in asymptomatic eye with visual acuity of 20/20. (**b**) Steep angle of VMT (*arrow*) with distortion of the foveal architecture and an intraretinal cyst in a symptomatic eye with visual acuity of 20/70. (**c**) Concurrent VMT with temporally directed tractional forces in an eye with cystoid macular edema following cataract extraction and a history of dry age-related macular degeneration with visual acuity of 20/40. (**d**) Broad area of VMT with significant distortion of the retinal architecture with cystic intraretinal fluid and anteriorly directed tractional forces in a symptomatic eye with vision of 20/100 (Unless stated otherwise all SD-OCT images acquired with by Cirrus SD-OCT, Carl Zeiss Meditec, Inc., Dublin, CA)

ple, focal VMT tends to distort the foveal surface, elevate the foveal floor, and form pseudocysts within the central macula that can diminish visual acuity and cause visual distortion (Haouchine et al. 2001). In contrast, broad VMT can cause a wider area of macular thickening, macular schisis, cystoid macular edema, and vascular leakage on fluorescein angiography. The SD-OCT appearance of VMT informs the optimal choice of management and the patient's prognosis with treatment. OCT can also be used to sequentially follow VMT over time to detect resolution of the traction or, in some cases, progression to FTMH (Fig. 19.3). "Symptomatic VMA" is a clinical diagnosis with OCT showing VMT with or without concurrent macular hole and clinical complaints attributable to the retinal architectural changes (Stalmans et al. 2013). VMA and VMT may alter the pathophysiology of other retinal diseases including neovascular or wet age-related macular degeneration (wAMD) and diabetic macular edema (DME). In one meta-analysis, VMA was found to be 2.15 times more likely in the eyes with wAMD than controls and 2.54 times more likely than the eyes with dry AMD (Jackson et al. 2013). Some studies suggest that the presence of VMA impacts wAMD patients' functional outcomes with treatment, as well as the frequency of retreatment (Waldstein et al. 2014). In patients with PVD, a lower treatment frequency of intravitreal ranibizumab may be feasible, whereas patients with VMA or recent release of vitreomacular contact may benefit from more intensive retreatment (Mayr-Sponer et al. 2013). Other studies have found an association between DME and both VMA and VMT

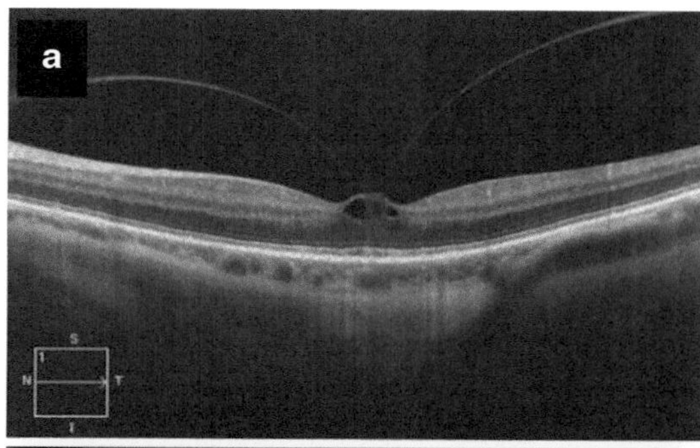

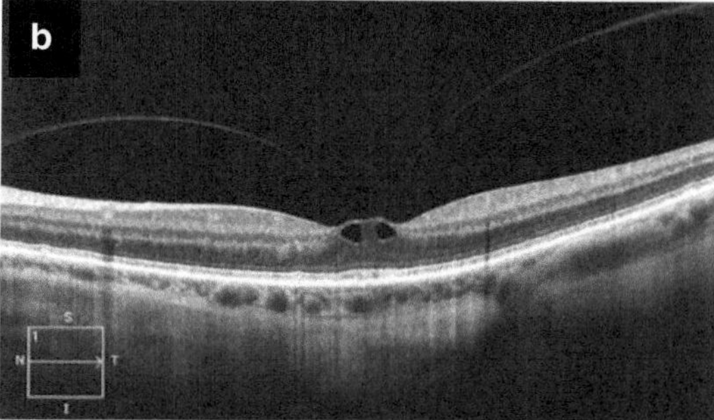

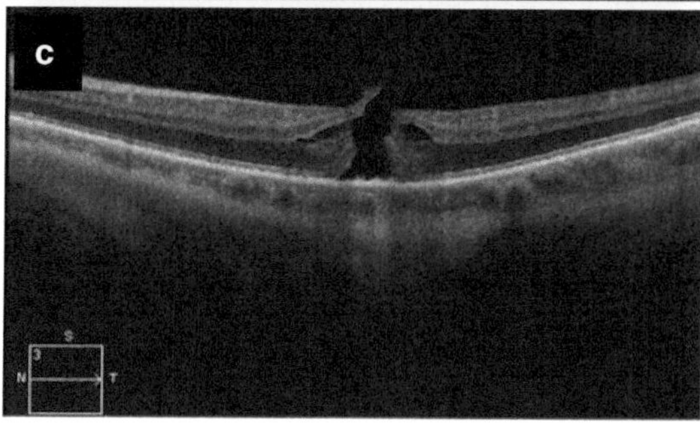

Fig. 19.3 Progression of vitreomacular traction to full-thickness macular hole. (**a**) Focal VMT on presentation with anteriorly directed vitreous traction causing intraretinal cyst formation in an asymptomatic eye with visual acuity of 20/25. (**b**) Focal VMT 6 months later with persistent anteriorly directed vitreous traction and intraretinal cysts in an eye with minimal symptoms and visual acuity of 20/40. (**c**) Focal VMT 12 months after presentation with small full-thickness macular hole in a symptomatic eye with visual acuity of 20/70 (Unless stated otherwise all SD-OCT images acquired with by Cirrus SD-OCT, Carl Zeiss Meditec, Inc., Dublin, CA)

(Jackson et al. 2013; Ophir et al. 2010). In one study, macular edema resolved spontaneously more frequently in the eyes with vitreomacular separation than in eyes with persistent vitreomacular adhesion (Hikichi et al. 1997). Asymptomatic VMA may increase the risk of diffuse DME by greater than three times as compared with diabetic patients with a complete PVD or complete vitreoretinal attachment (Lopes de Faria et al. 1999). Additional studies with SD-OCT are needed to determine the optimal treatment strategies for patients with concurrent VMA or VMT with other retinal diseases.

19.5 Epiretinal Membrane (ERM)

OCT has also led to a better understanding of the connection between PVD and the formation of epiretinal membranes. Anatomic autopsy studies have demonstrated that residual vitreous remains on the surface of the retina in nearly half of all eyes with PVD (Kishi et al. 1986). This finding called vitreoschisis can also be observed on OCT. The residual vitreous may proliferate to form an epiretinal membrane (ERM) during or after vitreous separation. This observation is supported by studies, which show a high incidence of apparent PVD in the eyes with macular pucker (Snead et al. 2008). The vitreous remnants form a scaffold for glial cells and laminocytes to attach and proliferate leading to contracture and stress on the underlying foveal architecture (Gandorfer et al. 2002).

OCT helps the physician judge whether the patient's symptoms match the alterations in the retinal anatomy caused by ERM (Wilkins et al. 1996). This understanding allows for the most appropriate intervention given the limitations of clinical biomicroscopy. In the phase III studies of enzymatic vitreolysis with ocriplasmin, SD-OCT was found to be significantly better at detecting ERMs as compared with TD-OCT (Folgar et al. 2012). Interestingly, a clear benefit of SD-OCT over TD-OCT was not observed in the analysis of VMA or FTMHs.

There is a wide range of pathology from ERMs that can be visualized by SD-OCT (Figs. 19.4 and 19.5). A thin ERM may cause minimal alteration of the underlying retinal architecture with only a slight change in the foveal contour. However, ERMs can also result in a complete loss of the foveal contour with cystoid intraretinal fluid and marked thickening of the retina. More subtle findings on SD-OCT can

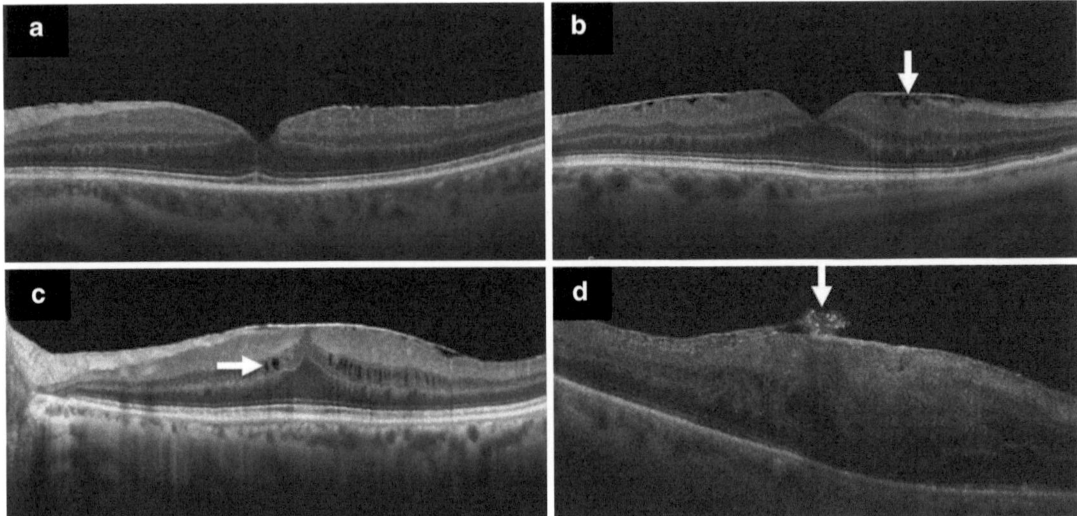

Fig. 19.4 Range of pathology of epiretinal membrane. (**a**) Trace ERM with slight distortion of the foveal architecture in a minimally symptomatic eye with vision of 20/40. (**b**) ERM with nonreflective pockets between the ERM and the internal limiting membrane (*arrows*) in the parafoveal macula in a minimally symptomatic eye with vision of 20/25. (**c**) ERM with loss of foveal contour and intraretinal cysts (*arrow*) in a symptomatic eye with vision of 20/100. (**d**) ERM in a patient with a history of macula involving retinal detachment repair with counting fingers vision. *Arrow* indicates elevation of ERM that could be used to initiate surgical membrane peel (Unless stated otherwise all SD-OCT images acquired with by Cirrus SD-OCT, Carl Zeiss Meditec, Inc., Dublin, CA)

include hypo-reflective cystic spaces visualized between the ERM and the internal limiting membranes (ILM).

The thickness of the ERM and degree of macular distortion and pseudocyst formation can help prognosticate the benefit of vitrectomy with membrane peel or prompt investigation of other causes for the patient's symptoms. This is a frequently encountered situation in patients with concurrent epiretinal membranes and cataracts. The SD-OCT findings may be useful to inform whether the visual symptoms are primarily due to the cataract, the epiretinal membrane, or both and inform the management accordingly. The appearance of the bands corresponding to the photoreceptors in the outer retina (variably defined as the inner segment/outer segment (IS/OS) junction or the ellipsoid layer) is particularly useful to prognosticate visual acuity in patients undergoing vitrectomy with membrane peel or in the eyes with spontaneous release of epiretinal membranes (Inoue et al. 2011; Suh et al. 2009; Yang et al. 2014). Other studies have correlated edema of the inner nuclear layer (INL) on SD-OCT in the eyes with epiretinal membranes and metamorphopsia (Watanabe et al. 2009). These findings may be useful to the retina surgeon in determining who may benefit from removal of epiretinal membranes and in the preoperative counseling of patients.

19.6 Macular Pseudohole

Macular pseudohole is a clinical diagnosis made at the slit lamp with a contact or a noncontact lens. It is a clinical descriptive term for a finding that appears to be a full-thickness retinal defect, but subsequent OCT proves that the outer retina is intact. Clinically, what is most often seen is a discrete, reddish, round, or oval lesion in the fovea simulating the appearance of a full-thickness macular hole (Haouchine et al. 2004). OCT with multiple foveal line scans is critical to differentiate between a true full-thickness macular hole and a pseudohole. On OCT, the pseudohole has no loss of foveal tissue and central foveal thickness is normal or slightly thin (Haouchine et al. 2004). The IVTS further defined a macular

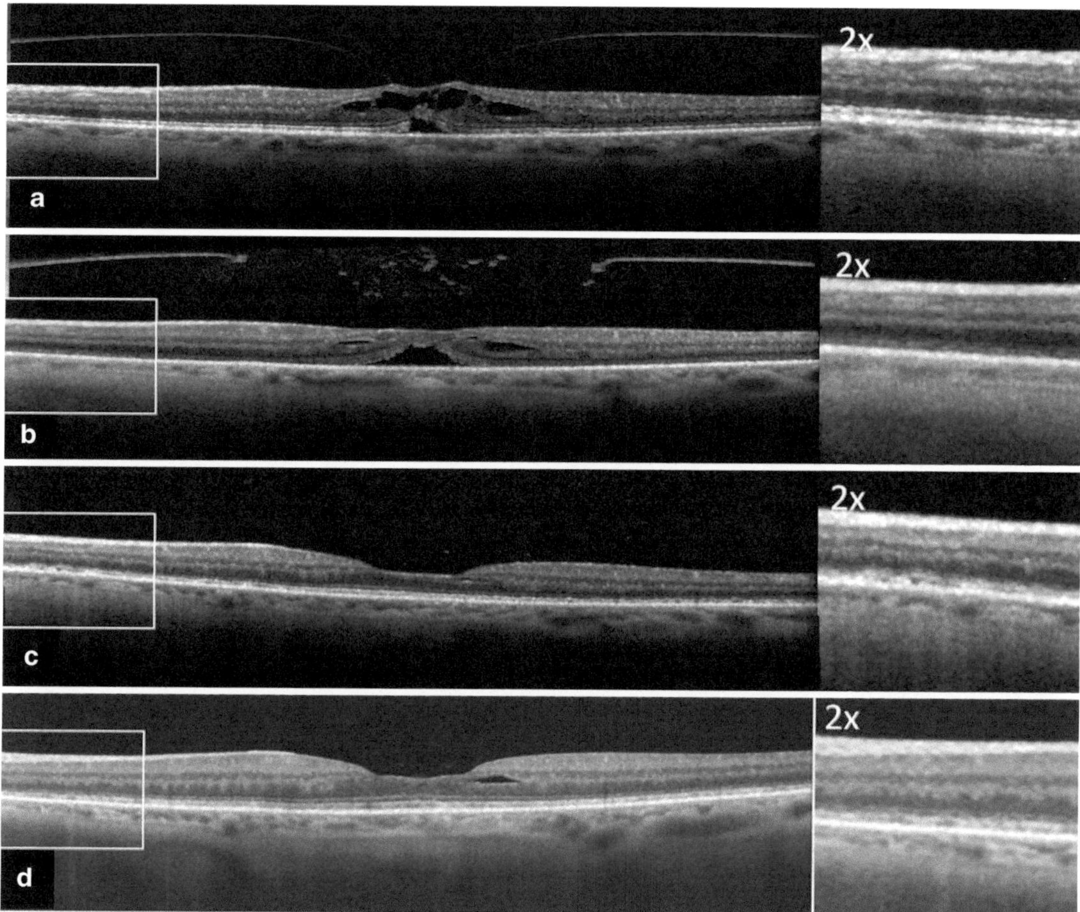

Fig. 19.5 Vision improvement after ocriplasmin injection for vitreomacular traction. (**a**) On presentation, there is vitreomacular traction (VMT) with distortion of the foveal contour with cystic changes in the inner and outer retina in an eye with visual acuity of 20/60. A 2× magnified area of the nasal macula shows an intact ellipsoid layer. (**b**) The day following treatment, the VMT has released and there is a decrease in the cystic changes in the inner retina. The vision decreased to 20/200. A 2× magnified area in the nasal macula shows a near disappearance of the ellipsoid layer. (**c**) Two months after treatment, there is resolution of the VMT and cystic changes in the retina with an improvement in the continuity of the IS/OS junction. Vision improved to 20/50 at this exam. A 2× magnified area of the nasal macula shows improvement in the IS/OS (ellipsoid) layer; however, it remains irregular (*arrow*). (**d**) Four months after treatment, there is persistent discontinuity of the IS/OS junction (ellipsoid) line. Vision improved to 20/40 at this visit. A 2× magnified area of the nasal macula shows this more clearly (*arrow*) (Adapted with permission from Tibbetts et al. 2014 (Images **a**–**c** acquired by Heidelberg Spectralis SD-OCT, Heidelberg Engineering, Heidelberg, Germany and image D acquired by Cirrus SD-OCT, Carl Zeiss Meditec, Inc., Dublin, CA). (Unless stated otherwise all SD-OCT images acquired with by Cirrus SD-OCT, Carl Zeiss Meditec, Inc., Dublin, CA))

pseudohole based on four OCT characteristics (Duker et al. 2013):

1. Invaginated or heaped foveal edges
2. Concomitant ERM with central opening
3. Steep macular contour to the central fovea with near-normal central foveal thickness
4. No loss of retinal tissue

Based on the observations from biomicroscopic examination and OCT, an ERM is thought to be causative with contraction pulling the underlying retinal tissue toward the center of the fovea. This process results in invagination of the perifoveal retina into a shape that resembles a hole with no loss of tissue. Most patients with pseudohole are minimally symptomatic and can be observed. If the associated ERM causes a decrease in vision, the ERM can be removed by surgical membrane peel.

19.7 OCT-Guided Surgical Management of Vitreomacular Interface Disease

OCT is now considered the gold standard for the preoperative and postoperative management of the diseases of the VMI (Goldberg et al. 2014). OCT is necessary for an accurate diagnosis and guides preoperative decision-making and surgical planning. In one study, six vitreoretinal specialists examined patients with slit lamp biomicroscopy to diagnose ERM or VMT and determine whether surgery was indicated (Do et al. 2006). The clinical findings were then compared to the results of time domain (TD) OCT. The TD-OCT was more sensitive than the clinical exam, particularly for VMT. The higher resolution of SD-OCT further enhances the clinician's ability to make an accurate diagnosis and manage the patient accordingly. SD-OCT is helpful to guide the management of VMT. The size of the vitreous adhesion can inform the patient's prognosis with vitrectomy to relieve macular traction. In one study, the eyes with focal VMT had a significantly greater improvement in vision with vitrectomy compared with the eyes with broad VMT (Sonmez et al. 2008). The anatomical distortion of the retina can also inform the patient's prognosis. In another study of patients undergoing vitrectomy for VMT, a lamellar separation between the inner and outer fovea was not associated with a significant improvement in vision, whereas cystoid macular edema and perifoveal traction were associated with improved vision (Witkin et al. 2010).

SD-OCT is also helpful to determine the thickness and extent of an ERM to inform surgical planning and predict the difficulty of ERM removal (Kim et al. 2012). Surgical difficulty of ERM removal is strongly associated with more extensive adherence as observed on SD-OCT (Kim et al. 2012). SD-OCT findings may also inform the surgeon's decision to peel the ILM (Chang et al. 2013; Seidel et al. 2013). In one study, the greater extent of ERM elevation above the retina and thickness was predictive of ILM persistence after ERM peel (Seidel et al. 2013). Only peeling the ERM (and not ILM) results in a greater proportion of the eyes with residual ERM, yet one study revealed no differences in postoperative visual acuity between single and double peeling (Chang et al. 2013). SD-OCT can also guide the surgeon as to where to initiate the membrane peel based on the elevation above the retina, thickness, and the presence of an identifiable edge (Hirano et al. 2010; Kim et al. 2012). These insights may make the surgery easier and potentially reduce operating times. Retinal surface EN FACE OCT holds promise to further guide surgical planning of ERM by determining morphological changes on the retinal surface and areas devoid of ILM secondary to ERM contraction (Rispoli et al. 2012).

SD-OCT is also helpful to inform the patient's prognosis with ERM peeling. Multiple studies of the eyes with ERM have demonstrated that the preoperative integrity of the IS/OS junction band on OCT helps prognosticate postoperative visual acuity (Falkner-Radler et al. 2010; Inoue et al. 2011; Suh et al. 2009). In the eyes with a disrupted IS/OS prior to surgery, none had a normal appearing IS/OS junction on SD-OCT after indocyanine green (ICG)-assisted internal limited membrane (ILM) peeling when followed up to 1 year postoperatively (Inoue et al. 2011). There was no correlation between preoperative central foveal thickness, presence of a macular pseudohole, and presence of retinal cysts with the postoperative visual acuity (Inoue et al. 2011).

Postoperative SD-OCT can also provide insights on the outcome of surgery. In particular, SD-OCT may be helpful in evaluating poor visual outcomes that may be attributable to subretinal or intraretinal fluid, disruptions to the RPE or photoreceptors, or recurrence of the ERM. These findings may guide treatment of postoperative cystoid macular edema or help determine if repeat surgery is indicated.

19.8 OCT-Guided Management of Vitreoretinal Interface Disease with Pharmacologic Vitreolysis

The approval of ocriplasmin (Jetrea, ThromboGenics, Iselin, New Jersey) for “symptomatic vitreomacular adhesion” in October 2012 opened a new era in the management of vitreoretinal interface disease (FDA 2012). Ocriplasmin is a recombinant protease with activity against components of the vitreoretinal interface including fibronectin and laminin. In phase III, MIVI-TRUST studies, 652 eyes were randomized with 464 receiving 125 μg of ocriplasmin by intravitreal injection and 188 receiving a placebo injection of saline (Stalmans et al. 2012). VMA resolved in 26.5 % of ocriplasmin-injected eyes compared to 10.1 % of placebo-injected eyes at 28 days after injection. This primary endpoint was determined by TD-OCT. Therefore, ocriplasmin is the first drug to be approved by the FDA based on an OCT analysis rather than a visual acuity or other functional outcome. Additional findings from the original trials included higher rate of closure of macular holes (40.6 % of ocriplasmin-injected eyes versus 10.6 % of placebo-injected eyes) and a higher percentage of patients with three lines of visual acuity gains (12.3 % of eyes injected with ocriplasmin versus 6.4 % of eyes injected with placebo). SD-OCT is critical to determine the ideal candidates for pharmacologic vitreolysis. In phase III trials, a higher rate of VMA resolution was found in patients without epiretinal membranes (37.4 % in the ocriplasmin group as compared with 14.3 % in the placebo group). Of patients with epiretinal membrane, VMA resolution occurred in just 8.7 % with ocriplasmin compared with 1.5 % with placebo. These data suggest that the proteolytic action of ocriplasmin is not as effective in the presence of ERMs. The careful examination of the OCT to determine if an ERM is present can inform the clinician's choice of optimal therapy.

The clinical trials also demonstrated that phakic eyes had a higher rate of VMA resolution as compared to pseudophakic patients after treatment with ocriplasmin (34.2 % of phakic eyes compared to 13.4 % of pseudophakic eyes). This finding supports previous observations that cataract surgery with or without subsequent posterior capsulotomy often induces PVD (Mirshahi et al. 2009; Sheard et al. 2003). The pseudophakic eyes with persistent VMA were likely to have a tighter vitreoretinal adhesion and therefore less likely to respond to enzymatic vitreolysis.

The predictor criteria for a higher rate of success based on the MIVI-TRUST and subsequent studies can be summarized as follows (Singh et al. 2014; Stalmans et al. 2012):

- No ERM at baseline
- VMA diameter <1500 μm
- Phakic lens status
- Age younger than 65

SD-OCT has also been helpful to explain patient's symptoms post-ocriplasmin. In phase III trials, 68.4 % of patients in the ocriplasmin group and 53.5 % of patients in the placebo group had ocular adverse events (Stalmans et al. 2012). These events primarily included vitreous floaters and photopsia, but 5.4 % of patients reported visual impairment compared to 1.6 % with placebo. In addition, the Jetrea package insert notes that 2 % of patients reported yellowing of their vision (dyschromatopsia) with half of these patients also having a decrease of a- and b-wave amplitudes on ERG (Jetrea 2012). Since clinical use of ocriplasmin began in 2013, multiple reports have documented patient's complaints of dyschromatopsia and nyctalopia (Fahim et al. 2014; Freund et al. 2013; Tibbetts et al. 2014). These symptoms have been correlated with the loss of the photoreceptor bands (IS/OS or ellipsoid layer) throughout the retina on SD-OCT. Given that the phase III MIVI-TRUST studies were performed with lower-resolution TD-OCT, it is likely that these findings were not observed. The case reports have also demonstrated suppression of electroretinography (ERG) amplitudes with rod greater than cone dysfunction up to 4 months after treatment, as well as pupillary abnormalities and visual field constriction (Fahim et al. 2014; Tibbetts et al. 2014).

Given that ocriplasmin is a protease, a proposed mechanism for these panretinal changes is enzymatic cleavage of intraretinal laminin (Fahim et al. 2014). Laminin is present in the interphotoreceptor matrix, and therefore cleavage of laminin may explain the disruption in the IS/OS band visualized on SD-OCT (Libby et al. 2000). This theory is supported by animal studies, which demonstrate an effect of ocriplasmin on fibronectin and laminin in the outer retina (Chen et al. 2009). Interestingly, the loss of the IS/OS has been correlated with a higher rate of VMA release. In one small study, 75 % of responders (6 of 8 patients) demonstrated loss of the IS/OS band on SD-OCT as compared to only 11 % of nonresponders (1 of 9 patients) (Singh et al. 2014). The IS/OS changes were transient with an average resolution by 29 days, but the long-term effect on retinal function is unknown. In planned phase IV post-marketing studies, SD-OCT should provide further insights into the effects of ocriplasmin on the retina.

Conclusion

SD-OCT has revolutionized the understanding of vitreoretinal interface anatomy and disease. The IVTS has provided a framework to accurately identify, describe, and distinguish normal anatomical progression of a PVD and VMA from diseases of the VMI including VMT, ERM, and FTMH. SD-OCT is now essential to the preoperative evaluation of these diseases both to confirm the diagnosis and direct the most appropriate management. The insights from SD-OCT guide the choice of observation, pharmacologic vitreolysis, or vitrectomy with membrane peel to achieve the best outcomes for patients. Future advances in OCT technology including swept source OCT, en face imaging, and intraoperative OCT will further enhance the understanding of the VMI in the years ahead.

References

Bishop PN (2000) Structural macromolecules and supramolecular organisation of the vitreous gel. Prog Retin Eye Res 19:323–344

Chang S, Gregory-Roberts EM, Park S, Laud K, Smith SD, Hoang QV (2013) Double peeling during vitrectomy for macular pucker: the Charles L. Schepens Lecture. JAMA ophthalmol 131:525–530. doi:10.1001/jamaophthalmol.2013.2176

Chen W, Mo W, Sun K, Huang X, Zhang YL, Song HY (2009) Microplasmin degrades fibronectin and laminin at vitreoretinal interface and outer retina during enzymatic vitrectomy. Curr Eye Res 34:1057–1064. doi:10.3109/02713680903308487

de Faria JM L, Jalkh AE, Trempe CL, McMeel JW (1999) Diabetic macular edema: risk factors and concomitants. ActaophthalmologicaScandinavica 77:170–175

DeCroos FC, Toth CA, Folgar FA, Pakola S, Stinnett SS, Heydary CS, Burns R, Jaffe GJ (2012) Characterization of vitreoretinal interface disorders using OCT in the interventional phase 3 trials of ocriplasmin. Invest Ophthalmol Vis Sci 53:6504–6511. doi:10.1167/iovs.12-10370

Do DV, Cho M, Nguyen QD, Shah SM, Handa JT, Campochiaro PA, Zimmer-Galler I, Sung JU, Haller JA (2006) The impact of optical coherence tomography on surgical decision making in epiretinal membrane and vitreomacular traction. Trans Am Ophthalmol Soc 104:161–166

Duker JS, Kaiser PK, Binder S, de Smet MD, Gaudric A, Reichel E, Sadda SR, Sebag J, Spaide RF, Stalmans P (2013) The International Vitreomacular Traction Study Group classification of vitreomacular adhesion, traction, and macular hole. Ophthalmology 120:2611–2619. doi:10.1016/j.ophtha.2013.07.042

Fahim AT, Khan NW, Johnson MW (2014) Acute panretinal structural and functional abnormalities after intravitreous ocriplasmin injection. JAMA ophthalmol 132:484–486. doi:10.1001/jamaophthalmol.2013.8142

Falkner-Radler CI, Glittenberg C, Hagen S, Benesch T, Binder S (2010) Spectral-domain optical coherence tomography for monitoring epiretinal membrane surgery. Ophthalmology 117:798–805. doi:10.1016/j.ophtha.2009.08.034

FDA U (2012) FDA approves Jetrea for symptomatic vitreomacular adhesion in the eyes [press release]. Updated 18 Oct 2012. http://www.fda.gov/NewsEvents/Newsroom/PressAnnouncements/ucm324369.htm. Accessed 1 June 2014

Folgar FA, Toth CA, DeCroos FC, Girach A, Pakola S, Jaffe GJ (2012) Assessment of retinal morphology with spectral and time domain OCT in the phase III trials of enzymatic vitreolysis. Invest Ophthalmol Vis Sci 53:7395–7401. doi:10.1167/iovs.12-10379

Freund KB, Shah SA, Shah VP (2013) Correlation of transient vision loss with outer retinal disruption following intravitreal ocriplasmin. Eye 27:773–774. doi:10.1038/eye.2013.94

Gandorfer A, Rohleder M, Kampik A (2002) Epiretinal pathology of vitreomacular traction syndrome. Br J Ophthalmol 86:902–909

Gaudric A, Haouchine B, Massin P, Paques M, Blain P, Erginay A (1999) Macular hole formation: new data provided by optical coherence tomography. Arch Ophthalmol 117:744–751

Goldberg RA, Waheed NK, Duker JS (2014) Optical coherence tomography in the preoperative and postoperative management of macular hole and epiretinal membrane. Br J Ophthalmol 98:ii20–3. doi:10.1136/bjophthalmol-2013-304447

Haouchine B, Massin P, Gaudric A (2001) Foveal pseudocyst as the first step in macular hole formation: a prospective study by optical coherence tomography. Ophthalmology 108:15–22

Haouchine B, Massin P, Tadayoni R, Erginay A, Gaudric A (2004) Diagnosis of macular pseudoholes and lamellar macular holes by optical coherence tomography. Am J Ophthalmol 138:732–739. doi:10.1016/j.ajo.2004.06.088

Hikichi T, Fujio N, Akiba J, Azuma Y, Takahashi M, Yoshida A (1997) Association between the short-term natural history of diabetic macular edema and the vitreomacular relationship in type II diabetes mellitus. Ophthalmology 104:473–478

Hirano Y, Yasukawa T, Ogura Y (2010) Optical coherence tomography guided peeling of macular epiretinal membrane. Clin ophthalmol 5:27–29. doi:10.2147/OPTH.S16031

Inoue M, Morita S, Watanabe Y, Kaneko T, Yamane S, Kobayashi S, Arakawa A, Kadonosono K (2011) Preoperative inner segment/outer segment junction in spectral-domain optical coherence tomography as a prognostic factor in epiretinal membrane surgery. Retina 31:1366–1372. doi:10.1097/IAE.0b013e318203c156

Itakura H, Kishi S, Li D, Akiyama H (2013) Observation of posterior precortical vitreous pocket using swept-source optical coherence tomography. Invest Ophthalmol Vis Sci 54:3102–3107. doi:10.1167/iovs.13-11769

Jackson TL, Nicod E, Angelis A, Grimaccia F, Prevost AT, Simpson AR, Kanavos P (2013) Vitreous attachment in age-related macular degeneration, diabetic macular edema, and retinal vein occlusion: a systematic review and metaanalysis. Retina 33:1099–1108. doi:10.1097/IAE.0b013e31828991d6, Jetrea (2012) Iselin, NJ: ThromboGenics Inc

Johnson MW (2010) Posterior vitreous detachment: evolution and complications of its early stages. Am J Ophthalmol 149:371–382. doi:10.1016/j.ajo.2009.11.022

Kim JS, Chhablani J, Chan CK, Cheng L, Kozak I, Hartmann K, Freeman WR (2012) Retinal adherence and fibrillary surface changes correlate with surgical difficulty of epiretinal membrane removal. Am J Ophthalmol 153:692–697. doi:10.1016/j.ajo.2011.08.042

Kishi S, Demaria C, Shimizu K (1986) Vitreous cortex remnants at the fovea after spontaneous vitreous detachment. Int Ophthalmol 9:253–260

Koizumi H, Spaide RF, Fisher YL, Freund KB, Klancnik JM Jr, Yannuzzi LA (2008) Three-dimensional evaluation of vitreomacular traction and epiretinal membrane using spectral-domain optical coherence tomography. Am J Ophthalmol 145:509–517. doi:10.1016/j.ajo.2007.10.014

Libby RT, Champliaud MF, Claudepierre T, Xu Y, Gibbons EP, Koch M, Burgeson RE, Hunter DD, Brunken WJ (2000) Laminin expression in adult and developing retinae: evidence of two novel CNS laminins. J neurosci: the official journal of the Society for Neuroscience 20:6517–6528

Mayr-Sponer U, Waldstein SM, Kundi M, Ritter M, Golbaz I, Heiling U, Papp A, Simader C, Schmidt-Erfurth U (2013) Influence of the vitreomacular interface on outcomes of ranibizumab therapy in neovascular age-related macular degeneration. Ophthalmology 120:2620–2629. doi:10.1016/j.ophtha.2013.05.032

Mirshahi A, Hoehn F, Lorenz K, Hattenbach LO (2009) Incidence of posterior vitreous detachment after cataract surgery. J Cataract Refract Surg 35:987–991. doi:10.1016/j.jcrs.2009.02.016

Ophir A, Trevino A, Fatum S (2010) Extrafoveal vitreous traction associated with diabetic diffuse macular oedema. Eye 24:347–353. doi:10.1038/eye.2009.106

Puliafito CA, Hee MR, Lin CP, Reichel E, Schuman JS, Duker JS, Izatt JA, Swanson EA, Fujimoto JG (1995) Imaging of macular diseases with optical coherence tomography. Ophthalmology 102:217–229

Rispoli M, Le Rouic JF, Lesnoni G, Colecchio L, Catalano S, Lumbroso B (2012) Retinal surface en face optical coherence tomography: a new imaging approach in epiretinal membrane surgery. Retina 32:2070–2076. doi:10.1097/IAE.0b013e3182562076

Sebag J (1987) Age-related changes in human vitreous structure. Graefe's Arch Clin Exp Ophthalmol = Albrecht von GraefesArchiv fur klinische und experimentelleOphthalmologie 225:89–93

Sebag J (2004) Anomalous posterior vitreous detachment: a unifying concept in vitreo-retinal disease. Graefe's Arch Clin Exp Ophthalmol = Albrecht von GraefesArchiv fur klinische und experimentelleOphthalmologie 242:690–698. doi:10.1007/s00417-004-0980-1

Sebag J, Balazs EA (1989) Morphology and ultrastructure of human vitreous fibers. Invest Ophthalmol Vis Sci 30:1867–1871

Seidel G, Weger M, Stadlmuller L, Pichler T, Haas A (2013) Association of preoperative optical coherence tomography markers with residual inner limiting membrane in epiretinal membrane peeling. PLoS One 8:e66217. doi:10.1371/journal.pone.0066217

Sheard RM, Goodburn SF, Comer MB, Scott JD, Snead MP (2003) Posterior vitreous detachment after neodymium: YAG laser posterior capsulotomy. J Cataract Refract Surg 29:930–934

Singh RP, Li A, Bedi R, Srivastava S, Sears JE, Ehlers JP, Schachat AP, Kaiser PK (2014) Anatomical and visual outcomes following ocriplasmin treatment for symptomatic vitreomacular traction syndrome. Br J Ophthalmol 98:356–360. doi:10.1136/bjophthalmol-2013-304219

Snead DR, James S, Snead MP (2008) Pathological changes in the vitreoretinal junction 1: epiretinal membrane formation. Eye 22:1310–1317. doi:10.1038/eye.2008.36

Sonmez K, Capone A Jr, Trese MT, Williams GA (2008) Vitreomacular traction syndrome: impact of anatomical configuration on anatomical and visual outcomes. Retina 28:1207–1214. doi:10.1097/IAE.0b013e31817b6b0f

Spaide RF, Wong D, Fisher Y, Goldbaum M (2002) Correlation of vitreous attachment and foveal deformation in early macular hole states. Am J Ophthalmol 133:226–229

Stalmans P, Benz MS, Gandorfer A, Kampik A, Girach A, Pakola S, Haller JA, Group M-TS (2012) Enzymatic vitreolysis with ocriplasmin for vitreomacular traction and macular holes. N Engl J Med 367:606–615. doi:10.1056/NEJMoa1110823

Stalmans P, Duker JS, Kaiser PK, Heier JS, Dugel PU, Gandorfer A, Sebag J, Haller JA (2013) Oct-based interpretation of the vitreomacular interface and indications for pharmacologic vitreolysis. Retina 33:2003–2011. doi:10.1097/IAE.0b013e3182993ef8

Steel DH, Lotery AJ (2013) Idiopathic vitreomacular traction and macular hole: a comprehensive review of pathophysiology, diagnosis, and treatment. Eye 27(Suppl 1):S1–S21. doi:10.1038/eye.2013.212

Suh MH, Seo JM, Park KH, Yu HG (2009) Associations between macular findings by optical coherence tomography and visual outcomes after epiretinal membrane removal. Am J Ophthalmol 147:473–480. doi:10.1016/j.ajo.2008.09.020

Tibbetts MD, Reichel E, Witkin AJ (2014) Vision loss after intravitreal ocriplasmin: correlation of spectral-domain optical coherence tomography and electroretinography. JAMA ophthalmol 132:487–490. doi:10.1001/jamaophthalmol.2013.8258

Uchino E, Uemura A, Ohba N (2001) Initial stages of posterior vitreous detachment in healthy eyes of older persons evaluated by optical coherence tomography. Arch Ophthalmol 119:1475–1479

Waldstein SM, Ritter M, Simader C, Mayr-Sponer U, Kundi M, Schmidt-Erfurth U (2014) Impact of vitreomacular adhesion on ranibizumab mono- and combination therapy for neovascular age-related macular degeneration. Am J Ophthalmol 158:328–336.e1. doi:10.1016/j.ajo.2014.04.02

Watanabe A, Arimoto S, Nishi O (2009) Correlation between metamorphopsia and epiretinal membrane optical coherence tomography findings. Ophthalmology 116:1788–1793. doi:10.1016/j.ophtha.2009.04.046

Wilkins JR, Puliafito CA, Hee MR, Duker JS, Reichel E, Coker JG, Schuman JS, Swanson EA, Fujimoto JG (1996) Characterization of epiretinal membranes using optical coherence tomography. Ophthalmology 103:2142–2151

Witkin AJ, Patron ME, Castro LC, Reichel E, Rogers AH, Baumal CR, Duker JS (2010) Anatomic and visual outcomes of vitrectomy for vitreomacular traction syndrome. Ophthalmic Surg Lasers Imaging : the official journal of the International Society for Imaging in the Eye 41:425–431. doi:10.3928/15428877-20100525-07

Worst JG (1977) Cisternal systems of the fully developed vitreous body in the young adult. Trans Ophthalmol Soc U K 97:550–554

Yamada N, Kishi S (2005) Tomographic features and surgical outcomes of vitreomacular traction syndrome. Am J Ophthalmol 139:112–117. doi:10.1016/j.ajo.2004.08.055

Yang HS, Hong JW, Kim YJ, Kim JG, Joe SG (2014) Characteristics of spontaneous idiopathic epiretinal membrane separation in spectral domain optical coherence tomography. Retina 34:20179–20187. doi:10.1097/IAE.0000000000000199

Macular Hole

20

Alain Gaudric and Aude Couturier

Contents

A. Gaudric, MD (✉) • A. Couturier, MD
Department of Ophthalmology, Université Paris 7-Diderot. Sorbonne Paris Cité, and Hôpital Lariboisière, AP-HP, Paris, France
e-mail: agaudric@gmail.com

20.1 Introduction

Macular hole (MH) is a round full-thickness opening in the foveal center. Idiopathic MH, i.e., due to abnormal vitreofoveal traction, is the most common presentation. The role of the vitreous cortex in the pathogenesis of MH has begun to be better understood with the biomicroscopic observations of JDM Gass (Gass 1988). The advent of optical coherence tomography (OCT), which showed the partially detached posterior hyaloid (PH), has clarified the understanding of MH formation. Spectral domain OCT (SD-OCT) has subsequently provided more detailed views of the initial foveal changes induced by the vitreofoveal traction. MH classification has been recently simplified and combines the hole diameter and the presence or absence of a residual vitreous traction on its edge (Duker et al. 2013). The terminology used in this chapter to describe OCT images complies with the lexicon proposed by the international OCT consensus (Staurenghi et al. 2014).

20.2 Impending Macular Hole and Vitreomacular Traction in the Fellow Eye

When the vitreous is completely attached to the retina at the posterior pole, the posterior vitreous cortex is barely visible, but the presence of a

C.H. Meyer et al. (eds.), *Spectral Domain Optical Coherence Tomography in Macular Diseases*,
DOI 10.1007/978-81-322-3610-8_20

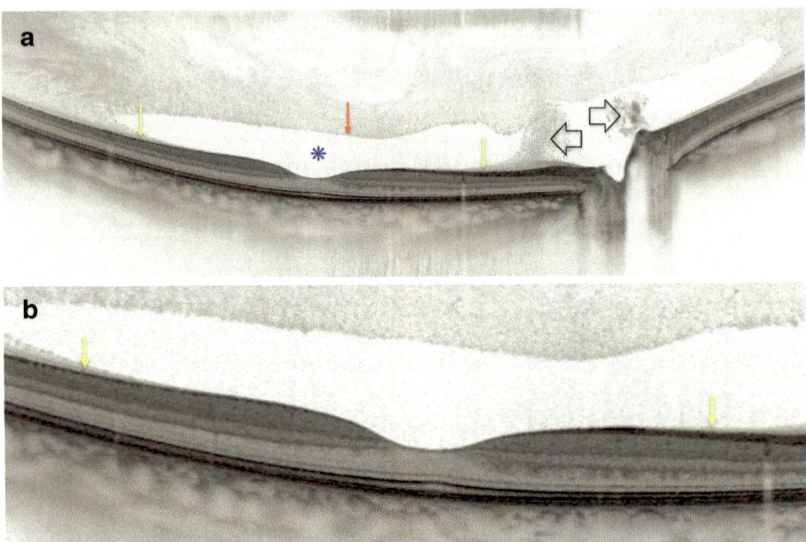

Fig. 20.1 Normal posterior vitreous in the normal eye of a 30-year old woman. Horizontal 12-mm B-scan. (**a**) The vitreous cortex is completely attached to the retinal surface of the posterior pole but is only visible on the margin of the macula (*yellow arrows*). The bursa premacularis (*asterisk*) is an optically empty space over the macula. Its anterior wall is well visible (*red arrow*). The wall of Cloquet's canal (*large arrows*) is in connection with the vitreous cortex. (**b**) Detail showing the progressive thinning of the vitreous cortex on the edge of the fovea

premacular vitreous pocket indicates that the posterior vitreous cortex is still attached to the macula (Pang et al. 2014; Schaal et al. 2014) (Fig. 20.1).

The initial stage of impending MH is usually visible when it occurs in a patient with an MH in the other eye. The symptoms are mild or absent, and the impending MH can only be detected by OCT of the fellow eye. When early signs of vitreomacular traction (VMT) are diagnosed in an eye without anomaly, there are no specific signs in the other eye indicating that the evolution will turn to an MH rather than to a more advanced VMT without hole. The vitreous cortex normally starts to detach from the surface of the macula in the fifth decade of life, and this process progressively progresses with age (Johnson 2010, 2012; Ma et al. 2014; Uchino et al. 2001) (Fig. 20.2).

Impending MHs have been described by Gass (1995) and classified into two stages (1A and B) based on biomicroscopy findings. The role of the perifoveal vitreous separation as well as the formation of intrafoveal cysts have subsequently been identified by time domain OCT (TD-OCT) (Gaudric et al. 1999; Haouchine et al. 2001).

SD-OCT has shown various degrees of foveal surface alterations more or less combined with microstructural intrafoveal changes, which constitute the spectrum of impending MHs, and the Gass classification is no longer useful. The earliest signs of vitreofoveal traction observed in a fellow eye of MH are minute changes in the curvature of the foveal pit. These anomalies could be only a part of the normal process of age-related vitreomacular detachment but have a special significance in the context of an MH in the other eye (Ma et al. 2014) (Fig. 20.3).

More frequently, surface anomalies are associated with various degrees of foveal microstructural changes. They may be a simple discrete elevation of the ellipsoid zone (EZ), a change in the reflectivity of the foveal center, an inner foveal cyst, a central split in the fovea, an outer foveal cavitation, or a combination thereof (Takahashi et al. 2011a, b). Moreover, these anomalies may evolve overtime (Fig. 20.4). It is also of note that some anomalies are very small and may be present on only one B-scan even when tight rasters are used (Fig. 20.5).

When the foveal floor is elevated due to the traction exerted by the posterior hyaloid on its center, a foveal cyst may occur (Gaudric et al. 1999; Haouchine et al. 2001). The retinal outer

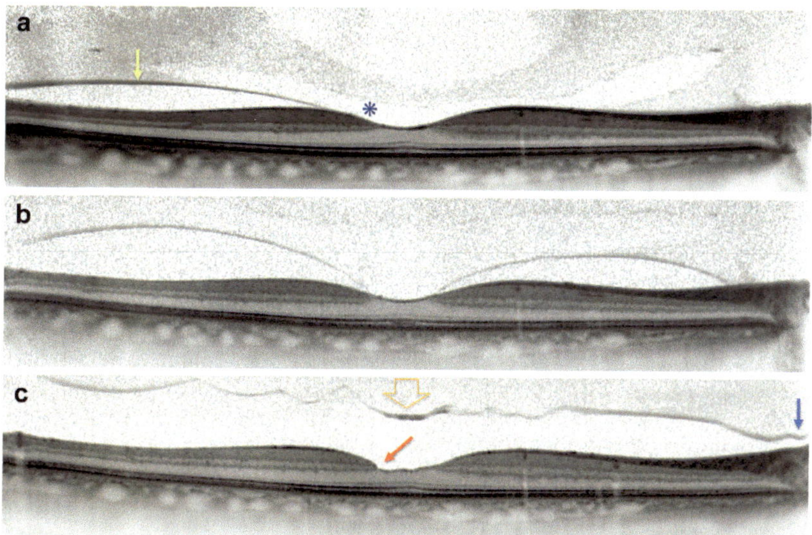

Fig. 20.2 Uncomplicated natural history of a posterior vitreous detachment (PVD) in a fellow eye of a macular hole. (**a**) May 2010, partial detachment of the posterior vitreous cortex in temporal of the macula (*arrow*). The presence of the premacular bursa (*asterisk*) in front of the macula shows that the vitreous still adheres to the macular surface. (**b**) April 2011, the posterior vitreous cortex is now detached all around the foveal center and only adheres at the foveal pit. (**c**) June 2011, the posterior vitreous cortex is now completely detached from the posterior pole but not from the optic disc (OD) (*blue arrow*). There is a condensation in the plane of the detached vitreous cortex (*large arrow*) probably due to an avulsion of the foveal surface; the foveal pit is slightly irregular (*red arrow*)

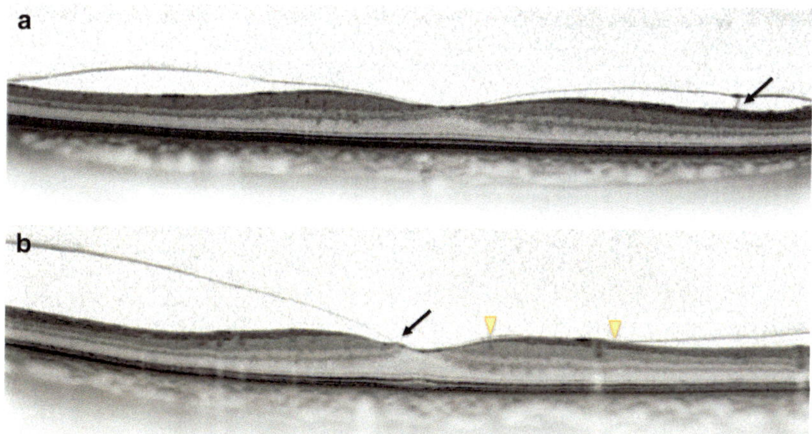

Fig. 20.3 Asymptomatic perifoveal posterior vitreous detachment in the fellow eye of a macular hole. (**a**) Horizontal B-scan showing the adherence of the posterior hyaloid to the foveal center without change in its curvature. Note an adherence between the posterior hyaloid and the retinal surface near the optic disc (*arrow*). (**b**) Vertical B-scan showing a discrete focal elevation of the foveal curvature (*arrow*) at the attachment point of the posterior hyaloid below the foveal center. The posterior hyaloid adheres more widely to the upper part of the macular surface (*arrowheads*)

layers may be intact (Haouchine et al. 2001; Takahashi et al. 2011b). However, SD-OCT has shown that, more frequently than previously thought, the photoreceptor IS/OS layer may be elevated or even disrupted at the foveal center. The yellow spot visible on fundus examination, which may be associated with the inner foveal cyst, is probably due to the foveolar detachment of the cone outer segments (Takahashi et al. 2011a) (Figs. 20.6 and 20.7).

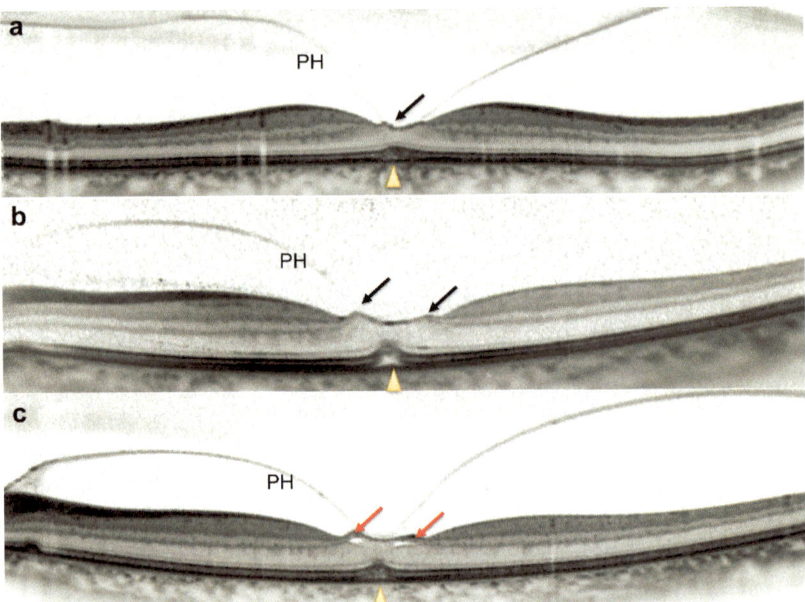

Fig. 20.4 Various degrees of tractional anomalies in the fovea of fellow eyes of macular holes. (**a**) Discrete elevation and irregularity of the foveal floor (*black arrow*) at the junction with the partially detached posterior hyaloid (PH). Note the slight elevation of the ellipsoid and interdigitation zones at the foveal center (*arrowhead*). (**b**) More marked foveal floor elevation (*arrows*) due to the traction of the posterior hyaloid (PH). The elevation of the central photoreceptors, ellipsoid, and interdigitation zones is more marked (*arrowhead*). (**c**) In addition to the elevation of the foveal floor by traction of the posterior hyaloid (PH) and elevation of the central photoreceptors (*arrowhead*), there are also small cystic spaces in the inner part of the fovea

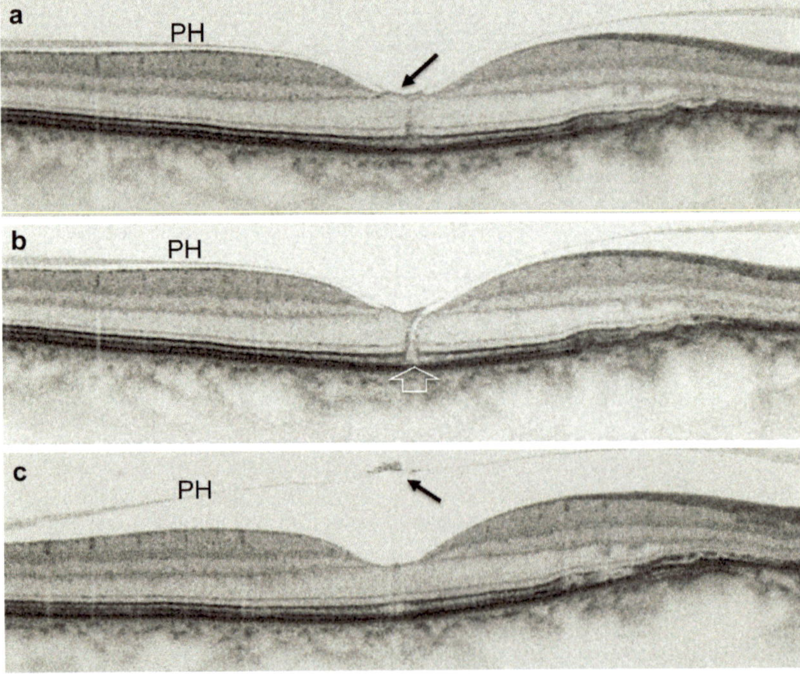

Fig. 20.5 Vitreomacular traction and spontaneous resolution (raster of 5 B-scans spaced by 75 μm). (**a**) Shallow posterior hyaloid (PH) detachment with discrete elevation of the foveal floor (*arrow*). (**b**) On the adjacent B-scan distant from 75 μm, there is a narrow full-thickness micro-hole (*large arrow*), visible only on this B-scan. (**c**) Three months later, the posterior hyaloid (PH) is detached from the macula and contains an operculum (*arrow*). The micro-hole is now closed

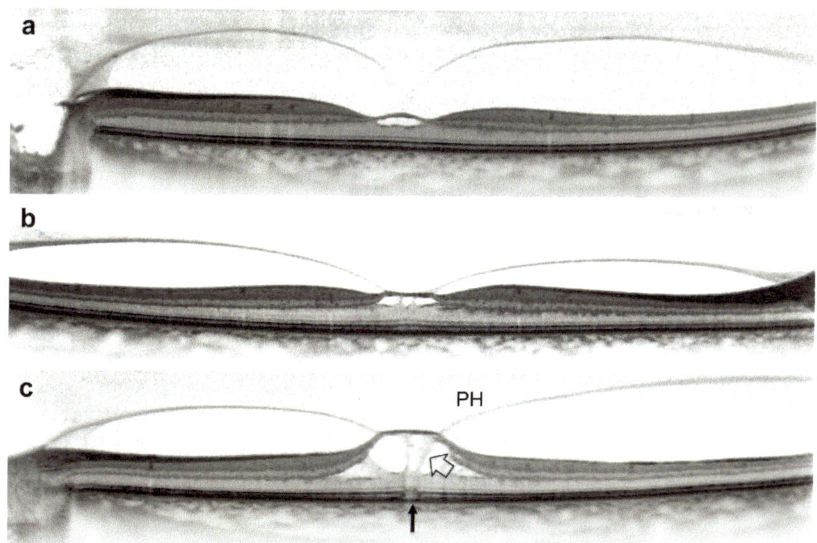

Fig. 20.6 Three different cases of vitreomacular traction with inner foveal cysts, in fellow eyes of macular holes. (**a**) Vitreomacular traction on the foveal center resulting in the formation of an inner foveal cyst. The outer retina is intact. (**b**) The inner foveal cyst is larger than in (**a**), but the outer retina is also intact. (**c**) Voluminous tractional cystoid spaces in the inner part of the fovea. There is a defect in the ellipsoid line (*black arrow*) which seems in continuity with the posterior hyaloid (PH) and the septa separating cystoid spaces (*large arrow*)

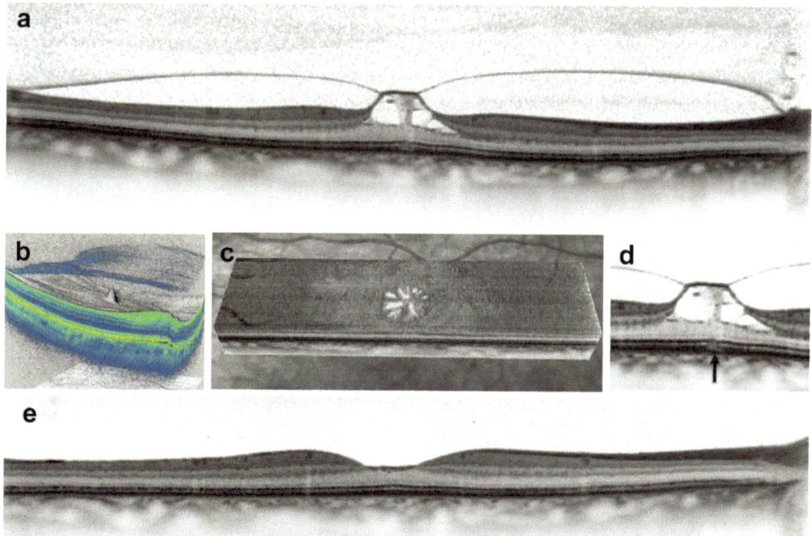

Fig. 20.7 Vitreomacular traction with inner foveal cystic spaces and central alteration of the interdigitation zone. (**a**) Horizontal 9-mm B-scan showing the traction of the posterior hyaloid (PH) on the roof of the foveal cystic spaces. (**b**) Three dimensional reconstructions showing the focal adhesion of the posterior hyaloid to the cystic foveal center. (**c**) En-face OCT showing the radial distribution of the foveal cystoid spaces. (**d**) Detail of the B-scan showing a small interruption of the continuity of the interdigitation zone; the ellipsoid zone is intact. (**e**) One year later, normalization of the macular profile after spontaneous release of the vitreomacular traction

Inner foveolar cysts may also communicate with an outer retinal cavitation forming an “occult” MH (Gass 1995). The retinal layers are disrupted in the whole thickness of the fovea except at a very superficial layer containing the inner limiting membrane (ILM) on which the posterior hyaloid is still attached (Gaudric et al. 1999; Haouchine et al. 2001; Michalewski et al. 2011; Takahashi et al. 2011a, b). In this regard, some impending MHs (former stage 1B) are true occult MHs. At any stage of impending MH, a complete resolution is possible if the VMT decreases or spontaneously releases (Figs. 20.8 and 20.9).

However, there is a significant risk of evolution toward a full-thickness macular hole (FTMH). There are few data on the risk of MH in a fellow eye when a VMT is associated or not with structural intrafoveal anomalies. According to recent publications, the risk could range between 30 and 50% (Kumagai et al. 2011; Takahashi et al. 2011b) (Fig. 20.10).

20.3 Full-Thickness Macular Holes

The recent international classification (Duker et al. 2013) proposes to differentiate MHs according to the presence of a vitreomacular adhesion and the hole diameter (Table 20.1).

20.3.1 Macular Hole with Persistent Vitreous Traction

MH with persistent vitreous traction includes what has been called stage 2 MH. Stage 2 MH has

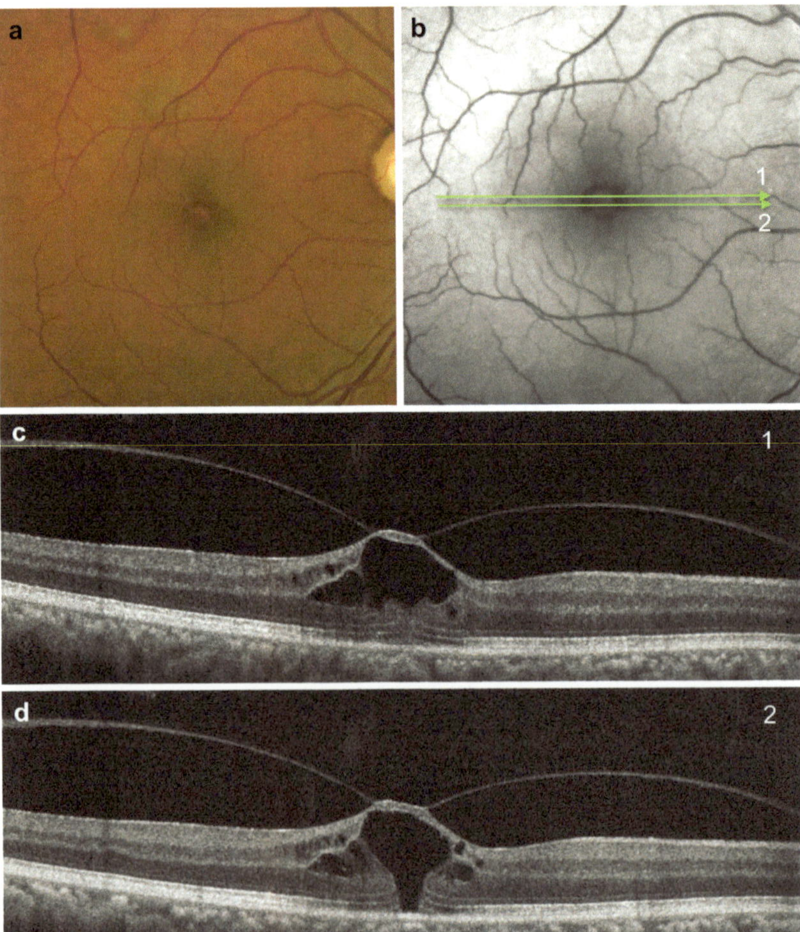

Fig. 20.8 Vitreomacular traction with outer retinal break in a fellow eye of a macular hole. (**a**) Fundus color photo showing a yellow spot in the foveal center. (**b**) Red-free photograph on which *green lines 1 and 2* refer to the two B-scans displayed in c and d and separated by 75 µm. (**c**) B-scan 1 mainly shows a voluminous inner foveal cyst and an outer retina which seem intact. (**d**) B-scan 2 shows that in fact there is a central break in the outer retina

been described as an eccentric oval, crescent, or horseshoe-shaped retinal defect inside the edge of the yellow ring and a diameter of less than 400 μm (Johnson and Gass 1988; Gass 1995). OCT has subsequently shown that the incompletely detached operculum is pulled in an oblique direction by the traction of the posterior hyaloid (Gaudric et al. 1999; Hee et al. 1995) (Fig. 20.11).

Moreover, recent observations by Takahashi et al. (2010, 2011a, b) have shown that the neuronal elements formed a constitutive part of the operculum at least in some cases (Fig. 20.12). This observation corroborates the histological findings of Ezra, who has shown the presence of cone components in two-thirds of the opercula he examined (Ezra et al. 2001) (Fig. 20.13).

Small MHs may close spontaneously when the VMT spontaneously releases, but this event is rare (Privat et al. 2007). OCT shows that MH with persistent vitreous traction may present various profiles and a large range of diameters from the extra small break to a large foveal opening greater than 400 μm, although small holes are the majority.

20.3.2 Macular Hole with Released Vitreous Traction

According to international classification (Duker et al. 2013), this category includes all the cases in which the posterior hyaloid is detached from the hole edge regardless of whether the vitreous is also detached or not from the optic disc. In the Gass definition, stage 3 MH was a central round retinal defect with a diameter greater than 400 μm, a rim of elevated retina, with or without prefoveolar pseudo-operculum, and without a Weiss ring.

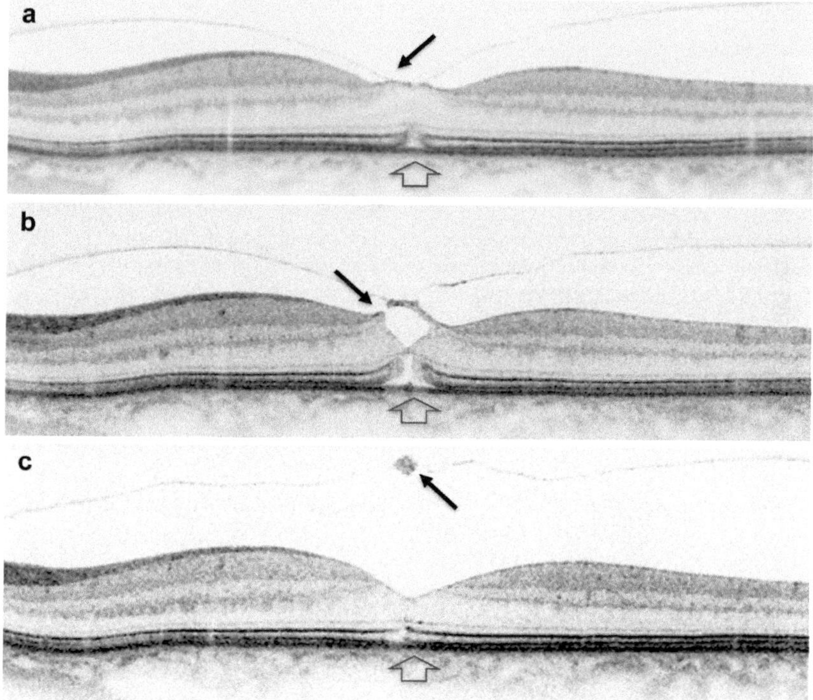

Fig. 20.9 Worsening and spontaneous resolution of an impending macular hole. (**a**) Vitreomacular traction with small elevation of the foveal floor (*black arrow*). The interdigitation and ellipsoid zones are slightly elevated or focally disrupted (*large arrow*). (**b**) Six months later, formation of an inner foveal cyst whose roof is disrupted (*black arrow*) by the posterior hyaloid traction. Elevation of the foveal photoreceptors with disruption of the ellipsoid zone (*large arrow*). (**c**) Six months later, spontaneous release of the vitreous traction with avulsion of an operculum (*black arrow*). Reattachment of the central photoreceptors but the continuity of the ellipsoid zone is not yet complete (*large arrow*)

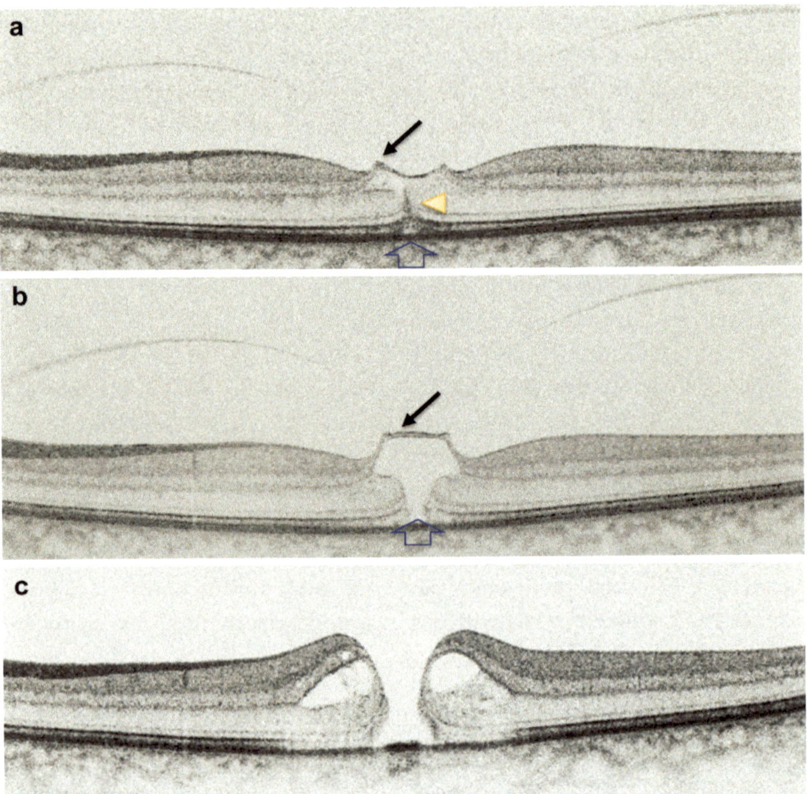

Fig. 20.10 Evolution of a vitreomacular traction toward a full-thickness macular hole. (**a**) Vitreomacular traction with focal elevation of the foveal floor and microcystic space (*black arrow*), elevation of the central photoreceptors (*large arrow*) and vertical hyperreflective line (*arrow head*). (**b**) Four months later, worsening of the vitreomacular traction with elevation of the foveal floor (*black arrow*) which forms the roof of a large foveal cyst. Breakdown of the photoreceptor layer (*large arrow*). This case can be considered as an "occult" macular hole. (**c**) Three months later, the vitreous has detached, but a full-thickness macular hole is present

Table 20.1 Comparison of the classification commonly used for macular holes, adapted from Gass classification, with the international VMT study classification

Classification commonly used for full-thickness MH	International VMT study
Stage 2: small hole	Small or medium FTMH with VMT
Stage 3: large hole	Medium or large FTMH with VMT
Stage 4: FTMH with PVD	Small, medium, or large FTMH without VMT

Adapted from Duker et al. (2013)
FTMH full-thickness macular hole, *VMT* vitreomacular traction, *PVD* posterior vitreous detachment

The presence of a Weiss ring defined the stage 4. Subsequently, OCT has shown that even when the vitreous was not detached from the optic disc, it could be completely detached from the retinal surface over the posterior pole and not connected to the hole edge.

20.3.2.1 Diameter of the Macular Hole and Vitreomacular Status

Moreover, the precise measurement of the hole diameter on OCT scans has shown that the size of MH with and without VMT varies greatly. Although the diameter of stage 2 MHs generally tends to be smaller than that of stage 3 MHs; large stage 2 and small stage 3 MHs are in fact not uncommon (Privat et al. 2007; Takahashi et al. 2011b).

In a recent study conducted on 100 consecutive idiopathic full-thickness macular holes

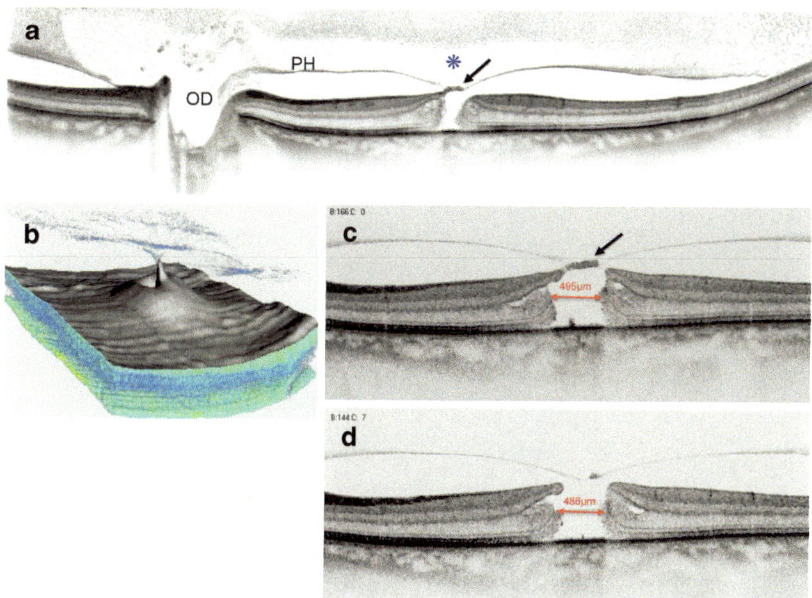

Fig. 20.11 Large full-thickness macular hole with vitreomacular traction. (**a**) Montage of horizontal B-scans showing the traction of the posterior hyaloid (PH) on the operculum (*arrow*) of the macular hole. The vitreous is still attached to the optic disc (OD). The bursa premacularis (*asterisk*) is elevated with partial detachment of the vitreous. (**b**) Three-dimensional OCT showing the adherence of the vitreous on the operculum. (**c**) Horizontal B-scan showing the operculum still attached to the edge of the hole (*arrow*). The diameter of the hole on this B-scan is 495 μm. (**d**) Horizontal B-scan, distant of 75 μm from the scan in c. The posterior hyaloid (PH) seems detached from the retina. However, the shape of double arc converging toward the fovea does not fit with a PH completely detached from the macular surface. The diameter of the hole on this B-scan is 488 μm

(FTMH), we have found that the mean preoperative hole diameter was not significantly different according to the presence or absence of a VMT: 339 ± 134 μm in eyes with VMT and 423 ± 191 μm in eyes without VMT ($p = 0.057$). Only 13 % of cases had a diameter of 400 μm or less, and 6 % had a diameter of 250 μm or less (Philippakis 2015) (Fig. 20.14).

20.3.2.2 Method for Measuring Macular Hole Diameter

The aperture size is measured using the caliper function on SD-OCT devices. The minimum hole width is measured at the narrowest hole point in the mid-retina, using the OCT caliper function, as a line parallel to the retinal pigment epithelium (RPE) (Duker et al. 2013). Empirically, it corresponds to a line drawn between the terminations of the detached photoreceptor outer segments. Other methods have also been studied (Wakely et al. 2012; Xu et al. 2013), but the minimum hole width tends to be a standard. The accurate measurement of the MH size has several practical consequences. MHs of 250 μm or less have a likelihood of about 50 % to be closed by intravitreal ocriplasmin injection (Stalmans et al. 2012). MHs of 400 μm or less have an increased likelihood to be closed surgically than larger ones (Ip et al. 2002; Tadayoni et al. 2006). ILM peeling could be only needed in MH larger than 400 μm (Chang 2012; Tadayoni et al. 2006, 2009) (Fig. 20.15).

20.4 Macular Hole and Epiretinal Membrane

A noncontractile epiretinal membrane (ERM) may cover the macular surface around the hole. It is especially well visualized on blue reflectance photographs (Blain et al. 1998). The frequency of the formation of an ERM increases with the stage,

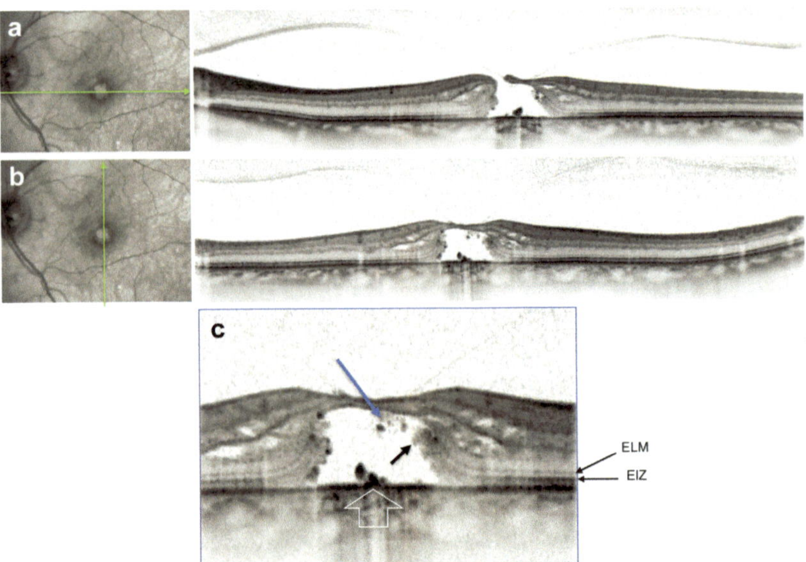

Fig. 20.12 Full-thickness macular hole with vitreomacular traction. (**a**) Horizontal B-scan showing the vitreomacular traction on the operculum attached to the hole edge. (**b**) The vertical B-scan does not pass through the marginal opening of the operculum, and the case may be misinterpreted as an impending macular hole. (**c**) Detail of the scan above: the external limiting membrane (ELM) and the ellipsoid zone (EZ) are detached in the area of the hole. The photoreceptor outer segments are also detached (*black arrow*) and elongated. Note also debris of photoreceptors at the posterior face of the operculum (*blue arrow*). Proliferation of the retinal pigment epithelium in the area of the hole (*large arrow*)

duration, and size of the hole (Blain et al. 1998; Cheng et al. 2000, 2002). However, this does not affect the surgical prognosis once the membrane has been peeled off during surgery (Fig. 20.16).

20.5 Differential Diagnosis

Differentiating a full-thickness MH from other roundish anomalies of the fovea is no longer a problem since the advent of OCT, which clearly shows the characteristic profiles of lamellar MHs and macular pseudoholes. However, foveal cysts of various origins as well as micro-holes may be more difficult to differentiate from idiopathic FTMH.

20.5.1 Lamellar Macular Hole

The term of lamellar macular hole (LMH) has been coined by Gass in 1975 to characterize a macular lesion resulting from the opening of the central cyst of a cystoid macular edema. The term lamellar hole has been used to describe both the end stage of a cystoid macular edema (Frangieh et al. 1981) and the aborted process of formation of a MH (Haouchine et al. 2001, 2004).

Lamellar MHs, i.e., defects in the inner fovea due to the avulsion of the roof of a foveal cyst (either tractional or due to a cystoid macular edema), are characterized on OCT by an irregular thinning of the foveal floor, a cleavage between the inner and outer retina at the lamellar hole edge and the absence of a contractile ERM (Haouchine et al. 2004) (Figs. 20.17 and 20.18).

It is common that an epiretinal proliferation occurs at the surface of the retina, around the lamellar hole, well visible on SD-OCT on the ILM. On en-face OCT, this proliferation is amorphous, noncontractile and well differentiated from contractile ERMs, causing a macular thickening (Compera et al. 2015; Gaudric et al. 2013; Pang et al. 2015).

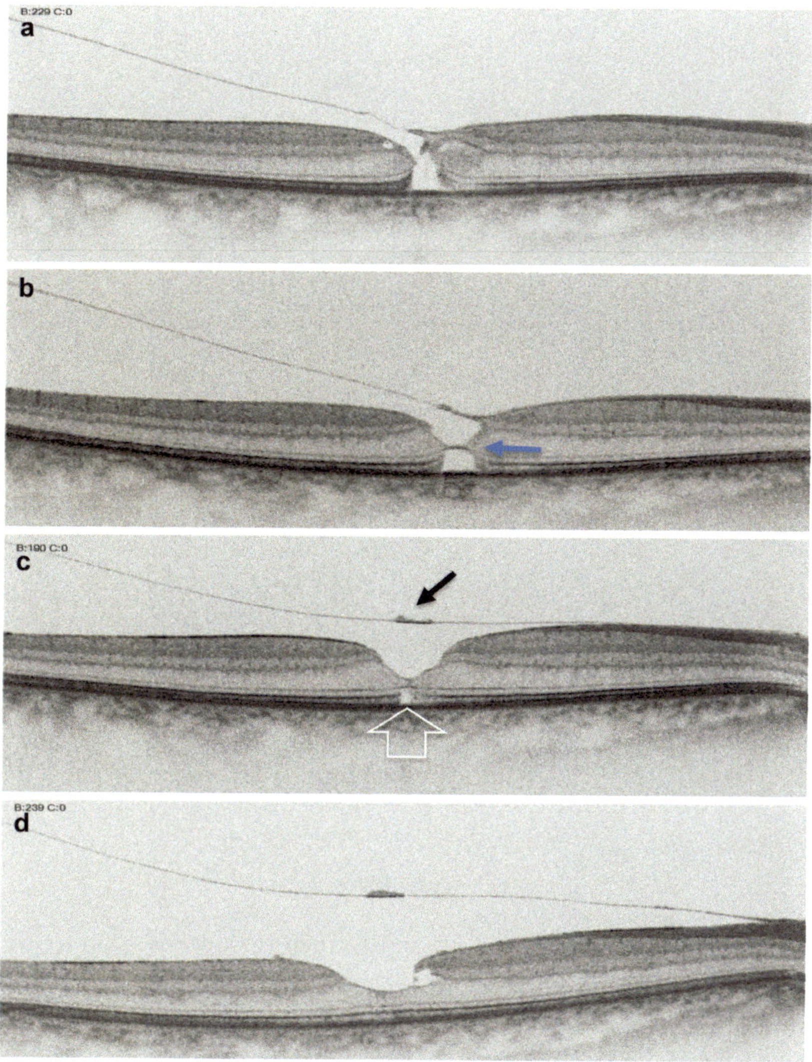

Fig. 20.13 Spontaneous closure of a small macular hole with vitreomacular traction. (**a**) Small macular hole (diameter of 133 μm) with vitreomacular traction on a small operculum. (**b**) Three months later, increase in the vitreous traction on the operculum. At the same time, a diaphragm closes the hole in its middle (*arrow*). (**c**) After 5 months, the posterior hyaloid has detached from the macula with the operculum (*black arrow*), and the healing process has closed the hole, leaving only a small interruption in the ellipsoid zone (*large arrow*). (**d**) Two years later, remodeling of the fovea: there is no more defect in the ellipsoid zone. A discrete cleavage is present in the nasal edge of the fovea

20.5.2 Foveal Cysts of Various Origins

OCT and fluorescein angiography facilitate the differentiation of full-thickness MHs from foveal cysts occurring in pathologies other than MH, such as cystoid macular edema, X-linked retinoschisis, or foveal cysts of type 2 macular telangiectasia.

20.6 Non-idiopathic Macular Holes

20.6.1 High Myopia

The pathogenesis of high myopic MH may be different from that of non-myopic eyes because of anomalies associated with posterior

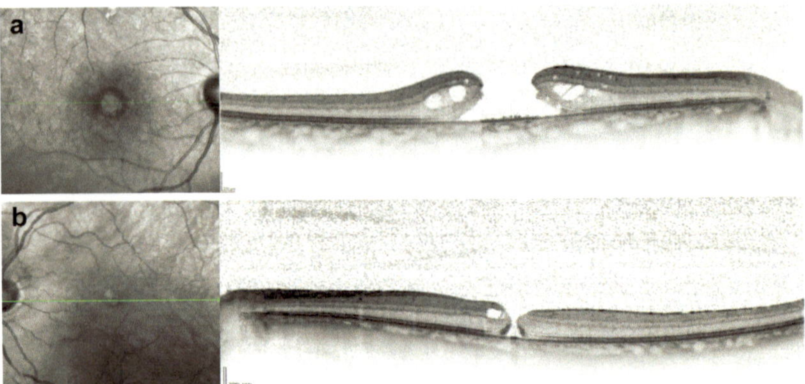

Fig. 20.14 Variations in diameter of macular holes without vitreomacular traction. (**a**) Horizontal scan of a large macular hole (880 µm). (**b**) Horizontal scan of a small macular hole (75 µm)

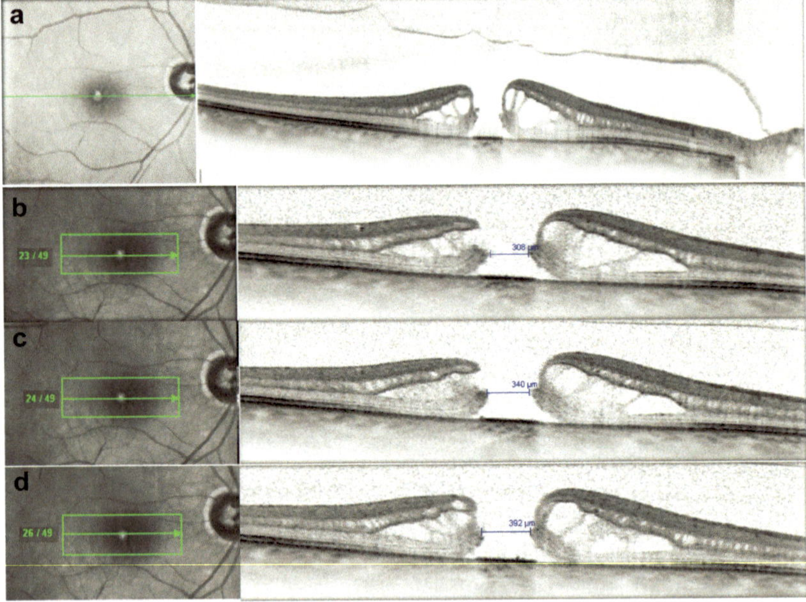

Fig. 20.15 Accurate measurement of the macular hole diameter (aperture size). (**a**) Horizontal 9-mm B-scan showing a full-thickness macular hole without vitreomacular traction. (**b**–**d**) Horizontal 6-mm B-scan raster (**b**) and (**c**) are spaced by 50 µm and (**c**) and (**d**) by 100 µm. The diameter of the hole aperture is measured at the narrowest hole point in the mid-retina using the OCT caliper as a line parallel to the retinal pigment epithelium. It corresponds to the end of the photoreceptor outer segments (*blue bar*). In this example, the size may vary from 308 to 392 µm depending on the location of the scan. Due to the instable fixation of these eyes, a raster of several tight B-scans should be obtained. The largest value corresponds to the exact diameter of the hole aperture (macular hole size)

staphyloma and because the vitreous cortex often remains adherent to the retinal surface. In general, the adherence of the posterior vitreous cortex to the retinal surface around the hole is wider than in idiopathic MHs, and MH staging cannot be exactly applied to high myopic MHs (Fig. 20.19).

Myopic foveoschisis is an anteroposterior distension of the retina due to the combined effects of the progressive deepening of the staphyloma and the stiffness of the retinal surface due to changes in the adherent vitreous cortex (Ikuno et al. 2004; Spaide and Fisher 2005; Takano and Kishi 1999) (Figs. 20.20 and 20.21).

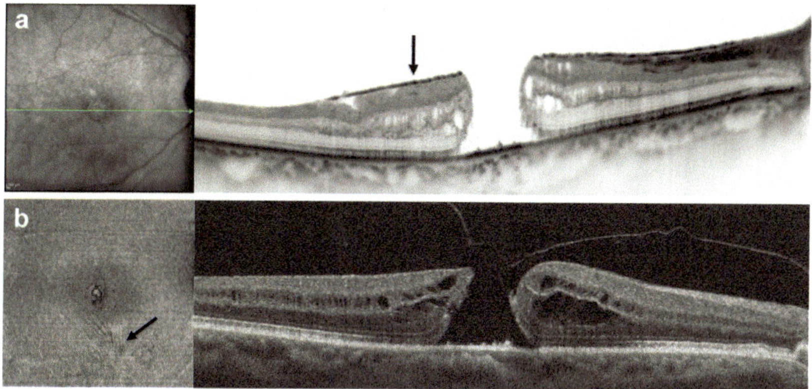

Fig. 20.16 Epiretinal membrane associated with macular holes. (**a**) The epiretinal membrane is not visible on the fundus image (*left*) but is present on the OCT B-scan on the right (*arrow*). (**b**) The epiretinal membrane induces some stellar superficial folds on the en-face OCT image on the left (*arrow*) but is not visible on the horizontal OCT B-scan (*right*)

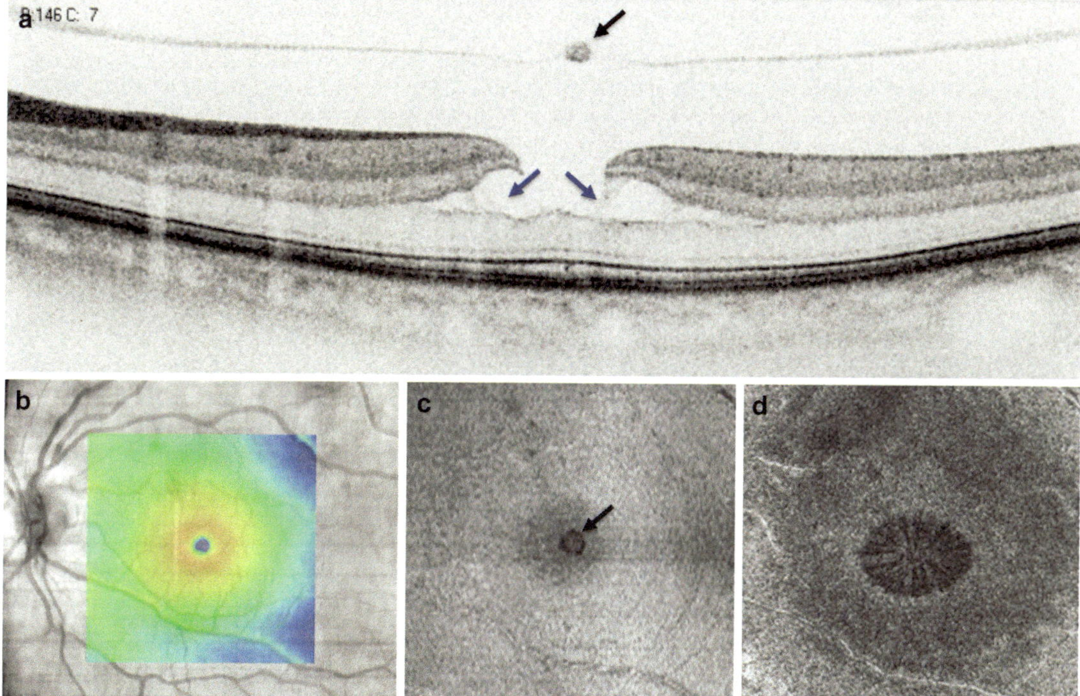

Fig. 20.17 Lamellar macular hole after opening of a foveal cyst, in a fellow eye of full-thickness macular hole. (**a**) Horizontal B-scan showing an operculum in the plane of the detached posterior hyaloid (*black arrow*). Cleavage between the inner and outer retinas on the edge of the fovea with persistence of septa between cystic formations (*blue arrows*). (**b**) OCT map showing a near normal macular thickness. (**c**) En-face OCT with segmentation at the inner limiting membrane: no epiretinal membrane, no folds. Presence of a central round defect (*arrow*). (**d**) En-face OCT with segmentation at the inner nuclear layer: note the radial pattern of the cystic spaces around the central defect

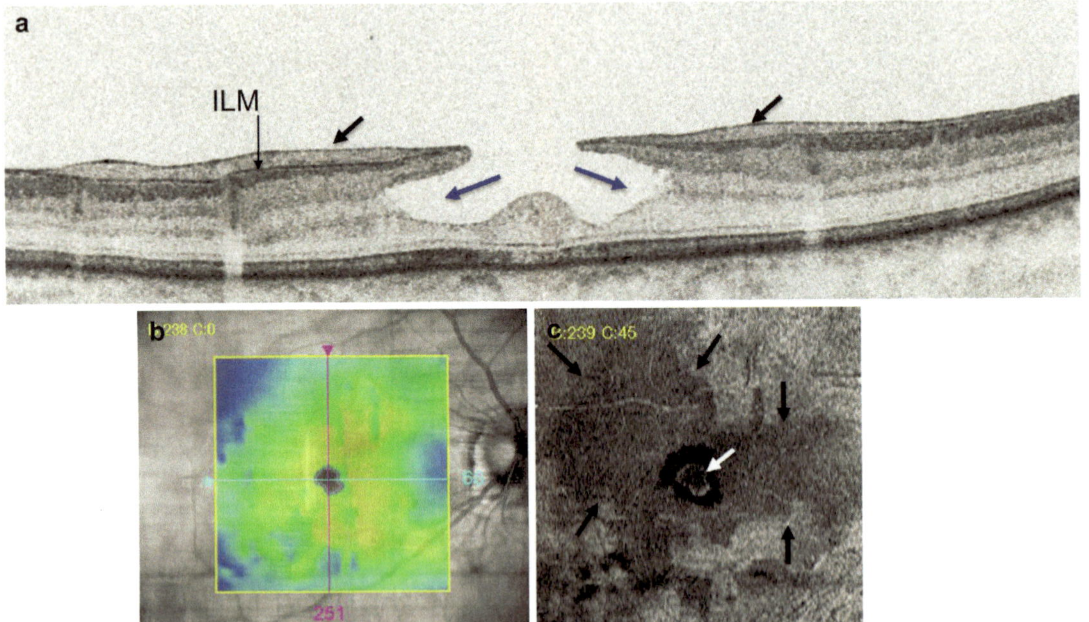

Fig. 20.18 Lamellar macular hole with epiretinal proliferation. (**a**) Cleavage between the inner and outer retinas on the edge of the fovea with persistence of septa between cystic formations (*blue arrows*). Epiretinal proliferation (*black arrows*) on the inner limiting membrane (ILM). (**b**) OCT map showing a moderate irregular thickening of the macular area. (**c**) En-face OCT with segmentation at the macular surface: presence of a central round defect (*white arrow*) and abnormal reflectivity of the epiretinal proliferation without any retinal fold (*black arrows*)

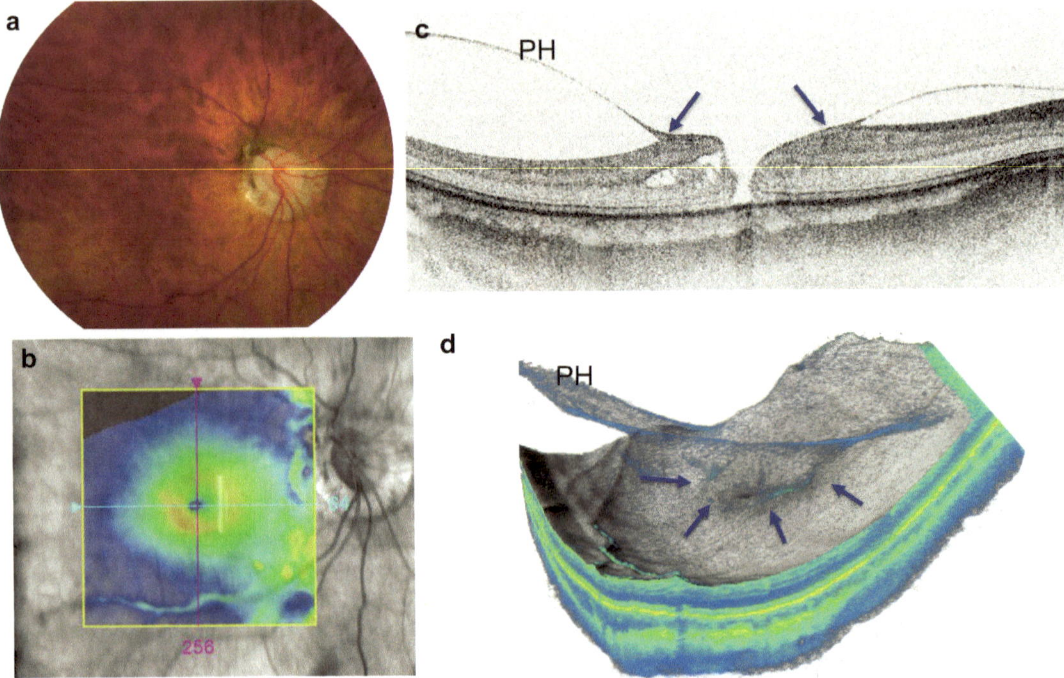

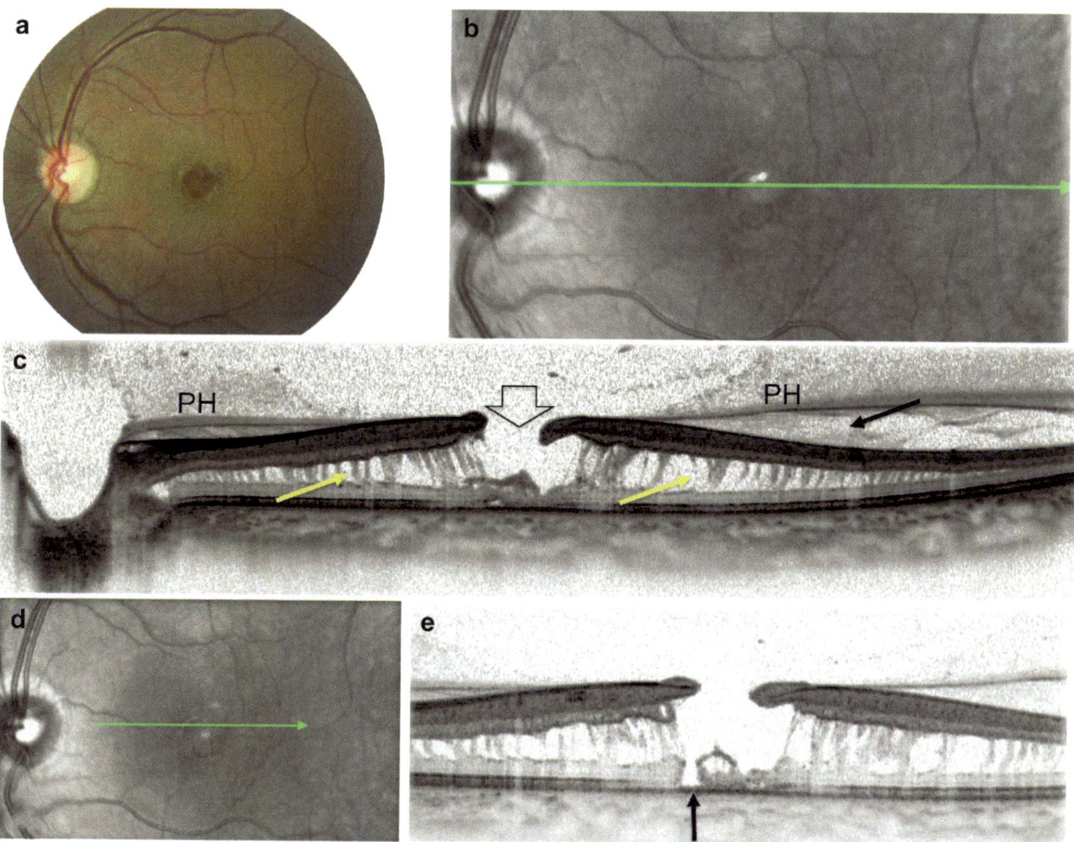

Fig. 20.20 Small macular hole in a myopic foveoschisis. (**a**) Fundus color photo showing an aspect of macular hole. (**b**) Scanning laser ophthalmoscope image of the same fundus with the direction of the B-scan in c (*green line*). (**c**) The B-scan shows that the aspect of macular hole seen on color photo is mainly due to a lamellar hole (*large arrow*) in a foveoschisis (*yellow arrows*). The posterior hyaloid (PH) (posterior vitreous cortex) is delaminated in a vitreoschisis (*black arrows*) but still adherent to the retinal surface. (**d**) Direction of another B-scan (*green line*) just adjacent to that shown in (b). (**e**) This B-scan shows a photoreceptor disruption at the bottom of the lamellar macular hole (*arrow*)

Some of these MHs occur after a progressive decrease in vision due to the worsening of foveoschisis (Gaucher et al. 2007; Shimada et al. 2008). Others may be asymptomatic and only revealed by OCT examination of the fundus (Coppe et al. 2005). In general, the occurrence of a foveal detachment (FD) and even more a breakdown in the photoreceptor layer associated with a myopic foveoschisis are at high risk of MH (Shimada et al. 2008).

20.6.2 Posttraumatic Macular Holes

These MHs usually occur in children and young male adults as accidents at work or in the home

Fig. 20.19 Macular hole with vitreomacular traction in a highly myopic eye. (**a**) Fundus color photo showing the myopic conus around the optic disc. (**b**) OCT map showing the elevation of the macular edge. (**c**) OCT B-scan showing a small macular hole with a posterior hyaloid (PH) completely attached to the hole edge (*arrows*) but partly detached from the retinal surface of the posterior pole. (**d**) Three-dimensional OCT showing the surface of the traction (*arrows*) of the posterior hyaloid (PH) around the hole

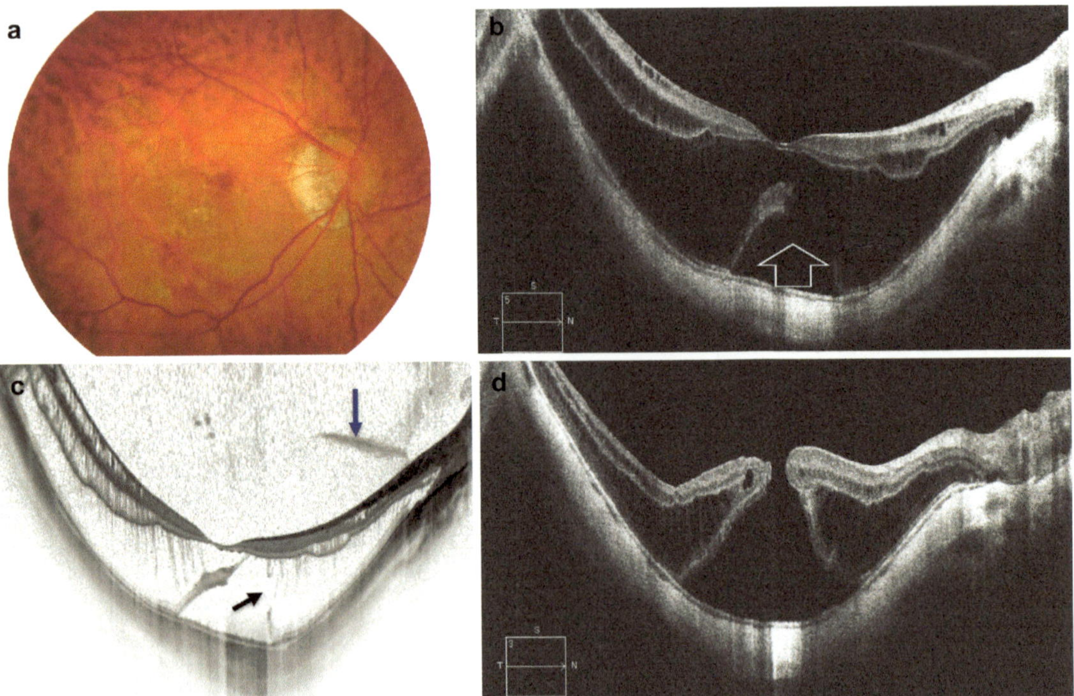

Fig. 20.21 Evolution of a myopic foveoschisis toward a macular hole. (**a**) Fundus color photo showing the characteristic myopic tessellation. (**b**) OCT B-scan (Cirrus, Zeiss) showing the foveoschisis with a foveal detachment (*arrow*). (**c**) OCT B-scan (Spectralis, Heidelberg), same day, showing a breakdown in the photoreceptor layer (*black arrow*). Note that the posterior hyaloid is still attached to the retina, at least near the optic disc (*blue arrow*). (**d**) Full-thickness macular hole occurred 4 months later

or during ball games (Atmaca and Yilmaz 1993; Shakin and Yannuzzi 1987). They are due to the sudden axial compression of the eye resulting in equatorial expansion and retinal rupture of the fovea. The hole may be combined with other fundus lesions such as choroidal or the Bruch membrane disruption, commotio retinae, sclopetaria, or peripheral breaks. The visual prognosis depends not only on the closure of the hole but also on the topography of the other lesions. If a choroidal disruption passes through the fovea or if the post-contusive RPE atrophy includes the foveal center, the visual prognosis will be poor. Unlike what occurs in idiopathic MH, the vitreous is not detached at all from the posterior pole. Surgery is usually successful, but a traumatic MH may also sometimes close spontaneously within the first weeks of its occurrence (Barreau et al. 1997; Kusaka et al. 1997; Parmar et al. 1999) (Fig. 20.22).

20.7 Surgery of Macular Holes

20.7.1 Preoperative Optical Coherence Tomography During Macular Hole Surgery

Intraoperative OCT (iOCT) may provide new insights into the physiopathology of vitreomacular diseases, by imaging some retinal microstructure alterations occurring during the surgical procedure. Indeed, the PIONEER Study has reported the feasibility and the potential usefulness of iOCT for surgical decision (Ehlers et al. 2014a). Regarding MH surgery, iOCT has not shown significant retinal thickness changes during the procedure, including after ILM removal (Ray et al. 2011). MH closure has not been observed at the end of the surgical procedure (Ehlers et al. 2014b; Ray et al. 2011).

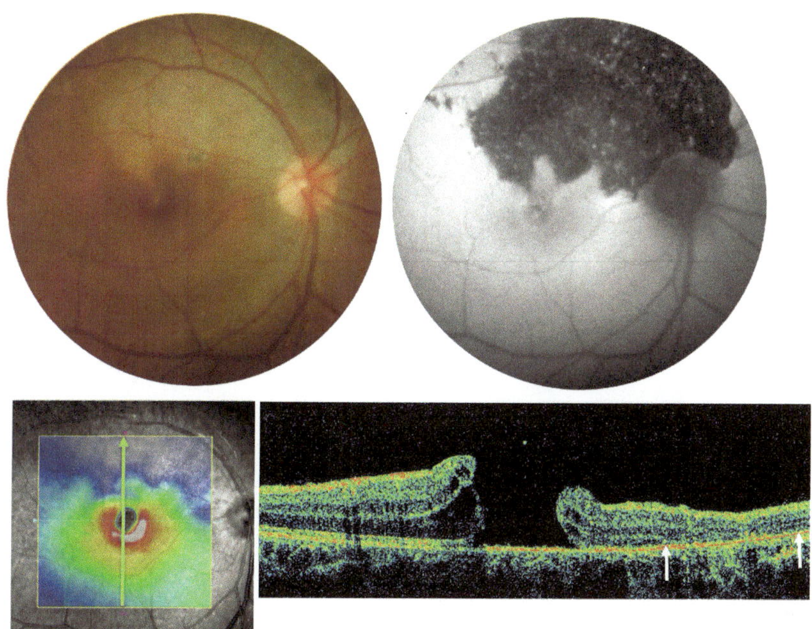

Fig. 20.22 Posttraumatic macular hole due to tennis ball contusion, 3 weeks after the trauma. (**a**) Color fundus photograph showing a pale area of retinal pigment epithelium atrophy in the superior part of the posterior pole. (**b**) Fundus autofluorescence showing the severe hypoautofluorescence of the contusion area of the retinal pigment epithelium. (**c**) OCT macular map showing that the hypoautofluorescence also corresponds to an area of retina atrophy (*deep blue*). The *green line* indicates the direction of the B-scan shown in (d). (**d**) Vertical B-scan (time domain OCT) showing a large macular hole. Note that the superior edge is less edematous than the inferior one; the outer retina becomes atrophic superior to the macular hole (*arrows*)

Using iOCT, a new subfoveal hyporeflectivity due to the expansion of the space between the IS/OS band and the RPE after ERM peeling has been described in MH and ERM and may be associated with visual acuity (VA) recovery and MH closure (Ray et al. 2011) (Fig. 20.23).

20.7.2 Optical Coherence Tomography of Closed Macular Holes

20.7.2.1 Macular Hole Closure After Surgery

Vitrectomy and gas tamponade associated or not with ILM peeling is the gold standard for the treatment of most MHs. Since the first OCT examinations at the end of the 1990s, the understanding of the healing process of MH closure after surgery has considerably improved. Several reports have described hyporeflective defects of the outer fovea in the early postoperative period following MH closure, named outer foveal defects, outer foveal cysts, foveal detachment, or foveal bridge depending on the authors (Bottoni 2011; Kang 2010; Takahashi 2000). These hyporeflective defects of the outer fovea can be classified into two groups which can also be combined: disruptions of the EZ and foveal detachment (FD) characterized by the elevation of the photoreceptor layers.

Foveal detachment should be distinguished from EZ disruptions, which are more frequent and can persist for more than 12 months after surgery (Kawano 2011). The rate of persistent FD is variable in the literature, ranging from 10 to 40 % 1 month after surgery (Bottoni 2011; Chang

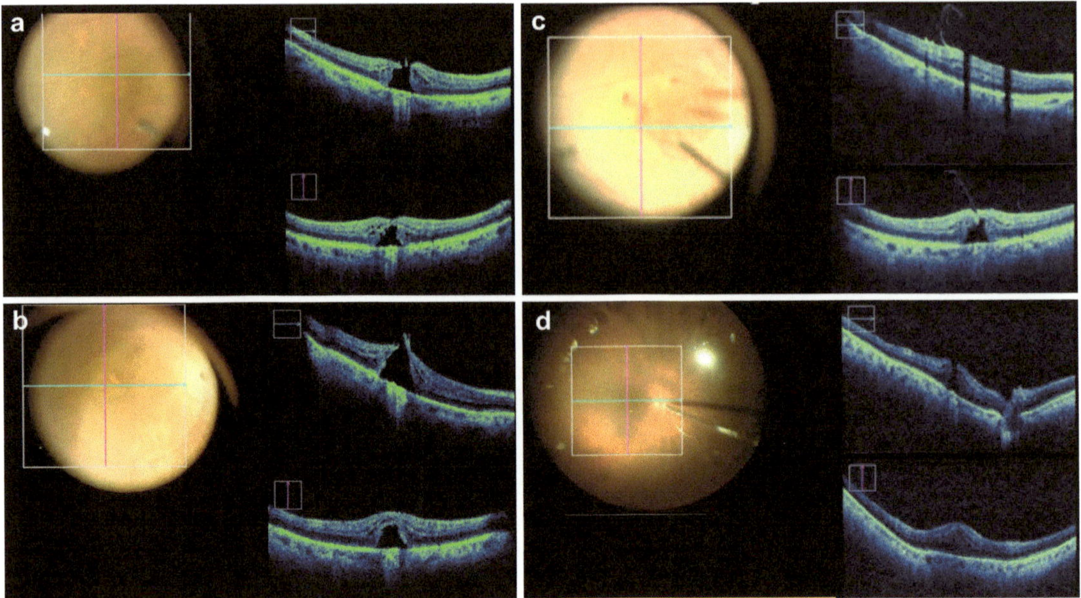

Fig. 20.23 Intraoperative optical coherence tomography during macular hole surgery. (**a**) Intraoperative imaging of the MH at the beginning of the surgical procedure. (**b**) During hyaloid separation, an acute traction is exerted on the retinal surface by the vitreous probe, and the retina is stretched but returned immediately in place. (**c**) During the ILM peeling, the edge of the ILM could be seen easily on iOCT. Analysis of MH dimensions did not show significant difference in minimal horizontal MH diameter and MH base diameter after hyaloid elevation and/or ILM peeling compared to initial diameters before surgical maneuvers. (**d**) After fluid-air exchange, the diameter of the MH decreased slightly, but no MH closure was observed

2015; Kawano 2011; Sano 2009; Ko 2006; Wakabayashi 2010).

The hyporeflective defects of the outer fovea seem to occur mostly in small MH (Kang 2010; Kawano 2011; Rahman 2013). Kang et al. have assumed that the healing process in large MHs was characterized by glial cell proliferation above the RPE with closure from the outer retina first, unlike small MHs which were characterized by an early closure from the inner retina first. Most FDs resolved 6 months after surgery, and the final visual outcome of these hyporeflective defects was similar (Kawano 2011; Rahman 2013; Sano 2009) (Fig. 20.24).

20.7.2.2 Macular Hole Closure After Ocriplasmin Injection

Subretinal fluid and outer retina changes seem to be a common finding after ocriplasmin injection and are more often seen in case of successful ocriplasmin treatment (Fahim et al. 2014; Quezada-Ruiz et al. 2015). FD occurring after intravitreal ocriplasmin may be due to a direct pharmacological effect of the enzyme on the outer retina (Johnson et al. 2015) (Fig. 20.25).

20.7.3 Inner Retina After Internal Limiting Membrane Peeling

20.7.3.1 Dissociated Optic Nerve Fiber Layer

Peeling of the ILM is commonly used in MH surgery to improve the closure rate at least in large MHs but more often in all types of MH. The ablation of the ILM results in the dissociation of the optic nerve fiber layer (DONFL) visible on blue reflectance photographs (Tadayoni et al. 2001)

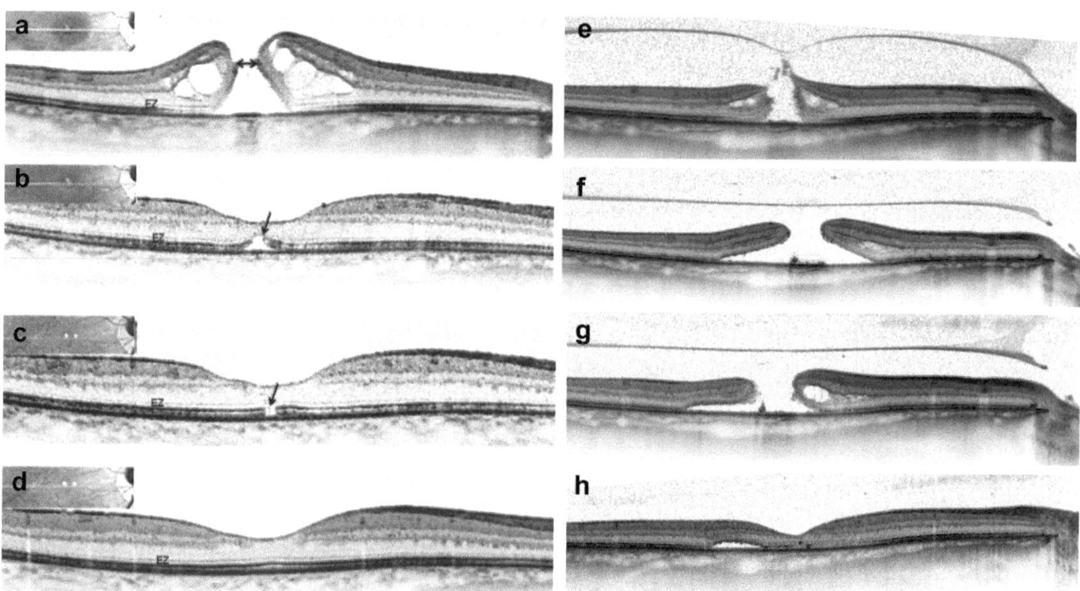

Fig. 20.24 Dynamic macular hole (MH) healing closure process after macular hole treatment. (**a–d**) MH healing closure process after surgery in the right eye (RE) of a 64-year old woman. (**a**) Preoperative OCT B-scan shows a full-thickness MH without vitreomacular traction. The MH diameter was of 231 μm (*arrow*), and the Snellen visual acuity (VA) was 20/80. (**b**) One month after surgery: persistent foveal detachment associated with disruption of the ellipsoid zone (EZ). The VA was 20/30. (**c**) Three months after surgery: persistent foveal disruption of the EZ. The VA was only 20/50 because of secondary cataract. (**d**) Six months after surgery: recovery of the photoreceptor layer integrity. The final VA after cataract surgery was 20/25. (**e–h**) Foveal detachment (FD) after ocriplasmin injection in the right eye of a 58-year old woman. (**e**) Initial OCT B-scan shows a full-thickness macular hole (MH) with vitreomacular traction (VMT). The MH diameter was of 381 μm, and the Snellen visual acuity (VA) was 20/125. (**e**) One month after the injection: persistent FD with a base diameter measured at 2205 μm, MH base diameter measured at 515 μm and stable VA at 20/125. (**g**) Three months after the injection: persistent FD with a base diameter measured at 1813 μm, MH base diameter measured at 536 μm, and stable VA at 20/125. (**h**) One month after secondary surgery: MH closure and parafoveolar FD with a base diameter measured at 670 μm. The postoperative VA was 20/100

and on en-face OCT as arcuate striae of the macular surface in the area of ILM peeling. They correspond to dimples into the retinal nerve fiber layer on OCT B-scan (Kishimoto et al. 2011; Spaide 2012). The observation of DONFL after MH surgery means that the ILM has been peeled off (Figs. 20.26 and 20.27).

20.7.3.2 Ganglion Cell Layer

Several studies have shown that the thickness of the retinal ganglion cell layer-inner plexiform layer (GCL-IPL) was significantly reduced after ILM peeling (Seo et al. 2015; Shinoda et al. 2008). However, they have also used indocyanine green (ICG) to stain the ILM, and ICG has been shown to have dose-dependent cytotoxic effects both in vivo and in vitro on retinal ganglion cells (Iriyama et al. 2004).

In another study in which the ILM has been stained with brilliant blue G, a safe dye for ganglion cells (Iriyama et al. 2012), a thinning of the GCL has also been found (Fig. 20.28) which predominated at the temporal side of the macula (Baba et al. 2014).

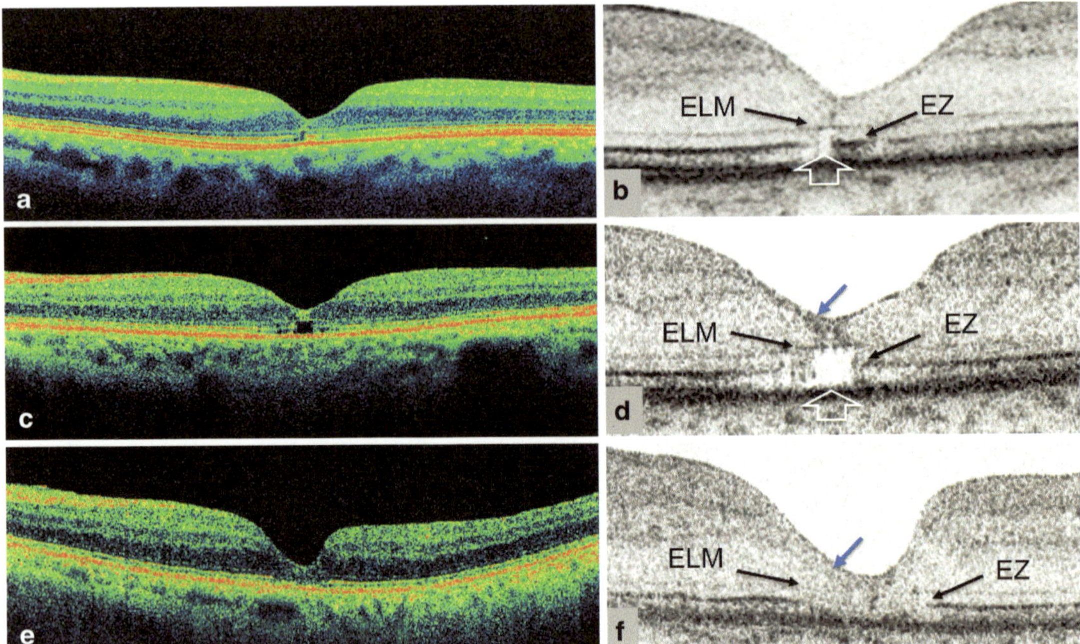

Fig. 20.25 Three examples of horizontal B-scans of macular holes closed 3 months after surgery. (**a**) Closed macular hole, with a slight asymmetry in the shape of the foveal contour. (**b**) Detail of (**a**): the continuity of the external limiting membrane (ELM) is reestablished (*arrow*). The ellipsoid zone (EZ) is still discontinuous with a small gap in the foveal center (*large arrow*). (**c**) Closed macular hole with thin retinal scar and persistent outer cavitation. (**d**) Detail of c: the external limiting membrane (ELM) is probably still disrupted in the foveal center. The hyperreflectivity could be only due to an effect of interface (*arrow*). The ellipsoid zone (EZ) remains disrupted, and a large outer cavitation persists (*large arrow*). (**e**) Closed macular hole with foveal scar. (**f**) Detail of e: thinning of the foveal center (*blue arrow*). The external limiting membrane (ELM) is incomplete. The ellipsoid zone (EZ) is largely disrupted

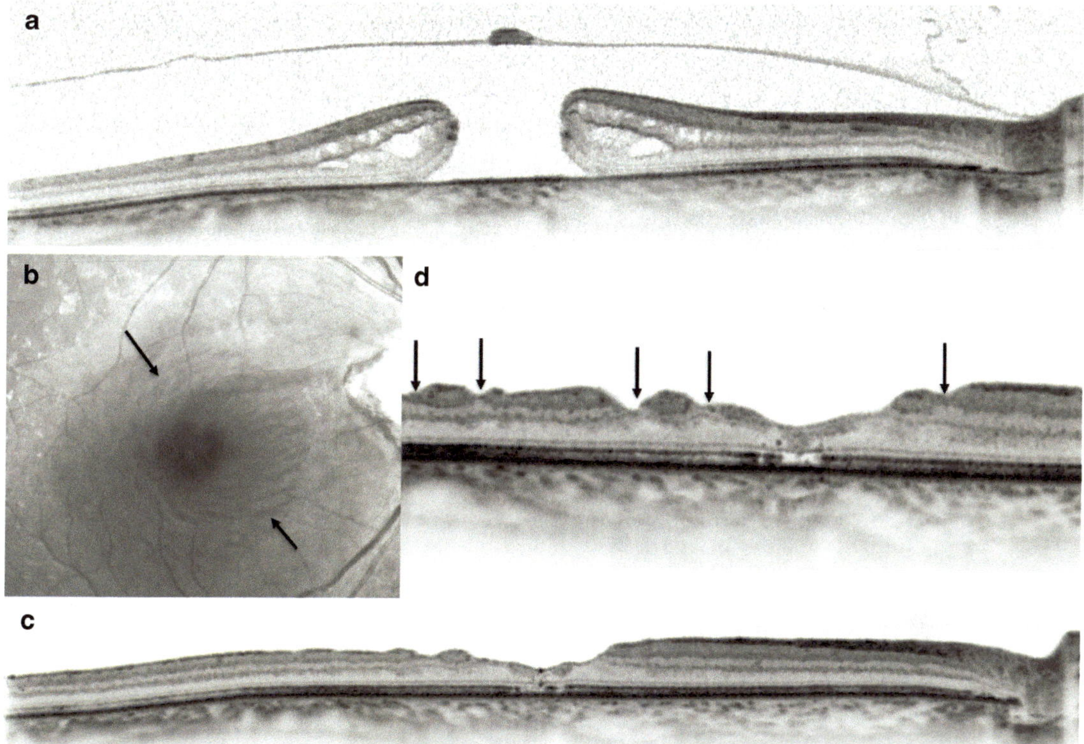

Fig. 20.26 Dissociated optic nerve fiber layer (DONFL) after surgical closure of a macular hole with internal limiting membrane (ILM) peeling. (**a**) B-scan OCT prior to surgery. (**b**) Blue reflectance photo of the fundus 3 months after surgical hole closure. Note the arcuate striae of the DONFL (*arrows*). (**c**) OCT B-scan after surgery, the hole is closed. (**d**) Detail of (**c**): deep dimples in the retinal nerve fiber layer (*arrows*) corresponding to the DONFL

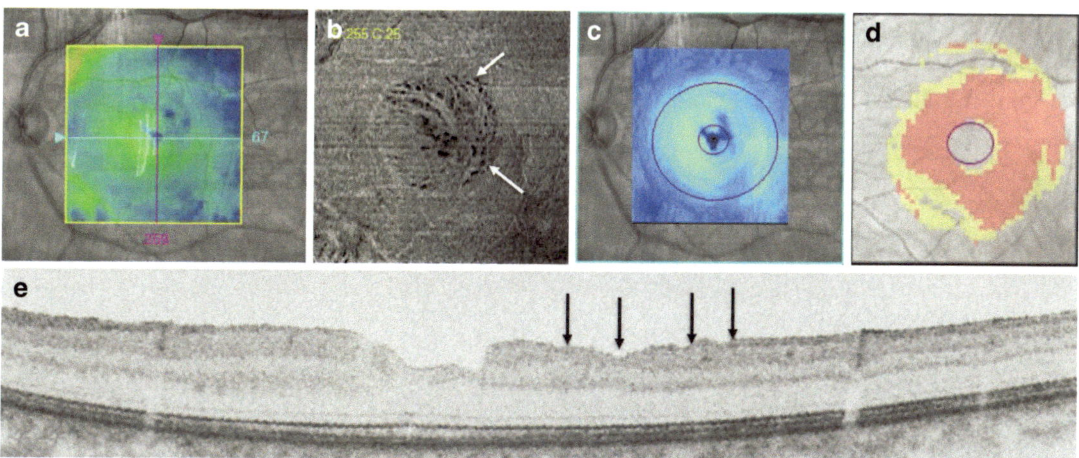

Fig. 20.27 Dissociated optic nerve fiber layer (DONFL) after surgical closure of a macular hole with internal limiting membrane (ILM) peeling. (**a**) OCT map showing the irregularities of the retinal surface. (**b**) En-face OCT image showing the fenestrations (*arrows*) in the retinal nerve fiber layer corresponding to the dimples seen in Figs. 20.20, 20.21, 20.22, 20.23, 20.24, 20.25, and 20.26. (**c**) Map of the ganglion cell thickness and (**d**) difference compared to normal in red, showing a decrease in ganglion cell layer thickness. (**e**) OCT B-scan showing the dimples in the retinal nerve fiber layer (*arrows*)

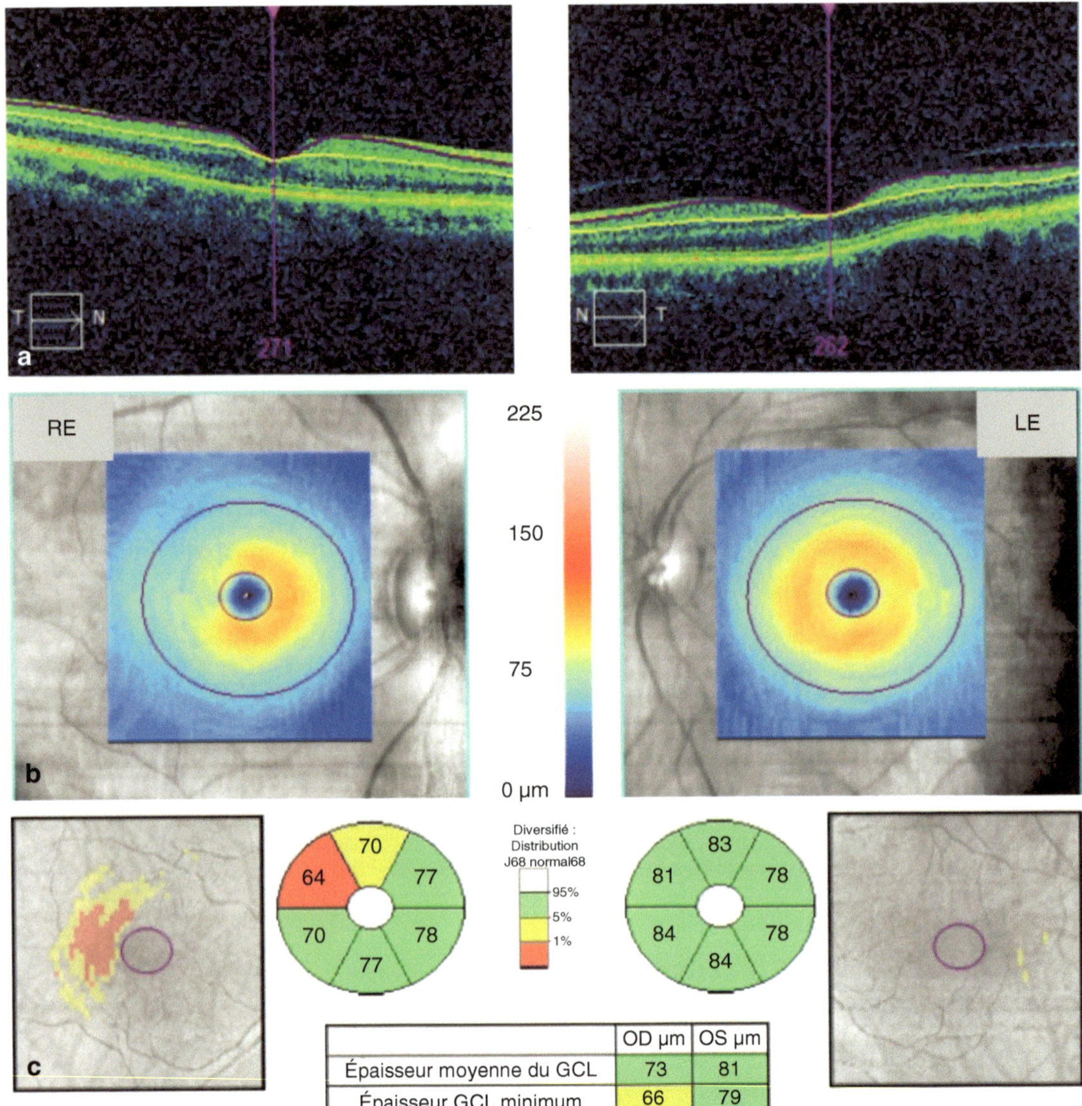

Fig. 20.28 Ganglion cell thinning after ILM peeling with brilliant blue G staining. (**a**) Horizontal SD-OCT B-scans showing the lines used to assess the retinal GCL-IPL thickness. Cell-inner plexiform layer (CIPL) thickness map showing a thinning at the superotemporal side of the fovea in the right eye (RE). (**b**) Retinal ganglion. (**c**) Deviation map to normative data and sector map showing the thinning of the retinal GCL-IPL in the superotemporal sector t (minus 64 µm) and the superior sector (minus 70 µm). Mean retinal GCL-IPL thickness is 73 µm in the RE versus 81 µm in the LE. Values are compared to normative data

References

Atmaca LS, Yilmaz M (1993) Changes in the fundus caused by blunt ocular trauma. Ann Ophthalmol 25:447–452

Baba T, Sato E, Oshitari T, et al (2014). "Regional reduction of ganglion cell complex after vitrectomy with internal limiting membrane peeling for idiopathic macular hole." J Ophthalmol 2014:372589

Barreau E, Massin P, Paques M, Santiago PY, Gaudric A (1997) Surgical treatment of post-traumatic macular holes. J Fr Ophtalmol 20:423–429

Blain P, Paques M, Massin P, Erginay A, Spielmann AC, Santiago PY, Gaudric A (1998) Epiretinal membranes surrounding idiopathic macular holes. Retina 18:316–321

Bottoni F, De Angelis S, Luccarelli S, et al (2011) The dynamic healing process of idiopathic macular holes after surgical repair: a spectral-domain optical coherence tomography study. Invest Ophthalmol Vis Sci 52:4439–46

Chang S (2012) Controversies regarding internal limiting membrane peeling in idiopathic epiretinal membrane and macular hole. Retina 32 Suppl 2:S200–S203; discussion S203–204. doi:10.1097/IAE.0b013e31825bc02b

Chang Y-C, Lin W-N, Chen K-J, et al (2015) Correlation Between the Dynamic Postoperative Visual Outcome and the Restoration of Foveal Microstructures After Macular Hole Surgery. Am J Ophthalmol 160:100–6

Cheng L, Freeman WR, Ozerdem U, Song MK, Azen SP (2000) Prevalence, correlates, and natural history of epiretinal membranes surrounding idiopathic macular holes. Virectomy for Macular Hole Study Group. Ophthalmol 107:853–859

Cheng L, Azen SP, El-Bradey MH, Toyoguchi M, Chaidhawangul S, Rivero ME, Scholz BM, Freeman WR (2002) Effects of preoperative and postoperative epiretinal membranes on macular hole closure and visual restoration. Ophthalmology 109:1514–1520

Compera D, Entchev E, Haritoglou C, Scheler R, Mayer WJ, Wolf A, Kampik A, Schumann RG (2015) Lamellar hole-associated epiretinal proliferation in comparison to epiretinal membranes of macular pseudoholes. Am J Ophthalmol 160:373–384 e371. doi:10.1016/j.ajo.2015.05.010

Coppe AM, Ripandelli G, Parisi V, Varano M, Stirpe M (2005) Prevalence of asymptomatic macular holes in highly myopic eyes. Ophthalmology 112:2103–2109

Duker JS, Kaiser PK, Binder S, de Smet MD, Gaudric A, Reichel E, Sadda SR, Sebag J, Spaide RF, Stalmans P (2013) The international vitreomacular traction study group classification of vitreomacular adhesion, traction, and macular hole. Ophthalmology 120:2611–2619

Ehlers JP, Dupps WJ, Kaiser PK, Goshe J, Singh RP, Petkovsek D, Srivastava SK (2014a) The Prospective Intraoperative and Perioperative Ophthalmic ImagiNg with Optical CoherEncE TomogRaphy (PIONEER) Study: 2-year results. Am J Ophthalmol 158:999–1007

Ehlers JP, Xu D, Kaiser PK, Singh RP, Srivastava SK (2014b) Intrasurgical dynamics of macular hole surgery: an assessment of surgery-induced ultrastructural alterations with intraoperative optical coherence tomography. Retina 34:213–221

Ezra E, Fariss RN, Possin DE, Aylward WG, Gregor ZJ, Luthert PJ, Milam AH (2001) Immunocytochemical characterization of macular hole opercula. Arch Ophthalmol 119:223–231

Fahim AT, Khan NW, Johnson MW (2014) Acute panretinal structural and functional abnormalities after intravitreous ocriplasmin injection. JAMA Ophthalmol 132:484–486

Frangieh GT, Green WR, Engel HM (1981) A histopathologic study of macular cysts and holes. Retina 1:311–336

Gass JD (1988) Idiopathic senile macular hole. Its early stages and pathogenesis. Arch Ophthalmol 106:629–639

Gass JD (1995) Reappraisal of biomicroscopic classification of stages of development of a macular hole. Am J Ophthalmol 119:752–759

Gaucher D, Haouchine B, Tadayoni R, Massin P, Erginay A, Benhamou N, Gaudric A (2007) Long-term follow-up of high myopic foveoschisis: natural course and surgical outcome. Am J Ophthalmol 143:455–462

Gaudric A, Haouchine B, Massin P, Paques M, Blain P, Erginay A (1999) Macular hole formation: new data provided by optical coherence tomography. Arch Ophthalmol 117:744–751

Gaudric A, Aloulou Y, Tadayoni R, Massin P (2013) Macular pseudoholes with lamellar cleavage of their edge remain pseudoholes. Am J Ophthalmol 155:733–742, 742 e731–734. doi:10.1016/j.ajo.2012.10.021

Haouchine B, Massin P, Gaudric A (2001) Foveal pseudocyst as the first step in macular hole formation: a prospective study by optical coherence tomography. Ophthalmology 108:15–22

Haouchine B, Massin P, Tadayoni R, Erginay A, Gaudric A (2004) Diagnosis of macular pseudoholes and lamellar macular holes by optical coherence tomography. Am J Ophthalmol 138:732–739

Hee MR, Puliafito CA, Wong C, Duker JS, Reichel E, Schuman JS, Swanson EA, Fujimoto JG (1995) Optical coherence tomography of macular holes. Ophthalmology 102:748–756

Ikuno Y, Sayanagi K, Ohji M, Kamei M, Gomi F, Harino S, Fujikado T, Tano Y (2004) Vitrectomy and internal limiting membrane peeling for myopic foveoschisis. Am J Ophthalmol 137:719–724

Ip MS, Baker BJ, Duker JS, Reichel E, Baumal CR, Gangnon R, Puliafito CA (2002) Anatomical outcomes of surgery for idiopathic macular hole as determined by optical coherence tomography. Arch Ophthalmol 120:29–35

Iriyama A, Uchida S, Yanagi Y, et al (2004). "Effects of indocyanine green on retinal ganglion cells." Invest Ophthalmol Vis Sci 45: 943–947

Iriyama A, Kadonosono K, Tamaki Y, et al (2012). "Effect of Brilliant Blue G on the retinal ganglion cells of rats." Retina 32: 613–616

Johnson MW (2010) Posterior vitreous detachment: evolution and complications of its early stages. Am J Ophthalmol 149:371–382–e371

Johnson MW (2012) Posterior vitreous detachment: evolution and role in macular disease. Retina 32 Suppl 2:S174–S178. doi:10.1097/IAE.0b013e318(b)ef62

Johnson RN, Gass JD (1988) Idiopathic macular holes. Observations, stages of formation, and implications for surgical intervention. Ophthalmology 95:917–924

Johnson MW, Fahim AT, Rao RC (2015) Acute ocriplasmin retinopathy. Retina 35:1055–1058

Kang SW, Lim JW, Chung SE, Yi C-H (2010) Outer foveolar defect after surgery for idiopathic macular hole. Am J Ophthalmol 150:551–7

Kawano H, Uemura A, Sakamoto T (2011) Incidence of outer foveal defect after macular hole surgery. Am J Ophthalmol 151:318–22.

Kishimoto H, Kusuhara S, Matsumiya W, Nagai T, Negi A (2011) Retinal surface imaging provided by Cirrus high-definition optical coherence tomography prominently visualizes a dissociated optic nerve fiber layer appearance after macular hole surgery. Int Ophthalmol 31:385–392

Ko TH, Witkin AJ, Fujimoto JG, et al (2006) Ultrahigh-resolution optical coherence tomography of surgically closed macular holes. Arch Ophthalmol 124:827–36.

Kumagai K, Hangai M, Larson E, Ogino N (2011) Vitreoretinal interface and foveal deformation in asymptomatic fellow eyes of patients with unilateral macular holes. Ophthalmology 118(8):1638–1644

Kusaka S, Fujikado T, Ikeda T, Tano Y (1997) Spontaneous disappearance of traumatic macular holes in young patients. Am J Ophthalmol 123:837–839

Ma F, Arcinue CA, Barteselli G, Cheng L, Ezon I, Lee SN, Freeman WR (2014) Optical coherence tomography findings of the vitreoretinal interface in asymptomatic fellow eyes of patients with acute posterior vitreous detachment. Retina 34:447–454

Michalewski J, Michalewska Z, Dziegielewski K, Nawrocki J (2011) Evolution from macular pseudohole to lamellar macular hole – spectral domain OCT study. Graefes Arch Clin Exp Ophthalmol 249:175–178

Pang CE, Freund KB, Engelbert M (2014) Enhanced vitreous imaging technique with spectral-domain optical coherence tomography for evaluation of posterior vitreous detachment. JAMA Ophthalmol 132:1148–1150

Pang CE, Spaide RF, Freund KB (2015) Comparing functional and morphologic characteristics of lamellar macular holes with and without lamellar hole-associated epiretinal proliferation. Retina 35:720–726

Parmar DN, Stanga PE, Reck AC, Vingerling JR, Sullivan P (1999) Imaging of a traumatic macular hole with spontaneous closure. Retina 19:470–472

Philippakis E, Amouyal F, Couturier A et al (2015) Size and vitreomacular attachment of full thickness macular hole. Invest Ophthalmol Vis Sci 56:1221

Privat E, Tadayoni R, Gaucher D, Haouchine B, Massin P, Gaudric A (2007) Residual defect in the foveal photoreceptor layer detected by optical coherence tomography in eyes with spontaneously closed macular holes. Am J Ophthalmol 143:814–819

Quezada-Ruiz C, Pieramici DJ, Nasir M, Rabena M, Steinle N, Castellarin AA, Dhoot D, Couvillion S, See RF, Avery RL (2015) Outer retina reflectivity changes on sd-oct after intravitreal ocriplasmin for vitreomacular traction and macular hole. Retina 35:1144–1150

Rahman R, Oxley L, Stephenson J (2013) Persistent outer retinal fluid following non-posturing surgery for idiopathic macular hole. Br J Ophthalmol 97:1451–4

Ray R, Baranano DE, Fortun JA, Schwent BJ, Cribbs BE, Bergstrom CS, Hubbard GB 3rd, Srivastava SK (2011) Intraoperative microscope-mounted spectral domain optical coherence tomography for evaluation of retinal anatomy during macular surgery. Ophthalmology 118:2212–2217

Sano M, Shimoda Y, Hashimoto H, Kishi S (2009) Restored photoreceptor outer segment and visual recovery after macular hole closure. Am J Ophthalmol 2147:313–8.

Schaal KB, Pang CE, Pozzoni MC, Engelbert M (2014) The premacular bursa's shape revealed in vivo by swept-source optical coherence tomography. Ophthalmology 121:1020–1028

Seo KH, Yu SY, Kwak HW (2015) "Topographic Changes in Macular Ganglion Cell-Inner Plexiform Layer Thickness after Vitrectomy with Indocyanine Green-Guided Internal Limiting Membrane Peeling for Idiopathic Macular Hole." Retina. 35:1828–35

Shakin JL, Yannuzzi LA (1987) Posterior segment manifestations of orbital trauma. Adv Ophthalmic Plast Reconstr Surg 6:115–135

Shinoda H, Shinoda K, Satofuka S et al (2008) "Visual recovery after vitrectomy for macular hole using 25-gauge instruments." Acta Ophthalmol 86:151–155

Shimada N, Ohno-Matsui K, Yoshida T, Sugamoto Y, Tokoro T, Mochizuki M (2008) Progression from macular retinoschisis to retinal detachment in highly myopic eyes is associated with outer lamellar hole formation. Br J Ophthalmol 92:762–764

Spaide RF (2012) "Dissociated optic nerve fiber layer appearance" after internal limiting membrane removal is inner retinal dimpling. Retina 32:1719–1726

Spaide RF, Fisher Y (2005) Removal of adherent cortical vitreous plaques without removing the internal limiting membrane in the repair of macular detachments in highly myopic eyes. Retina 25:290–295

Stalmans P, Benz MS, Gandorfer A, Kampik A, Girach A, Pakola S, Haller JA, Group M-TS (2012) Enzymatic vitreolysis with ocriplasmin for vitreomacular traction and macular holes. N Engl J Med 367:606–615

Staurenghi G, Sadda S, Chakravarthy U, Spaide RF, International Nomenclature for Optical Coherence Tomography P (2014) Proposed lexicon for anatomic landmarks in normal posterior segment spectral-domain optical coherence tomography: the IN*OCT consensus. Ophthalmology 121:1572–1578

Tadayoni R, Paques M, Massin P, Mouki-Benani S, Mikol J, Gaudric A (2001) Dissociated optic nerve fiber layer appearance of the fundus after idiopathic epiretinal membrane removal. Ophthalmology 108:2279–2283

Tadayoni R, Gaudric A, Haouchine B, Massin P (2006) Relationship between macular hole size and the potential benefit of internal limiting membrane peeling. Br J Ophthalmol 90:1239–1241

Tadayoni R, Creuzot-Garcher C, Korobelnik J-F, Le Mer Y, Massin P, Vicaut E, Gaudric A (2009) Internal limiting membrane peeling for large macular holes: a randomized, multicentric, and controlled clinical trial. Invest Ophthalmol Vis Sci 50:5206

Takahashi H, Kishi S (2000) Tomographic features of early macular hole closure after vitreous surgery. Am J Ophthalmol 130:192–6

Takahashi A, Nagaoka T, Ishiko S, Kameyama D, Yoshida A (2010) Foveal anatomic changes in a progressing stage 1 macular hole documented by spectral-domain optical coherence tomography. Ophthalmology 117:806–810

Takahashi A, Nagaoka T, Yoshida A (2011a) STAGE 1-A macular hole: a prospective spectral-domain optical coherence tomography study. Retina 31:127–147

Takahashi A, Yoshida A, Nagaoka T, Kagokawa H, Kato Y, Takamiya A, Sato E, Yokota H, Ishiko S, Hirokawa H (2011b) Macular hole formation in fellow eyes with a perifoveal posterior vitreous detachment of patients with a unilateral macular hole. Am J Ophthalmol 151(6):981–989.e4

Takano M, Kishi S (1999) Foveal retinoschisis and retinal detachment in severely myopic eyes with posterior staphyloma. Am J Ophthalmol 128:472–476

Uchino E, Uemura A, Ohba N (2001) Initial stages of posterior vitreous detachment in healthy eyes of older persons evaluated by optical coherence tomography. Arch Ophthalmol 119:1475–1479

Wakabayashi T, Fujiwara M, Sakaguchi H, et al (2010) Foveal microstructure and visual acuity in surgically closed macular holes: spectral-domain optical coherence tomographic analysis. Ophthalmology 117:1815–24

Wakely L, Rahman R, Stephenson J (2012) A comparison of several methods of macular hole measurement using optical coherence tomography, and their value in predicting anatomical and visual outcomes. Br J Ophthalmol 96:1003–1007

Xu D, Yuan A, Kaiser PK, Srivastava SK, Singh RP, Sears JE, Martin DF, Ehlers JP (2013) A novel segmentation algorithm for volumetric analysis of macular hole boundaries identified with optical coherence tomography. Invest Ophthalmol Vis Sci 54:163–169

Retinal Detachment

21

Ali Dirani and Thomas J. Wolfensberger

Contents

A. Dirani, MD • T.J. Wolfensberger, MD, MBA (✉)
Department of Ophthalmology, University of Lausanne, Hôpital Ophtalmique Jules Gonin, Lausanne, Switzerland
e-mail: thomas.wolfensberger@fa2.ch

21.1 Introduction

Although optical coherence tomography (OCT) was first introduced to investigate and characterize primarily macular diseases, clinical studies rapidly started to address the use of OCT in the diagnosis and management of retinal detachment. Before that time, the pre- and postoperative evaluation of the detached retina were entirely clinical, but even so, this yielded some useful data as early as 1937, when Algernon Reese hypothesized for the first time that poor postoperative visual acuity after retinal detachment repair may be related to the presence of a cystic macular degeneration as observed preoperatively in the detached macula (Reese 1937). What Reese could observe by ophthalmoscopy almost 80 years ago was eventually confirmed using OCT by looking at retinal detachments both pre- and postoperatively (Hagimura et al. 2002; Wolfensberger and Gonvers 2002). This chapter summarizes the current literature on the role of OCT in the diagnosis and the management of retinal detachment.

21.2 Clinical Evaluation of Preoperative Macular Microanatomy

Several tools have been proposed to evaluate macular microanatomy before and after surgery for macula-off retinal detachments. Clinical

C.H. Meyer et al. (eds.), *Spectral Domain Optical Coherence Tomography in Macular Diseases*, DOI 10.1007/978-81-322-3610-8_21

examination of the macula (direct and indirect ophthalmoscopy) remains an important and easily performed technique to ascertain macular integrity, and as Reese has showed, microanatomical details can be gleaned if ophthalmoscopy is performed with an expert's eye. Other clinical tools, which have been proposed to evaluate visual recovery, include the Amsler grid (Kreissig et al. 1981), contrast sensitivity, as well as color vision testing (Liem et al. 1994). Fundus reflection densitometry has also been employed by measuring macular photopigment density, which is an indirect indicator of photoreceptor-RPE complex recovery after surgery (Liem et al. 1994). However, since its discovery (Huang et al. 1991), OCT has superseded most of these investigational tools to establish itself as the gold standard for the rapid noncontact evaluation of the macula in retinal detachment patients (Hee et al. 1995). This novel technique is able to detect with precision both pre- and postoperative microanatomical changes such as preoperative intraretinal edema as well as clinically and angiographically silent subfoveal fluid accumulation (Hagimura et al. 2002; Wolfensberger and Gonvers 2002) and other microanatomical changes described below. These observations can help to characterize the retinal detachment and the prediction of visual acuity recovery (Hagimura et al. 2000).

21.3 Preoperative Optical Coherence Tomography Examination of Retinal Detachment

21.3.1 Macular Edema in Detached Macula

Macular edema in the detached retina has been implicated in limited visual recovery after macula-off retinal detachment for many years. Following on from the prescient report by Reese who described a cystic retinal degeneration in the detached macula of 12 eyes with simple macula-off retinal detachment, the advent of OCT has enabled a much more detailed look at these changes. Morphological changes such as retinal splitting and undulation of the outer retina have been reported in eyes with a highly detached macula, and these findings were associated with impaired postoperative visual recovery (Hagimura et al. 2002). The authors also showed that the presence of retinal separation or a wavy external layer before surgery is associated with an unfavorable final visual acuity. A further study which examined 16 patients with OCT preoperatively and 1, 6, and 10–12 months after buckle surgery for macula-off retinal detachment showed four categories of morphological macular changes (Fig. 21.1) including two categories of macular edema – one with an intact foveal depression and one without. There was a trend that the more edema was found in the detached macula, the worse postoperative visual acuity recovery was (Wolfensberger and Gonvers 2002). Although other authors later reported the absence of a correlation between the final postoperative visual acuity, the height of the retinal detachment, the extent of structural changes in the detached retina, and the preoperative distance from the central fovea to the nearest undetached retina on OCT (Lecleire-Collet et al. 2006) have been confirmed by several more recent studies to be important for visual recovery. Others have corroborated the previous findings that visual acuity 6 months after surgery was indeed worse for the eyes with preoperative edema of the outer nuclear layer than for the eyes with a normal retinal architecture before surgery (Matsui et al. 2013). In addition, preoperative visual acuity was also correlated with the existence of intraretinal separation (IRS) along with outer layer undulation (OLU) (Nakanishi et al. 2009).

21.3.2 Changes at Ellipsoid Zone

The preoperative microstructural changes (IRS and OLU) in the detached macula appeared to be negatively correlated with postoperative recovery of the photoreceptor layer (as assessed by Ellipsoid Zone (EZ) integrity and external limiting membrane (ELM) status). It was furthermore shown that a preoperative foveal loss of EZ in the region of the detached macula was

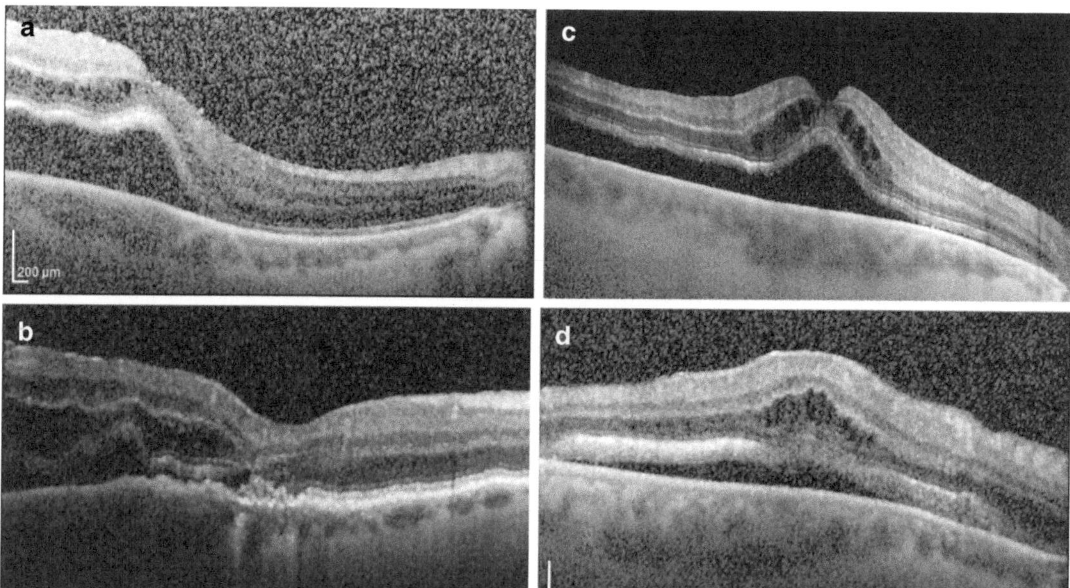

Fig. 21.1 Preoperative images of retinal detachment. (**a**) Class I: SD-OCT showing a detached macula with a retina of normal retinal and foveal thickness but the foveal depression is inverted. (**b**) Class II: SD-OCT showing a detached macula with relatively normal retinal thickness but with increasing loss of the foveal depression. (**c**) Class III: SD-OCT showing widespread edema in the external plexiform layer of the detached retina and a retained foveal depression. (**d**) Class IV: SD-OCT showing widespread retinal edema in the external plexiform layer with loss of the foveal depression

significantly correlated with poor postoperative visual acuity (Nakanishi et al. 2009), whereas others demonstrated that the mean postoperative best-corrected visual acuity in the eyes with photoreceptor layer abnormalities (disruption EZ) was significantly lower than in the eyes without photoreceptor layer alterations (Gharbiya et al. 2012).

21.3.3 Height of Macular Detachment

The height of macular detachment may also interfere with visual recovery in a negative way. In accordance with observations made on experimental models, in which photoreceptor degeneration increased with greater distance of the detached retina from the RPE (Machemer 1968), the extent of macular elevation has been shown to correlate with impaired functional recovery (Ross et al. 2005). More recent studies using OCT have however for the first time allowed objective and quantitative measurements of retinal detachment height. In a prospective study of 25 patients with macula-off retinal detachment, preoperative visual acuity was negatively affected by the height of the retinal detachment as measured by OCT (Hagimura et al. 2000).

Several other studies have also confirmed that the visual outcome becomes worse as the height of retinal detachment increases. Matsui and others have reported that the preoperative and 6-month postoperative visual acuity of eyes with a preoperative height of the retinal detachment ≥1000 μm were worse than the eyes with a preoperative height of the retinal detachment <1000 μm (Matsui et al. 2013; Joe et al. 2013). This observation can be explained by the fact that the greater the distance between the foveal cones and the RPE layer becomes, the less likely it is that the cones will receive adequate oxygenation and nutrition from the choriocapillaris and epithelial layer via diffusion across the subretinal space (Linsenmeier and Padnick-Silver 2000; Machemer 1968).

21.3.4 Duration of the Retinal Detachment

The exact duration of retinal detachment and its potential impact on visual acuity recovery has for decades remained a matter of debate (Burton 1982; Reese 1937). In a large retrospective study, which included several hundred patients, a maximal delay of 5 days for retinal detachment repair was determined adequate clinically without incurring undue risks for visual acuity recovery. A more recent large prospective study of 100 cases with macula-off retinal detachment compared three groups of patients operated between 1 and 2 days, 3 and 4 days, and 5 and 7 days after macular detachment, with a mean follow-up of 10.5 months, but no statistical difference in visual recovery between groups was found (Ross et al. 2005). Using OCT more detailed information has recently become available showing that an increase in duration of the macula-off retinal detachment was significantly associated with reduced postoperative restoration of the IS/OS and the external limiting membrane (ELM). Some preoperative variables (intraretinal separation and outer layer undulation) were not significantly associated with duration of the macular detachment but with the height of the detached macula (Joe et al. 2013).

21.4 Preoperative Optical Coherence Tomography Examination of Retinal Detachment

Very recently an experimental intraoperative OCT device has been investigated, which allows to obtain intraoperative OCT images (Binder et al. 2011). This novel technique could be potentially useful in the intraoperative evaluation of the detached macula in case of vitreous hemorrhage or other vitreous opacities which preclude a detailed preoperative evaluation of the detached macula. Intraoperative OCT could also help in the differentiation between a large macular cyst and a macular hole in the detached macula, which would directly influence the surgical management (Ehlers et al. 2013).

21.5 Postoperative Optical Coherence Tomography Examination of Retinal Detachment

21.5.1 Surgical Technique Influencing Postoperative Retinal Anatomy on Optical Coherence Tomography

The choice for the use of a specific surgical technique for retinal detachments is in general dictated by the type and severity of the retinal detachment to ensure optimal anatomical and functional outcome. It has thus come with some surprise that a recent report using OCT has found that the incidence of postoperative residual subretinal fluid affecting the macular region varies after different surgical techniques. Residual fluid accumulation is significantly higher after scleral buckling with a residual macular detachment occurring in 63 % after transscleral surgery and only in 13 % after vitrectomy (Kambara et al. 2000). Looking at the long-term evolution of this fluid, it was shown that there is an incidence of subretinal fluid in 69 % at 1 month, 50 % at 3 months, and 13 % at 12 months follow-up (Wolfensberger and Gonvers 2002) (Fig. 21.2). However, when looking at patients who had been operated on using vitrectomy, cryotherapy, and fluid-gas exchange, no postoperative persistent subretinal fluid as evaluated by OCT at 1 month after surgery was observed (Wolfensberger 2004). The order of this relationship was also confirmed in two larger studies using both pars plana vitrectomy (Benson et al. 2006) and episcleral buckle surgery (Benson et al. 2007) whereby the subfoveal fluid accumulation occurred in 15 % after vitrectomy and in 55 % after buckle surgery at 6 weeks follow-up. In the most recent study on the subject, postoperative subretinal fluid was noted in 86 % after scleral buckling versus 33 % after vitrectomy at 3 months postoperatively (Matsui et al. 2013). This difference is very likely to be explained by the fact that during vitrectomy, the subretinal space is inadvertently washed out by the continuous flow through the infusion line if the retinal breaks are

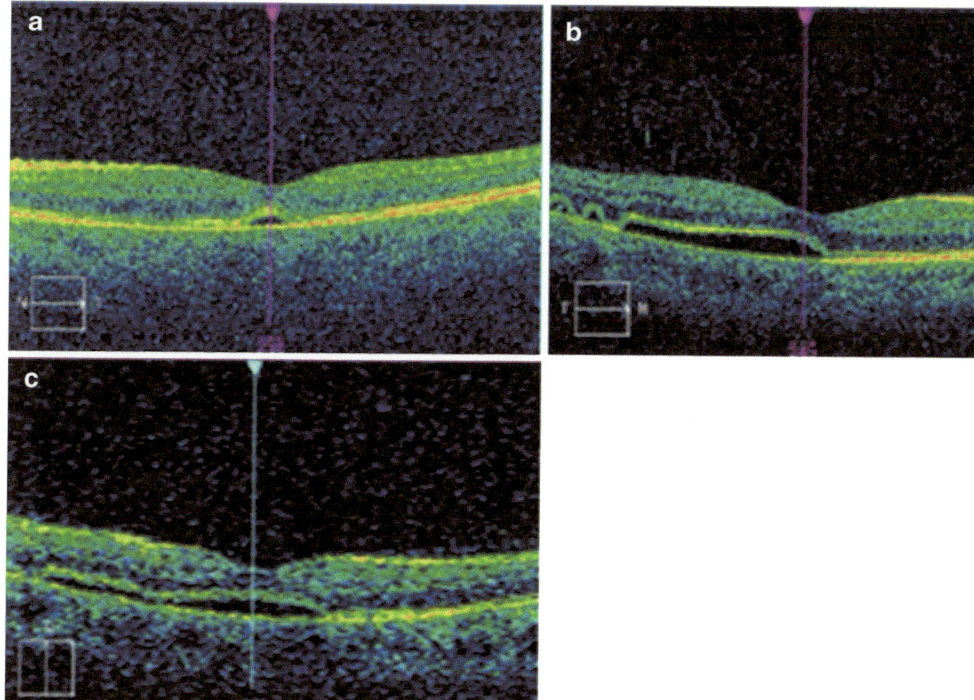

Fig. 21.2 Postoperative images of retinal detachment. (**a**) SD-OCT showing persistent single subretinal foveal bleb at 6 months in a patient successfully treated for a retinal detachment with pars plana vitrectomy. (**b**) SD-OCT showing persistent multiple subretinal foveal blebs at 3 months in a patient successfully treated for a retinal detachment with vitrectomy. (**c**) SD-OCT showing persistent flat subretinal fluid at 3 months in a patient successfully treated for a retinal detachment with vitrectomy

of sufficient size. Simple transscleral drainage of subretinal fluid will always leave a narrow slither of potentially viscous subretinal fluid, which will take a long time to resolve (Veckeneer et al. 2012).

21.5.2 Postoperative Factors

It has been known for many decades that several gross macular abnormalities, such as cystoid macular edema, epiretinal membrane formation, retinal folds, and pigment migration, can occur after successful surgery for retinal. In some cases, no clinically detected macular changes are however observed, and the reduced postoperative VA remained unexplained. With the advent of OCT, many of these cases could be related to clinically silent modification of macular area, which are described below.

21.5.2.1 Cystoid Macular Edema

Although cystoid macular edema appeared historically to be a frequent postoperative macular complication, which was correlated with partial visual recovery after retinal surgery (Sabates et al. 1989), it disappears spontaneously in the majority of cases (Bonnet et al. 1983). More recent OCT-guided investigations have not confirmed an important role of classic cystoid macular edema in the postoperative phase after retinal detachment (Wolfensberger and Gonvers 2002).

21.5.2.2 Retention of Subretinal Fluid

Subretinal fluid retention after macula-off retinal detachment can occur in two different types of pattern. The most common appearance is a small subfoveal bleb, which has been reported by several authors using postoperative OCT examination. It appears that prolonged fluid retention for more than 3 months after retinal detachment surgery may be one of the causes of delayed restoration of visual acuity (Hagimura et al. 2002; Wolfensberger and Gonvers 2002; Lecleire-Collet et al. 2005; Matsui et al. 2013). On the other hand, other authors have indicated that subretinal fluid finally resolved at 1 year without influencing final visual acuity in 44 eyes after successful scleral buckling for acute macula-off rhegmatogenous retinal detachment (Soe et al. 2008; Delome et al 2012). These fluid blebs may also appear in multiple clusters, which have been linked to intraoperative reattachment of the retina (Kim et al. 2004).

The less common pattern of subretinal fluid accumulation is a diffuse layer of fluid under the macula, which is usually linked to highly myopic eyes in young patients with long-standing asymptomatic inferior retinal detachment (Abouzeid et al. 2009). This fluid may linger for many months despite intraoperative transscleral drainage during buckle surgery (Fig. 21.3). Looking at the long-term evolution of this fluid, it was shown that there is an incidence of diffuse accumulation in 12 % at 1 month, 6 % at 3 months, and total disappearance at 12 months follow-up (Wolfensberger and Gonvers 2002).

21.5.2.3 Postoperative Foveal Thickness

Decreased postoperative foveal thickness as measured with OCT has been implicated as a factor for reduced visual acuity recovery in a study following patients with both macula-on and macula-off retinal detachments. However, the correlation between the reduced postoperative ONL thickness and postoperative best-corrected visual acuity was lower in the macula-off group suggesting that the visual acuity is primarily related to the preoperative state of the macula which leads to a higher chance of cone cell loss and subsequent ONL thickness decrease (Gharbiya et al. 2012). A direct analysis of the central foveal thickness failed to demonstrate a correlation with visual acuity outcome in successfully repaired retinal detachments (Wakabayashi et al. 2009).

21.5.2.4 Postoperative Foveal Microstructure

Apart from the persistent subretinal fluid accumulation, the discontinued Ellipsoid Zone (EZ) is the most frequent lesion seen in the eyes operated for macula-off retinal detachments. In several studies, it was found in 40–82 % of patients, and it was described as a marker for poor visual prognosis (Fig. 21.4) (Lai et al. 2010; Nakanishi et al. 2009; Shimoda et al. 2010; Smith et al. 2008; Wakabayashi et al. 2009). It has been reported that the presence of one or more abnormalities among the ELM and the EZ was correlated with poor postoperative visual acuity (Lai et al. 2010). Others have shown that IS/OS lesions were detected in 53.3 % of the eyes, lesions which were not significantly correlated with visual recovery but rather with low macular sensitivity and reduced photoreceptor outer segment thickness (Delome et al. 2012). Furthermore, it was noted that a disrupted EZ was present in 43 % of 51 macula-off eyes and that the integrity of both the ELM and the EZ was significantly associated with better visual outcome (Wakabayashi et al.

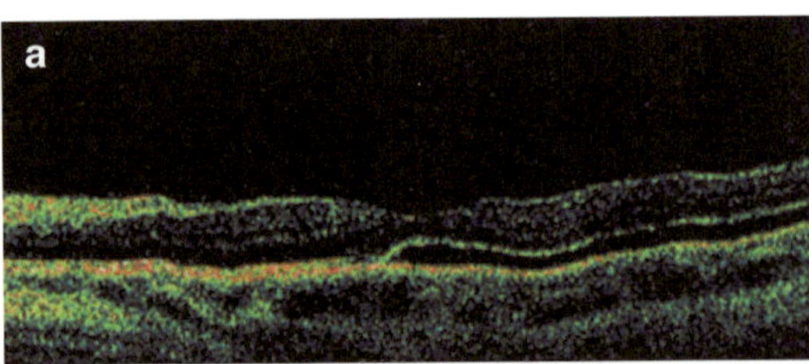

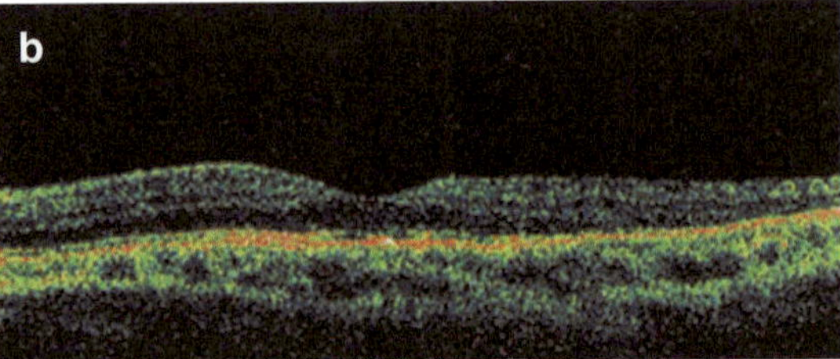

Fig. 21.3 Retinal detachment treated with buckle surgery and external fluid drainage. (**a**) SD-OCT of a young patient, 1 month after inferior retinal detachment treated with buckle surgery and external fluid drainage, shows a diffuse shallow elevation of the retina. (**b**) SD-OCT shows final complete reattachment of the fovea at 17 months after surgery; the attachment occurred between 6 and 9 months after surgery (Reproduced from Abouzeid et al. (2009), with permission of Acta Scandinavica)

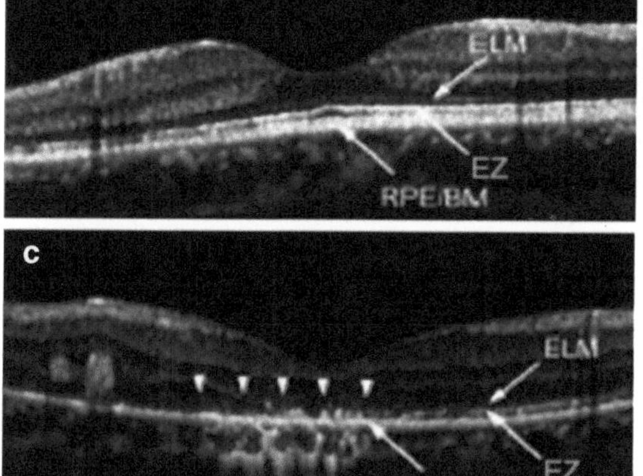

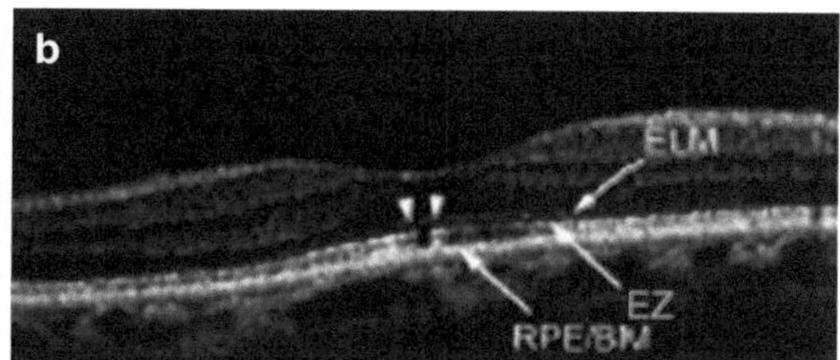

Fig. 21.4 Patterns of the photoreceptor and ellipsoid zone after rhegmatogenous retinal detachment repair. (**a**) SD-OCT shows an intact ellipsoid zone (EZ) and external limiting membrane (ELM) obtained from a 23-year-old man 19.5 months after macula-off RRD repair. The visual acuity (VA) is 20/12.5. (**b**) SD-OCT shows an OCT image with disruption (*arrowheads*) of the EZ junction at the fovea. The ELM is preserved. The image is from a 67-year-old woman 22.5 months after macula-off RRD repair. The VA is 20/50. (**c**) SD-OCT shows an image obtained from a 28-year-old man 25 months after macula-off RRD repair; it shows disruption of both the EZ junction and ELM at the fovea (*arrowheads*). The VA is 20/67. *RPE/BM* retinal pigment epithelium/Bruch's membrane (Reproduced from Wakabayashi et al. (2009), with permission of Ophthalmology)

2009). It has also been suggested that the improvement of vision after reattachment of the retina was correlated with a decrease of EZ disruption and that the resolution of ELM disruption was a prerequisite for restoration of the EZ (Kawashima et al. 2011). These findings were confirmed by others, who showed that visual acuity at 6 months postoperatively was better if there was EZ continuity at both 3 and 6 months after surgery compared to if this was not the case. In addition, the rate of achieving EZ continuity was higher, and the visual acuity 6 months postoperatively was better in the eyes, which had developed ELM continuity 3 months after surgery (Matsui et al. 2013; Shimoda et al. 2010). A more detailed analysis of the ELM and the EZ revealed eyes with photoreceptor layer disruption ≥200 μm had a significantly worse postoperative best-corrected visual acuity than those who presented less extensive disruptions ≤200 μm. Multivariate analysis showed that the outer nuclear layer thickness and the status of the intermediate line were the most important predictors of visual outcome (Gharbiya et al. 2012). The preoperative microstructural changes (IRS and OLU) in the detached macula also appeared to be negatively correlated with postoperative recovery of the photoreceptor layer [as assessed by the EZ integrity and external limiting membrane (ELM) status] in a reattached macula (Joe et al. 2013).

Conclusion

The advent of OCT and its use in the pre-, intra- and postoperative phase has brought a new dimension to the diagnosis and management of retinal detachment. The main preoperative advantage of this novel technology is to classify the amount of microanatomical changes in the detached retina and to use this information for the prediction of visual acuity recovery. Intraoperative OCT can potentially be used to make an OCT-based assessment of the detached macula in the case of preoperative vitreous hemorrhage or other major opacities, and it may help to make surgical decisions concerning the status of the macula and ensuing potential surgical maneuvers. The postoperative evaluation of the macula can again shed a lot of light on the microanatomical status of the different retinal layers, in particular the ELM and the EZ junction. The combination of these OCT findings will help us in determining their influence on postoperative visual recovery.

Despite this progress, there will still be patients in the future who show limited visual recovery in whom none of the described OCT changes can be seen. Further development of OCT resolution may be useful in the future, but also the recent advent of novel imaging technology such as adaptive optics could potentially help us in analyzing changes at the cellular level such as the density of remaining cones (Saleh et al. 2014). Finally, in addition to microanatomical changes, which can be evaluated with OCT, we should also consider that damaged macula may have undergone molecular and biochemical changes which cannot be detected with conventional investigational methods. These changes will only be unmasked when newer molecular assays reflecting sublethal cellular suffering will be available for clinical use.

References

Abouzeid H, Becker K, Holz FG et al (2009) Submacular fluid after encircling buckle surgery for inferior macula-off retinal detachment in young patients. Acta Ophthalmol 87:96–99

Benson SE, Schlottmann PG, Bunce C et al (2006) Optical coherence tomography analysis of the macula after vitrectomy surgery for retinal detachment. Ophthalmology 113:1179–1183

Benson SE, Schlottmann PG, Bunce C et al (2007) Optical coherence tomography analysis of the macula after scleral buckle surgery for retinal detachment. Ophthalmology 114:108–112

Binder S, Falkner-Radler C, Hauger C et al (2011) Feasibility of intrasurgical spectral-domain optical coherence tomography. Retina 31:1332–1336

Bonnet M, Bievelez B, Noel A et al (1983) Fluorescein angiography after retinal detachment microsurgery. Graefes Arch Clin Exp Ophthalmol 221:35–40

Burton TC (1982) Recovery of visual acuity after retinal detachment involving the macula. Trans Am Ophthalmol Soc 80:475–497

Delome MP, Dugas B, Nicot F et al (2012) Anatomical and functional macular changes after rhegmatogenous retinal detachment with macula off. Am J Ophthalmol 153:128–136

Ehlers JP, Ohr MP, Kaiser PK et al (2013) Novel microarchitectural dynamics in rhegmatogenous retinal detachments identified with intraoperative optical coherence tomography. Retina 33:1428–1434

Gharbiya M, Grandinetti F, Scavella V et al (2012) Correlation between spectral domain optical coherence tomography findings and visual outcome after primary rhegmatogenous retinal detachment repair. Retina 32:43–53

Hagimura N, Suto K, Iida T et al (2000) Optical coherence tomography of the neurosensory retina in rhegmatogenous retinal detachment. Am J Ophthalmol 129:186–190

Hagimura N, Iida T, Suto K et al (2002) Persistent foveal retinal detachment after successful rhegmatogenous retinal detachment surgery. Am J Ophthalmol 133:516–520

Hee MR, Izatt JA, Swanson EA et al (1995) Optical coherence tomography of the human retina. Arch Ophthalmol 113:325–332

Huang D, Swanson EA, Lin CP et al (1991) Optical coherence tomography. Science 254:1178–1181

Joe SG, Kim YJ, Chae JB et al (2013) Structural recovery of the detached macula after retinal detachment repair as assessed by optical coherence tomography. Korean J Ophthalmol 27:178–185

Kambara C, Inoda S, Shimizu Y et al (2000) Optical coherence tomographic features after surgery for rhegmatogenous retinal detachment with macular involvement. Jpn J Clini Ophthalmol 3:327–330

Kawashima H, Mizukawa K, Watanabe I et al (2011) Evaluation of recovery process of photoreceptor outer segment after retinal detachment repair. Nippon Ganka Gakkai Zasshi 115:374–381

Kim YK, Ahn J, Woo SJ et al (2004) Multiple subretinal fluid blebs after successful retinal detachment surgery: incidence, risk factors, and presumed pathophysiology. Am J Ophthalmol 157:834–841

Kreissig I, Lincoff H, Witassek B et al (1981) Colour vision and other parameters of macular function after retinal reattachment. Dev Ophthalmol 2:77–85

Lai WW, Leung GY, Chan CW et al (2010) Simultaneous spectral domain OCT and fundus autofluorescence imaging of the macula and microperimetric correspondence after successful repair of rhegmatogenous retinal detachment. Br J Ophthalmol 94:311–318

Lecleire-Collet A, Muraine M, Ménard JF et al (2005) Predictive visual outcome after macula-off retinal detachment surgery using optical coherence tomography. Retina 25(1):44–53

Lecleire-Collet A, Muraine M, Ménard JF et al (2006) Evaluation of macular changes before and after successful retinal detachment surgery using stratus optical coherence tomography. Am J Ophthalmol 142:176–179

Liem ATA, Keunen JEE, van Meel GJ et al (1994) Serial foveal densitometry and visual function after RD surgery with macular involvement. Ophthalmology 101:1945–1952

Linsenmeier RA, Padnick-Silver L (2000) Metabolic dependence of photoreceptors on the choroid in the normal and detached retina. Invest Ophthalmol Vis Sci 41:3117–3123

Machemer R (1968) Experimental RD in the owl monkey. II. Histology of retina and pigment epithelium. Am J Ophthalmol 66:396–410

Matsui A, Toshida H, Honda R et al (2013) Preoperative and postoperative optical coherence tomography findings in patients with rhegmatogenous retinal detachment involving the macular region. ISRN Ophthalmol. doi:10.1155/2013/426867

Nakanishi H, Hangai M, Unoki N et al (2009) Spectral-domain optical coherence tomography imaging of the detached macula in rhegmatogenous retinal detachment. Retina 29:232–242

Reese AB (1937) Defective central vision following successful operations for detachment of the retina. Am J Ophthalmol 20:591–598

Ross W, Lavina A, Russell M et al (2005) The correlation between height of macular detachment and visual outcome in macula-off retinal detachments of<or=7 days' duration. Ophthalmology 112:1213–1217

Sabates NR, Sabates FN, Sabates R et al (1989) Macular changes after retinal detachment surgery. Am J Ophthalmol 108:22–29

Saleh M, Debellemanière G, Meillat M et al (2014) Quantification of cone loss after surgery for retinal detachment involving the macula using adaptive optics. Br J Ophthalmol 98:1343–1348

Shimoda Y, Sano M, Hashimoto H et al (2010) Restoration of photoreceptor outer segment after vitrectomy for retinal detachment. Am J Ophthalmol 149:284–290

Smith AJ, Telander DG, Zawadzki RJ et al (2008) High-resolution Fourier-domain optical coherence tomography and microperimetric findings after macula-off retinal detachment repair. Ophthalmology 115:1923–1929

Soe JH, Woo JS, Park KH et al (2008) Influence of persistent submacular fluid on visual outcome after successful scleral buckle surgery for macula-off retinal detachment. Am J Ophthalmol 145:915–922

Veckeneer M, Derycker L, Lindstedt EW et al (2012) Persistent subretinal fluid after surgery for rhegmatogenous retinal detachment: hypothesis and review. Graefes Arch Clin Exp Ophthalmol 250:795–802

Wakabayashi T, Oshima Y, Fujimoto H et al (2009) Foveal microstructure and visual acuity after retinal detachment repair: imaging analysis by Fourier-domain optical coherence tomography. Ophthalmology 116:519–528

Wolfensberger TJ (2004) Foveal reattachment after macula-off retinal detachment occurs faster after vitrectomy than after buckle surgery. Ophthalmology 111:1340–1343

Wolfensberger TJ, Gonvers M (2002) Optical coherence tomography in the evaluation of incomplete visual acuity recovery after macula-off retinal detachments. Graefe's Arch Clin Exp Ophthalmol 240:85–89

22 Myopic Macular Pathologies

Yasushi Ikuno

Contents

Y. Ikuno, MD
Department of Ophthalmology,
Osaka University Medical School, Osaka, Japan
e-mail: ikuno@ophthal.med.osaka-u.ac.jp

22.1 Introduction

Pathological myopia, characterized by elongation of the axial length, is a common cause of social blindness worldwide, especially in East Asian countries. The incidence of high myopia is 5.5 % (>−6.0 diopters [D]) in Japan (Sawada et al. 2008) and 3.3 % (<−5.0D) in China (Xu et al. 2007). Pathological myopia causes various kinds of macular diseases including macular holes with or without retinal detachment, myopic foveoschisis, choroidal neovascularization (CNV), and chorioretinal atrophy.

Diagnosing these pathologies was extremely challenging before the advent of optical coherence tomography (OCT), because the atrophic fundus reduces the contrast during the fundus examination. For instance, previously the presence of a persistent macular hole postoperatively was uncertain; however, OCT identified a very low rate of anatomic success (Ikuno et al. 2003). OCT is not simply a diagnostic tool but also a research modality in micropathology. Thus, OCT is contributing greatly to advancing retinal practice in high myopia in several ways.

However, time-domain OCT was not a good modality for evaluating myopia because of signal attenuation. It was often stressful for examiners to obtain clear images. Spectral-domain (SD) OCT has a much higher scanning speed and provides higher-resolution and improved images. SD-OCT makes it possible to see more detailed architecture

C.H. Meyer et al. (eds.), *Spectral Domain Optical Coherence Tomography in Macular Diseases*,
DOI 10.1007/978-81-322-3610-8_22

in these eyes. This chapter provides the background information on myopic macular diseases including clinical manifestations and pathogenesis, and SD-OCT images are presented and discussed.

22.2 Basic Principles of Optical Coherence Tomography in High Myopia

Pathological myopia is characterized by axial length elongation, and OCT shows several differences between pathological myopia and non-myopic eyes. The light path courses a long distance inside the eye, which attenuates the OCT signal from the fundus. Highly myopic eyes often have a subtle cataract or corneal opacification. The curve of the eye wall is steep posteriorly, and the edge of the OCT image often fall offs or is inverted (Fig. 22.1). Generally, it is difficult to obtain an entire scan in the desired direction in an image. SD-OCT is known to have theoretical signal decay. Normally, the signal is attenuated at the bottom of the images, and thus the area of interest must be located in the middle to the upper half of the image.

Because of relatively small pathology and unstable fixation, multiple scans are recommended for better screening using SD-OCT. We investigated 21 eyes using both a five-line raster scan and a three-dimensional scan at the same visit and compared the detection rate (Sayanagi et al. 2010). The three-dimensional scanning mode of SD-OCT tended to be superior to both the one- and five-line raster scanning modes for detecting the inner and outer segments, epiretinal membranes (ERMs), macular holes, paravascular microholes, and internal limiting membranes (ILMs). Thus, the three-dimensional scan mode of SD-OCT must be checked when small pathology is suspected in highly myopic eyes.

22.3 Choroid/Scleral Thinning and Posterior Staphyloma

Posterior eye wall stretching causes choroidal and scleral tissue thinning in highly myopic eyes. The foveal thickness is similar to that in emmetropic eyes; however, the choroid and the sclera are extremely thin (Fig. 22.2). The average thickness of the subfoveal choroid in emmetropic eyes

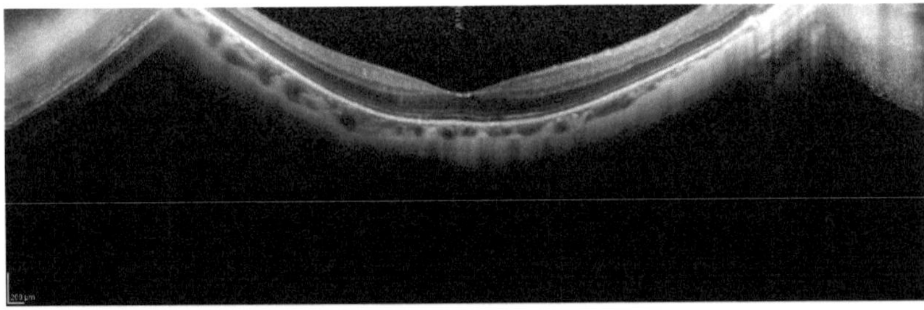

Fig. 22.1 Myopic staphyloma. SD-OCT showing deep posterior staphyloma. Both edges of the structure are inverted and delineated as an inverted image

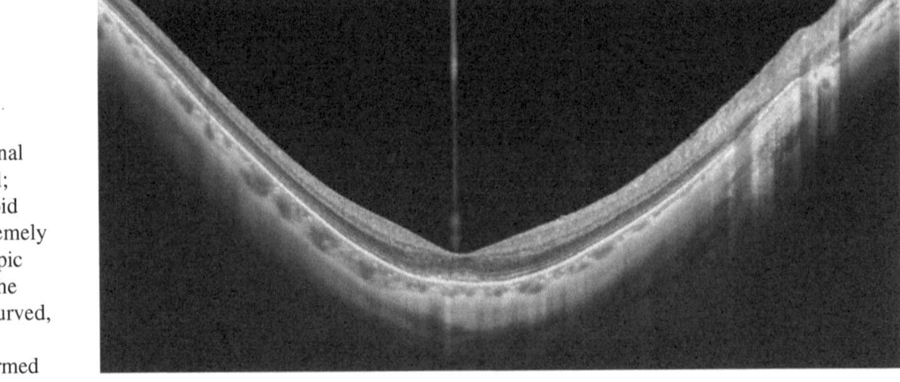

Fig. 22.2 The retinal thickness is normal; however, the choroid and sclera are extremely thin in highly myopic eyes. In addition, the wall is markedly curved, and a posterior staphyloma has formed

is about 287 μm (Margolis and Spaide 2009) while that in highly myopic eyes is about 100 μm (Ikuno and Tano 2009). The choroidal thickness is associated significantly with the axial length or refractive error and age. The subfoveal, inferior, and nasal areas are relatively thinner than the superior and temporal areas around the fovea (Ikuno and Tano 2009). The sclera is also 200–300 μm thick in highly myopic eyes (Maruko et al. 2012).

Axial length elongation does not simply promote expansion of the eye wall of the entire globe but disproportional scleral protrusion, also called posterior staphyloma. There are wide variations in the shapes of posterior staphylomas. Curtin (1977) classified the shapes into ten types depending on the area and location of the protrusion. Posterior staphylomas normally are delineated as U shaped on OCT when the macula is centered. However, there are some exceptional shapes when the optic nerve head is more posterior than the macula. The presence of posterior staphylomas makes it difficult to focus the OCT image on the location of interest because of the signal decay in SD-OCT.

22.4 Myopic Foveoschisis

22.4.1 Pathogenesis

Myopic foveoschisis is characterized by retinoschisis and subsequent retinal detachment specific to highly myopic eyes. Myopic foveoschisis was first described in the 1950s (Phillips 1958) and was so common as to be found in 10 of 32 highly myopic eyes (Takano and Kishi 1999). However, this pathology is challenging to diagnose correctly without OCT. Myopic foveoschisis is substantially a tractional disease that is generated from various components. The vitreous cortex is one causes of the inward retinal traction. ERMs often develop and also generate traction. The rigidity of ILMs and the retinal vascular traction are unique and both are new idea of pathogeneses. ILM detachment from the other retinal layer often is observed on OCT images (Sayanagi et al. 2006) (Fig. 22.3). This indicates that the ILM is less flexible than the other retinal layers and exerts inward traction on those layers. Retinal vascular traction is postulated based on a unique OCT finding, i.e., retinal microfolds (Ikuno et al. 2005; Sayanagi et al. 2005). The retinal microfolds appear on OCT images as small peaks in the inner retina and are typical findings after vitrectomy performed to treat myopic foveoschisis (Fig. 22.4). The retinal vessels, especially the retinal arterioles, are less flexible and cannot be stretched as much as the other retinal components. Thus, myopic foveoschisis is caused by multiple factors and can be regarded as a split between the flexible outer retina and the inflexible inner retina.

22.4.2 Natural Course

OCT has demonstrated a more detailed mechanism related to myopic foveoschisis. Myopic foveoschisis starts with retinoschisis but ultimately leads to a macular hole via a

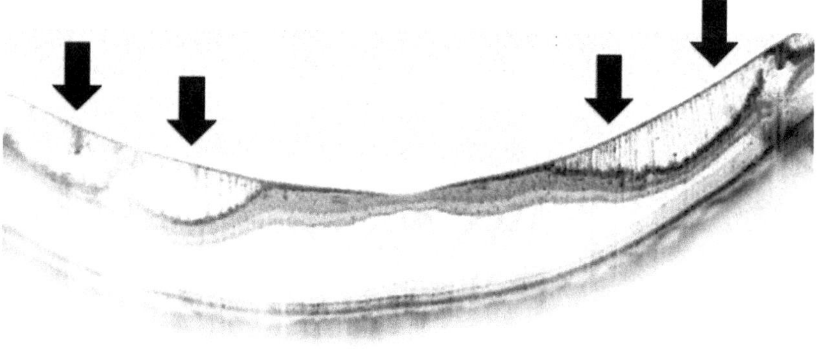

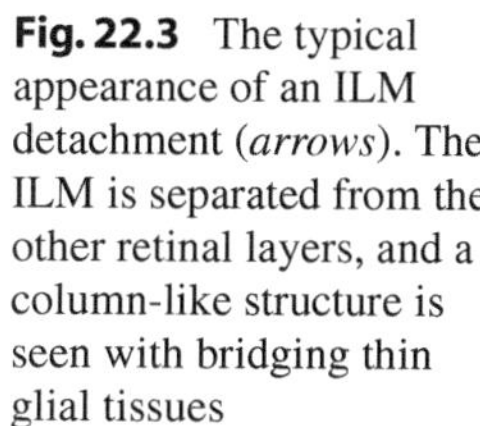

Fig. 22.3 The typical appearance of an ILM detachment (*arrows*). The ILM is separated from the other retinal layers, and a column-like structure is seen with bridging thin glial tissues

focal retinal detachment (Ikuno et al. 2008). The natural course of myopic foveoschisis is poor (Gaucher et al. 2007; Shimada et al. 2013), and 11–50 % of patients have a retinal detachment and/or macular hole formation within 2–3 years of follow-up without treatment. The high risk of severe visual loss from macular holes with retinal detachments is a surgical indication.

22.4.3 Clinical Manifestations and Diagnosis

Myopic foveoschisis occurs mainly in middle-aged to older women. OCT shows various appearances of myopic foveoschisis including lamellar holes and retinal cysts (Benhamou et al. 2002). Myopic foveoschisis begins as retinoschisis without a retinal detachment, i.e., the retinoschisis type. A retinal detachment can start at the fovea after several months or years if there is sufficient traction, i.e., the foveal detachment type (Fig. 22.5) (Ikuno et al. 2008).

22.4.4 Treatment

Vitrectomy is the most common treatment for myopic foveoschisis (Ishikawa et al. 2001; Kobayashi and Kishi 2003; Ikuno et al. 2004). The surgical goal is release of all retinal traction in order to reattach and reconstruct the normal structure. There are several subtypes; however, the subtypes with the best surgical indications are controversial. We investigated the surgical results and found that eyes with a foveal detachment are good surgical candidates for visual improvement (Ikuno et al. 2008). Other investigators also have reported that a foveal detachment is a positive predictive factor for favorable visual outcomes (Kumagai et al. 2010). However, there is no consensus about the surgical indication, and any type of pathology can be an indication for surgery. The ILM

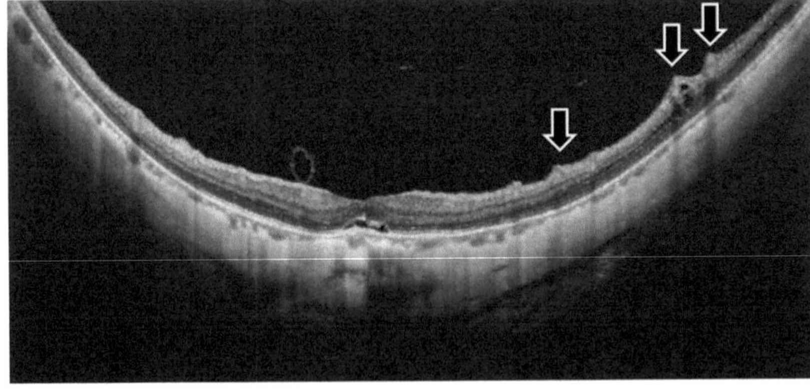

Fig. 22.4 The typical appearance of a vascular microfold after vitrectomy for myopic foveoschisis (*arrows*). The arterioles are elevated because of vascular traction and appear as a tent-like shape on an OCT image

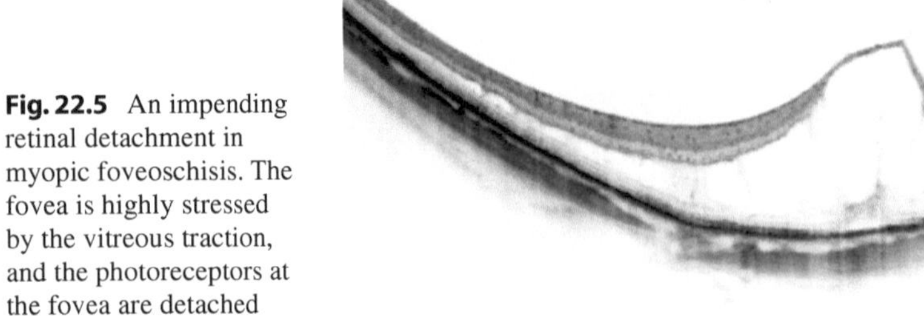

Fig. 22.5 An impending retinal detachment in myopic foveoschisis. The fovea is highly stressed by the vitreous traction, and the photoreceptors at the fovea are detached

is peeled and injecting a vital dye and gas tamponade are performed frequently to enhance retinal reattachment.

22.4.5 Outcome

The recovery of visual functional is correlated highly with the OCT findings (Fig. 22.6). We investigated the SD-OCT appearance of 17 eyes with myopic foveoschisis and in relation to visual acuity (VA) (Fujimoto et al. 2013). The mean preoperative central foveal thickness was 470.8 μm. The mean postoperative retinal thicknesses decreased significantly and were 310.4 μm at 1 month, 251.8 μm at 3 months, 218.2 μm at 6 months, and 218.7 μm at 12 months. The preoperative best-corrected VA (BCVA), final integrity of the inner segment/outer segment (IS/OS) junction, and the external limiting membrane (ELM) were associated significantly with the final BCVA. Interestingly, the integrity of the IS/OS and ELM lines were attenuated at 1 month and then started to improve in most cases. This behavior was associated with the mean VA, which decreased temporarily 1 month postoperatively.

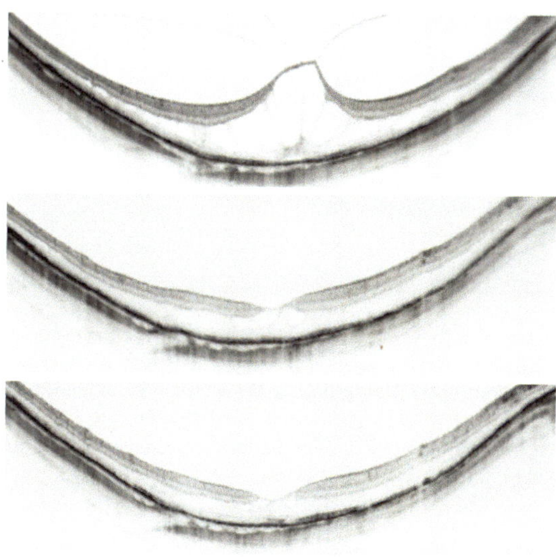

Fig. 22.6 OCT images of the case in Fig. 22.5 (*top*) that was treated successfully by vitrectomy. The retina reattached slowly after 1 month (*middle*) and 3 months postoperatively (*bottom*). The retinal schisis has almost resolved; however, cystic changes remain around the fovea

We reported that about 50 % of patients with the retinoschisis type of macular hole obtained visual improvement 6 months postoperatively as did 80 % of those with the foveal detachment type and 30 % with the macular hole type (Ikuno et al. 2008). Other investigators reported similar results, i.e., the final vision in the foveal detachment group and non-foveal detachment group improved in 70 % and 42 %, was unchanged in 26 % and 33 %, and worsened in 4 % and 25 % of the eyes, respectively (Kumagai et al. 2010).

Macular hole formation is one of the most severe postoperative complications, with an incidence of about 20 % (Gaucher et al. 2007). To identify the risk factors for secondary full-thickness macular holes after pars plana vitrectomy with ILM peeling, we retrospectively reviewed patients who had undergone those procedures to treat myopic foveoschisis (Gao et al. 2013). A macular hole developed postoperatively in eight (19.0 %) of 42 eyes. No significant association between age, axial length, VA, foveal status, posterior staphylomas, or chorioretinal atrophy was found in patients with and without macular holes. Only the percentage of eyes with an IS/OS junction defect was significantly higher (Fig. 22.7).

The pathogenesis of secondary macular holes after vitrectomy for macular foveoschisis remains unclear. Gass (1995) hypothesized that the Müller cell cone supplies structural support to the fovea and plays a critical role in the pathogenesis of macular holes. Potential trauma to the underlying Müller cells may be a possi-

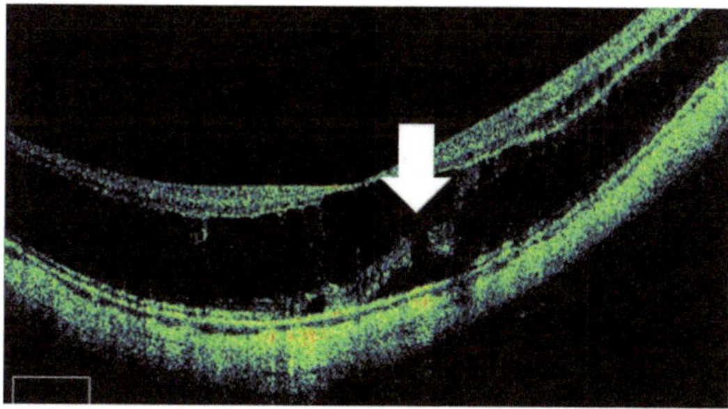

Fig. 22.7 An IS/OS defect on an OCT image (*arrow*), indicating discontinuity of the outer part of the retina. This indicates a higher risk of development of a macular hole after surgery to treat myopic foveoschisis

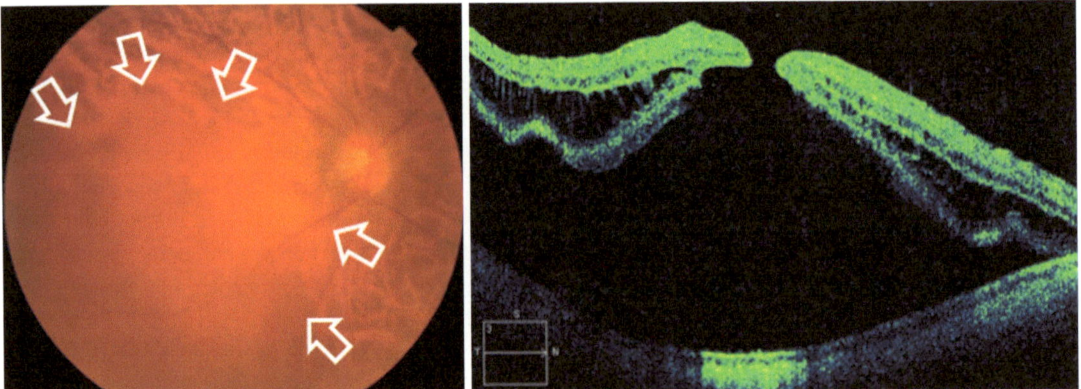

Fig. 22.8 A fundus photograph and OCT image of the localized macular hole with a retinal detachment. The area of the detachment (*arrows*) is localized to the posterior pole. The OCT image clearly shows a macular hole and surrounding retinal detachment

ble explanation for postoperative macular holes. ILM peeling may result in loss of Müller cell end feet in the area from which the ILM was peeled and weakening of the macular glial structure.

22.5 Macular Hole with or Without Retinal Detachment

22.5.1 Pathogenesis

Macular holes often lead to retinal detachments in highly myopic eyes. Histologic studies of specimens obtained during vitrectomy have shown that a retinal detachment results from the tangential traction of the vitreous cortex and/or thin ERMs adhering to the retinal surface (Bando et al. 2005; Ishida et al. 2000).

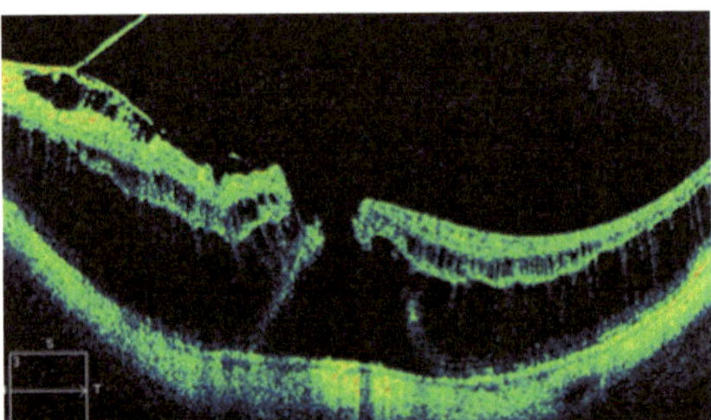

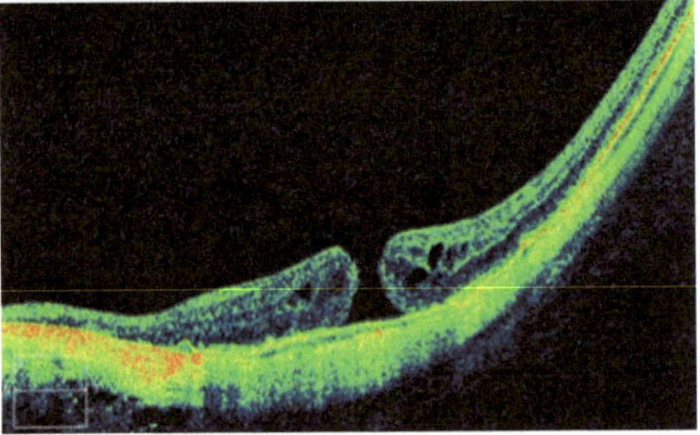

Fig. 22.9 Two types of myopic foveoschisis are seen on the OCT images (*top*). The retinoschisis type is characterized only by retinoschisis, and no retinal detachment has started (*bottom*). The foveal detachment type is more advanced, and the photoreceptors are separated from the pigment epithelium

22.5.2 Clinical Manifestations and Diagnosis

The areas of macular holes with a retinal detachment vary widely. Some patients are stable and the pathology is localized for months within the posterior staphyloma (Fig. 22.8); however, most patients develop an extensive detachment beyond the edge of the staphyloma. A small hole is seen in the central macular area on ophthalmoscopy and can be confirmed by OCT, which generally shows a detached retina and a hole with or without surrounding retinoschisis.

Interestingly, two types of macular holes are seen on OCT in high myopia (Fig. 22.9), and they have distinctly different prognoses (Jo et al. 2012). We investigated 22 eyes that underwent vitrectomy for highly myopic macular holes and the SD-OCT images. Ten eyes had retinoschisis around the macular hole and 12 did not. The patients in the schisis group were significantly older and had a worse VA and higher posterior staphyloma. Preoperative OCT images must be interpreted carefully to determine the surgical results.

22.5.3 Treatment

Regarding the basic surgical techniques, see Sect. 4.4. The only difference is the duration of the gas tamponade. A longer period of gas tamponade with perfluoropropane normally is needed to enhance the reattachment (Lim et al. 2014).

22.5.4 Outcome

The prognosis of macular holes with a retinal detachment is relatively poor. The postoperative VA is an average of 20/200 or less, and retinal reattachment occurs in about 70 % of cases after the initial surgery (Nakanishi et al. 2008). In addition, the macular holes do not close in more than 50 % of cases (Ikuno et al. 2003). Macular buckling, which can be considered when the retina is resistant, converts the vector force on the retinal surface and pushes the retina onto the retinal pigment epithelium (RPE), which is why this procedure normally has a higher success rate of over 90 % compared with vitrectomy (Ripandelli et al. 2001).

22.6 Myopic Choroidal Neovascularization

22.6.1 Pathogenesis

The pathogenesis remains controversial; however, the consensus is that local production of vascular endothelial growth factor (VEGF) is somehow upregulated, which leads to CNV growth. The pre-existing lacquer crack is thought to be a risk, and it is found in most cases with myopic CNV (mCNV) (Neelam et al. 2012). A recent OCT study reported that choroidal thinning at the fovea is a risk factor. For instance, our study found that eyes with unilateral mCNV had a significantly thinner choroid under the fovea compared with healthy, myopic, fellow eyes (Ikuno et al. 2010a). The association between choroidal thinning and upregulated VEGF production is not understood fully; however, a circulatory disturbance was reported around the macular area in mCNV (Wakabayashi and Ikuno 2010). Choroidal ischemia is supposed to increase the local VEGF concentration, which leads to VEGF production.

22.6.2 Clinical Manifestations and Diagnosis

mCNV is normally small and grayish at the macula or adjacent to the crescent of the optic nerve head. This lesion is often pigmented, the so-called Förster-Fuchs spot. The Verteporfin in Photodynamic Therapy (VIP) study (2001) reported that more than 70 % of cases had the classic type, and in 65 % the lesion was subfoveal. Occult CNV and pigment epithelial detachment (PED) are rarely present. mCNV is sometimes accompanied by a small hemorrhage between the photoreceptors and RPE. Fluorescein angiography (FA) is helpful for diagnosis. mCNV appears as hyperfluorescence in the early phase and fluorescein leakage in the late stage. Indocyanine green angiography (ICGA) provides additional information about the RPE and Bruch's membrane. The location of lacquer cracks also can be more clearly depicted on ICGA images. SD-OCT is also useful for diagnosis, monitoring, and treatment decision-making. mCNV normally grows from the choroid and migrates into the subretinal space. Fibrin reaction and subretinal fluid (SRF) are observed when mCNV is active (Fig. 22.10).

22.6.3 Natural Course

A histologic study showed that chorioretinal atrophy is augmented by photoreceptor loss and choroidal vascular obstruction and replacement with fibrous tissue (Ohno 1983). More than 90 % of the eyes had a VA over 20/200 at the

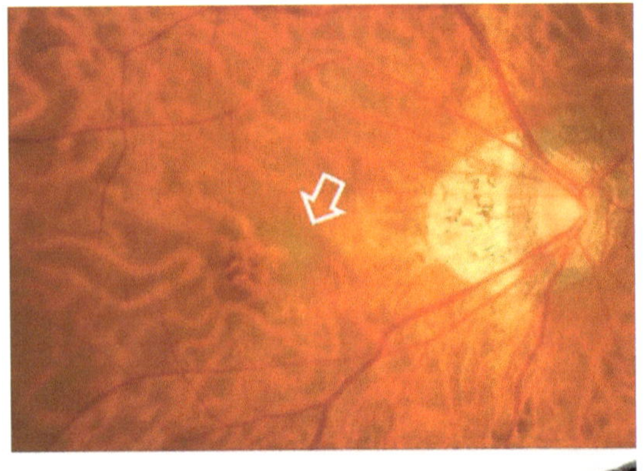

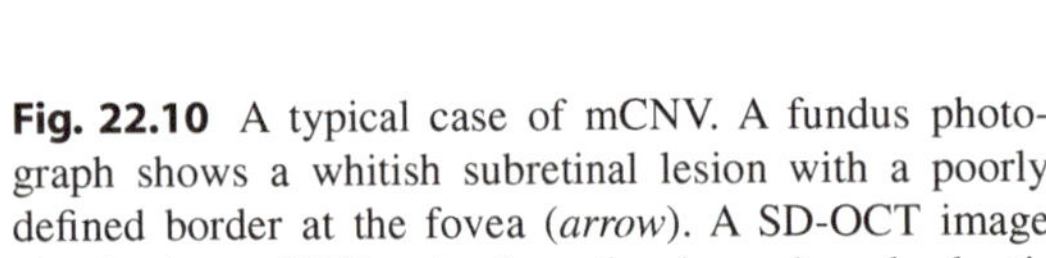

Fig. 22.10 A typical case of mCNV. A fundus photograph shows a whitish subretinal lesion with a poorly defined border at the fovea (*arrow*). A SD-OCT image clearly shows CNV under the retina (*arrow*), and subretinal fluid, which is a sign of activity

onset; however, the vision was preserved in less than 10% after 5 or 10 years (Yoshida et al. 2003). mCNV-associated atrophy usually grows around the CNV and typically appears as a white scar where the choroid is almost absent. OCT shows loss of photoreceptors and enhancement of the OCT signal (shadow) at the corresponding area because loss of the photoreceptors and RPE strengthen the signal into the deep tissue (Fig. 22.11).

22.6.4 Related Conditions

22.6.4.1 Dome-Shaped Macula

A dome-shaped macula is characterized by the convex shape of the posterior sclera and is often accompanied by a serous retinal detachment at the macula (Gaucher et al. 2008). The mechanism of the detachment remains hypothetical, and choroidal thinning at the fovea and scleral thickening of the surrounding area are thought to

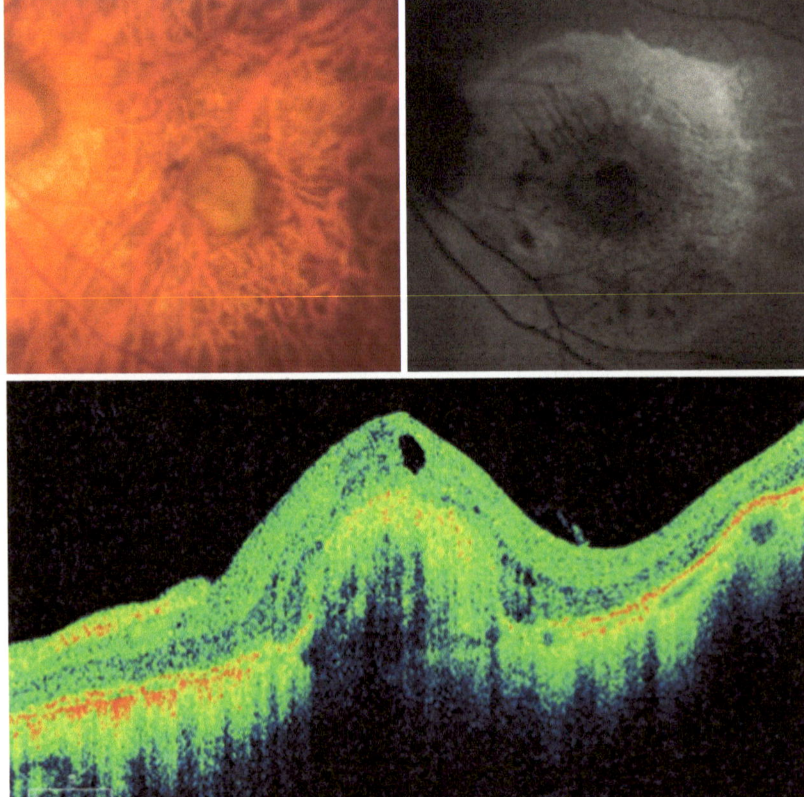

Fig. 22.11 An old case of mCNV shows pigment epithelial atrophy around the fovea. A fundus photo shows a subtle color change, but fundus autofluorescence more clearly shows a hypofluorescent area corresponding to it. The OCT shows no SRF, and the mCNV is no longer active. The penetration of the OCT signal around the CNV seems to be increased because of photoreceptor and RPE loss

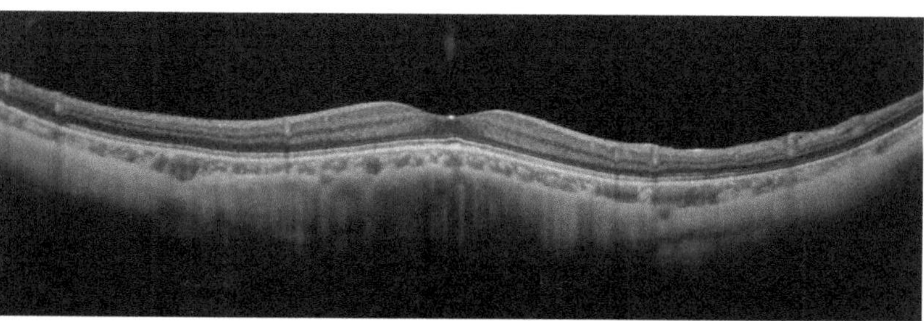

Fig. 22.12 The typical appearance of a dome-shaped macula. The macula appears convex, and this sometimes complicates mCNV or a serous retinal detachment

cause some circulatory problems in the choroid and a resultant increase in choroidal pressure. The dome-shaped macula often is mistaken for mCNV, because of the presence of SRF. However, the FA normally does not present dye leakage but a window defect from the RPE degeneration. ICGA also shows loss of choriocapillaris but not like CNV or typical lacquer cracks. Therefore, the FA findings are key for the differential diagnosis. No effective treatment has been established for this condition, and patients usually are observed without treatment (Fig. 22.12).

Interestingly, some eyes with a dome-shaped macula are often complicated by mCNV, and care must be taken when diagnosing. We investigated the morphologic characteristics of macular complications of dome-shaped macula (Ohsugi et al. 2014) and found that the central scleral thickness was significantly negatively correlated with age and axial length. We classified the eyes into three groups: six eyes with CNV, eight eyes with aPED, and five eyes with a serous retinal detachment; 35 eyes had no complications. The patients in the CNV group were significantly older and had a longer axial length than the other groups. The central choroidal thickness was significantly thinner in the CNV group than in the group with no complications. Thus, scleral thinning due to long-term changes may cause mCNV.

22.6.4.2 Polypoidal Choroidal Vasculopathy

Polypoidal Choroidal Vasculopathy (PCV) is often accompanied by high myopia (Mauget-Faÿsse et al. 2006), which is sometimes confused with mCNV. An abnormal choroidal vascular network and polyp formation are the hallmarks of PCV. It also can cause a serous detachment with a RPE detachment. PCV typically shows a steep PED; however, that is unlikely with mCNV. Thus, the presence of a PED rules out PCV. ICGA is also useful for elucidating choroidal pathologies. PCV generally is characterized by polyp formation, which is well imaged in the middle to late phase of ICGA. In addition, the presence of an associated abnormal vascular network is another hallmark of PCV. PCV is generally treated with a combination therapy of PDT and intravitreal anti-VEGF injection.

22.6.4.3 Submacular Hemorrhage Without Choroidal Neovascularization

High myopia sometimes causes a subretinal hemorrhage at the macula even without CNV (mSH). This is normally seen in younger patients based on axial length elongation, and the hemorrhage results from a break in Bruch's membrane or RPE because of the posterior eye wall elongation. The hemorrhage is not accompanied by SRF, and OCT shows a uniform intensity under the retina, while mCNV shows varying degrees of intensity inside (Fig. 22.13).

The SD-OCT appearance of this condition is interesting (Asai et al. 2014). We retrospectively investigated 13 consecutive eyes with mSH that were followed for 6 months. The hemorrhages resolved in 12 (92.3 %) eyes by 6 months. The tops of the hemorrhages reached the outer nuclear layer (ONL) in three (23 %) eyes, the ILM in five (38 %) eyes, and between the two layers in five (39 %) eyes. At 6 months, the intraretinal hyperreflective sign was seen in all (100 %) eyes and extended into the ONL in five (38 %) eyes, to the ILM in four (31 %) eyes, and between the two layers in four (31 %) eyes. The location of the

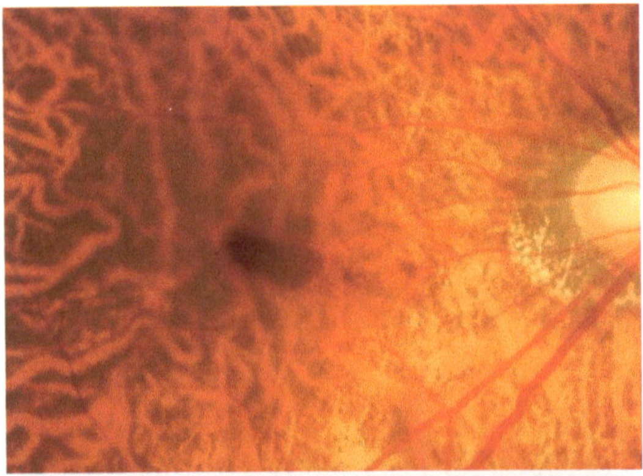

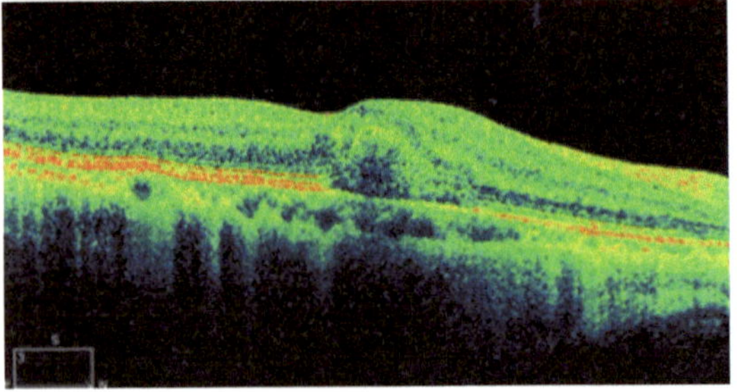

Fig. 22.13 A typical fundus photograph and OCT image of a myopic subretinal hemorrhage without CNV. The hemorrhage appears as a uniform lesion under the retina. In addition, the SRF and fibrin formation is minimal, which is important to rule out

hyperreflective signs at 6 months coincided with the ruptured retinal layers at baseline in all eyes. Thus, the subretinal hemorrhage invades the inner retinal layers, which can be recognized as thin hyperreflective lines between the synapses and across the retina over the long term.

22.6.5 Treatment

22.6.5.1 Photodynamic Therapy (PDT) with Verteporfin

PDT was accepted widely as a treatment for mCNV. The VIP study (2001), a randomized, prospective, clinical trial to test the safety and efficacy of treating mCNV, found a significantly better visual outcome at 12 months; however, that results were no longer significant at 24 months (VIP Study Group 2003), indicating the questionable long-term efficacy. PDT leads to choroidal vascular thrombosis (Schmidt-Erfurth and Hasan 2000), which is a major concern in such an atrophic choroid in patients with high myopia. Reduced-fluence PDT might be considered; however, the safety and efficacy have not been established to date.

22.6.5.2 Anti-VEGF Therapy

The anti-VEGF therapy is currently the most popular and promising (Fig. 22.14). Bevacizumab (Avastin, Genentech Inc., South San Francisco, CA) is the first anti-VEGF drug used to treat mCNV, and several large case series have described 60–70 % significant (2 lines or more) visual improvement and a mean of two to three lines visual improvement (Chan et al. 2009; Ikuno et al. 2009). Several prospective and retrospective investigations have shown that anti-VEGF therapies provide better visual outcomes compared with PDT (Ikuno et al. 2010b; Hayashi et al. 2009). Recently, the RADIANCE study, a prospective, double-masked, randomized, controlled, multicenter study of the safety and efficacy of ranibizumab (Lucentis, Genentech Inc.) for treating mCNV confirmed the significant effect on vision and anatomy over 12 months (Wolf et al. 2014).

22.6.6 Outcome

The RADIANCE study reported 14.4 letters of mean visual improvement, and 65.7 % of patients attained complete resolution of leakage from mCNV at 12 months, which was significantly better than that of the control group. The central retinal thickness decreased quickly in response to treatment. Thus, anti-VEGF is effective for mCNV.

Small and new cases of mCNV typically respond quickly to anti-VEGF. The SRF decreases 1 week after intravitreal injection. The CNV shrinks and the SRF sometimes resolves after a month. Encapsulation of the RPE is the important process that controls the CNV. The RPE grows from the outside of the CNV and into the center. OCT clearly and dramatically delineates this process. The hyper scattering line, presumed to be the RPE, starts to extend over the CNV, and ultimately the CNV is fully covered by this line. Accompanying this process, the CNV changes in color from reddish to a darker color, indicating that the CNV is covered by the pigmented RPE.

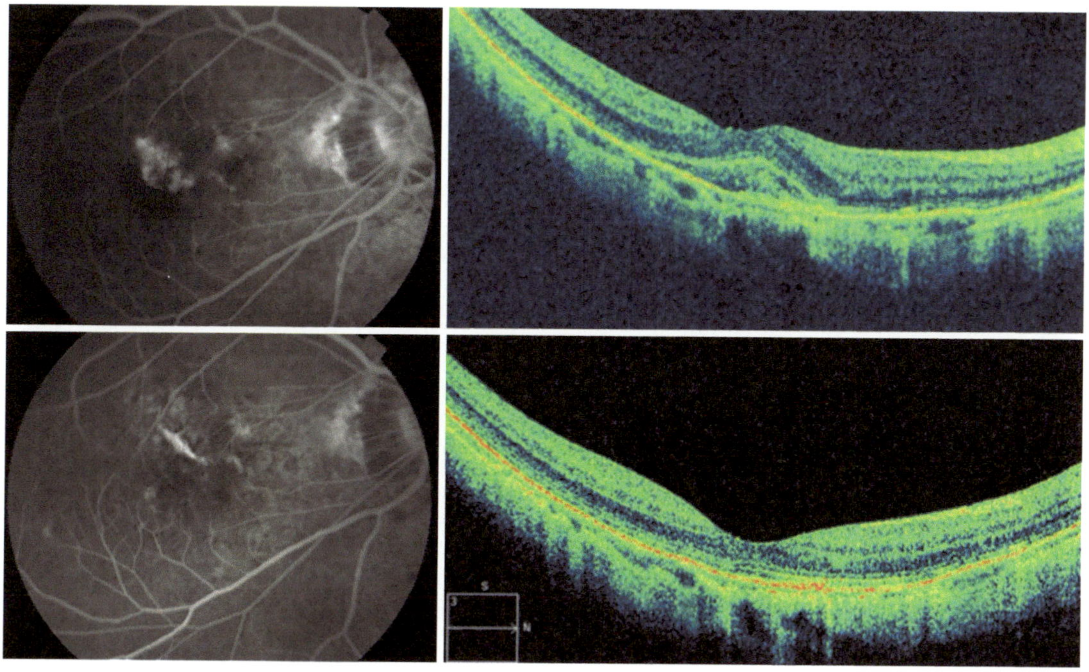

Fig. 22.14 The FA and OCT appearances of mCNV before and after treatment with anti-VEGF therapy. OCT shows that the SRF and fibrin tissue have resolved completely. FA also shows shrinkage of the mCNV, which is thin. The CNV has regressed from the fovea, and no CNV is seen at the subfoveal lesion

Although most cases respond well to treatment, some are refractory. Studies in which bevacizumab was administered have shown that cases with large and established lesions are unlike to respond. These cases typically have minimal SRF and sometimes atrophic changes around the CNV. Careful interpretation of the OCT findings allows an estimation of the response to anti-VEGF therapy. The best indicator of visual recovery is a small lesion with SRF.

mCNV can sometimes recur and is accompanied by recurrent SRF; in some cases, the capsule of the CNV ruptures. In those cases, patients normally report a visual disturbance. With repeated intravitreal injections of an anti-VEGF drug, the SRF normally recurs in fewer cases.

22.7 Closing Remarks

This chapter reviewed myopic foveoschisis, macular holes with or without retinal detachment, and mCNV in relation to the OCT findings. All are major macular diseases in patients with high myopia. OCT is a useful tool in daily practice for detecting micropathologies in highly myopic eyes and has disclosed a variety of underlying pathologies. We must be aware of the latest information because this field advances rapidly. Further investigation is needed to completely understand the detailed disease processes.

References

Asai T, Ikuno Y, Nishida K (2014) Macular microstructures and prognostic factors in myopic subretinal hemorrhages. Invest Ophthalmol Vis Sci 55:226–232

Bando H, Ikuno Y, Choi JS et al (2005) Ultrastructure of internal limiting membrane in myopic foveoschisis. Am J Ophthalmol 139:197–199

Benhamou N, Massin P, Haouchine B et al (2002) Macular retinoschisis in highly myopic eyes. Am J Ophthalmol 133:794–800

Chan WM, Lai TY, Liu DT et al (2009) Intravitreal bevacizumab (Avastin) for myopic choroidal neovascularisation: 1-year results of a prospective pilot study. Br J Ophthalmol 93:150–154

Curtin BJ (1977) The posterior staphyloma of pathologic myopia. Trans Am Ophthalmol Soc 75:67–86

Fujimoto S, Ikuno Y, Nishida K (2013) Postoperative optical coherence tomographic appearance and relation to visual acuity after vitrectomy for myopic foveoschisis. Am J Ophthalmol 156:968–973

Gao X, Ikuno Y, Fujimoto S et al (2013) Risk factors for development of full-thickness macular holes after pars plana vitrectomy for myopic foveoschisis. Am J Ophthalmol 155:1021–1027

Gass JD (1995) Reappraisal of biomicroscopic classification of stages of development of a macular hole. Am J Ophthalmol 119:752–759

Gaucher D, Haouchine B, Tadayoni R et al (2007) Long-term follow-up of high myopic foveoschisis: natural course and surgical outcome. Am J Ophthalmol 143:455–462

Gaucher D, Erginay A, Lecleire-Collet A et al (2008) Dome-shaped macula in eyes with myopic posterior staphyloma. Am J Ophthalmol 145:909–914

Hayashi K, Ohno-Matsui K, Teramukai S et al (2009) Comparison of visual outcome and regression pattern of myopic choroidal neovascularization after intravitreal bevacizumab or after photodynamic therapy. Am J Ophthalmol 148:396–408

Ikuno Y, Tano Y (2009) Retinal and choroidal biometry in highly myopic eyes with spectral-domain optical coherence tomography. Invest Ophthalmol Vis Sci 50:3876–3880

Ikuno Y, Sayanagi K, Oshima T et al (2003) Optical coherence tomographic findings of macular holes and retinal detachment after vitrectomy in highly myopic eyes. Am J Ophthalmol 136:477–481

Ikuno Y, Sayanagi K, Ohji M et al (2004) Vitrectomy and internal limiting membrane peeling for myopic foveoschisis. Am J Ophthalmol 137:719–724

Ikuno Y, Gomi F, Tano Y (2005) Potent retinal arteriolar traction as a possible cause of myopic foveoschisis. Am J Ophthalmol 139:462–467

Ikuno Y, Sayanagi K, Soga K et al (2008) Foveal anatomical status and surgical results in vitrectomy for myopic foveoschisis. Jpn J Ophthalmol 52:269–276

Ikuno Y, Sayanagi K, Soga K et al (2009) Intravitreal bevacizumab for choroidal neovascularization attributable to pathological myopia: one-year results. Am J Ophthalmol 147:94–100

Ikuno Y, Jo Y, Hamasaki T et al (2010a) Ocular risk factors for choroidal neovascularization in pathologic myopia. Invest Ophthalmol Vis Sci 51:3721–3725

Ikuno Y, Nagai Y, Matsuda S et al (2010b) Two-year visual results for older Asian women treated with photodynamic therapy or bevacizumab for myopic choroidal neovascularization. Am J Ophthalmol 149:140–146

Ishida S, Yamazaki K, Shinoda K et al (2000) Macular hole retinal detachment in highly myopic eyes: ultrastructure of surgically removed epiretinal membrane and clinicopathologic correlation. Retina 20:176–183

Ishikawa F, Ogino N, Okita K et al (2001) Vitrectomy for macular detachment without macular hole in highly myopic eyes. J Eye (AtarashiiGanka) 18:953–956

Jo Y, Ikuno Y, Nishida K (2012) Retinoschisis: a predictive factor in vitrectomy for macular holes without retinal detachment in highly myopic eyes. Br J Ophthalmol 96:197–200

Kobayashi H, Kishi S (2003) Vitreous surgery for highly myopic eyes with foveal detachment and retinoschisis. Ophthalmology 110:1702–1707

Kumagai K, Furukawa M, Ogino N et al (2010) Factors correlated with postoperative visual acuity after vitrectomy and internal limiting membrane peeling for myopic foveoschisis. Retina 30:874–880

Lim LS, Tsai A, Wong D et al (2014) Prognostic factor analysis of vitrectomy for retinal detachment associated with myopic macular holes. Ophthalmology 121:305–310

Margolis R, Spaide RF (2009) A pilot study of enhanced depth imaging optical coherence tomography of the choroid in normal eyes. Am J Ophthalmol 147:811–815

Maruko I, Iida T, Sugano Y et al (2012) Morphologic analysis in pathologic myopia using high-penetration optical coherence tomography. Invest Ophthalmol Vis Sci 53:3834–3838

Mauget-Faÿsse M, Cornut PL, Quaranta El-Maftouhi M et al (2006) Polypoidal choroidal vasculopathy in tilted disk syndrome and high myopia with staphyloma. Am J Ophthalmol 142:970–975

Nakanishi H, Kuriyama S, Saito I et al (2008) Prognostic factor analysis in pars plana vitrectomy for retinal detachment attributable to macular hole in high myopia: a multicenter study. Am J Ophthalmol 146:198–204

Neelam K, Cheung CM, Ohno-Matsui K et al (2012) Choroidal neovascularization in pathological myopia. Prog Retin Eye Res 31:495–525

Ohno H (1983) Electron microscopic studies of myopic retinochoroidal atrophies 1. Choroidal changes (in Japanese). Fol Ophthalmol Jpn 43:1244–1253

Ohsugi H, Ikuno Y, Oshima K et al (2014) Morphologic characteristics of macular complications of a dome-shaped macula determined by swept-source optical coherence tomography. Am J Ophthalmol 158(1):162–170.e1

Phillips CI (1958) Retinal detachment at the posterior pole. Br J Ophthalmol 42:749–753

Ripandelli G, Coppé AM, Fedeli R et al (2001) Evaluation of primary surgical procedures for retinal detachment with macular hole in highly myopic eyes: a comparison of vitrectomy versus posterior episcleral buckling surgery. Ophthalmology 108:2258–2264

Sawada A, Tomidokoro A, Araie M et al.; Tajimi Study Group (2008) Refractive errors in an elderly Japanese population: the Tajimi study. Ophthalmology 115:363–370

Sayanagi K, Ikuno Y, Gomi F et al (2005) Retinal vascular microfolds in highly myopic eyes. Am J Ophthalmol 139:658–663

Sayanagi K, Ikuno Y, Tano Y (2006) Tractional internal limiting membrane detachment in highly myopic eyes. Am J Ophthalmol 142:850–852

Sayanagi K, Morimoto Y, Ikuno Y et al (2010) Spectral-domain optical coherence tomographic findings in myopic foveoschisis. Retina 30:623–628

Schmidt-Erfurth U, Hasan T (2000) Mechanisms of action of photodynamic therapy with verteporfin for the treatment of age-related macular degeneration. Surv Ophthalmol 45:195–214

Shimada N, Tanaka Y, Tokoro T et al (2013) Natural course of myopic traction maculopathy and factors associated with progression or resolution. Am J Ophthalmol 156:948–957

Takano M, Kishi S (1999) Foveal retinoschisis and retinal detachment in severely myopic eyes with posterior staphyloma. Am J Ophthalmol 128:472–476

Verteporfin in Photodynamic Therapy Study Group (2001) Photodynamic therapy of subfoveal choroidal neovascularization in pathologic myopia with verteporfin.1-year results of a randomized clinical trial – VIP Report No.1. Ophthalmology 108:841–852

VIP Study Group (2003) Verteporfin therapy of subfoveal choroidal neovascularization in pathologic myopia: 2-year results of a randomized clinical trial – VIP Report No. 3. Ophthalmology 110:667–673

Wakabayashi T, Ikuno Y (2010) Choroidal filling delay in choroidal neovascularisation due to pathological myopia. Br J Ophthalmol 94:611–615

Wolf S, Balciuniene VJ, Laganovska G et al.; RADIANCE Study Group (2014) RADIANCE: a randomized controlled study of ranibizumab in patients with choroidal neovascularization secondary to pathologic myopia. Ophthalmology 121:682–692

Xu L, Li Y, Wang S et al (2007) Characteristics of highly myopic eyes: the Beijing Eye Study. Ophthalmology 114:121–126

Yoshida T, Ohno-Matsui K, Yasuzumi K et al (2003) Myopic choroidal neovascularization: a 10-year follow-up. Ophthalmology 110:1297–1305

Optic Disc Pit

23

Edmund Y.M. Wong and Vicky H.J. Lu

Contents

E.Y.M. Wong, MMed, FRCSEd (✉) • V.H.J. Lu
Singapore National Eye Center, Singapore, Singapore
e-mail: edwong39@yahoo.com.sg

23.1 Introduction

Optic disc pit is a rare congenital anomaly first described in 1882 by Wiethe (1882). It is reported to have an incidence of 1 in 11,000 seen in an ophthalmic setting (Krivoy et al. 1996) and is unilateral in the majority of cases (Greear 1942; Lincoff et al. 1993) with no gender predilection. It is characterized by an excavation within the optic disc (Fig. 23.1). It is considered part of the spectrum of congenital disc anomalies with morning glory anomaly, juxtapapillary staphyloma and optic disc coloboma (Gass 1987) which are associated with juxtapapillary and macular retinopathy.

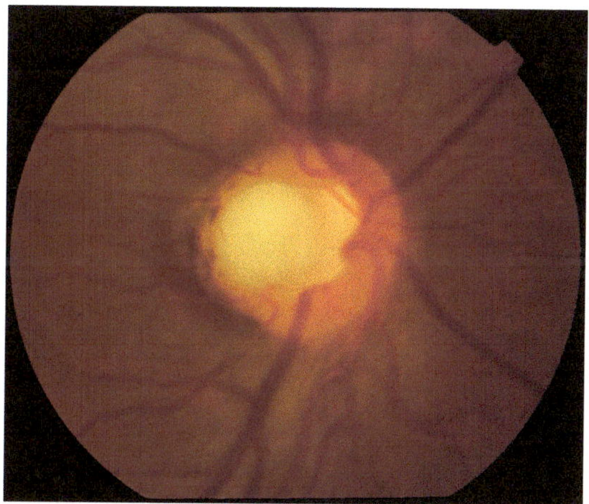

Fig. 23.1 Colour photograph of optic disc pit

C.H. Meyer et al. (eds.), *Spectral Domain Optical Coherence Tomography in Macular Diseases*,
DOI 10.1007/978-81-322-3610-8_23

23.2 Aetiology

Optic disc pits are congenital anomalies that most likely occur during the first trimester of pregnancy. They are known as 'atypical colobomas' due to incomplete closure of the embryonic fissure that would normally have surrounded the disc (Apple and Rabb 1998; Sugar 1962). Some argue, however, that optic disc pits are separate entities in that they are usually unilateral and rarely associated with systemic anomalies. Gass has suggested that optic disc pits are due to abnormal development of primordial optic nerve papillae and failure of complete resolution of peripapillary neuroectodermal folds, rather than being true colobomata from incomplete fissure closure (Gass 1969). Optic disc pit and other anomalies have been described in renal coloboma syndrome, with variable inheritance patterns (predominantly autosomal dominant) (Dureau et al. 2001). Mutations of the PAX2 gene, involved in the development of the optic and otic vesicles, genitourinary tracts and central nervous system, have been previously described (Eccles and Schimmenti 1999; Samimi et al. 2008).

23.3 Clinical Features

Optic disc pits may vary in size, occupying up to half the disc diameter. The morphology of the pit may also vary from localized distinct pit-like invaginations to excavated cuplike structures (Choi et al. 2014; Gregory Roberts et al. 2013; Kritzinger and Beaumont 1986; Waldstein et al. 2015). The pit may appear grey and white or sometimes be mistaken for cupping in glaucomatous optic neuropathy. The depression is frequently situated in the temporal or infra-temporal region of the optic disc. There have been reports of up to two to three depressions, although in the majority there is only one pit per optic disc (Kritzinger and Beaumont 1986). Peripapillary chorioretinal atrophy with pigmentary change is seen in almost all cases where the pit is situated near the optic disc margin. In 60 % of cases, a cilioretinal artery can be identified arising from the periphery of the pit (Krivoy et al. 1996).

Visual acuity may remain normal unless associated maculopathy develops. As many as 75 % of optic disc pits are associated with serous macula detachments (Brown et al. 1980; Gass 1969; Kritzinger and Beaumont 1986; Kranenberg 1960; Spencer 1986). These are usually related to larger pits located temporally in the disc and may present during childhood: however, these are more commonly present between the second and fourth decade of life (Krivoy et al. 1996). With the advent of ocular imaging (particularly optical coherence tomography), maculopathy can consist of intraretinal fluid and/or retinoschisis and/or macula serous detachment (Lincoff et al. 1988). Lamellar macular holes are usually in the outer retinal layers. Resolution of macular detachment without inducing full-thickness macular hole can result in good visual acuity; however, redetachment and delayed resolution are typical of optic disc pit maculopathies.

23.4 Clinical Investigations

23.4.1 Optical Coherence Tomography (OCT)

The use of optical coherence tomography (OCT) has indeed expanded our understanding of optic disc pit-associated maculopathy and corroborated with earlier histopathological findings and hypotheses (Jain and Johnson 2014). This non-invasive tool has helped demonstrate ultrastructural characteristics of optic disc pit-associated maculopathy and in the evaluation of outcome following intervention (Gregory Roberts et al. 2013; Ehlers et al. 2011).

Various papers in the recent years investigate the use of spectral-domain OCT(SD-OCT) (OCT 4000 Cirrus Carl Zeiss Meditec, Dublin, CA, USA; Spectralis OCT, Heidelberg Engineering, Heidelberg, Germany) with enhanced depth imaging (EDI SD-OCT) and the newer swept-source OCT (SS-OCT) (SS-OCT; DRI OCT-1; Topcon, Tokyo, Japan) in this condition, including intraoperative use (Bioptigen, Research Triangle Park, North Carolina). SD-OCT and SS-OCT have similar signal depth penetration.

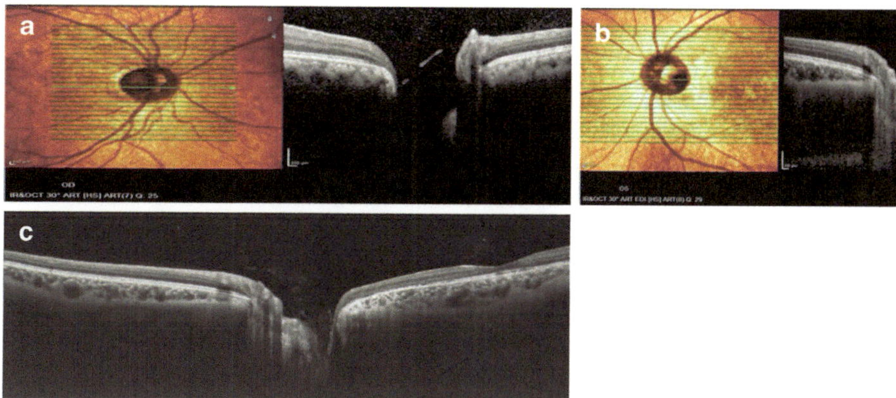

Fig. 23.2 (**a**) SD-OCT showing the membrane overlying the optic disc region. Details of the base of the optic disc pit cannot be seen. (**b**, **c**) Comparison of (**b**) SD-OCT (EDI) and (**c**) SS-OCT of the same patient showing similar cuts through the fovea of optic disc and vitreous matter entering the optic disc pit

However, while the SD-OCT shows superior contrast of choroidal vasculature, SS-OCT has a much faster scanning speed (up to 100-fold), with less sensitivity roll-off (Waldstein et al. 2015). These developments in technology allow for faster scanning speeds compared with previous OCT, higher resolution and the ability for three-dimensional reconstruction (Fig. 23.2). These high-resolution OCTs are invaluable in the characterization of optic disc pit morphology (Gregory Roberts et al. 2013) and its contents and membranes that cover and line the optic disc pit in order to better understand this rare condition and guide its management.

Morphology of the pit varies from localized distinct pit-like invaginations to deep excavated cuplike structures (Choi et al. 2014; Ehlers et al. 2011; Gregory Roberts et al. 2013). Small case series examined with EDI SD-OCT and SS-OCT were able to image choroidal and post-laminar structures with sufficient resolution to demonstrate defects in the lamina cribrosa and/or sclera and the track of fluid between perineural space and intraretinal/subretinal spaces, confirming previous histopathological findings (Ferry 1963; Gowdar et al. 2015; Irvine et al. 1986; Ohno-Matsui et al. 2013).

Herniation of dysplastic retina tissue into the optic disc pit can also be demonstrated (Aggio et al. 2007). Vitreous strands and glial tissue can sometimes be seen on SD-OCT or SS-OCT within the content of the pits, again correlating with histopathological understanding of this condition (Chang et al. 2012; Gregory Roberts et al. 2013; Ohno-Matsui et al. 2013; Theodossiadis et al. 2007). A hyperreflective diaphanous membrane is often demonstrated overlying the excavated disc anomaly (Fig. 23.3) (Chang et al. 2012; Gregory Roberts et al. 2013; Ohno-Matsui et al. 2013). Doyle suggested this was a protective barrier against vitreous entry to the pit, intraretinal space and thus maculopathy (Doyle et al. 2009). With advancements in SD-OCT and SS-OCT resolution and ability to visualize this membrane in slices several microns thin, this membrane is now seen to be porous and unlikely to serve this function. Similarly, a membrane lining the base of the optic disc pit does not seem to have prognostic value. This appears to represent pia mater (Ohno-Matsui et al. 2013), although histopathologically it has been reported as the

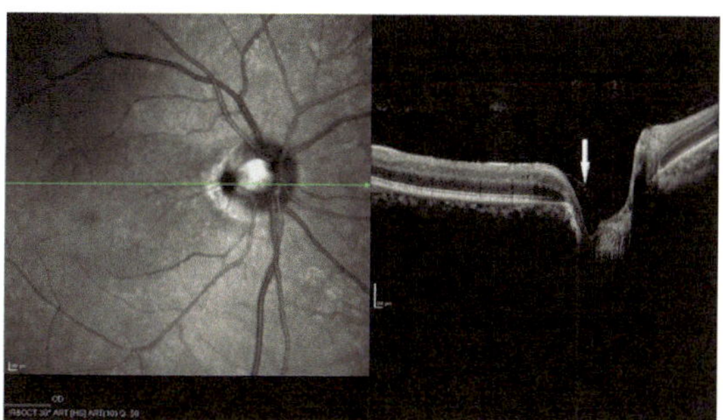

Fig. 23.3 SD-OCT showing the membrane overlying optic disc pit temporally (*arrow*), minimal intraretinal fluid and posterior vitreous detachment over macula region

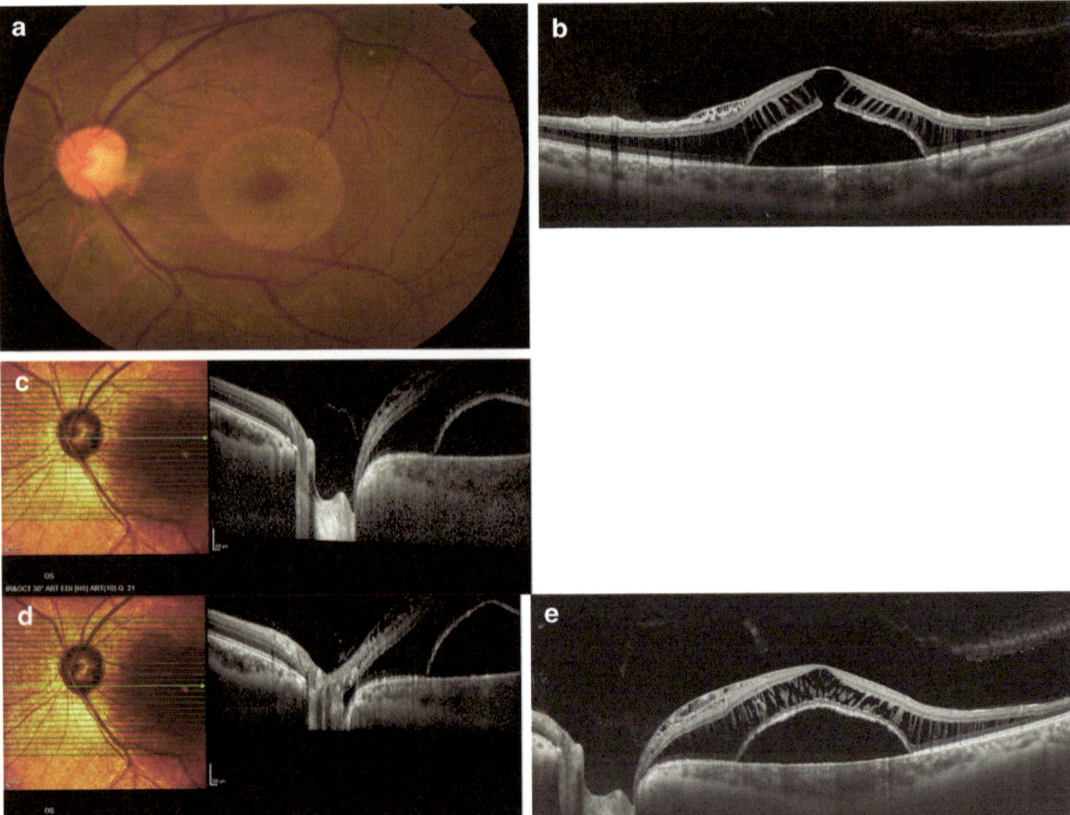

Fig. 23.4 (**a**) Fundus photograph of patient with optic disc pit. Lamellar hole and lipofuscin associated with chronic fluid can be seen. Macula elevation (correlating with intraretinal fluid) with an area of taut swelling centrally (subretinal fluid) can be seen. (**b**) SS-OCT of the macula showing outer retinal lamellar hole and intraretinal and subretinal fluid. (**c, d**) SD-OCT (EDI) two cuts in the same patient. (**c**) Through the optic pit and (**d**) at the inferior edge of the optic disc pit showing fluid track in continuity with intraretinal fluid. Note there is intraretinal fluid in both outer and inner retina, in addition to subretinal fluid. (**e**) SS-OCT similar cut to 4c showing optic disc pit, intraretinal fluid (inner and outer retina) and subretinal fluid. Incomplete posterior vitreous detachment can be noted

continuation of the internal limiting membrane over the disc representing rudimentary retinal tissue (Ferry 1963). The fluid in the perineural space posterior to this can also now be visualized (Michalewski et al. 2014).

Although aetiology of the retinal fluid associated with this rare condition is still under debate, SD-OCT and SS-OCT allow better visualization of the fluid, the level of the retina it is predominantly affecting and associations in each case with perineural and vitreous space. Fluid has been noted in various permutations with involvement of outer and/or inner plexiform layer and subretinal macula, with and without tracks emanating from the disc anomaly demonstrated (Fig. 23.4) (Krivoy et al. 1996; Michalewski et al. 2014; Hotta et al. 1999; Rutledge et al. 1996). SD-OCT and SS-OCT have also negated the importance of posterior hyaloid on the pathogenesis of optic disc pit maculopathy. Vitreomacular traction was not demonstrated in many cases with maculopathy contrary to previous beliefs (Chang et al. 2012; Hirakata et al. 2005; Imamura et al. 2010; Pham et al. 2007). In addition, maculopathy can recur following surgical development of posterior vitreous detachment (Jain and Johnson 2014).

Intraoperative SD-OCT (Bioptigen, Research Triangle Park, North Carolina) has also aided our understanding of this rare condition with serial real-time, high-resolution images of the optic nerve head and macula. It has been performed to show no improvement of optic disc pit-associated retinoschisis following induction of posterior vitreous detachment. However, following fluid air exchange (and return to fluid), intraoperative SD-OCT was able to demonstrate a reduction in the retinoschisis (Ehlers et al. 2011). The possibility raised by this immediate, intraoperative reduction of retinoschisis fluid is that there is some communication with the vitreous cavity or subarachnoid/perineural space.

High aspiration at optic disc pit with partial collapse of the retinoschisis even in the absence of connecting channels on OCT also suggests a sieve-like connection between the vitreous cavity and the intraretinal space at the pit, suggesting a rhegmatogenous component to the fluid accumulation (Ehlers et al. 2011). How vitrectomy procedures reduce and collapse macular schisis spaces are not well understood, but may be related to this operative finding. Further, SD-OCT and SS-OCT can be used in the evaluation of intervention – namely, progress of maculopathy, any resolution of intraretinal fluid and confirmation of the creation of intraretinal barrier to fluid migration with laser photocoagulation (Jain and Johnson 2014). In cases of recurrence, it can also be useful in visualizing persistent tracks of communication between the optic disc pit and macula.

23.4.2 Visual Field

Numerous visual field defects also exist. Reported changes included centrocecal defects, paracentral scotomas, arcuate defects, enlarged blind spots and nasal or temporal defects. Enlarged blind spots

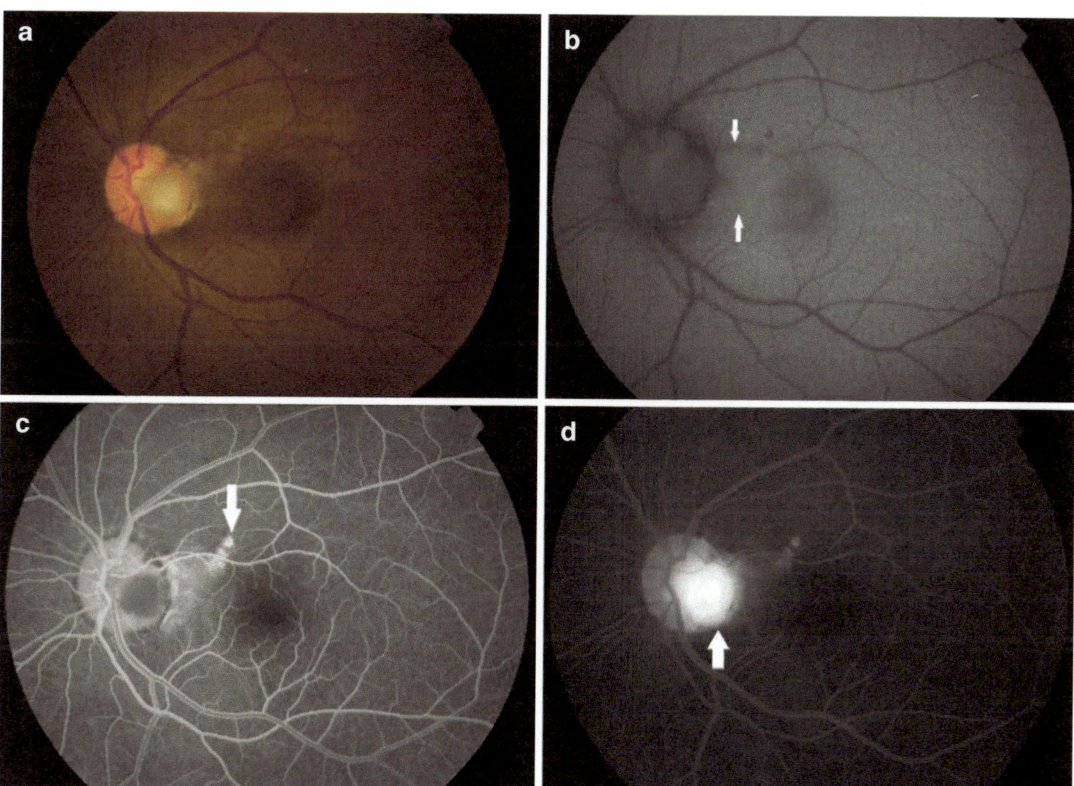

Fig. 23.5 Optic disc pit with serous macular detachment. (**a**) Colour photograph of optic disc pit with serous macular detachment. (**b**) Fundus autofluorescence. Slight masking of papillomacular area autofluorescence (*arrows*) due to serous detachment. Fairly normal appearance elsewhere over the macula. (**c**) Fluorescein angiography at 27 s. Hypofluorescence over optic disc pit. Oblique hyperfluorescence under superotemporal macular vessel due to retinal pigment epithelium (RPE) transmission defect (*arrow*). (**d**) Fluorescein angiography at 8 min. Staining of optic disc pit (*arrow*). RPE transmission defect showing reduced hyperfluorescence with waning phase of angiogram

and arcuate scotomas were the most commonly reported defects (Gass 1969).

23.4.3 Fluorescein and Indocyanine Green Angiography

Angiography of optic disc pits and maculopathies has been reported. Fluorescein angiography showed early hypofluorescence and late staining of the optic pit (Fig. 23.5). Indocyanine green angiography showed absolute hypofluorescence of the optic disc. Both can be implemented to demonstrate pooling of fluorescence within the area of macula elevation (Gordon and Chatfield 1969).

23.5 Management

Treatment options at this point target reduction of macular schisis associated with optic disc pits. These include laser to the edge of the optic disc, macular buckling and pars plana vitrectomy with or without internal limiting membrane peeling and gas tamponade.

23.6 Summary

Optic disc pits are a congenital anomaly of the optic disc that are fairly well characterized at this time clinically. They tend to become clinically significant when the associated macular schisis causes a reduction of vision. Current spectral-domain and swept-source OCT techniques with their higher resolutions and even intraoperative use allow us to understand this rare entity better, giving greater insight into the pathogenesis of this condition.

References

Aggio FB et al (2007) New stratus oct findings in extrapapillary excavated anomaly and secondary macular complications. Retina 27:113–115

Apple DJ, Rabb MF (1998) Developmental anomalies. In: Ocular pathology: clinical applications and self-assessment, in ocular pathology: clinical applications and self-assessment. Mosby, St Louis, pp 24–26

Brown GC, Shields JA, Goldberg RE (1980) Congenital pits of the optic nerve head. II. Clinical studies in humans. Ophthalmology 87:51–65

Chang S, Roberts EG, Chen R (2012) Retinal detachment associated with optic disc colobomas and morning glory syndrome. Eye (Lond) 26:494–500

Choi YJ et al (2014) Microstructure of the optic disc pit in open-angle glaucoma. Ophthalmology 121:2098–2106–e2

Doyle E et al (2009) High-resolution optical coherence tomography demonstration of membranes spanning optic disc pits and colobomas. Br J Ophthalmol 93:360–365

Dureau P et al (2001) Renal coloboma syndrome. Ophthalmology 108:1912–1916

Eccles MR, Schimmenti LA (1999) Renal-coloboma syndrome: a multi-system developmental disorder caused by PAX2 mutations. Clin Genet 56:1–9

Ehlers JP et al (2011) Analysis of pars plana vitrectomy for optic pit-related maculopathy with intraoperative optical coherence tomography: a possible connection with the vitreous cavity. Arch Ophthalmol 129:1483–1486

Ferry AP (1963) Macular detachment associated with congenital pit of the optic nerve head. pathologic findings in two cases simulating malignant melanoma of the choroid. Arch Ophthalmol 70:346–357

Gass JD (1969) Serous detachment of the macula. Secondary to congenital pit of the optic nerve head. Am J Ophthalmol 67:821–841

Gass JDM (1987) Stereoscopic atlas of macular diseases: diagnosis and treatment. Mosby, St Louis, p 732

Gordon R, Chatfield RK (1969) Pits in the optic disc associated with macular degeneration. Br J Ophthalmol 53:481–489

Gowdar JP et al (2015) An insight into the pathogenesis of optic disc pit-associated maculopathy with enhanced depth imaging. JAMA Ophthalmol 133:466–469

Greear JNJ (1942) Pits, or crater-like holes, in the optic disk. Arch Ophthalmol 28:467–483

Gregory Roberts EM et al (2013) Optic disk pit morphology and retinal detachment: optical coherence tomography with intraoperative correlation. Retina 33:363–370

Hirakata A, Okada AA, Hida T (2005) Long-term results of vitrectomy without laser treatment for macular detachment associated with an optic disc pit. Ophthalmology 112:1430–1435

Hirakata A et al (2012) Vitrectomy without laser treatment or gas tamponade for macular detachment associated with an optic disc pit. Ophthalmology 119:810–818

Hotta K, Hirakata A, Hida T (1999) Retinoschisis associated with disc coloboma. Br J Ophthalmol 83:124

Imamura Y et al (2010) High-resolution optical coherence tomography findings in optic pit maculopathy. Retina 30:1104–1112

Irvine AR, Crawford JB, Sullivan JH (1986) The pathogenesis of retinal detachment with morning glory disc and optic pit. Retina 6:146–150

Jain N, Johnson MW (2014) Pathogenesis and treatment of maculopathy associated with cavitary optic disc anomalies. Am J Ophthalmol 158:423–435

Kranenberg EW (1960) Crater-like holes in the optic disc and central serous retinopathy. Arch Ophthalmol 64:132–144

Kritzinger EE, Beaumont HM (1986) A colour atlas of optic disc abnormalities. Wolfe Medical Publications, London, p 332

Krivoy D et al (1996) Imaging congenital optic disc pits and associated maculopathy using optical coherence tomography. Arch Ophthalmol 114:165–170

Lincoff H et al (1988) Retinoschisis associated with optic nerve pits. Arch Ophthalmol 106:61–67

Lincoff H et al (1993) Improvement in visual function after displacement of the retinal elevations emanating from optic pits. Arch Ophthalmol 111:1071–1079

Michalewski J, Michalewska Z, Nawrocki J (2014) Spectral domain optical coherence tomography morphology in optic disc pit associated maculopathy. Indian J Ophthalmol 62:777–781

Ohno-Matsui K et al (2013) Evaluation of congenital optic disc pits and optic disc colobomas by swept-source optical coherence tomography. Invest Ophthalmol Vis Sci 54:7769–7778

Pham TQ et al (2007) Optical coherence tomography findings of acute traumatic maculopathy following motor vehicle accident. Am J Ophthalmol 143:348–350

Rutledge BK et al (1996) Optical coherence tomography of macular lesions associated with optic nerve head pits. Ophthalmology 103:1047–1053

Samimi S et al (2008) Bilateral macular detachment caused by bilateral optic nerve malformation in a papillorenal syndrome due to a new PAX2 mutation. Eur J Ophthalmol 18:656–658

Spaide RF, Costa DL, Huang SJ (2003) Macular schisis in a patient without an optic disk pit optical coherence tomographic findings. Retina 23:238–240

Spaide RF, Koizumi H, Pozzoni MC (2008) Enhanced depth imaging spectral-domain optical coherence tomography. Am J Ophthalmol 146:496–500

Spencer WH (1986) Ophthalmic pathology: an atlas and textbook. Saunders, Philadelphia, pp 2355–2357

Sugar HS (1962) Congenital pits in the optic disc with acquired macular pathology. Am J Ophthalmol 53:307–311. Am J Ophthalmol 53:307–311

Sugar HS (1964) An explanation for the acquired macular pathology associated with congenital pits of the optic disc. Am J Ophthalmol 54:833–835

Theodossiadis PG et al (2007) Vitreous findings in optic disc pit maculopathy based on optical coherence tomography. Graefes Arch Clin Exp Ophthalmol 245:1311–1318

Waldstein SM et al (2015) Comparison of penetration depth in choroidal imaging using swept source vs spectral domain optical coherence tomography. Eye (Lond) 29:409–415

Wiethe T (1882) Ein Fall von angeborener Difformität der Sehnervenpapille. Arch Augenheilkd 11:14–19

Part IV
Miscellaneous

Retinal Dystrophies and Degenerations

24

Anna C.S. Tan and Gemmy Cheung

Contents

24.1 Introduction

Retinal dystrophies comprise of a broad group of disorders which affect the retina and often lead to significant vision loss. This group of inherited diseases is characterised by progressive photoreceptor loss. The underlying genetic defect has been identified in many of these conditions, leading to a better understanding of the pathogenesis and the possibility of novel therapy (Bird 1995; Francis 2006; Hamel 2007). The high resolution of spectral domain optical coherence tomography (SD-OCT) images allows detailed examination of the retinal structure in many diseases. Detailed examination by SD-OCT offers much better ability to correlate with symptoms and progression, compared to fundus examination.

In this chapter, we will cover how SD-OCT is particularly valuable as an adjunct imaging tool in the management of patients with retinal dystrophies and degeneration.

24.2 Retinitis Pigmentosa/Rod-Cone Dystrophy

Retinitis pigmentosa (RP) is the most common retinal dystrophy, affecting about 1 in 3000 people (Bundey and Crews 1984; Bunker et al. 1984). This group of conditions is characterised by retinal degeneration and progressive loss of rod photoreceptors, which may be accompanied by variable degree of cone photoreceptor loss.

A.C.S. Tan, MMed • G. Cheung, MBBS, FRCOphth (✉)
Singapore Eye Research Institute,
Singapore National Eye Center, Singapore, Singapore
e-mail: gemmy.cheung.c.m@snec.com.sg

C.H. Meyer et al. (eds.), *Spectral Domain Optical Coherence Tomography in Macular Diseases*,
DOI 10.1007/978-81-322-3610-8_24

The age of disease onset, progression and severity of visual loss is variable but can be related to the genetic inheritance of this disease, with autosomal dominantly inherited RP generally having less severe visual loss and X-linked recessive RP having the worst prognosis (Fishman 1978).

Early symptoms of RP include nyctalopia and visual loss, which typically begin in the peripheral visual field and progress towards the centre (Hartong et al. 2006; Marshall 1988). Central vision is generally preserved until the late stage. However complications like cystoid macular oedema (CMO), epiretinal membrane growth and macular hole formation can affect the central vision in some cases (Hajali et al. 2008; Hagiwara et al. 2011; Sahel et al. 2010). Other associated diseases such as the development of cataract can also reduce the visual acuity (Fishman et al. 1985). Clinical characteristics of RP include retinal pigment epithelial (RPE) atrophy and arteriolar attenuation in the early stages (Fig. 24.1a). Bony spicules and waxy disc pallor appear in the later stages of this disease (Berson et al. 1985; Marshall 1988).

In the early stages of RP, a patient may experience symptoms in the absence of clear clinical signs. Diagnosis of RP in these cases may be possible with electrophysiological testing. In the early stage of the disease, the rod photoreceptors are predominantly affected, resulting in abnormal scotopic responses, with relatively preserved photopic responses. In the later stages, both the rod and cone photoreceptors may be involved resulting in abnormalities in photopic responses in addition to abnormalities in scotopic responses. In advanced stages of RP, however, when there is extensive photoreceptor loss, both scotopic and photopic responses may become undetectable (Fishman 1985; Goura and Carr 1964). Progressive concentric visual field loss is the most common pattern of progression. In advanced stages of the disease, only a small island of residual central visual field (Fig. 24.1c) may remain. This may be associated with a small peripheral island (Grover et al. 1998; Holopigian et al. 1996).

Fundus autofluorescence (FAF) is another useful imaging tool to monitor the progression of RP in addition to fundoscopy examination. RP changes on FAF have been previously correlated with findings on optical coherence tomography (OCT) and electrophysiology. An abnormal hyper-autofluorescent ring surrounding a normal fovea has been observed in 54–94 % of patients with RP (Fig. 24.2a). This ring corresponds to a loss in the inner segment ellipsoid zone (EZ) previously known as the inner/outer segment border seen on SD-OCT. This ring has been thought to represent dysfunction of both the RPE and the photoreceptor cells, and the progressive constriction of this ring can be associated with a decreased area of intact photoreceptors (Robson et al. 2006). Outside this ring, differing patterns of normal autofluorescence to areas of decreased autofluorescence can be observed. This corresponds to the generalised loss of the EZ line and the external limiting membrane (ELM) (Fig. 24.2b) (Murakami et al. 2008; Wakabayashi et al. 2010).

24.2.1 Optical Coherence Tomography

Spectral domain-OCT can be used to monitor RP-related changes in the retinal layers including the photoreceptor layers (represented by the

Fig. 24.1 Retinitis pigmentosa/rod-cone dystrophy. (**a**) A fundus photo of a 65-year-old male with retinitis pigmentosa showing early changes which include vessel attenuation and retinal pigment epithelium atrophy. (**b**) The corresponding spectral domain OCT showing (1) generalised thinning of the inner retinal layer in the peripheral retina, (2) loss of the inner segment ellipsoid layer (EZ) and external limiting membrane (ELM) in the mid-peripheral region, with relative preservation at the centre of the fovea. These findings are consistent with a reasonable central vision of 6/15 with peripheral field losses seen on the Goldmann visual field (GVF) (*below*), (3) patchy loss of the inner segment EZ with thinning of the outer nuclear layer (ONL) and (4) a thickened retinal nerve fibre layer (RNFL) was also observed. (5) Choroidal thinning was observed in some areas of patients with retinitis pigmentosa (RP). (**c**) Goldmann visual field (GVF) which showed the loss of the peripheral visual field with a residual "tubular" visual field

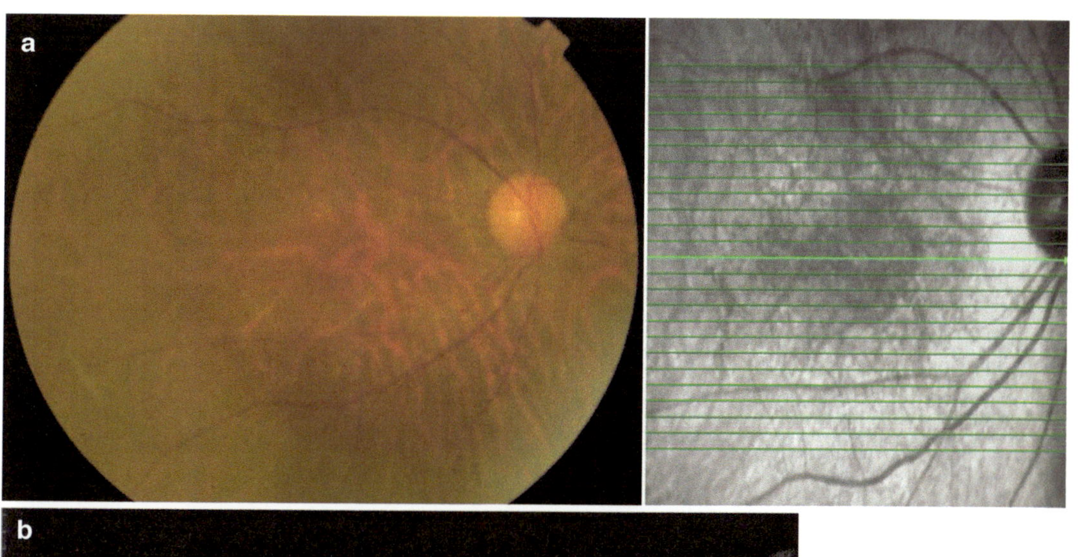
a

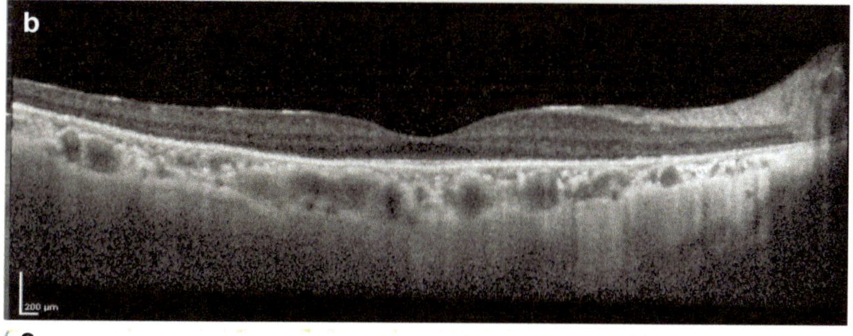
b
200 µm

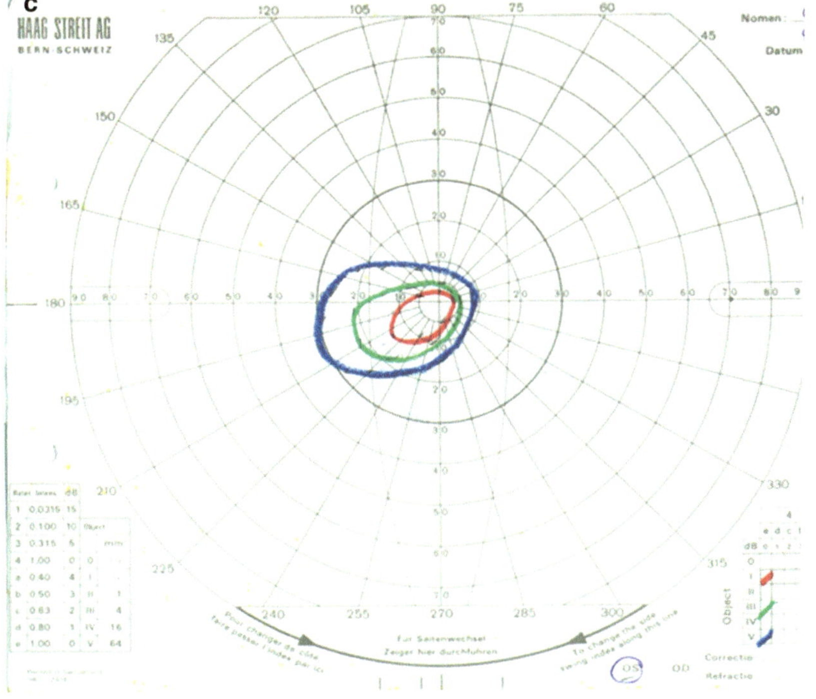
c
HAAG STREIT AG
BERN·SCHWEIZ
Nomen :
Datum
120
105
90
75
60
135
45
150
30
165
180
195
210
225
240
255
270
285
300
315
330
Für Seitenwechsel
Zeiger hier durchführen
OS
OD
Object

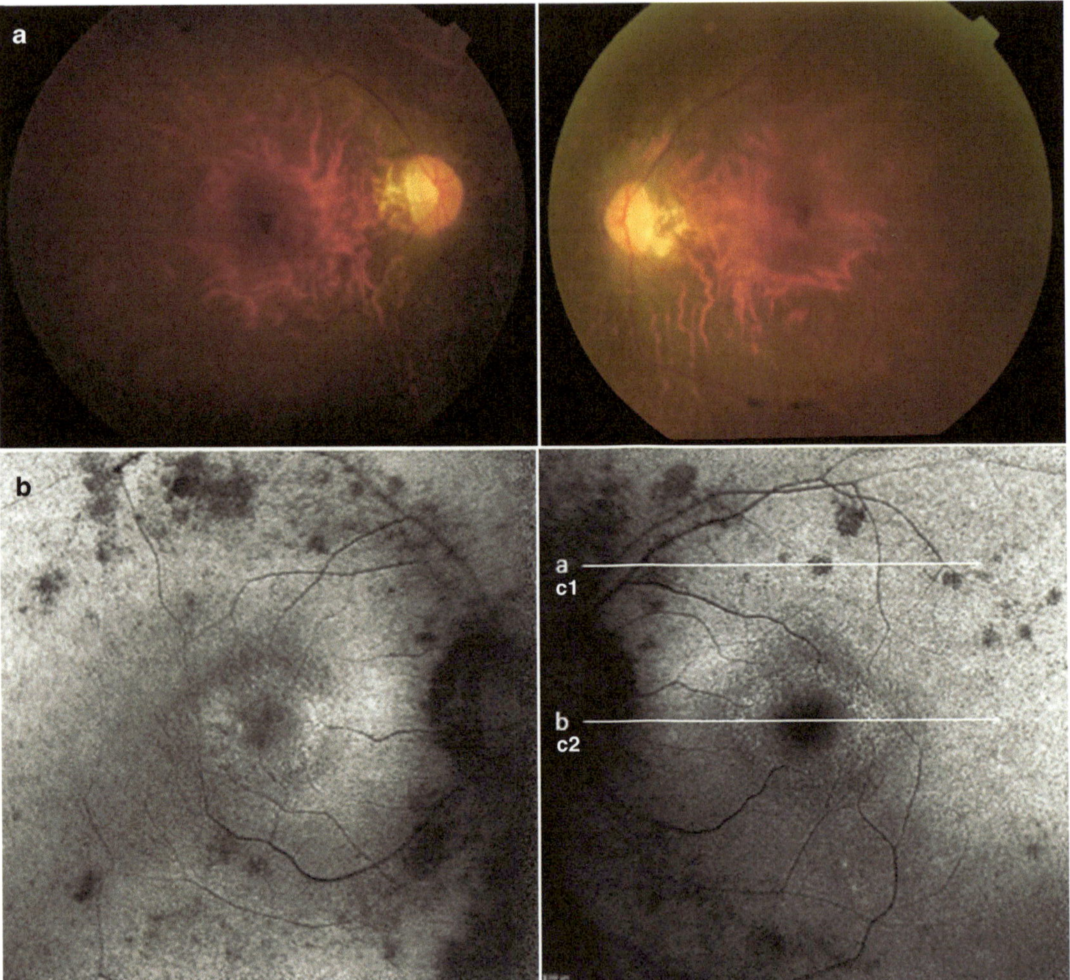

Fig. 24.2 Retinitis pigmentosa/rod-cone dystrophy. (**a**) Fundus photo (*above*) of a 49-year-old male with RP who presented with nyctalopia and a visual acuity of 6/30 on the right and 6/15 on the left, which showed arteriolar attenuation, RPE atrophy and bony spicules in the periphery. (**b**) Autofluorescent (AF) image (*below*) showed an abnormal hyper-autofluorescent ring surrounding the centre of the fovea and hypo-autofluorescent areas along the arcades corresponding to areas of retinal pigment epithelium (RPE) atrophy. (**c**) Spectral domain OCT of the patient above corresponding to the AF cross section c1 which showed (*1*) complete loss of EZ and ELM. (*2*) On the foveal cut OCT corresponding to the AF cross section c2, the extent of the EZ disruption corresponding to the inner boundary of the abnormal hyper-autofluorescent ring with generalised thinning of the EZ, ONL and ELM. (*3*) Choroidal thinning is also observed in the mid-peripheral retina. (**c**) Multifocal ERG showed reduced and delayed response throughout the macula, with some preservation of the central ring only. This functional assessment corresponds well with the structural changes seen on OCT and AF imaging

EZ), the ELM and the retinal nerve fibre layer (RNFL) (Hood et al. 2009; Triolo et al. 2013). A previous study demonstrated that the loss of the EZ can be directly related to the inner abnormal FAF border of the ring as well as visual field boundary. Ellipsoid zone loss may be patchy and incomplete in the early stages and become complete in the later stages. Correspondingly, in the early stages, the central cone photoreceptors may be spared. A loss of the ELM was also noted in some patients. In some cases thinning of the RPE/Bruch's membrane complex has also been

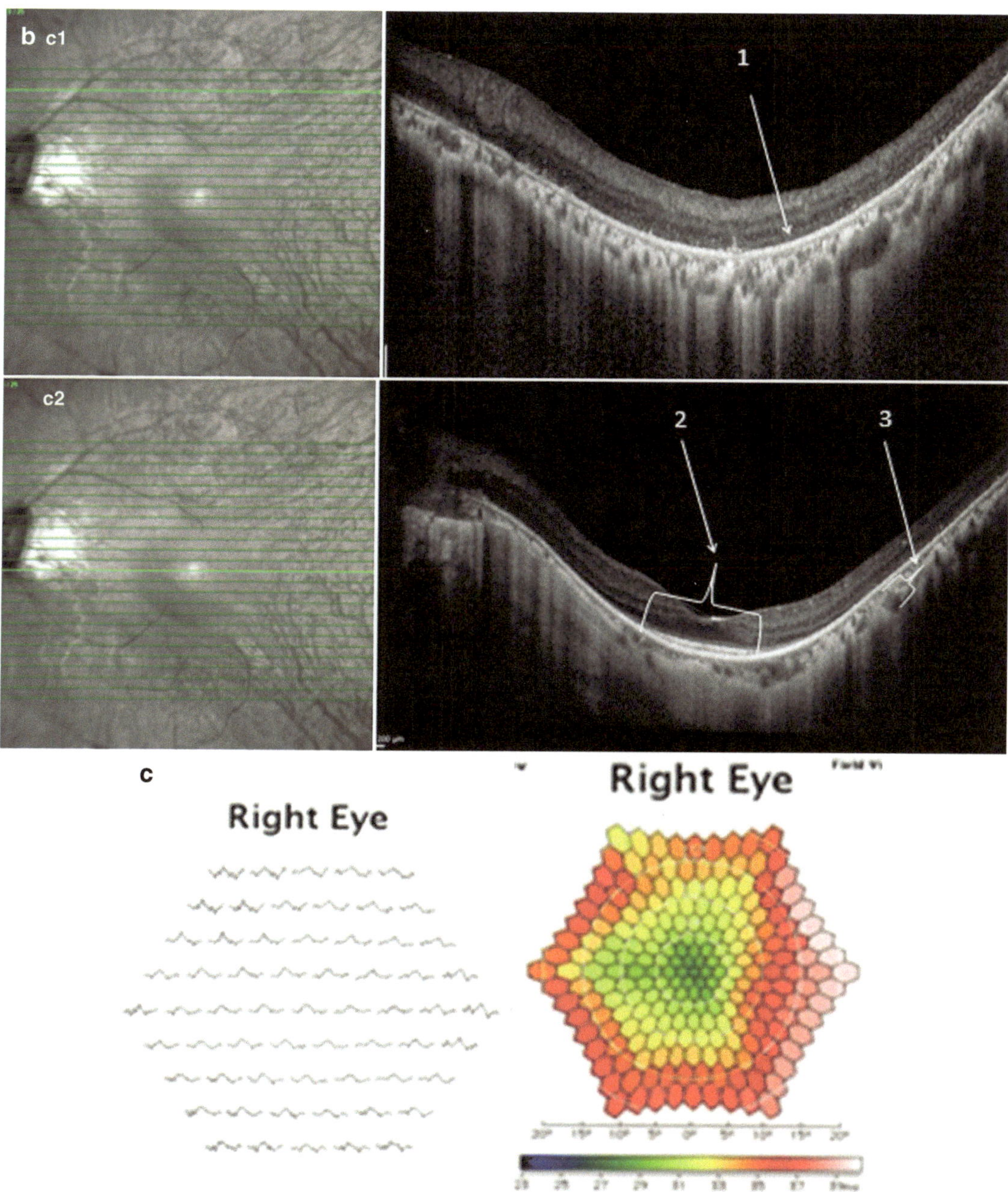

Fig. 24.2 (continued)

observed (Fig. 24.1b) (Hood et al. 2009; Hood et al. 2011a, b; Murakami et al. 2008; Triolo et al. 2013; Wakabayashi et al. 2010). Changes affecting the inner retina have also been reported: The RNFL has been noted to be thicker in RP patients when compared to controls (Fishman 1985). In addition, thinning of the inner retinal layers has also been found to occur at a faster rate in RP patients compared to normal subjects (Oishi et al. 2013).

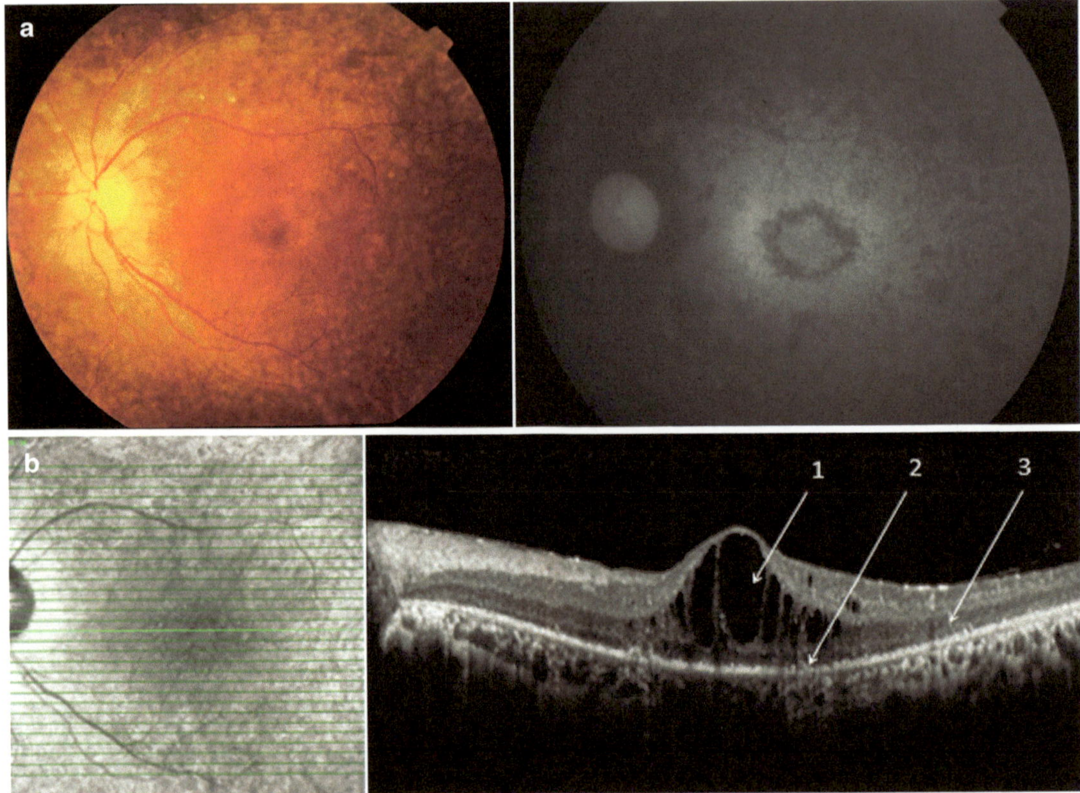

Fig. 24.3 Retinitis pigmentosa/rod-cone dystrophy. (**a**) A fundus photo (*left*) and AF image (*right*) of a 50-year-old female with RP who presented with right-eye blurring of vision and a visual acuity of 6/45. The fundus photo and AF show vessel attenuation, RPE atrophy and a bull's eye pattern of maculopathy. (**b**) Spectral domain OCT of the patient above that showed (*1*) cystoid macula oedema, (*2*) disruption in the EZ zone and loss of ELM which corresponds to impaired visual acuity, hyper-reflective foci (HFs) in the ONL and (*3*) HFs in the inner nuclear layer

Hyper-reflective foci in the inner nuclear layer (INL) in early stages followed by changes in the outer nuclear layer (ONL) in later stages have been described. These hyper-reflective foci are thought to be indicative of structural retinal changes (Figs. 24.3b and 24.4b) (Kuroda et al. 2014). Optical coherence tomography can aid in the detection of complications associated with RP, such as cystoid macular oedema (CMO), epiretinal membrane and macular hole formation. OCT can be used to monitor the response to treatment with medication or surgery (Hajali and Fishman 2009; Hajali et al. 2008; Hagiwara et al. 2011). In RP patients with severe CMO, visual impairment is strongly correlated to a disruption of the EZ (Fig. 24.3b) (Kim et al. 2013). After cataract surgery about 14 % of RP patients have macular oedema (Jackson et al. 2001). OCT is also useful to detect and monitor the response to treatment of CMO with acetazolamide (Chung et al. 2006).

Overall OCT imaging shows that disruption in the EZ, loss of the ELM and thinning of the inner retinal layers correlate to visual impairment in patients with RP. Choroidal thinning was also observed in both the subfoveal and peripheral retina; however there was no correlation to visual acuity (Dhoot et al. 2013). Optical coherence tomography imaging in combination with FAF imaging, electrophysiology and visual field testing are useful modalities to diagnose as well as monitor progression and response to treatment in patients with RP (Birch et al. 2013; Hood et al. 2011a, b).

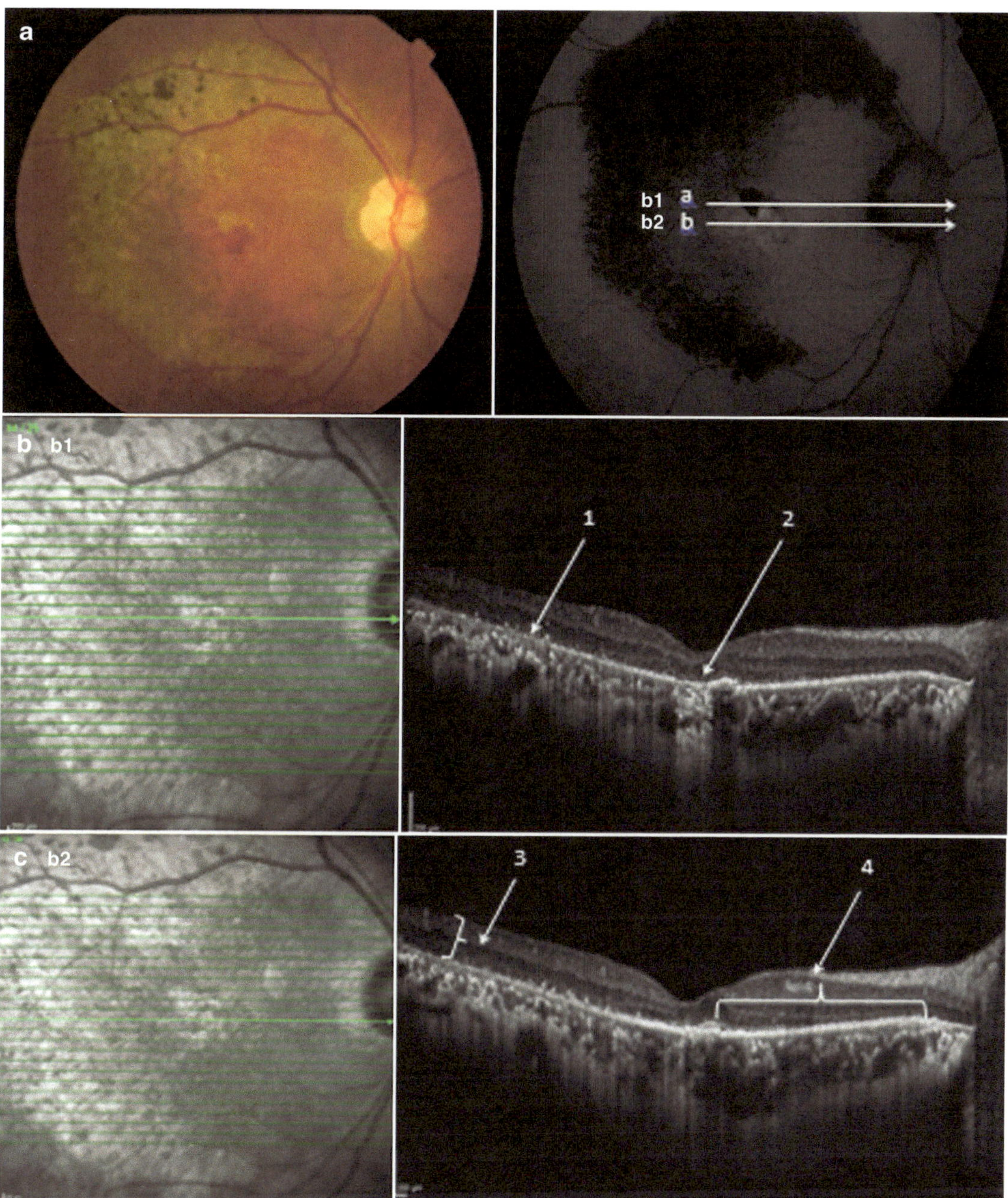

Fig. 24.4 Retinitis pigmentosa/rod-cone dystrophy. (**a**) A fundus photo (*left*) and AF image (*right*) of a 49-year-old male with pericentric RP and maculopathy who presented with blurring of vision and a visual acuity of 6/21. Fundus photo and AF show bony spicules and RPE atrophy in the mid-peripheral region and maculopathy. (**b**) Spectral domain OCT of the patient corresponding to the AF cut "b1" above which showed (*1*) loss of EZ and ELM and thinning in the ONL and RPE/Bruch's layer in these same areas with HFs in the outer nuclear layer and subretinal layer. (*2*) An area of RPE atrophy with increased transmission corresponding to the area of reduced AF. (**c**) Spectral domain OCT of the patient corresponding to the AF cut "b2" above showing (*3*) generalised thinning of the neurosensory retina in areas corresponding to RPE atrophy and bony spicules with (*4*) EZ disruption but preservation of the ELM and ONL corresponding to the areas of the normal retina between the disc and macula seen on the fundus photo and AF. (**d**) Multifocal ERG which showed reduced amplitude affecting the central three rings. (**e**) GVF of the same patient demonstrates central scotoma and relatively preserved peripheral vision

Fig. 24.4 (continued)

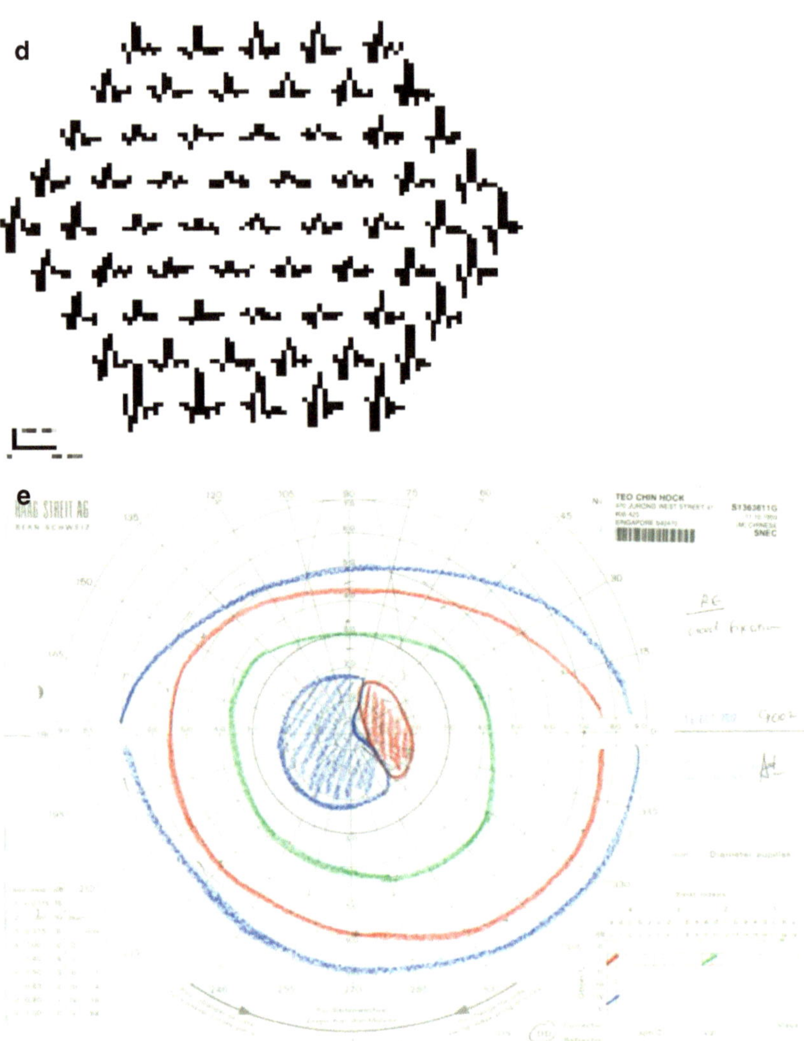

24.3 Cone Dystrophy

Cone dystrophy is a group of heterogenous conditions which predominantly affect the cone photoreceptors. Common symptoms include central vision loss, photophobia, dyschromatopsia and in some cases nystagmus (Michaelides et al. 2004a; Simunovic and Moore 1998). There are two types of cone dystrophy: stationary and progressive. Achromatopsia refers to early-onset cone dystrophy that is usually stationary. The majority of achromatopsia is inherited in an autosomal recessive manner. Blue cone monochromacy is a small subset of stationary cone dystrophy which is inherited in an X-linked recessive manner. Progressive cone dystrophy is most commonly inherited in an autosomal dominant manner. In the progressive form, visual acuity continues to deteriorate gradually, often resulting in legal blindness by adulthood (Jacobson et al. 1989; Ripps et al. 1987). Cone-rod dystrophy appears to involve only cones early in the disease, with progressive rod dysfunction developing later.

Characteristic clinical signs include the presence of a bull's eye appearance (Fig. 24.7a) with a dark central area at the fovea with surrounding pale zone (Grey et al. 1977). Other non-specific changes that may occur include macular retinal atrophy and pigment deposits. In the later stages, if there is rod

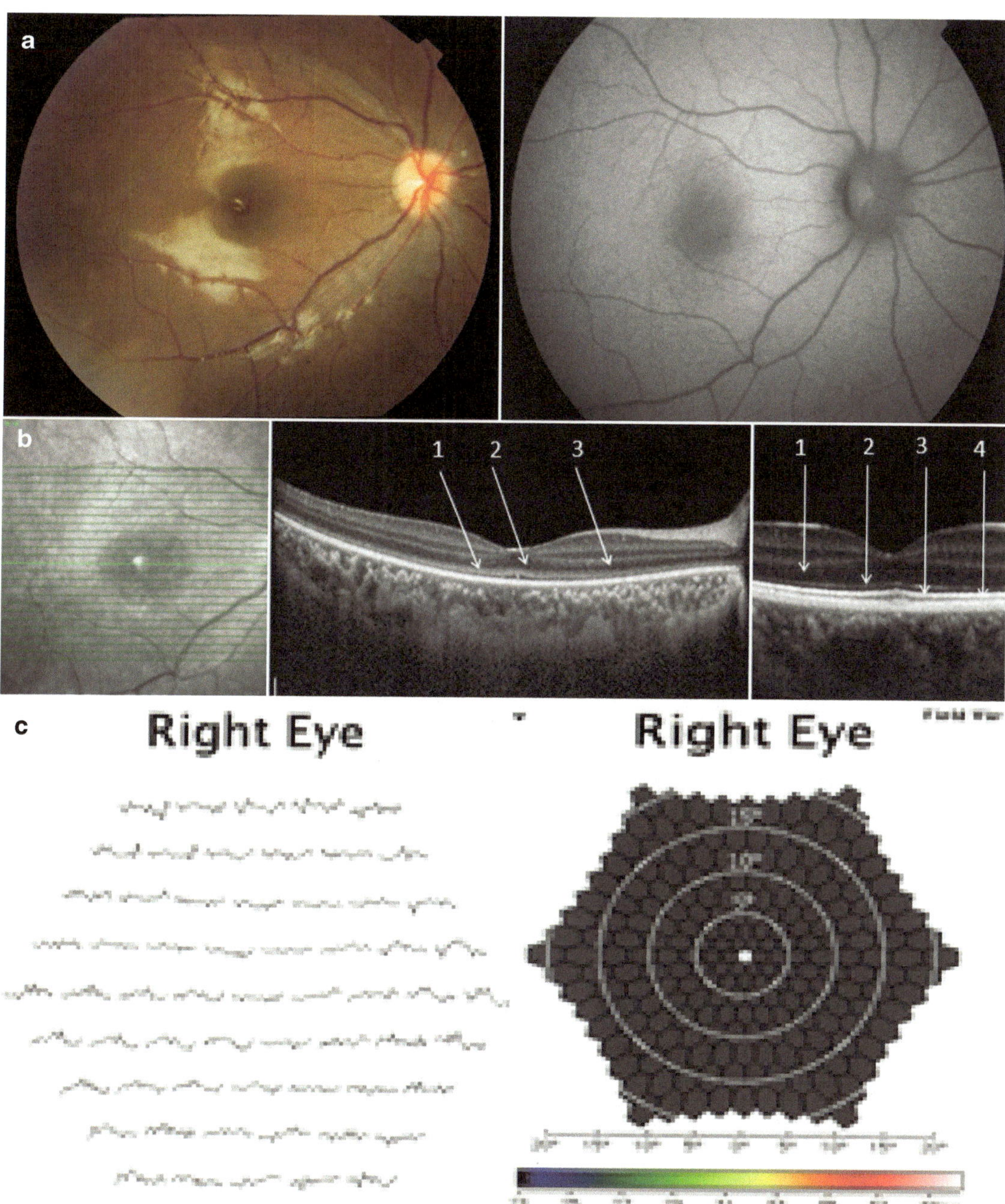

Fig. 24.5 Cone dystrophy. (**a**) A 12-year-old male with early cone dystrophy who presented with dyschromatopsia and visual acuity of 6/24 in both eyes. The fundus photo (*left*) and AF image (*right*) appear within normal limits. (**b**) Spectral domain OCT of the patient showed (*1*) a loss of the interdigitation zone (IZ) between the cone outer segments and the apical processes of the retinal pigment epithelium along the whole span of the cut but more marked in the foveal region and (*2*) foveal cavitation. (*3*) A less distinct border in the periphery between the EZ and the ELM with lower intensity and thinning of the EZ band is also observed. (*below*, *right*) A normal spectral domain OCT which showed four bands: (*1*) ELM, (*2*) inner segment ellipsoid zone (EZ), (*3*) interdigitation zone (IZ) and (*4*) RPE layer. (**c**) Reduced and delayed multifocal ERG responses which showed cone dysfunction despite no definite changes seen on the fundus photo

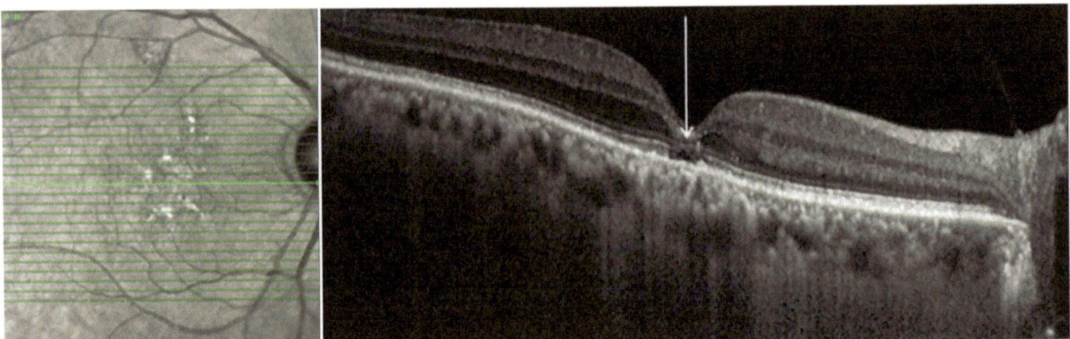

Fig. 24.6 Cone dystrophy. Another SD-OCT feature described in cone dystrophy: outer retinal layer loss with central retinal thinning and segmental foveal loss of the EZ band

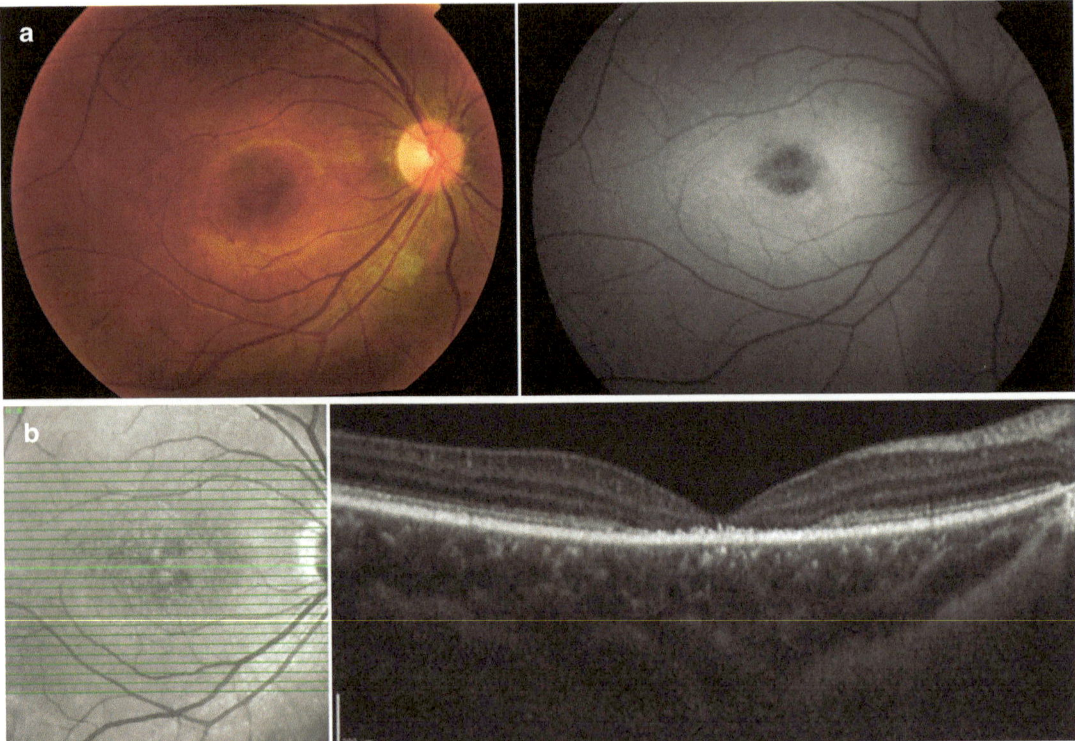

Fig. 24.7 Cone dystrophy. (**a**) A characteristic bull's eye pattern was seen in the fundus photo (*left*) of a 30-year-old male with cone dystrophy who presented with blurring of vision and visual acuity of 6/90. AF imaging (*right*) showed a ringlike area of hyper-autofluorescence surrounding a hypo-autofluorescent area of RPE atrophy. (**b**) (*middle*) Spectral domain OCT which showed complete loss of the EZ and ELM in the macular regions likely corresponding to the abnormal area on AF and multifocal ERG. (**c**) Multifocal ERG which showed localised abnormality affecting the centre three rings

involvement, vessel attenuation and bony spicule pigmentation in the periphery may develop. In advanced stages, severe diffuse chorioretinal atrophy, temporal disc pallor and even optic atrophy can occur (van Huet et al. 2013; Michaelides et al. 2004a, b; Simunovic and Moore 1998).

Visual symptoms may precede visible changes in the macula. Associated visual field defects include a central scotoma, an annular scotoma, a generalised sensitivity loss or uncommonly, a peripheral scotoma (Michaelides et al. 2004a, b; Sadowski and Zrenner 1997;

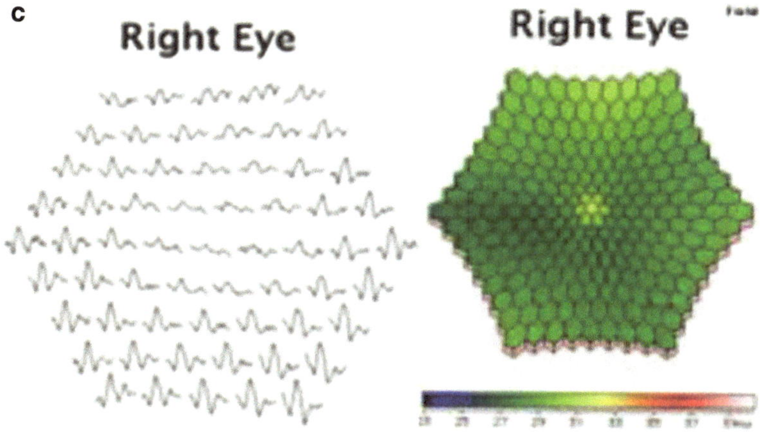

Fig. 24.7 (continued)

Zahlava et al. 2014). Typical electrophysiology findings in cone dystrophy include poor photopic and 30Hz flicker responses, with relatively preserved scotopic (rod-derived) responses. Multifocal electroretinogram also shows a reduction in the amplitude and delay in responses. Electroretinogram (ERG) findings are very informative as they may be abnormal even before any distinguishable clinical signs appear (Fig. 24.5). In the late stages of cone-rod dystrophy, completely undetectable waveforms maybe observed in both scotopic and photopic testing (Krill et al. 1973; Michaelides et al. 2004a, b; Ripps et al. 1987; Sadowski and Zrenner 1997; Simunovic and Moore 1998). Findings with FAF imaging can be variable, but a ring of hyper-autofluorescence surrounded by an area of macula RPE atrophy is commonly seen (Fig. 24.7a) (Robson et al. 2010).

24.3.1 Optical Coherence Tomography

Optical coherence tomography findings characteristic of cone dystrophy in the early stages may be subtle, such as loss of the interdigitation zone (IZ), with or without foveal cavitation (Fig. 24.5). There is a less distinct border in the periphery between the EZ and the ELM with lower intensity and thinning of the EZ zone. At the macula, the EZ zone can show irregular foveal loss or segmental foveal loss (Fig. 24.6). Another pattern of OCT abnormality that has been observed in cone dystrophy is central foveal thickening with irregular perifoveal loss of the EZ zone. In the later stages, the ELM and EZ may be completely lost at the macular region but preserved in the peripheral regions of the fundus (Fig. 24.7b). There is also generalised thinning of the RPE layer (Cho et al. 2013; Inui et al. 2014; Lima et al. 2013).

Overall, cone dystrophy and cone-rod dystrophy show characteristic changes on OCT that affects predominantly the macula area in the early stages and correlates with the level of visual impairment.

24.4 Stargardt Disease and Fundus Flavimaculatus

Stargardt disease and fundus flavimaculatus are variants of an inherited form of macular dystrophy. The recessive form caused by mutations in the *ABCA4* gene located on chromosome 1p13 is the most common form (Armstrong et al. 1998; Gerber et al. 1995; Hadden and Gass 1976). It has a prevalence of 1 in 10,000. Affected individuals usually present with visual loss in childhood to early teens and many progress to legal blindness by adulthood. A subset of these patients has the onset of disease at a later age, which is often associated with a better visual prognosis. Clinical symptoms include loss of central vision and dyschromatopsia. Fundus examination during the early stage of the disease can be normal, or show non-specific mottling only. As the disease progresses, loss of the foveal reflex and granulation in the RPE with a "snail slime" appearance can be seen (Figs. 24.8a and 24.9a). In the later stages, atrophy of the RPE may give rise to a "beaten bronze" appearance (Cibis et al. 1980; Eagle et al. 1980; Fujinami et al. 2013a, c; Michaelides et al. 2003; Rotenstreich et al. 2003). A characteristic finding of this disease is the bilateral white-yellowish deep retinal lesions (flecks) seen in the posterior pole which can extend to the mid-periphery (Fig. 24.8a). Flecks can vary in shape (e.g. pisciform), size and pattern (Armstrong et al. 1998).

Different FAF imaging patterns have been observed according to the stage of the disease and the rate of atrophy. During the early stages, increased autofluorescence can be seen within the flecks, which reflect the accumulation of autofluorescent material surrounded by a homogeneous background. This background signal can progress to become more heterogenous, developing numerous foci of abnormal signals. In later stage, with increasing atrophy, multiple areas of reduced autofluorescence in the posterior pole can be seen (Fig. 24.8a) (Fujinami et al. 2013a, b, c).

Electrophysiology testing demonstrates macular dysfunction in all cases. In addition, three patterns have been observed, which may have prognostic value: (1) severe abnormality on pattern ERG (macular function) with normal scotopic and photopic b-wave amplitudes, (2) reduced macular function with loss of photopic ERG responses (cone dysfunction) and (3) reduced photopic, scotopic and macular responses which showed global photoreceptor dysfunction of cones and rods (Lois et al. 1999). Long-term prognosis is worst in patients with global photoreceptor dysfunction in addition to maculopathy.

Fundus fluorescein angiography (FFA) shows a characteristic dark choroid with reduced visibility of the choroidal circulation. Newly formed flecks are not fluorescent as the lipofuscin is intracellular; however as the disease progresses, hyperfluorescence occurs due to a window defect in the preretinal and retinal phases (Anmarkrud 1979).

24.4.1 Optical Coherence Tomography

Findings on SD-OCT include a hyperplastic RPE with hyper-reflectivity seen in the fovea region. The residual neurosensory retina shows irregularity above the fovea and may be difficult to differentiate between the EZ and ELM layer in the parafoveal region (Fig. 24.8a) (Saxena et al. 2012). Retina flecks can be seen as hyper-reflective spots in the outer retinal layers and the RPE/Bruch's membrane complex. Flecks within the RPE (Fig. 24.9a) are associated with photoreceptor atrophy in the foveal region while flecks in the ONL (Figs. 24.8a and 24.9a) separate from the RPE may be a marker of possible evolution to foveal atrophy (Querques et al. 2009c).

Overall, OCT imaging allows quantitative, in vivo imaging of the photoreceptor layer and RPE in patients with Stargardt disease and fundus flavimaculatus. Flecks seen on the fundus can be seen in various layers of the retina on OCT and may be related to atrophic changes or progression of the disease. Choroidal thinning and atrophy is also observed in some cases (Yeoh et al. 2010). Therefore, SD-OCT allows detailed characterisation of this disease and the correlation with visual function, which other imaging modalities cannot achieve (Querques et al. 2006; Querques et al. 2009a, b, c; Saxena et al. 2012).

24.5 Bietti Crystalline Dystrophy

Bietti crystalline dystrophy (BCD) is a rare type of chorioretinal degeneration, characterised by yellow-white dot crystalline deposits seen in the paracentral and peripapillary retina occasionally associated with similar crystalline deposits in the cornea. Other retinal changes include progressive atrophy of the RPE and choroid with pigment clumping (Fig. 24.10a) (Bernauer and Daicker 1992; Mansour et al. 2007; Mauldin and O'Connor

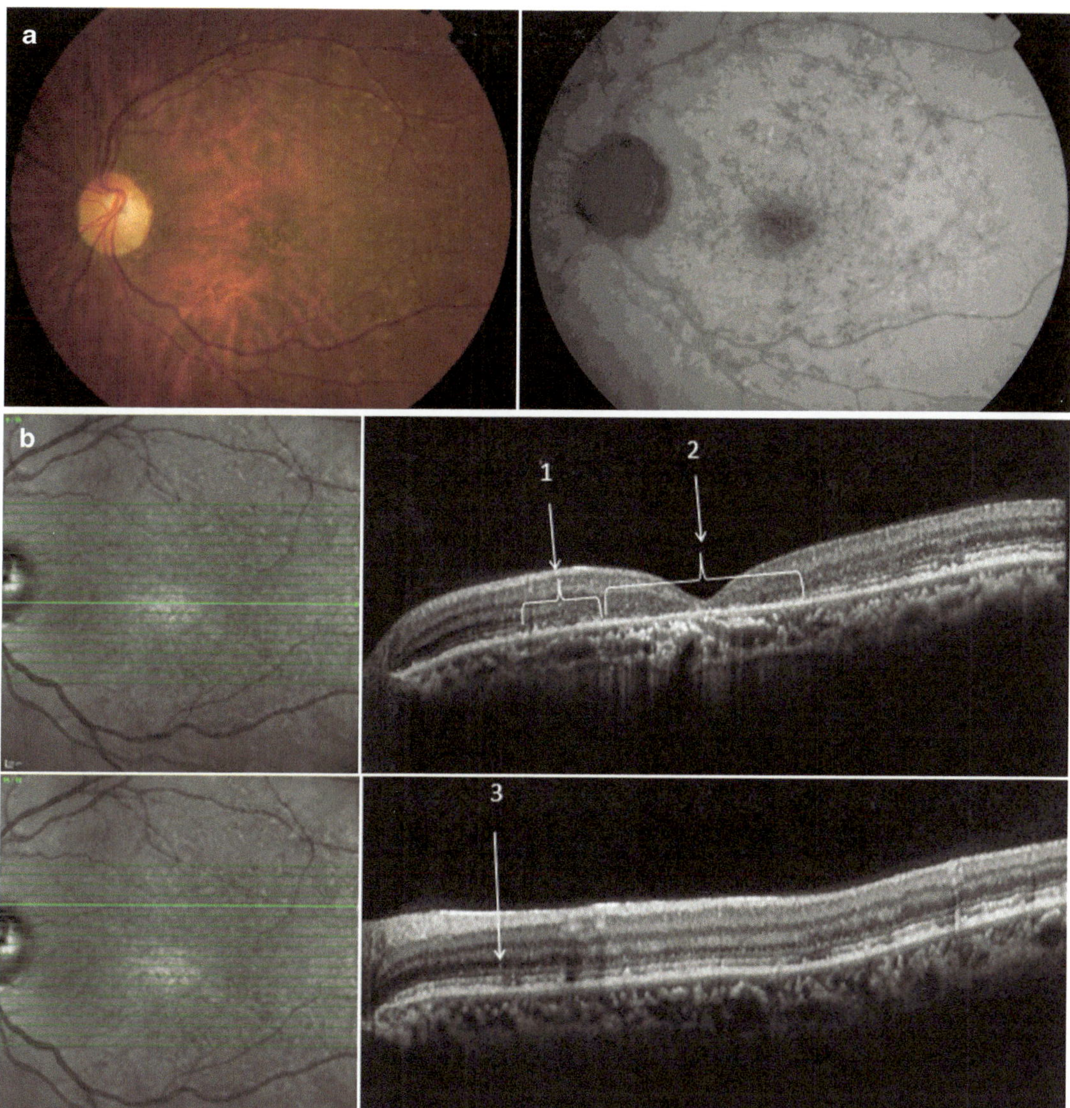

Fig. 24.8 Stargardt disease and fundus flavimaculatus. (**a**) A fundus photo (*left*) and AF image (*right*) of a 38-year-old male with Stargardt disease who presented with long-standing poor vision and a visual acuity of 6/90. Pisciform flecks can be seen on the posterior pole with macula atrophy. The area of macula atrophy appears hypo-AF whereas flecks showed varying degree of autofluorescence. (**b**) Stargardt disease and fundus flavimaculatus. Spectral domain OCT which showed (*above*) (*1*) demarcation of the parafoveal region where the EZ and ELM bands are poorly differentiated and (*2*) irregularity in the neurosensory retina with loss of the EZ and ELM bands affecting the centre of the fovea. Hyper-reflectivity of the RPE is noted throughout the macula. A peripheral SD-OCT image (*below*) showed (*3*) hyper-reflective spots in the ONL corresponding to the flecks

1981). Rarer complications include CMO, choroidal neovascular membrane and macula hole formation (Yin et al. 2014). Symptoms include nyctalopia, decreased visual acuity and a paracentral scotoma that usually presents between the second and fourth decades of life and often continue to progress to severe visual loss, constricted visual fields and legal blindness later in life (Chen et al. 2013; Kojima et al. 2012; Yin et al. 2014). Bietti crystalline dystrophy has been reported to be more common among the oriental race in East Asia and is caused by mutations in the CYP4V2

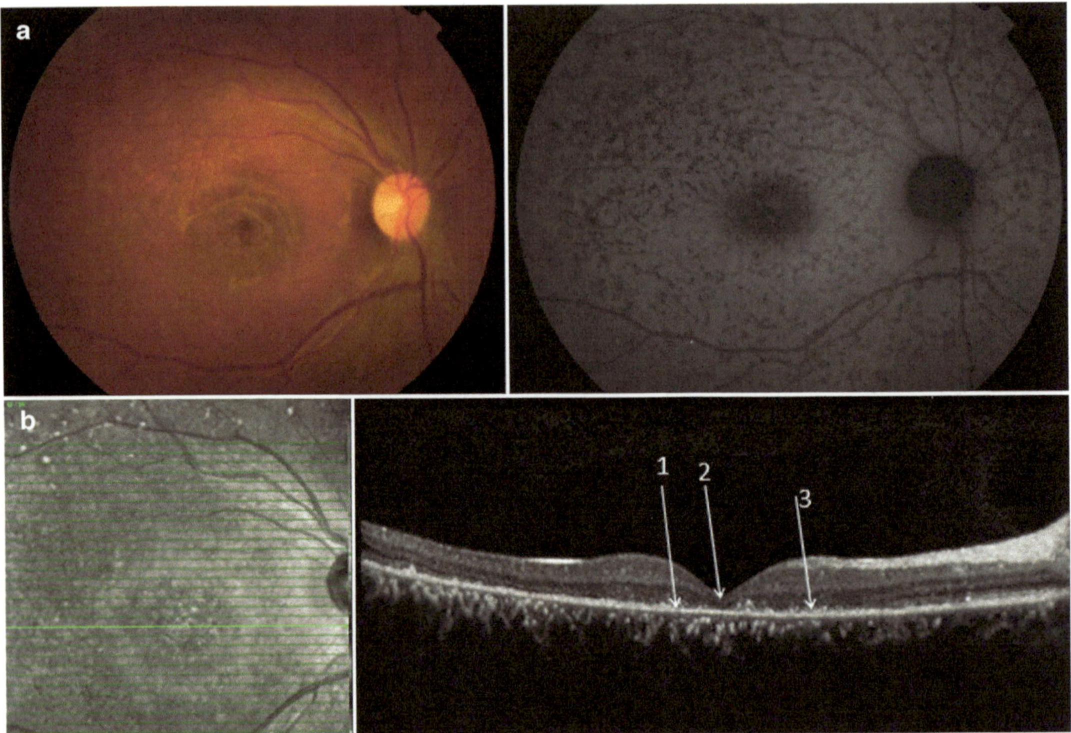

Fig. 24.9 Stargardt disease and fundus flavimaculatus. (**a**) A fundus photo (*left*) and AF image (*right*) of a 14-year-old male with Stargardt disease who presented with 6 months of poor vision and visual acuity of 6/120. Multiple greyish white flecks are seen on the posterior pole with snail slime like appearance of the macula. Hypo-autofluorescence seen in area of macula atrophy and flecks. (**b**) Spectral domain OCT which showed (*1*) hyper-reflective foci seen in the RPE corresponding to a fleck with, (*2*) a hyper-reflective RPE with loss of the EZ and ELM layer and marked thinning of the neurosensory retina. (*3*) Hyper-reflective foci can also be seen in the outer nuclear layer that was separate from the RPE corresponding to a fleck

gene, which causes abnormal lipid metabolism (Kaiser-Kupfer et al. 1994; Rossi et al. 2013; Toto et al. 2013; Yin et al. 2014).

Fundus autofluorescence imaging shows the presence of hypo-autofluorescent areas corresponding to areas of atrophy in the RPE and choroid (Fig. 24.10a). Hyper-autofluorescent spots are seen in the areas of the crystalline deposits only in some cases (Halford et al. 2014). Electrophysiology testing shows decreased amplitudes in both the scotopic and photopic responses with less-affected implicit times. However, there have also been reports of full-field ERG responses remaining normal even in the later stages of the disease. Multifocal ERG can show decreased amplitude in all rings. Visual field loss is also variable and may be in the form of ring, paracentral or central scotoma (Rossi et al. 2013; Sen et al. 2011). Indocyanine green angiography (ICGA) shows disruption in the choroidal circulation with delayed choroidal filling (Fong 2009).

24.5.1 Optical Coherence Tomography

Spectral domain OCT shows that most of the crystalline deposits are located at the level of the RPE/Bruch's membrane complex in portions of the retina that were spared from patchy degeneration (Fig. 24.10b) (Halford et al. 2014; Kojima et al. 2012; Toto et al. 2013). One study with serial imaging showed that the disappearance of the crystals was associated with severe disruption and thinning of the RPE/Bruch's membrane (Halford et al. 2014; Yeoh

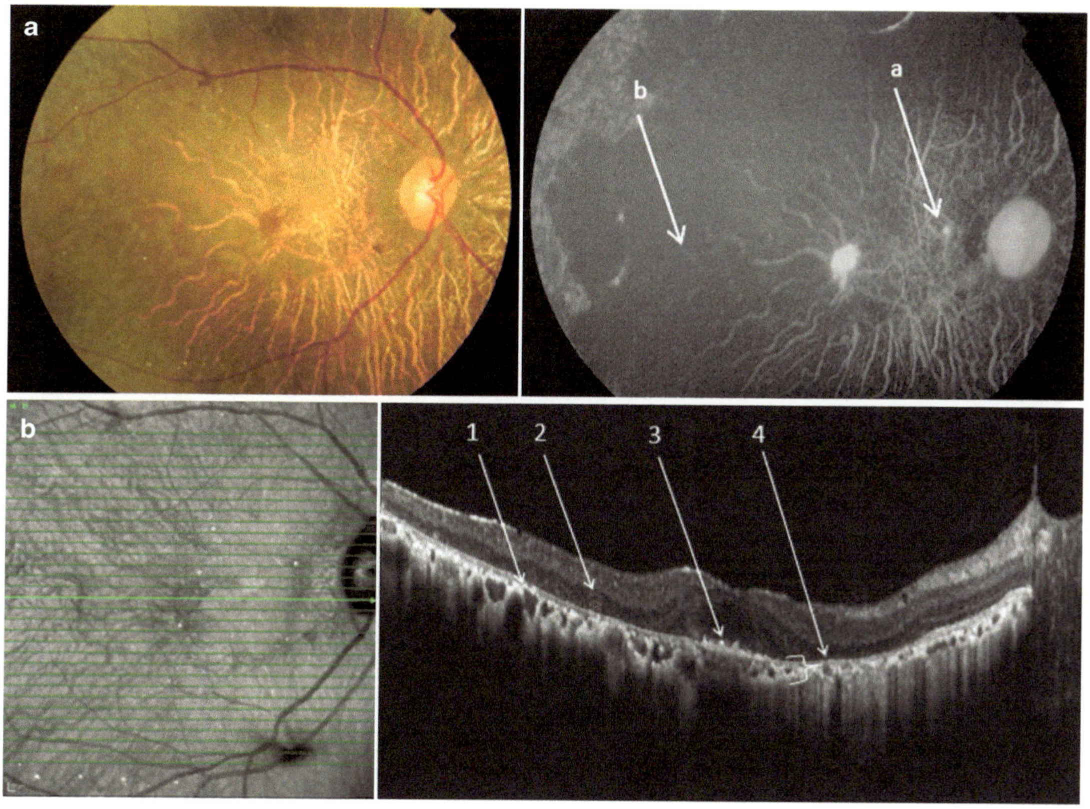

Fig. 24.10 Bietti crystalline dystrophy. (**a**) A fundus photo (*left*) of a 72-year-old lady with Bietti's crystalline dystrophy (BCD) and bilateral visual acuity of counting finger which showed widespread choroid and RPE atrophy with crystalline deposits in the mid-periphery. AF imaging showed that (*a*) some crystals appeared as hyper-autofluorescent spots and (*b*) widespread hypo-autofluorescence corresponded to areas of retinal atrophy. (**b**) Spectral domain OCT which showed (*1*) Crystalline deposits that were located in the layer of the RPE/Bruch's membrane complex. (*2*) Spherical structures in the ONL that have been associated with suspected areas of ongoing retinal degeneration, (*3*) Crystalline deposits located at the fovea, and (*4*) Severe chorio-retinal atrophy with complete loss of the EZ, ELM and severe thinning of the choroid (Figures reprinted with permission from Dr Lee Shu Yen)

et al. 2010). In the ONL, hyper-refractive, spherical structures are associated with suspected areas of ongoing retinal degeneration (Kojima et al. 2012).

24.6 Best's Vitelliform Macular Dystrophy

Best's vitelliform macular dystrophy (BVMD) is an autosomal dominant inherited condition with a variable penetrance. Patients with BVMD typically present in the first and second decades with metamorphopsia and progressive impairment of their central vision. Functional visual acuity is usually able to be preserved in at least one eye even in adulthood (Fishman et al. 1993; Mohler and Fine 1981; Ponjavic et al. 1999; Sohn et al. 2009). Mutations in the *Best1* gene on chromosome 11q12–q13 have been found to cause changes in the bestrophin-1 protein located in the RPE. This defective protein expresses properties of Ca^{2+}-activated Cl^{-} channels, which may explain the underlying pathogenesis of this disease (Rosenthal et al. 2006; Sun et al. 2002).

Juvenile BVMD has been characterised by the deposition of subretinal lipofuscin-rich material in the macula. Five stages have been observed as the disease progresses: (1) previtelliform stage (normal macula or subtle RPE changes), (2) vitelliform stage (Fig. 24.11a, right) (well-defined "egg yolk" lesion), (3) pseudohypopyon stage (Fig. 24.12a, right) (the yellow material settles

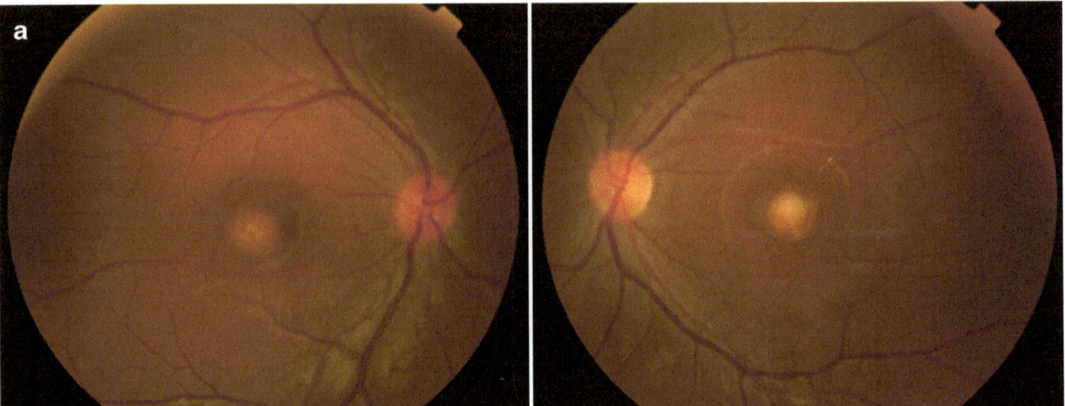

Fig. 24.11 Best's vitelliform macular dystrophy. (**a**) A fundus photo of a 10-year-old boy with Best's vitelliform macula dystrophy (BVMD) which showed the vitelliform stage (*right*) and a secondary choroidal neovascularisation (CNV) (*left*). This patient presented with left blurring of vision with a visual acuity of 6/9 on the right and 6/120 on the left. (**b**) AF imaging which showed hyper-autofluorescent material in the areas of the vitelliform lesion (*right*), central area of hypo-autofluorescence corresponding to the CNV with a ring of hyper-autofluorescence of vitelliform material. (**c**) (*above*) Spectral domain OCT (SD-OCT) image of the right eye of the patient above, which showed the vitelliform stage with (*1*) a dome-shaped accumulation of hyper-reflective material between the RPE layer and the photoreceptor layer. (*2*) The ONL is thinned over the contour of the elevation, and (*3*) the middle highly reflective layer (HRL) was seen to be elevated at the margins of the dome with thickening and fragmentation above the dome elevation but intact and thickened along the rest of the retina. (**d**) (*middle*) Spectral domainOCT image of the left eye of the patient which showed (*1*) The disruption of both the middle HRL and EZ also extending to above the lesion, (*2*) Aneurosensory detachment surrounding (*3*) A secondary CNV and (*4*) Areas of thinning of the ONL over the lesion all the way to the margins. (**e**) (*below*) Multifocal ERG showed a mild delay in central responses corresponding to the vitelliform lesion on the right eye and a more marked reduction and delay in responses in the left corresponding to the area with the secondary CNV; the EOG Arden ratio was reduced in both eyes (RE 133 %, LE 123 %)

inferiorly), (4) vitelliruptive stage (Fig. 24.12a, left and 24.13a, left) (a scrambled egg lesion with partial resorption of the material) and (5) atrophic stage (macular atrophy) (Fig. 24.13a, right) (Gass 1977; Mohler and Fine 1981; Querques et al. 2009a). Rupture of the Bruch's membrane with the development of choroidal neovascularisation (CNV) (Fig. 24.11a, right) can also occur (Noble 1978). Treatment of these secondary choroidal neovascularisations with photodynamic therapy and intra-vitreal anti-vascular endothelial growth factor (Anti-VEGF) has been reported to achieve good results (Andrade et al. 2003; Chung et al. 2001; Querques et al. 2008). Multifocal vitelliform lesions have also been reported (Boon et al. 2007a, b; Querques et al. 2009b). Late stages include fibrosis and geographic atrophy (Mohler and Fine 1981; Querques et al. 2009a).

Electrophysiology testing is often useful in making the diagnosis. Abnormal electrooculogram (EOG) with an Arden ratio of <140 % is demonstrated in BVMD, even in the early pre-vitelliform stage (Fig. 24.11e) (Thorburn and Nordstrom 1978). Multifocal ERG response delay has been shown to correlate with the loss of foveal photoreceptors in the EZ and was associated with decreased vision (Schatz et al. 2010).

Fundus autofluorescence imaging shows characteristic hyper-autofluorescence of the vitelliform material. Fundus fluorescein angiography in the vitelliform stage shows blocked fluorescence at the macula with a hypofluorescent disc. During the pseudohypopyon stage, the lower part with the vitelliform material shows blocked fluorescence with a contrasting superior portion with absent vitelliform material that can have normal or hyperfluorescence. The vitelliruptive stage has variable hyper- or hypofluorescence according to the distribution of the vitelliform material. The atrophic stage shows typical hyperfluorescence

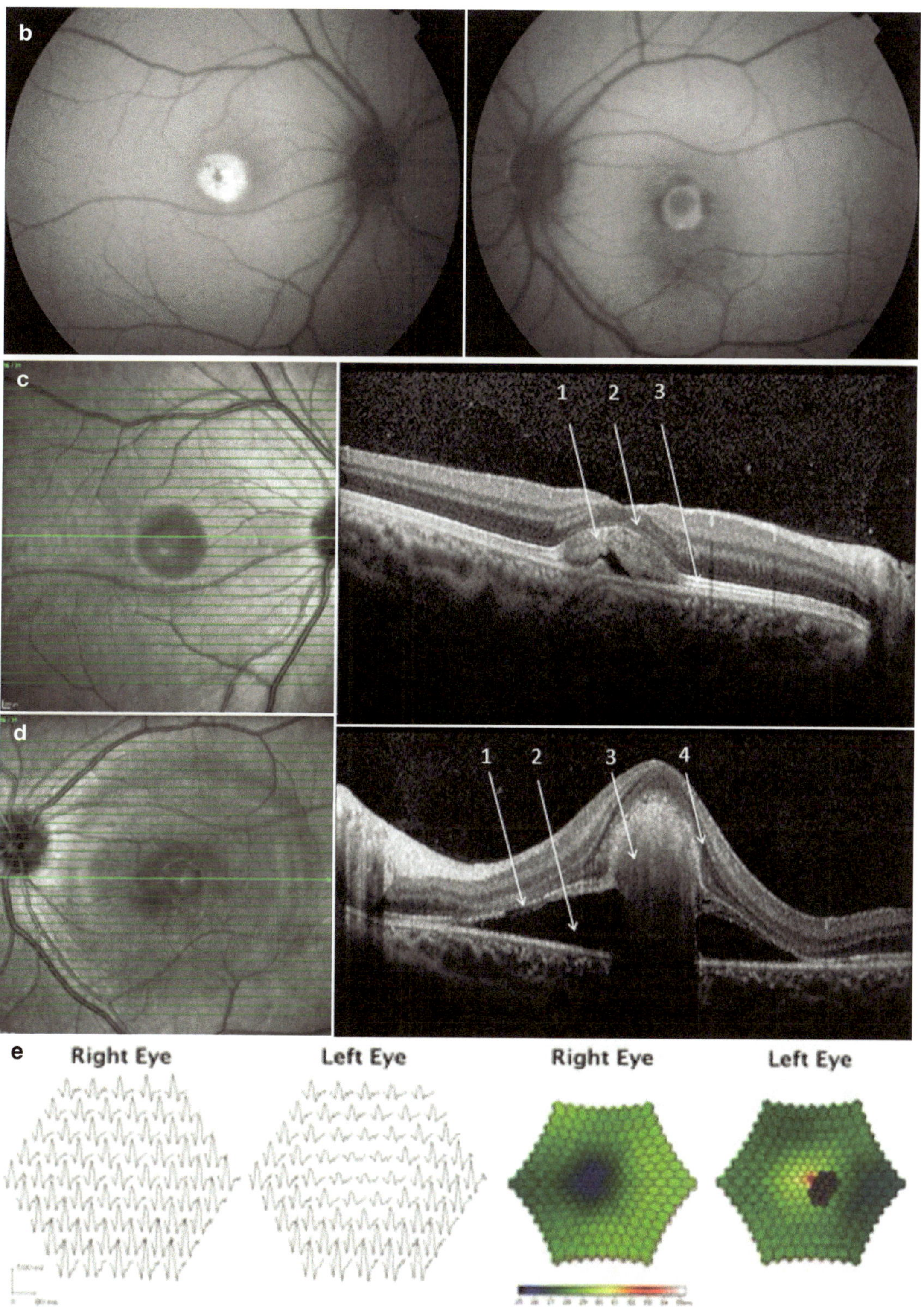

Fig. 24.11 (continued)

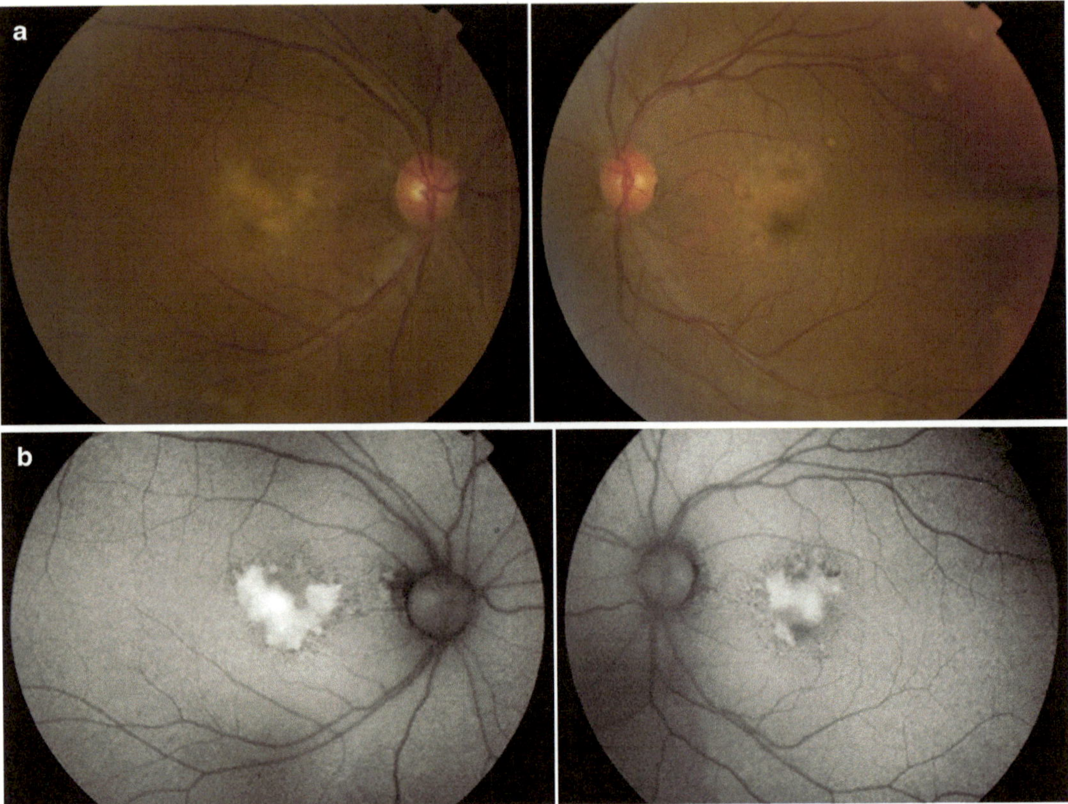

Fig. 24.12 Best's vitelliform macula dystrophy. (**a**) (*above*) A fundus photo of a 59-year-old lady with adult-onset foveomacular vitelliform dystrophy (AFVD) who was as symptomatic with a visual acuity of 6/7.5 on the right and 6/6 on the left. The right eye showed the pseudohypopyon stage with the accumulation of the yellowish material in the inferior part of the vitelliform lesion and the left eye showed the accumulation of vitelliform material inferiorly with partial resorption of the material and greyish clumps of subretinal tissue. (**b**) (*below*) AF imaging which showed hyper-autofluorescence of the vitelliform material in both eyes with areas of hypo-autofluorescence corresponding to areas of atrophy. (**c**) (*above*) (*a*) Spectral domain OCT (SD-OCT) image of right eye of the patient above of the vitelliform-like lesion which showed (*1*) a localised neurosensory retinal detachment with (*2*) clumps of hyper-reflective subretinal material seen at the base of this detachment. (*3*) The ONL was thinned with focal regions of heterogenous reflectivity and (*4*) a pigment epithelial detachment was observed. (*below*) (*b*) Spectral domain OCT image one year later which showed (*1*) increased vitelliform material accumulation and (*2*) focal areas of EZ disruption and irregular thickening of the middle HRL. (**d**) (*above*) (*a*) Spectral domain OCT image of left eye of the patient above which showed (*1*) irregular elongation of the outer segments of the photoreceptors causing an irregular middle HRL interspersed with focal areas of EZ disruption and (*2*) thinning of the ONL above the lesion. Two types of hyper-reflective mounds at the level of the RPE/Bruch's complex were observed. (*3*) The first type of mound was associated with shadowing of underlying choroidal structures. (*below*) (*b*) Spectral domain OCT image one year later which showed (*4*) a hyper-reflective spot of partially resorbed vitelliform material. (*5*) The second type of RPE mound that was associated with the overlying collapse of the outer retinal layers, hyper-reflectivity of the underlying choroid and (*6*) disruption of the EZ and middle HRL over the area of the lesion

due to an RPE window defect. Fibrotic changes in the late stages will stain early with intense hyperfluorescence. Fundus fluorescein angiography and ICGA can also be useful in the diagnosis and monitoring of secondary choroidal neovascularisation (Duncker et al. 2014; Ferrara et al. 2010; Gass 1977; Schatz et al. 2010).

24.6.1 Optical Coherence Tomography

Spectral domain OCT allows visualisation of changes in the retinal structure which can aid in monitoring of progression of BVMD (Ferrara et al. 2010; Querques et al. 2009a, b, c; Xu et al. 2013).

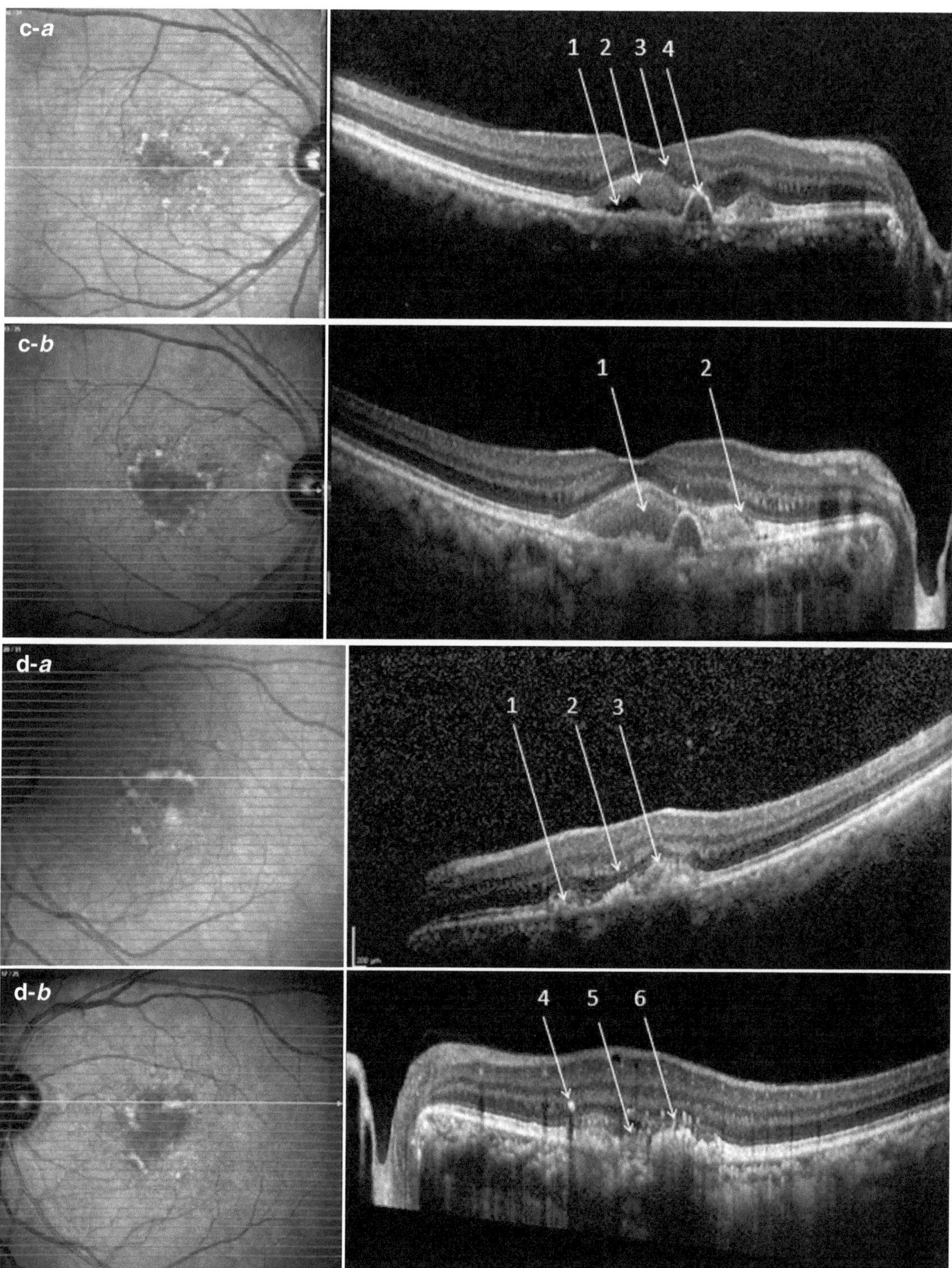

Fig. 24.12 (continued)

Previtelliform stage: A thickened middle highly reflective layer (HRL) between the RPE/Bruch's complex and the EZ can be observed even in early subclinical disease. The corresponding ONL starts to thin out at the fovea so the overall retinal thickness is maintained.

Vitelliform stage (Fig. 24.11c): A dome-shaped elevation can be seen at the fovea due to the accumulation of hyper-reflective material between the RPE layer and the photoreceptor layer. The middle HRL is seen to be elevated at the margins of the dome with thickening and fragmentation above the dome elevation. The ONL is thinned both over the contour of the elevation and even beyond the margins of the dome.

Pseudohypopyon stage (Fig. 24.12c): There is a localised neurosensory retinal detachment with clumps of hyper-reflective subretinal material seen at the base of this detachment. The ONL is thinned and there are focal regions of heterogenous reflectivity. There are focal areas of EZ disruption and irregular thickening of the middle HRL. There are small hyper-reflective mounds observed at the level of the RPE/Bruch's complex.

Vitelliruptive stage (Fig. 24.12d): A similar area of neurosensory detachment is seen with obvious thinning of the ONL. There is irregular elongation of the outer segments of the photoreceptors causing an irregular middle HRL interspersed with focal areas of EZ disruption. Greyish subretinal tissue is seen in the middle of these lesions which corresponded to two types of hyper-reflective mounds at the level of the RPE/Bruch's complex. The first type of mound is associated with shadowing of underlying choroidal structures. The second type is associated with collapse of the overlying outer retinal layers and hyper-reflectivity of the underlying choroid (Ferrara et al. 2010).

Atrophic stage: Overall thinning of the neurosensory layer may progress with further loss of photoreceptors. There is complete loss of the EZ and middle HRL with thinning of the overlying ONL associated with visual impairment. The RPE/Bruch's membrane complex is relatively well preserved.

24.7 Adult-Onset Foveomacular Vitelliform Dystrophy

Adult-onset foveomacular vitelliform dystrophy (AFVD) is an autosomal dominantly inherited disorder characterised by bilateral, round or oval, yellow, symmetrical, subretinal lesions similar to BVMD (Fig. 24.13a). However this disease has a later onset (after the fourth decade) with less severe visual impairment. Symptoms of this disease include a relative scotoma, metamorphopsia or sometimes can be detected on routine eye exam. Clinical signs can range from the typical bilateral deposition of lipofuscin-rich material within the RPE associated with photoreceptor loss to more subtle changes like satellite flecks. In some cases, it can mimic age-related degenerative diseases. Secondary choroidal neovascularisation and atrophy can be seen as this disease progresses (Brecher and Bird 1990; Gass 1974; Saito et al. 2003; Vine and Schatz 1980; Wiznia et al. 1981).

Electrooculogram findings can be normal or subnormal. Multifocal ERG responses are reduced in most cases especially in the central regions despite having good visual acuity. Fundus autofluorescence imaging shows similar hyper-autofluorescence of the vitelliform material to BVMD (Saito et al. 2003; Wiznia et al. 1981).

24.7.1 Optical Coherence Tomography

The SD-OCT findings show hyper-reflective clumps of vitelliform material within the ONL and outer plexiform layer (Fig. 24.13d). The EZ in some cases appeared to encase the dome-shaped portion of the highly reflective vitelliform material and in other eyes appeared irregular and disrupted. The RPE/Bruch's membrane complex is either normal, disappeared over the vitelliform lesion or became thickened and less well defined (Yeoh et al. 2010). One previous study showed choroidal thickening in AFVD compared to

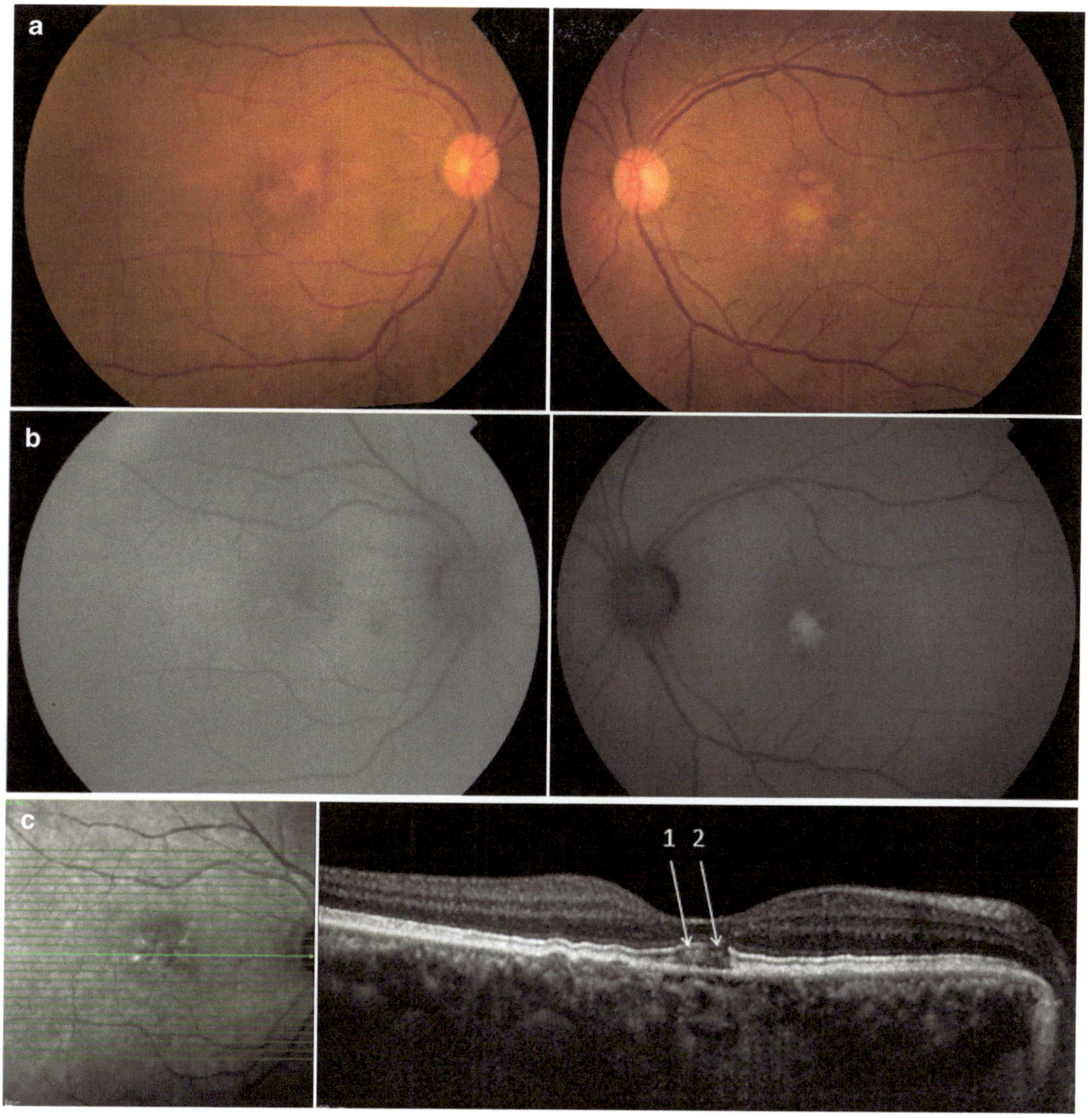

Fig. 24.13 Adult-onset foveomacular vitelliform dystrophy. (**a**) (*above*) A fundus photo of a 70-year-old lady with adult-onset foveomacular vitelliform dystrophy (AFVD) who presented with bilateral blurring of vision with visual acuity of 6/9 on the right eye and 6/21 on the left eye. The mild atrophic changes were shown on the right eye and a residual vitelliform-like lesion was shown on the left eye. (**b**) (*below*) AF imaging showed areas of hypo-autofluorescence corresponding to areas of atrophy on the right eye and areas of hyper-autofluorescence in the left eye corresponding to the partially resorbed vitelliform material. (**c**) (*above*) Spectral domain OCT image of the above patient of the atrophic stage which showed (*1*) preservation of the EZ and thickening and irregularity in the middle HRL which corresponds to good visual acuity of 6/9. An area of atrophy with (*2*) complete loss of the EZ and middle HRL away from foveal centre with thinning of the overlying ONL. The RPE/Bruch's membrane complex is relatively well preserved. (**d**) (*below*) Spectral domain OCT image of the above patient which showed (*1*) hyper-reflective clumps of vitelliform material within the outer plexiform layer, (*2*) an RPE mound was associated with shadowing of underlying choroidal structures and (*3*) pigment epithelial detachment

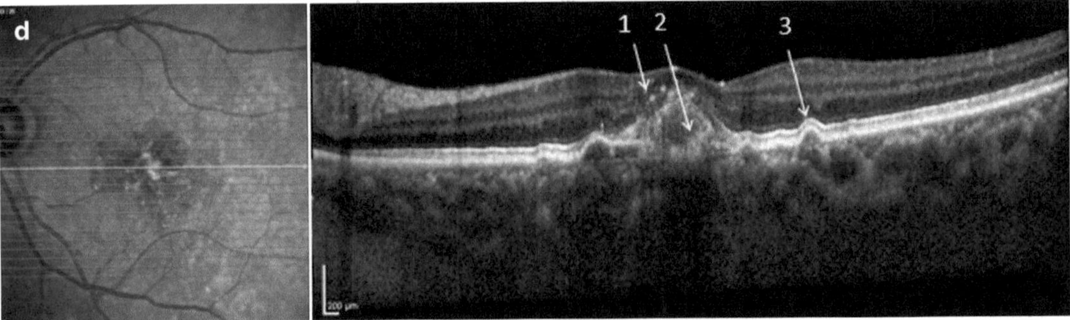

Fig. 24.13 (continued)

choroidal thinning observed in advanced age-related macular degeneration (AMD) (Coscas et al. 2014). The vitelliform material near the macula appeared as a highly reflective dome-shaped lesion located between the RPE and photoreceptor layer. In a small proportion of eyes, the macula lesion is hyporeflective. Retinal pigment mottling and discrete pigment epithelial detachments were also observed in some cases (Benhamou et al. 2003; Benhamou et al. 2004; Puche et al. 2010; Querques et al. 2011) (Fig. 24.13c).

24.8 X-Linked Retinoschisis

X-linked retinoschisis (XLRS) is an inherited vitreoretinal degeneration that is usually bilateral and symmetrical. In most cases there is characteristic macular involvement with splitting of the nerve fibre layer which sometimes may appear as a spoke-like pattern (Fig. 24.14). About half of these patients have peripheral schisis which most commonly occurs in the infero-temporal retina. The onset of symptoms is usually in the first decade, and affected males have moderate to severe visual impairment that worsens over the second and third decades and then stabilises (Apushkin et al. 2005; Gregori et al. 2013; Tantri et al. 2004). The RS1 gene is responsible for this disease codes for retinoschisis, a secreted protein that may be involved in cellular adhesion or interactions (Tantri et al. 2004). Electroretinogram findings reflect the predominant inner retina dysfunction, leading to reduction in the dark adapted b-wave amplitude with a relatively preserved a-wave (electronegative waveform) (Nakamura et al. 2001). Photopic 30Hz flicker ERG response has been reported to be delayed in some patients. S-cone ERGs have also been reported to be abnormal in 50 % of patients. Fundus autofluorescence imaging frequently demarcates the spoke-wheel pattern seen on the fundus (Vincent et al. 2013).

24.8.1 Optical Coherence Tomography

Foveal macula splitting can occur in any layer of the retina. It is most frequently seen between the deeper retinal layers i.e. between the inner and outer nuclear layer and can have characteristic cystoid spaces. A few smaller cysts have been observed in the parafoveal region at the ganglion cell layer and retinal nerve fibre layer. Peripheral schisis has also been reported to be more superficial, affecting the retinal nerve fibre layer (Urrets-Zavalía et al. 2006; Yu et al. 2010). The thinning of the temporal perifoveal inner retina, thickening of the inner fovea as well as changes in the outer segments of the photoreceptors may be correlated to visual acuity (Andreoli and Lim 2014; Yang et al. 2014). OCT also helps in the differentiation of peripheral schisis versus suspected retinal detachment which is important for management (Fig. 24.14).

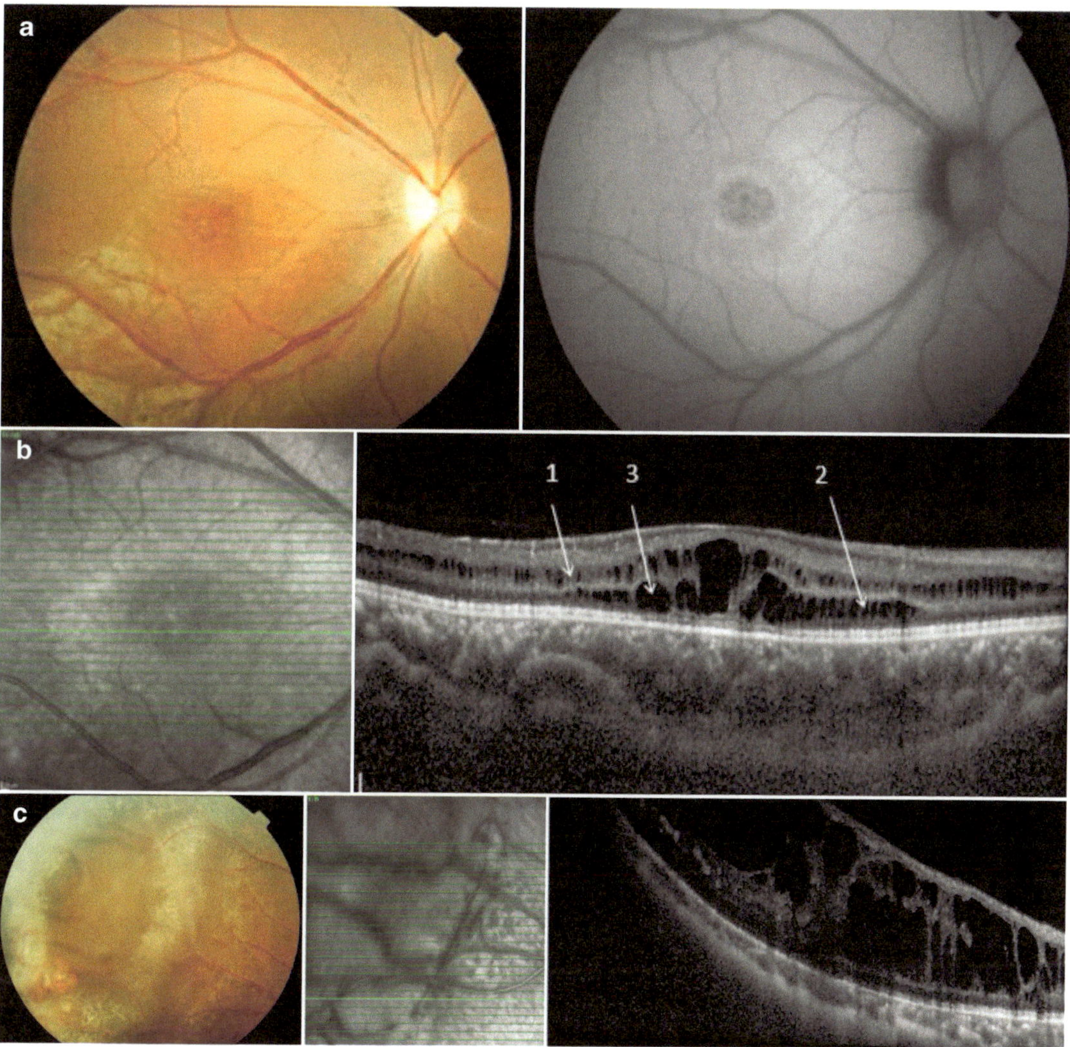

Fig. 24.14 X-linked retinoschisis. (**a**) (*above*) A right fundus photo (*left*) of an 18-year-old male with X-linked retinoschisis (XLRS) who presented with floaters in both eyes with visual acuity of 6/21 in both eyes. Bilateral foveal schisis is observed with a characteristic spoke-like pattern seen (*left eye similar*). AF imaging (*right*) showed corresponding areas of hypo-autofluorescence corresponding to the areas of foveal retinoschisis. (**b**) (*below*) Spectral domain OCT image showing foveal macula schisis affecting the (*1*) inner nuclear layer (INL) and (*2*) outer nuclear layer, with characteristic cystoids spaces (*3*). In this example, Outer nuclear layer schisis is more marked around the foveal macular region and less prominent in peripheral areas. (**c**) (*above*) Fundus image (*left*) showing an area of peripheral schisis and spectral domain OCT images showing cross-sectional images of the INL splitting (*right image*) (Contributed by Dr. Loh Boon Kwang (Singapore))

References

Andrade RE, Farah ME, Costa RA (2003) Photodynamic therapy with verteporfin for subfoveal choroidal neovascularization in best disease. Am J Ophthalmol 136:1179–1181

Andreoli MT, Lim JI (2014) Optical coherence tomography retinal thickness and volume measurements in X-linked retinoschisis. Am J Ophthalmol 158:567–573

Anmarkrud N (1979) Fundus fluorescein angiography in fundus flavimaculatus and Stargardt's disease. Acta Ophthalmol (Copenh) 57:172–182

Apushkin MA, Fishman GA, Rajagopalan AS (2005) Fundus findings and longitudinal study of visual acuity loss in patients with X-linked retinoschisis. Retina 25:612–618

Armstrong JD, Meyer D, Xu S et al (1998) Long-term follow-up of stargardt's disease and fundus flavimaculatus. Ophthalmology 105:448–457

Benhamou N et al (2003) Adult-onset foveomacular vitelliform dystrophy: a study by optical coherence tomography. Am J Ophthalmol 135:362–367

Benhamou N et al (2004) Adult-onset foveomacular vitelliform dystrophy with OCT 3. Am J Ophthalmol 138:294–296

Bernauer W, Daicker B (1992) Bietti's corneal-retinal dystrophy. A 16-year progression. Retina 12:18–20

Berson EL et al (1985) Natural course of retinitis pigmentosa over a three-year interval. Am J Ophthalmol 99:240–251

Birch DG et al (2013) Spectral-domain optical coherence tomography measures of outer segment layer progression in patients with X-linked retinitis pigmentosa. JAMA Ophthalmol 131:1143–1150

Bird AC (1995) Retinal photoreceptor dystrophies LI. Edward Jackson Memorial Lecture. Am J Ophthalmol 119:543–562

Boon CJ et al (2007a) Clinical and genetic heterogeneity in multifocal vitelliform dystrophy. Arch Ophthalmol 125:1100–1106

Boon CJ et al (2007b) Mutations in the peripherin/RDS gene are an important cause of multifocal pattern dystrophy simulating STGD1/fundus flavimaculatus. Br J Ophthalmol 91:1504–1511

Brecher R, Bird AC (1990) Adult vitelliform macular dystrophy. Eye (Lond) 4:210–215

Bundey S, Crews SJ (1984) A study of retinitis pigmentosa in the City of Birmingham. I Prevalence. J Med Genet 21:417–420

Bunker CH et al (1984) Prevalence of retinitis pigmentosa in Maine. Am J Ophthalmol 97:357–365

Chen H et al (2013) Functional and clinical findings in 3 female siblings with crystalline retinopathy. Doc Ophthalmol 116:237–243

Cho SC et al (2013) Morphologic characteristics of the outer retina in cone dystrophy on spectral-domain optical coherence tomography. Korean J Ophthalmol 27:19–27

Chung MM et al (2001) Visual outcome following subretinal hemorrhage in Best disease. Retina 21:575–580

Chung H et al (2006) Optical coherence tomography in the diagnosis and monitoring of cystoid macular edema in patients with retinitis pigmentosa. Retina 26:922–927

Cibis GW, Morey M, Harris DJ (1980) Dominantly inherited macular dystrophy with flecks (Stargardt). Arch Ophthalmol 98:1785–1789

Coscas F et al (2014) Comparison of macular choroidal thickness in adult onset foveomacular vitelliform dystrophy and age-related macular degeneration. Invest Ophthalmol Vis Sci 55:64–69

Dhoot DS et al (2013) Evaluation of choroidal thickness in retinitis pigmentosa using enhanced depth imaging optical coherence tomography. Br J Ophthalmol 97:66–69

Duncker T et al (2014) Quantitative fundus autofluorescence and optical coherence tomography in best vitelliform macular dystrophy. Invest Ophthalmol Vis Sci 55:1471–1482

Eagle RC, Lucier AC, Bernardino VB et al (1980) Retinal pigment epithelial abnormalities in fundus flavimaculatus: a light and electron microscopic study. Ophthalmology 87:1189–1200

Ferrara DC et al (2010) Multimodal fundus imaging in best vitelliform macular dystrophy. Graefes Arch Clin Exp Ophthalmol 248:1377–1386

Fishman GA (1978) Retinitis pigmentosa: visual loss. Arch Ophthalmol 96:1185–1188

Fishman GA (1985) Electrophysiology and inherited retinal disorders. Doc Ophthalmol 60:107–119

Fishman GA, Anderson RJ, Lourenco P (1985) Prevalence of posterior subcapsular lens opacities in patients with retinitis pigmentosa. Br J Ophthalmol 69:263–266

Fishman GA et al (1993) Visual acuity in patients with best vitelliform macular dystrophy. Ophthalmology 100:1665–1670

Fong AM et al (2009) Bietti's crystalline dystrophy in Asians: clinical, angiographic and electrophysiological characteristics. Int Ophthalmol 29:459–470

Francis PJ (2006) Genetics of inherited retinal disease. J R Soc Med 99:189–191

Fujinami K et al (2013a) A longitudinal study of stargardt disease: clinical and electrophysiologic assessment, progression, and genotype correlations. Am J Ophthalmol 155:1075–1088

Fujinami K et al (2013b) A longitudinal study of Stargardt disease: quantitative assessment of fundus autofluorescence, progression, and genotype correlations. Invest Ophthalmol Vis Sci 54:8181–8190

Fujinami K et al (2013c) Clinical and molecular analysis of Stargardt disease with preserved foveal structure and function. Am J Ophthalmol 156:487–501

Gass JD (1974) A clinicopathologic study of a peculiar foveomacular dystrophy. Trans Am Ophthalmol Soc 72:139–156

Gass JD (1977) Stereoscopic atlas of macular diseases: diagnosis and treatment. Mosby Inc., St. Louis

Gerber S, Rozet JM, Bonneau D et al (1995) A gene for late-onset fundus flavimaculatus with macular dystrophy maps to chromosome 1p13. Am J Hum Genet 56:396

Goura P, Carr RE (1964) Electrophysiological studies in early retinitis pigmentosa. Arch Ophthalmol 72:104–110

Gregori NZ, Lam BL, Gregori G et al (2013) Wide-field spectral-domain optical coherence tomography in patients and carriers of X-linked retinoschisis. Ophthalmology 120:169–174

Grey RH, Blach RK, Barnard WM (1977) Bull's eye maculopathy with early cone degeneration. Br J Ophthalmol 61:702–718

Grover S, Fishman GA, Brown J Jr (1998) Patterns of visual field progression in patients with retinitis pigmentosa. Ophthalmology 105:1069–1075

Hadden OB, Gass JD (1976) Fundus flavimaculatus and stargardt's disease. Am J Ophthalmol 82:527–539

Hagiwara A, Yamamoto S, Ogata K et al (2011) Macular abnormalities in patients with retinitis pigmentosa: prevalence on OCT examination and outcomes of vitreoretinal surgery. Acta Ophthalmol 89:122–125

Hajali M, Fishman GA (2009) The prevalence of cystoid macular edema on optical coherence tomography in retinitis pigmentosa patients without cystic changes on fundus examination. Eye (Lond) 23:915–919

Hajali M, Fishman GA, Anderson RJ (2008) The prevalence of cystoid macular edema in retinitis pigmentosa patients determined by optical coherence tomography. Br J Ophthalmol 92:1065–1068

Halford S, Liew G, Mackay DS et al (2014) Detailed phenotypic and genotypic characterization of Bietti crystalline dystrophy. Ophthalmology 121:1174–1184

Hamel CP (2007) Cone rod dystrophies. Orphanet J Rare Dis 2:7

Hartong DT, Berson EL, Dryja TP (2006) Retinitis pigmentosa. Lancet 368:1795–1809

Holopigian K, Greenstein V, Seiple W et al (1996) Rates of change differ among measures of visual function in patients with retinitis pigmentosa. Ophthalmology 103:398–405

Hood DC, Lin CE, Lazow MA et al (2009) Thickness of receptor and post-receptor retinal layers in patients with retinitis pigmentosa measured with frequency-domain optical coherence tomography. Invest Ophthalmol Vis Sci 50:2328

Hood DC, Ramachandran R, Holopigian K et al (2011a) Method for deriving visual field boundaries from OCT scans of patients with retinitis pigmentosa. Biomed Opt Express 2:1106–1114

Hood DC, Lazow MA, Locke KG, Greenstein VC et al (2011b) The transition zone between healthy and diseased retina in patients with retinitis pigmentosa. Invest Ophthalmol Vis Sci 52:101

Inui E, Oishi A, Oishi M et al (2014) Tomographic comparison of cone-rod and rod-cone retinal dystrophies. Graefes Arch Clin Exp Ophthalmol 252:1065–1069

Jackson H, Garway-Heath D, Rosen P et al (2001) Outcome of cataract surgery in patients with retinitis pigmentosa. Br J Ophthalmol 85:936–938

Jacobson DM, Thompson HS, Bartley JA (1989) X-linked progressive cone dystrophy. Clinical characteristics of affected males and female carriers. Ophthalmology 96:885–895

Kaiser-Kupfer MI, Chan CC, Markello TC et al (1994) Clinical biochemical and pathologic correlations in Bietti's crystalline dystrophy. Am J Ophthalmol 118:569–582

Kim YJ, Joe SG, Lee DH et al (2013) Correlations between spectral-domain OCT measurements and visual acuity in cystoid macular edema associated with retinitis pigmentosa SD-OCT measurements and visual acuity in RP with CME. Invest Ophthalmol Vis Sci 54:1303–1309

Kojima H, Otani A, Ogino K et al (2012) Outer retinal circular structures in patients with Bietti crystalline retinopathy. Br J Ophthalmol 96:390–393

Krill AE, Deutman AF, Fishman M (1973) The cone degenerations. Doc Ophthalmol 35:1–80

Kuroda M, Hirami Y, Hata M et al (2014) Intraretinal hyperreflective foci on spectral-domain optical coherence tomographic images of patients with retinitis pigmentosa. Clin Ophthalmol 8:435

Lima LH, Sallum JM, Spaide RF (2013) Outer retina analysis by optical coherence tomography in cone-rod dystrophy patients. Retina 33:1877–1880

Lois N, Holder GE, Fitzke FW et al (1999) Intrafamilial variation of phenotype in Stargardt macular dystrophy-Fundus flavimaculatus. Invest Ophthalmol Vis Sci 40:2668–2675

Mansour AM, Uwaydat SH, Chan CC (2007) Long-term follow-up in Bietti crystalline dystrophy. Eur J Ophthalmol 17:680–682

Marshall J (1988) Pathologic findings and putative mechanisms in retinitus pigmentosa. In: Heckenlively JR (ed) Retinitis pigmentosa. Lippincott, Philadelphia

Mauldin WM, O'Connor PS (1981) Crystalline retinopathy (Bietti's tapetoretinal degeneration without marginal corneal dystrophy). Am J Ophthalmol 92:640–646

Michaelides M, Hunt DM, Moore AT (2003) The genetics of inherited macular dystrophies. J Med Genet 40:641–650

Michaelides M, Hunt DM, Moore AT (2004a) The cone dysfunction syndromes. Br J Ophthalmol 88:291–297

Michaelides M, Aligianis IA, Ainsworth JR et al (2004b) Progressive cone dystrophy associated with mutation in CNGB3. Invest Ophthalmol Vis Sci 45:1975–1982

Mohler CW, Fine SL (1981) Long-term evaluation of patients with Best's vitelliform dystrophy. Ophthalmology 88:688–692

Murakami T, Akimoto M, Ooto S et al (2008) Association between abnormal autofluorescence and photoreceptor disorganization in retinitis pigmentosa. Am J Ophthalmol 145:687–694

Nakamura M, Ito S, Terasaki H et al (2001) Japanese X-linked juvenile retinoschisis: conflict of phenotype and genotype with novel mutations in the XLRS1 gene. Arch Ophthalmol 119:1553–1554

Noble KG, Scher BM, Carr RE (1978) Polymorphous presentations in vitelliform macular dystrophy: subretinal neovascularisation and central choroidal atrophy. Br J Ophthalmol 62:561–570

Oishi A, Ogino K, Nakagawa S et al (2013) Longitudinal analysis of the peripapillary retinal nerve fiber layer thinning in patients with retinitis pigmentosa. Eye (Lond) 27:597–604

Ponjavic V, Eksandh L, Andréasson S et al (1999) Clinical expression of Best's vitelliform macular dystrophy in Swedish families with mutations in the bestrophin gene. Ophthalmic Genet 20:251–257

Puche N, Querques G, Benhamou N et al (2010) High-resolution spectral domain optical coherence tomography features in adult onset foveomacular vitelliform dystrophy. Br J Ophthalmol 94:1190–1196

Querques G, Leveziel N, Benhamou N et al (2006) Analysis of retinal flecks in fundus flavimaculatus using optical coherence tomography. Br J Ophthalmol 90:1157–1162

Querques G, Angulo Bocco MC, Soubrane G et al (2008) Intravitreal ranibizumab (Lucentis) for choroidal neovascularization associated with vitelliform macular dystrophy. Acta Ophthalmol 86:694–695

Querques G, Zerbib J, Santacroce R et al (2009a) Functional and clinical data of Best vitelliform macular dystrophy patients with mutations in the BEST1gene. Mol Vis 15:2960

Querques G, Regenbogen M, Soubrane G et al (2009b) High-resolution spectral domain optical coherence tomography findings in multifocal vitelliform macular dystrophy. Surv Ophthalmol 54:311–316

Querques G, Prato R, Coscas G et al (2009c) In vivo visualization of photoreceptor layer and lipofuscin accumulation in stargardt's disease and fundus flavimaculatus by high resolution spectral-domain optical coherence tomography. Clin Ophthalmol 3:693

Querques G, Forte R, Querques L et al (2011) Natural course of adult-onset foveomacular vitelliform dystrophy: a spectral-domain optical coherence tomography analysis. Am J Ophthalmol 152:304–313

Ripps H, Noble KG, Greenstein VC et al (1987) Progressive cone dystrophy. Ophthalmology 94:1401–1409

Robson AG, Saihan Z, Jenkins SA et al (2006) Functional characterisation and serial imaging of abnormal fundus autofluorescence in patients with retinitis pigmentosa and normal visual acuity. Br J Ophthalmol 90:472–479

Robson AG, Webster AR, Michaelides M et al (2010) Cone dystrophy with supernormal rod electroretinogram: a comprehensive genotype/phenotype study including fundus autofluorescence and extensive electrophysiology. Retina 30:51–62

Rosenthal R, Bakall B, Kinnick T et al (2006) Expression of bestrophin-1, the product of the VMD2 gene, modulates voltage-dependent Ca2+ channels in retinal pigment epithelial cells. FASEB J 20:178–180

Rossi S, Testa F, Li A et al (2013) Clinical and genetic features in Italian Bietti crystalline dystrophy patients. Br J Ophthalmol 97:174–179

Rotenstreich Y, Fishman GA, Anderson RJ (2003) Visual acuity loss and clinical observations in a large series of patients with Stargardt disease. Ophthalmology 110:1151–1158

Sadowski B, Zrenner E (1997) Cone and rod function in cone degenerations. Vision Res 37:2303–2314

Sahel J, Bonnel S, Mrejen S et al (2010) Retinitis pigmentosa and other dystrophies. Dev Ophthalmol 47:160–167

Saito W, Yamamoto S, Hayashi M et al (2003) Morphological and functional analyses of adult onset vitelliform macular dystrophy. Br J Ophthalmol 87:758–762

Saxena S, Mishra N, Meyer CH (2012) Three-dimensional spectral domain optical coherence tomography in Stargardt disease and fundus flavimaculatus. J Ocul Biol Dis Infor 5:13–18

Schatz P, Bitner H, Sander B et al (2010) Evaluation of macular structure and function by OCT and electrophysiology in patients with vitelliform macular dystrophy due to mutations in BEST1. Invest Ophthalmol Vis Sci 51:4754–4765

Sen P, Ray R, Ravi P (2011) Electrophysiological findings in Bietti's crystalline dystrophy. Clin Exp Optom 94:302–308

Simunovic MP, Moore AT (1998) The cone dystrophies. Eye (Lond) 12:553–565

Sohn EH, Francis PJ, Duncan JL et al (2009) Phenotypic variability due to a novel Glu292Lys variation in exon 8 of the BEST1 gene causing best macular dystrophy. Arch Ophthalmol 127:913–920

Sun H, Tsunenari T, Yau W et al (2002) The vitelliform macular dystrophy protein defines a new family of chloride channels. Proc Natl Acad Sci U S A 99:4008–4013

Tantri A, Vrabec TR, Cu-Unjieng A et al (2004) X-linked retinoschisis: a clinical and molecular genetic review. Surv Ophthalmol 49:214–230

Thorburn W, Nordstrom S (1978) EOG in a large family with hereditary macular degeneration. (Best's vitelliform macular dystrophy) identification of gene carriers. Acta Ophthalmol 56:455–464

Toto L, Carpineto P, Parodi MB et al (2013) Spectral domain optical coherence tomography and in vivo confocal microscopy imaging of a case of Bietti's crystalline dystrophy. Clin Exp Optom 96:39–45

Triolo G, Pierro L, Parodi MB et al (2013) Spectral domain optical coherence tomography findings in patients with retinitis pigmentosa. Ophthalmic Res 50:160–164

Urrets-Zavalía JA, Venturino JP, Mercado J et al (2006) Macular and extramacular optical coherence tomography findings in X-linked retinoschisis. Ophthalmic Surg Lasers Imaging 38:417–422

vanHuet RA, Estrada-Cuzcano A, Banin E et al (2013) Clinical characteristics of rod and cone photoreceptor dystrophies in patients with mutations in the C8orf37 gene. Invest Ophthalmol Vis Sci 54:4683–4690

Vincent A, Robson AG, Neveu MM et al (2013) A phenotype–genotype correlation study of X-linked retinoschisis. Ophthalmology 120:1454–1464

Vine AK, Schatz H (1980) Adult-onset foveomacular pigment epithelial dystrophy. Am J Ophthalmol 89:680–691

Wakabayashi T, Sawa M, Gomi F et al (2010) Correlation of fundus autofluorescence with photoreceptor morphology and functional changes in eyes with retinitis pigmentosa. Acta Ophthalmol 88:e177–e183

Wiznia RA, Perina B, Noble KG (1981) Vitelliform macular dystrophy of late onset. Br J Ophthalmol 65:866–868

Xu H, Ying L, Lin P et al (2013) Optical coherence tomography for multifocal vitelliform macular dystrophy. Optom Vis Sci 90:94–99

Yang HS, Lee JB, Yoon YH et al (2014) Correlation between spectral-domain OCT findings and visual acuity in X-linked retinoschisis OCT characteristics of juvenile retinoschisis. Invest Ophthalmol Ves Sci 55:3029–3036

Yeoh J, Rahman W, Chen F et al (2010) Choroidal imaging in inherited retinal disease using the technique of enhanced depth imaging optical coherence tomography. Graefes Arch Clin Exp Ophthalmol 248:1719–1728

Yin H, Jin C, Fang X et al (2014) Molecular analysis and phenotypic study in 14 Chinese families with Bietti crystalline dystrophy. PLoS One 9:e94960

Yu J, Ni Y, Keane PA et al (2010) Foveomacular schisis in Juvenile X-linked retinoschisis: an optical coherence tomography study. Am J Ophthalmol 149:973–978

Zahlava J, Lestak J, Karel I (2014) Optical coherence tomography in progressive cone dystrophy. Biomed Pap Med Fac Univ Palacky Olomouc Czech Repub 158:628–634

Uveitis

25

Xavier Fagan, Weng Onn Chan, Lyndell Lim, and Jagjit S. Gilhotra

Contents

X. Fagan, MBBS, FRANZCO
Northern Eye Consultants, Melbourne, Australia

W.O. Chan, MB, ChB, MPhil • J.S. Gilhotra, MBBS, FRANZCO (✉)
South Australian Institute of Ophthalmology, Royal Adelaide Hospital, Adelaide, Australia
e-mail: jsgilhotra@gmail.com

L. Lim, MBBS, FRANZCO
Centre for Eye Research Australia, Royal Victorian Eye and Ear Hospital and Royal Melbourne Hospital, Melbourne, Australia

25.1 Introduction

Optical coherence tomography (OCT) provides fast, non-contact and reproducible high-resolution imaging of the posterior pole. With improving resolution down to 1 μm and the ability to clearly define anatomical layers, OCT plays an ever-increasing role in the management of uveitis. Diagnostically, the ability to observe alteration in the reflectivity, thickness and retinal architecture is invaluable in understanding the pathophysiology of some uveitic conditions. Whilst there are general agreements on anatomical layer and nomenclature of the inner retinal layers, the same is less so for the outer retinal layers. In 2014, the IN OCT group produced a consensus statement on the four distinct

C.H. Meyer et al. (eds.), *Spectral Domain Optical Coherence Tomography in Macular Diseases*,
DOI 10.1007/978-81-322-3610-8_25

hyper-reflective outer retinal bands (Staurenghi et al. 2014). From the outermost to the innermost are the retinal pigment epithelium (RPE)/Bruch's membrane complex, the interdigitation zone (IZ), the ellipsoid zone (EZ) and the external limiting membrane (ELM) (Staurenghi et al. 2014). The term 'zone' is used when tissues within a region cannot be clearly delineated with current technology. With enhanced depth imaging, choroidal vasculature and thickness can also be both qualitatively and quantitatively measured. This is particularly helpful in uveitic conditions such as Vogt-Koyanagi-Harada (VKH) syndrome, sympathetic ophthalmia (SO), Behcet's disease and choroidal granuloma.

From a management perspective, OCT is useful in documenting longitudinal changes and resolution of complications, e.g. cystoid macular oedema (CMO), subretinal fluid and choroidal neovascular membrane (CNVM). Specific OCT changes associated with uveitic conditions [e.g. hyper-reflectivity of the outer retina seen in acute posterior multifocal placoid pigment epitheliopathy (APMPPE)] often resolve with treatment, making OCT ideal for assessing treatment response. Prognostically, OCT can be used to predict visual outcome. Patients with disruption of EZ and thinning at the fovea are significantly associated with worse visual acuity (Forooghian et al. 2009). It can also be used to detect the presence of vitreomacular traction (VMT), epiretinal membrane (ERM), foveal atrophy and lamellar holes that can adversely affect the visual outcome.

The main limitation of OCT in uveitis is that any hyper-reflective structures will cast shadows and may mask underlying disorder. Additionally, media opacities (e.g. haemorrhage and vitritis) and movement artefacts can significantly degrade image quality. Finally compared to angiography, OCT can be falsely negative in the presence of leakage.

Whilst uveitic condition often presents with nonspecific inflammatory changes (Fig. 25.1), some have distinct manifestations on OCT. The following chapter will aim to highlight some of the prototypical changes associated with uveitic conditions.

25.2 Macular Oedema

Many uveitic conditions may cause vision loss through reactive macular oedema. Three patterns of macular oedema have been described (Markomichelakis et al. 2004):

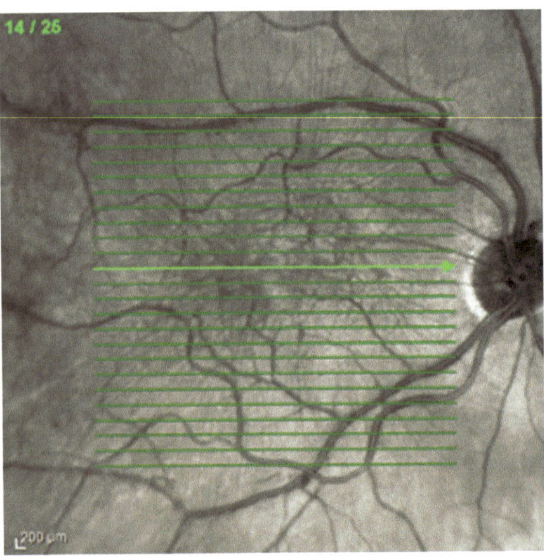

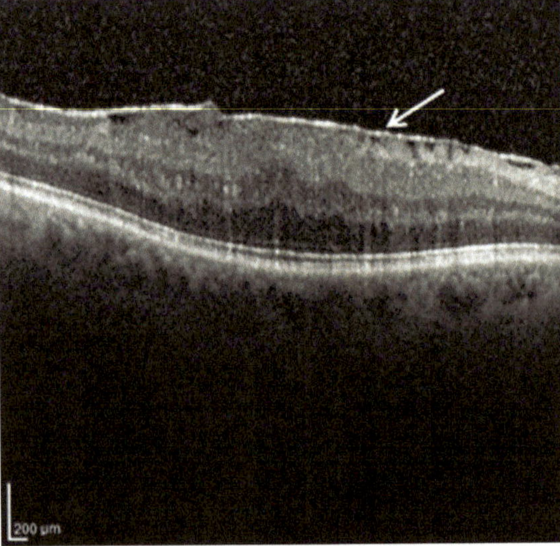

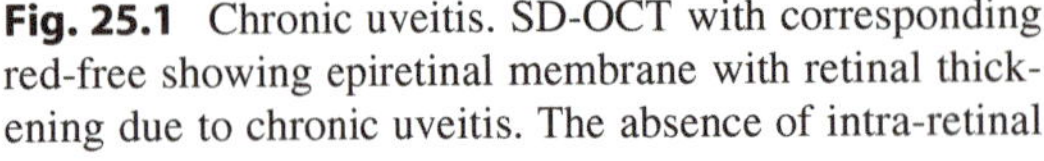

Fig. 25.1 Chronic uveitis. SD-OCT with corresponding red-free showing epiretinal membrane with retinal thickening due to chronic uveitis. The absence of intra-retinal hyporeflective spaces is useful in excluding cystic macular oedema. White arrow pointing to hyper-reflective and thickened epiretinal membrane

1. Diffuse – increased retinal thickness, multiple hyporeflective spaces and separation of retinal lamellae (Fig. 25.2)
2. Cystoid – well-defined intra-retinal cystoid spaces in the retina (Fig. 25.3)
3. Serous detachment – separation of the neurosensory retina from the underlying retinal pigment epithelial-Bruch's membrane complex

Vitreoretinal interface disorders are another potential complications of uveitis and can be seen on OCT as epiretinal membranes, vitreomacular traction or macular hole formation. The ability to detect and measure macular oedema through qualitative and quantitative measures has led to new study designs for the management of uveitic eye disease.

25.3 Idiopathic Inflammatory Chorioretinopathies

25.3.1 Multiple Evanescent White Dot Syndrome (MEWDS)

This transient disorder typically presents in young adults with photopsia and manifests fundoscopically as multiple small, white dots in the

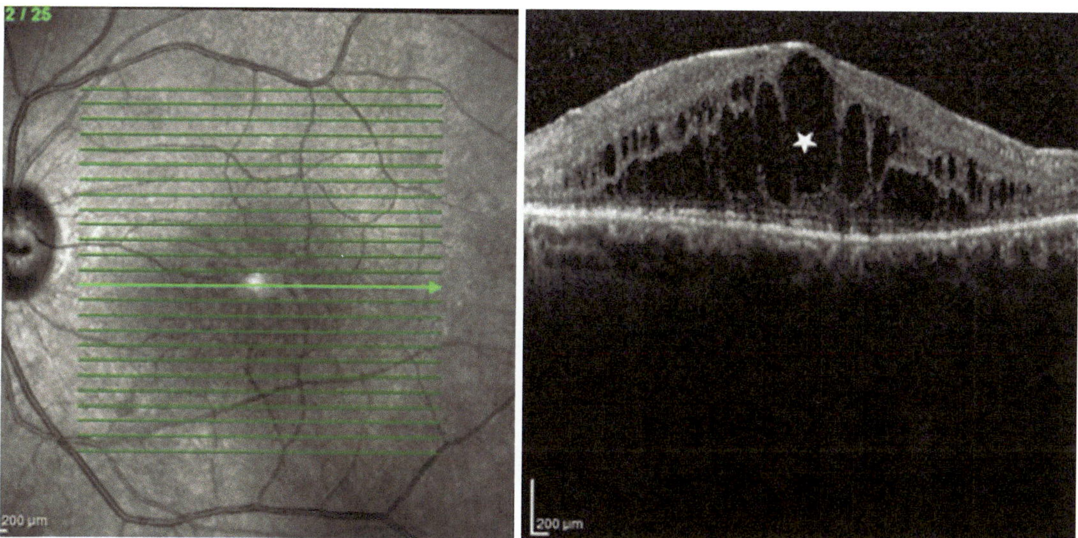

Fig. 25.2 Diffuse cystoid macular oedema (CMO). SD-OCT shows increased retinal thickness with hyporeflective spaces (*white star*) and splitting of the retinal lamellae

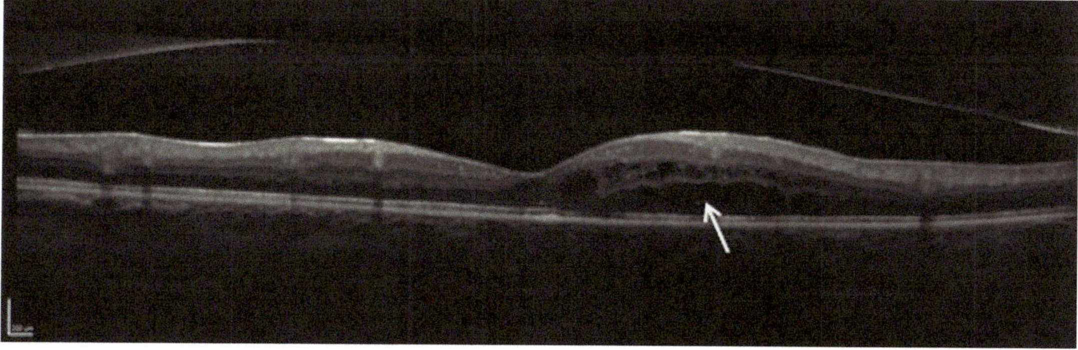

Fig. 25.3 Focal cystoid macular oedema. Focal CMO (*white arrow*) secondary to birdshot choroiditis

posterior pole. Acute presentations demonstrate disruption of the photoreceptor ellipsoid zone (EZ) and interdigitation zone (IZ) (Fig. 25.4a, b) (de Bats et al. 2014; Kanis and van Norren 2006). The disruption may either be diffuse or multifocal. This may be associated with choroidal thickening on enhanced depth imaging OCT (EDI-OCT) and small round hyper-reflective points in other layers such as the ganglion cell layer (de Bats et al. 2014). During follow-up, reconstitution of the EZ occurs gradually over several weeks to months (Li and Kishi 2009) (Fig. 25.5). In some cases, this occurs with an intermediary appearance of small dome-shaped hyper-reflective material that eventually flattens (Amin 2006; Hashimoto and Kishi 2015). En face OCT at the level of the ellipsoid zone may display large patchy areas of hyporeflection corresponding to the diffuse areas of EZ attenuation (de Bats et al. 2014).

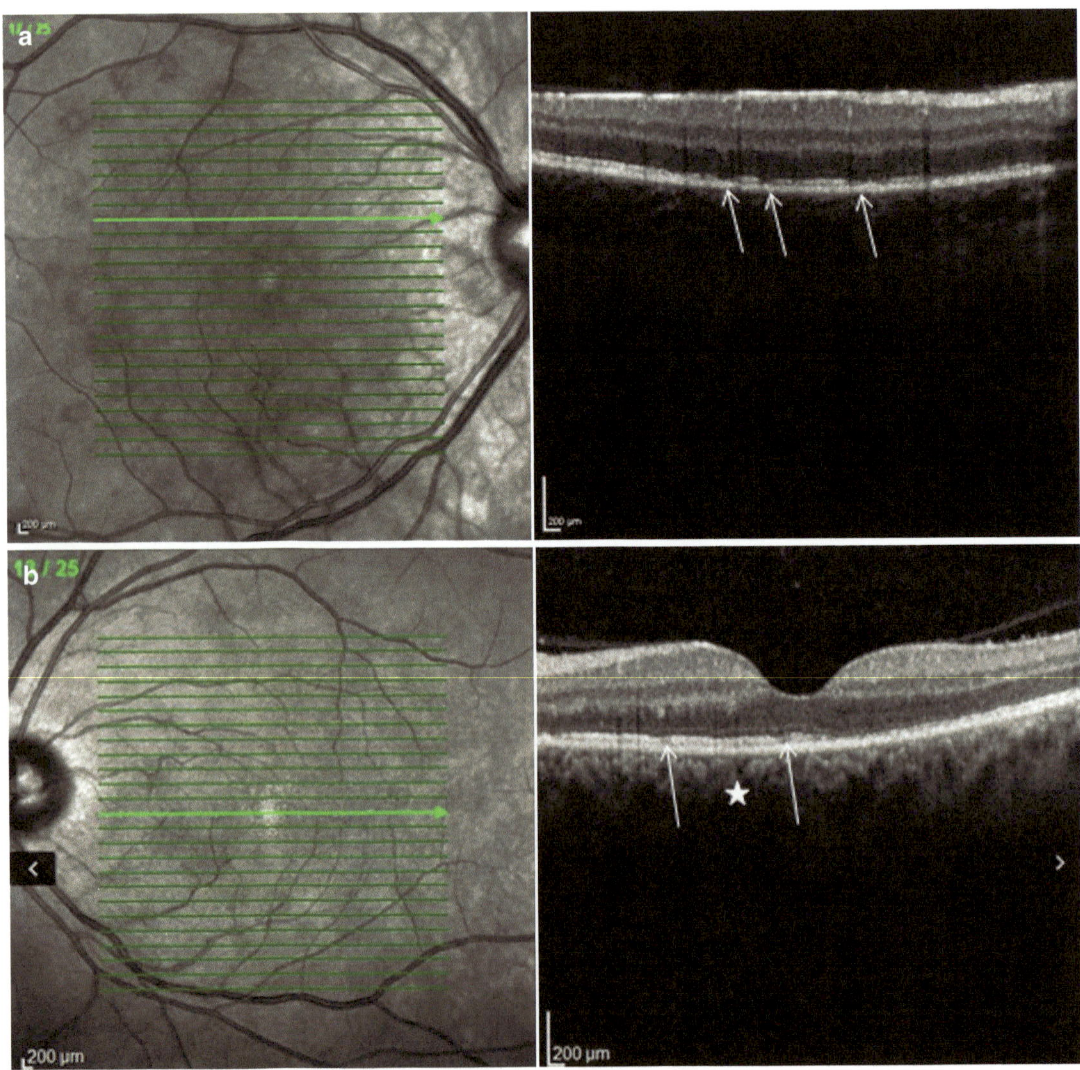

Fig. 25.4 Multiple evanescent white dot syndrome (MEWDS). (**a**) Spectral domain optical coherence tomography (SD-OCT) shows multifocal areas of ellipsoid and interdigitation zone disruption (*white arrows*) corresponding to hyporeflective lesions on the infrared scout map. (**b**) SD-OCT with corresponding red-free showing disruption at the ellipsoid layer (*white arrows*) with associated increased thickness of the choroid (*white star*)

25.3.2 Acute Posterior Multifocal Placoid Pigment Epitheliopathy (APMPPE)

Patients with this acute posterior multifocal placoid pigment epitheliopathy (APMPPE) present with multiple, deep, creamy-white plaques of ½ to 1 disc diameter in size in the posterior pole. Unilateral presentation may also occur. The creamy plaques may be represented on OCT as outer retinal hyper-reflective material with sparing of the middle and inner retina (Scheufele et al. 2005; Souka et al. 2006) (Fig. 25.6). Marked anterior displacement of the neurosensory retina and retinal pigment epithelium (RPE) due to choroidal inflammation may occur (Lim et al. 2006). Areas of turbid subretinal fluid with overlying hyper-reflective material on the RPE (Birnbaum et al. 2010; Lee et al. 2011) and large intra-retinal cysts (Montero et al. 2011) are also described in the acute phase (Fig. 25.7). Serous detachments may be so significant as to mimic Vogt-Koyanagi-Harada disease (Wickremasignhe and Lim 2010). The fluid may become loculated by dividing intra-retinal septa (Lee et al. 2011).

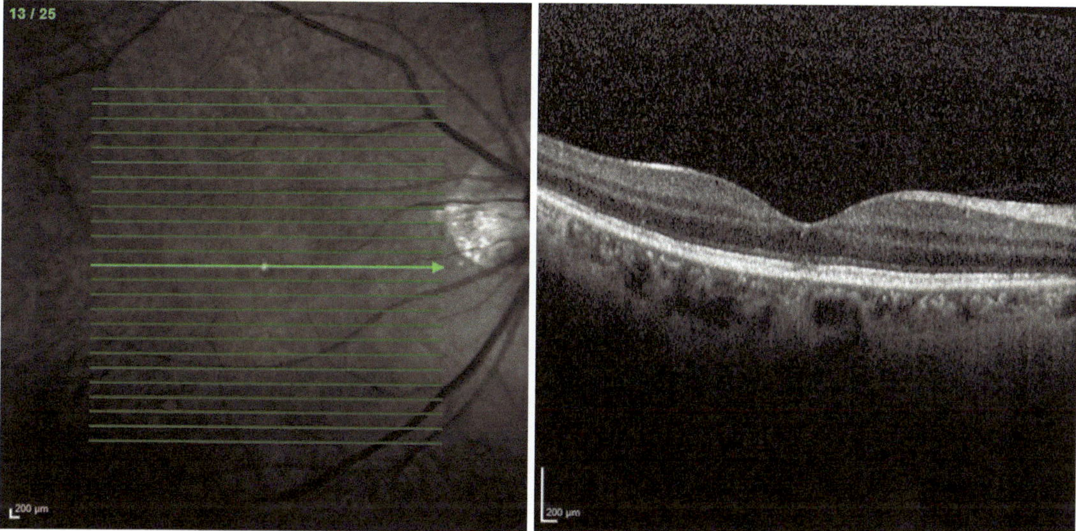

Fig. 25.5 Multiple evanescent white dot syndrome (MEWDS). SD-OCT showing partial reconstitution of the outer retina 2 weeks after onset in a patient with MEWDS

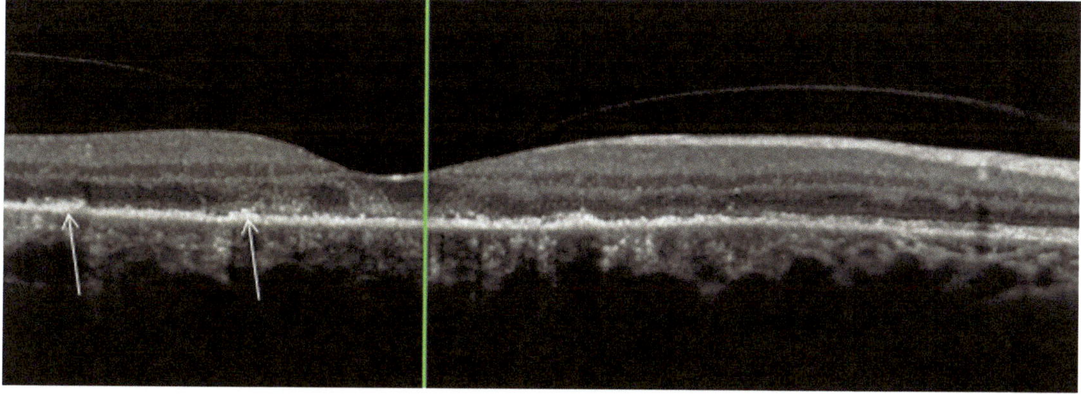

Fig. 25.6 Acute posterior multifocal placoid pigment epitheliopathy (APMPPE). SD-OCT shows outer retinal hyper-reflective material (*white arrows*) and disruption of outer retinal layers. Note sparing of the inner and middle retina

In the convalescent phase, there is rapid resolution of the intra-retinal and subretinal fluid (Birnbaum et al. 2010). This occurs in conjunction with disruption or loss of the IZ, EZ, ELM and outer nuclear layer (ONL). As further repair occurs, there is a variable restoration of outer retinal and RPE elements (Lee et al. 2011) with some cases displaying persistent thinning of the ONL, EZ attenuation and RPE atrophy (Scheufele et al. 2005) (Fig. 25.8).

25.3.3 Relentless Placoid Chorioretinopathy (RPC)

Relentless placoid chorioretinopathy (RPC) also known as ampiginous choroiditis is a related but distinct entity to APMPPE. Whilst initial presentation may be similar, patients with ampiginous choroiditis have prolonged clinical course marred with multiple recurrences. In the acute stages, OCT over the placoid lesions can show pigment epithelial detachment associated with hyperreflectivity of the ganglion cell layer and the inner and the outer nuclear layers (Amer and Florescu 2008) (Fig. 25.9). In the resolution phase, OCT over the placoid scar shows RPE atrophy with associated window defect. However, in contrast to serpiginous chorioretinopathy, retinal and choroidal thickness in RPC is preserved (Dolz-Marco et al. 2014) (Fig. 25.10).

25.3.4 Birdshot Chorioretinopathy

Birdshot chorioretinopathy (BCR) is a typically progressive posterior uveitis characterized by

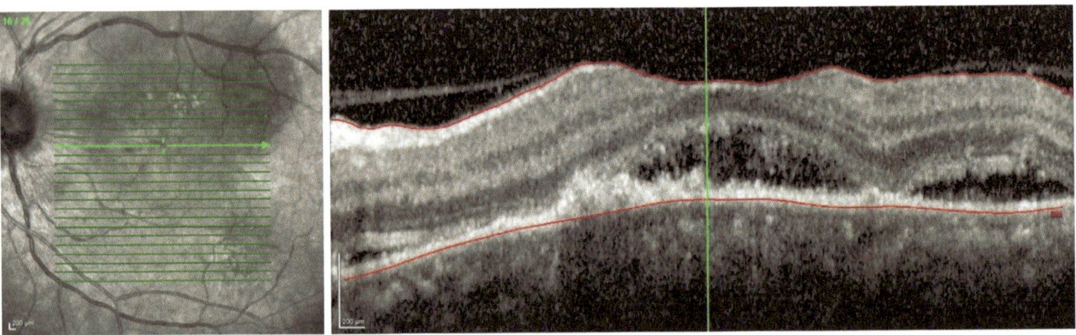

Fig. 25.7 Acute posterior multifocal placoid pigment epitheliopathy. SD-OCT shows subretinal fluid in acute APMPPE

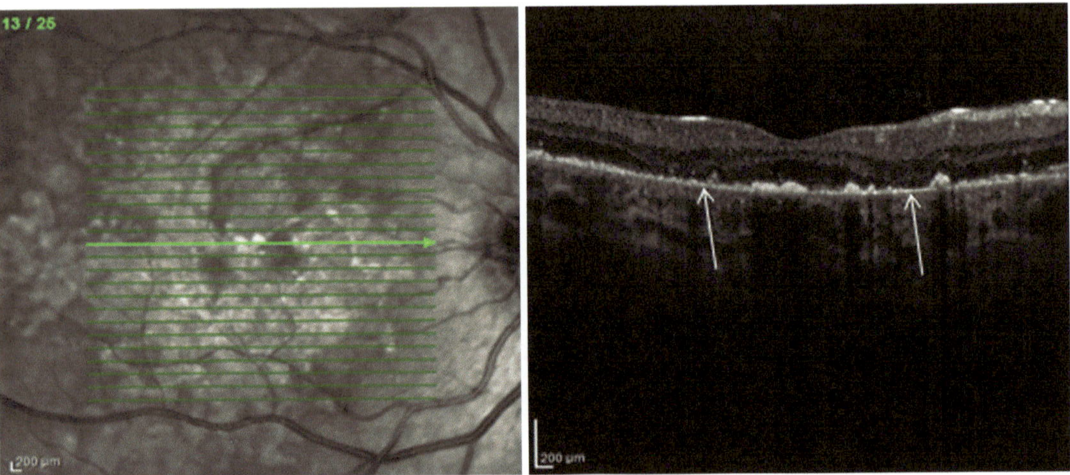

Fig. 25.8 Acute posterior multifocal placoid pigment epitheliopathy. SD-OCT shows loss of outer nuclear layer, interdigitation zone and gross disruption of RPE (*white arrows*) in a patient with previous APMPPE

vitritis, small non-pigmented yellow-white spots predominantly of the nasal fundus and vasculitis and complicated by cystoid macular oedema (CMO). Macular oedema is a common vision-threatening complication of BCR. As described in a previous section, the oedema may be cystoid, diffuse, subretinal fluid or related to epiretinal membrane (Monnet et al. 2007). Classic birdshot lesions can be subtly appreciated as increased transmission of OCT signal to the sclera through the RPE and choroid (Keane et al. 2013) (Fig. 25.11a). Vitritis may be seen as hyper-reflective foci in the lucent background of the vitreous cavity (Fig. 25.11b). Patients with BCR may have suprachoroidal fluid on EDI-OCT (enhanced depth imaging OCT), and there is evidence that the amount of fluid may correlate with photopsias (Birnbaum et al. 2014). Other features include EZ loss, RPE disruption, possible choroidal thinning and outer retinal hyper-reflective

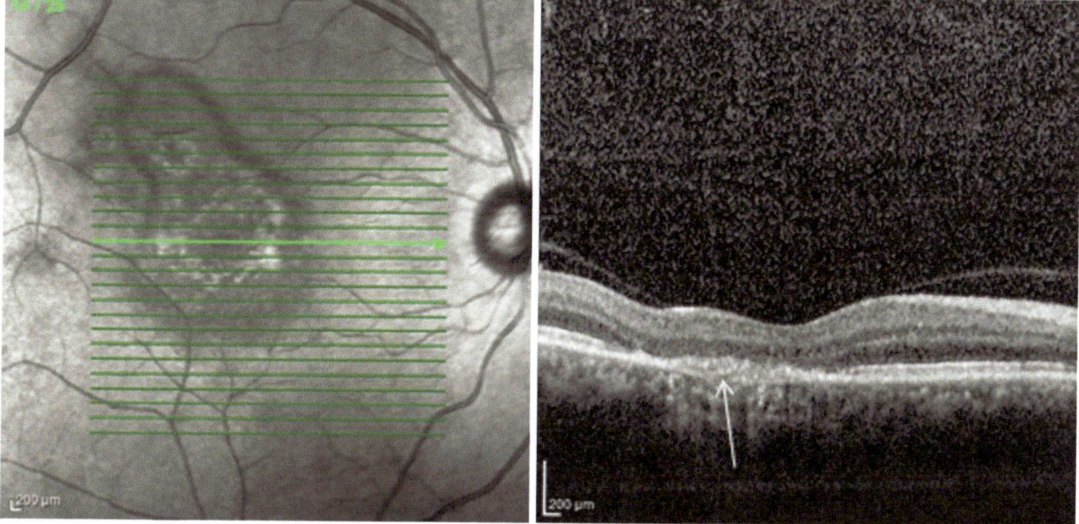

Fig. 25.9 Relentless placoid chorioretinopathy (acute phase). SD-OCT with corresponding red-free showing hyper-reflectivity of the irregular and disrupted outer retinal layers (*white arrow*)

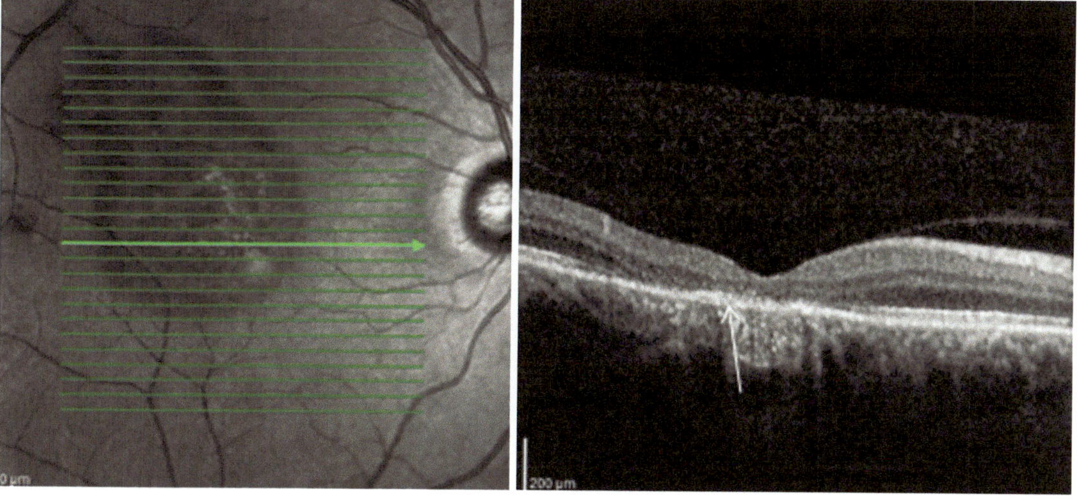

Fig. 25.10 Relentless placoid chorioretinopathy (resolution phase). SD-OCT with corresponding red-free showing disruption at the ellipsoid layer (*white arrow*) in resolution stages of RPC

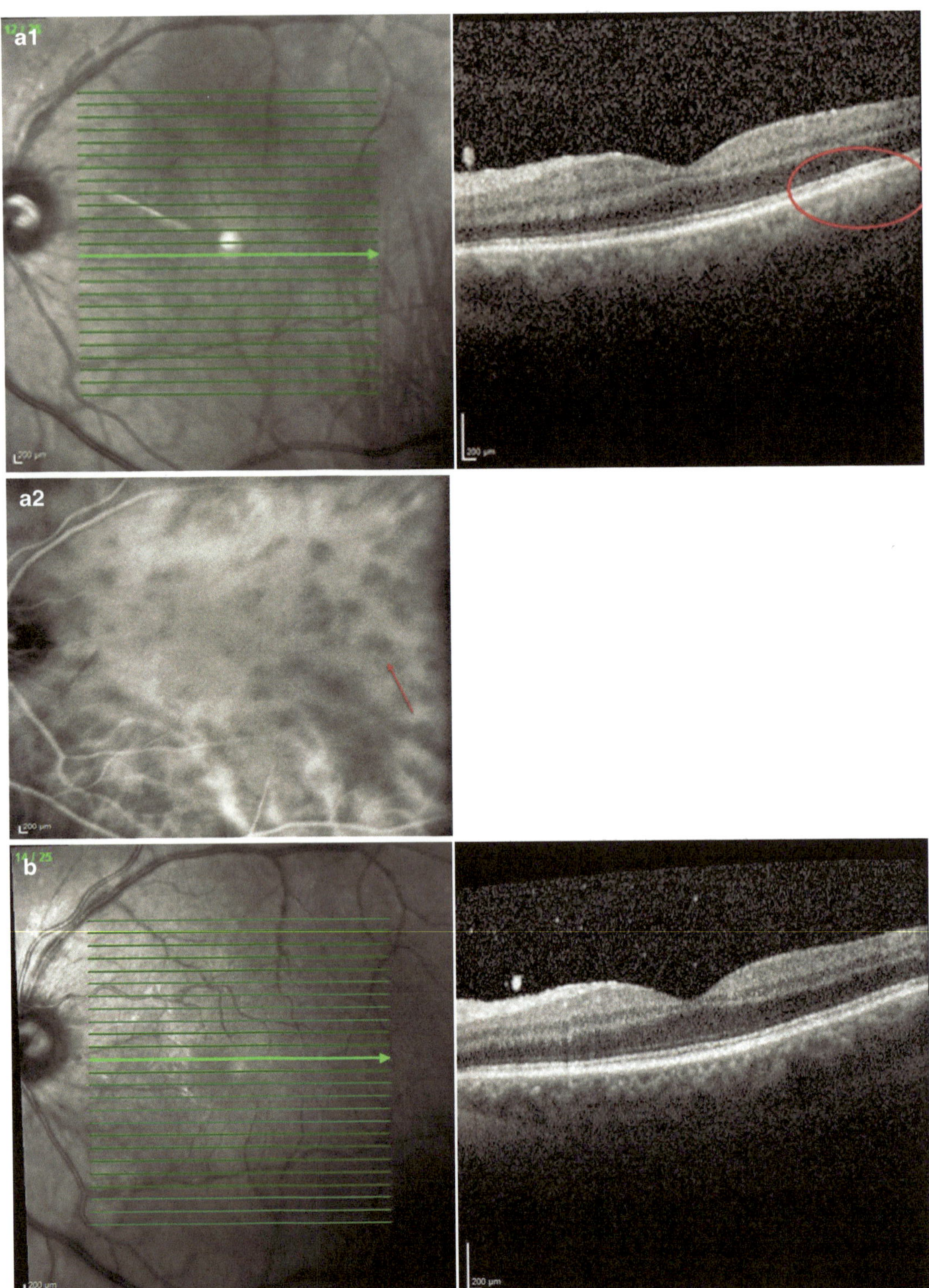

Fig. 25.11 Birdshot chorioretinopathy. (**ai**) SD-OCT with corresponding red-free showing hyper-reflectivity of the outer retinal layers (*red circle*). (**aii**) Indocyanine green angiography (ICG) shows corresponding area as hypofluorescent spot (*red arrow*). (**b**) SD-OCT showing BCR with associated vitritis manifesting as multiple hyper-reflective dots in the vitreous space

lesions or 'clumps' (Keane et al. 2013). Such changes may occur outside the macula and require extra-macular scanning to be detected.

25.3.5 Serpiginous Choroiditis

This disorder is typically characterized by a progressive and recurrent inflammation extending from the optic disc in a centrifugal manner. The active edge of inflammation is a creamy-white colour in the deep layers. The old lesions are seen as atrophic with variable pigment change. It may be complicated by choroidal neovascularization (CNV). Active lesions appear as hyper-reflectivities only in the outer retina (van Velthoven et al. 2006), disruption of the EZ and RPE (Arantes et al. 2011) (Fig. 25.12) or cystic macular oedema (Punjabi et al. 2008). En face OCT represents the new inflammation as hyper-reflectivity in the outer retina adjacent to the previous inflammation (van Velthoven et al. 2006). Atrophic, chronic lesions are characterized by subsistence of the retina due to loss of outer retinal elements such as the ONL, EZ and RPE (Arantes et al. 2011). Increased transmission through to the choroid is a secondary consequence. Lesions complicated by CNV will display OCT evidence of CNV (Punjabi et al. 2008) depending on the duration of the neovascularization and the involvement of the retina in the primary pathology.

Fundus autofluorescence is a useful adjunctive modality for identifying new lesions as hyper-autofluorescent and chronic lesions as hypo-autofluorescence or absent autofluorescence (Arantes et al. 2011).

25.3.6 Multifocal Choroiditis with Panuveitis and Punctate Inner Choroidopathy

Previously thought to be separate entities, it has been proffered that punctate inner choroidopathy (PIC) is indistinguishable from multifocal choroiditis (MFC) (Spaide et al. 2013). Both manifest multifocal white-yellow deep infiltrates that may become punched-out scars but had previously been separated by the presence of visible inflammatory cells, lesion size or refractive correction. For the purposes of this section, they will be considered together. Active lesions of MFC may appear as dome-shaped sub-RPE deposits, dehiscence of the RPE, subretinal infiltration and/or loss of the EZ (Channa et al. 2012; Spaide et al. 2013; Vance et al. 2011a). The choroid appears largely uninvolved on multimodal imaging including EDI-OCT (Spaide et al. 2013) but may have increased transmission defects

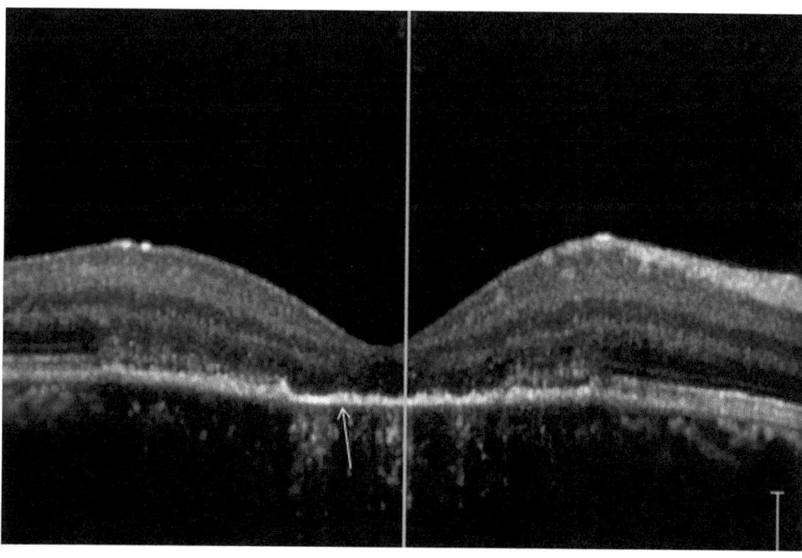

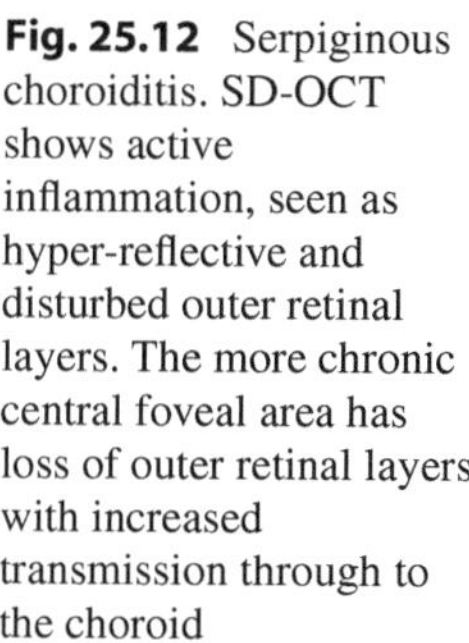

Fig. 25.12 Serpiginous choroiditis. SD-OCT shows active inflammation, seen as hyper-reflective and disturbed outer retinal layers. The more chronic central foveal area has loss of outer retinal layers with increased transmission through to the choroid

from RPE disruption (Vance et al. 2011a, b). Vitreal cells may be visible in the scans. Chronic lesions may show variable presence of the normal outer retinal lamellae or persistent elevation or the absence of the RPE (Channa et al. 2012; Spaide et al. 2013). CNV can complicate MFC and it may be difficult to distinguish it from a new acute MFC lesion. CNV may be associated with subretinal heterogeneous material and round hyporeflective structures suggestive of a vascular lumen (Spaide et al. 2013) (Fig. 25.13).

25.3.7 Acute Macular Neuroretinopathy (AMN)

Prior to OCT and infrared imaging, this condition was clinically detected as subtle, lobular macular red-brown retinal lesions in patients presenting with paracentral scotomas.

There are two subtypes of OCT appearance of acute macular neuroretinopathy (AMN):

A. Outer retinal AMN (Fig. 25.14)
B. Middle maculopathy (Fig. 25.15)

A. Outer retinal AMN was the first to be demonstrated with OCT. Time-domain OCT in the acute presentation showed hyper-reflectivity of the outer retina (Feigl and Haas 2000). On spectral domain OCT (SD-OCT) in the very early presentation, there may be outer retinal hyper-reflectivity followed by focal EZ, IZ and RPE disruption and ONL thinning on spectral domain machines (Monson et al. 2007; Fawzi et al. 2012; Hughes et al. 2009). The EZ re-establishes over time as the condition improves, but ONL thinning and IZ hyporeflectivity thinning may persist (Fawzi et al. 2012; Vance et al. 2011b).

B. Middle maculopathy was identified later in patients with the same demographics, clinical symptoms, fundoscopic findings and infrared reflectance patterns. OCT shows hyper-reflectivity of the INL with shadowing of

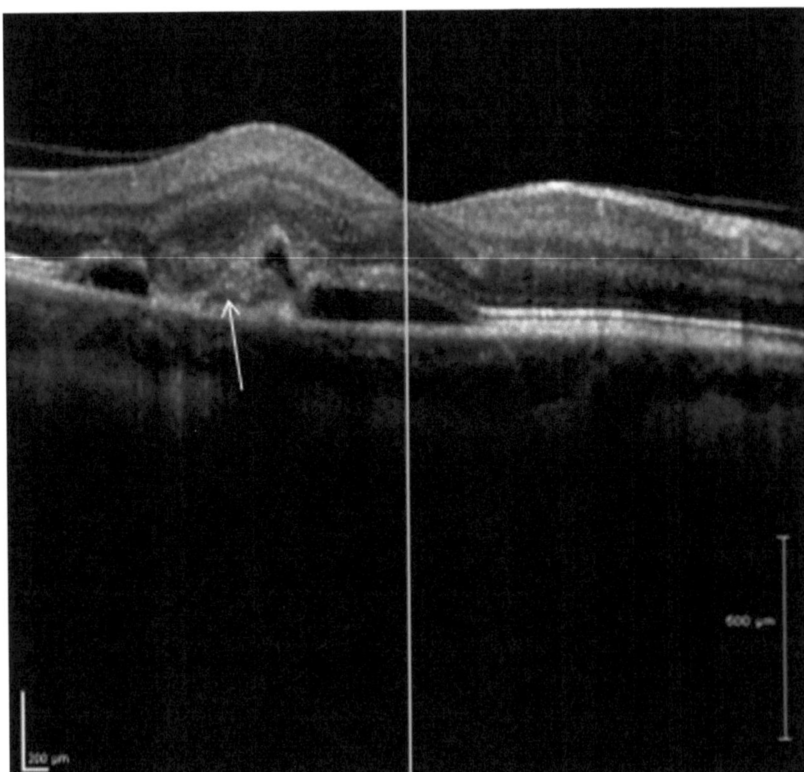

Fig. 25.13 Multifocal choroiditis. Choroidal neovascularization (CNV) (*white arrow*) complicating an old multifocal choroiditis (MFC) lesion. Note the subretinal fluid and heterogeneous material

deeper structures but no focal attenuation (Sarraf et al. 2013). Convalescent images displayed subsequent atrophy of the INL (Sarraf et al. 2013). Whilst it was originally thought that this middle maculopathy might be pathognomonic, it has since been demonstrated in retinal artery occlusion, central retinal vein occlusion, prolonged globe compression and haemoglobinopathies such as sickle cell disease, retinal vasculitis and Purtscher-like retinopathy (Chen et al. 2015; Rahimy et al. 2014; Yu et al. 2015).

It has been postulated that these two patterns represent capillary ischaemia from interruption of the superficial (inner) retinal capillary plexus or deep (outer) retinal capillary plexus (Yu et al. 2014).

25.3.8 Acute Zonal Occult Outer Retinopathy (AZOOR)

The definition of AZOOR is variable. This section refers to otherwise well patients with an initial presentation of photopsia or diminished night

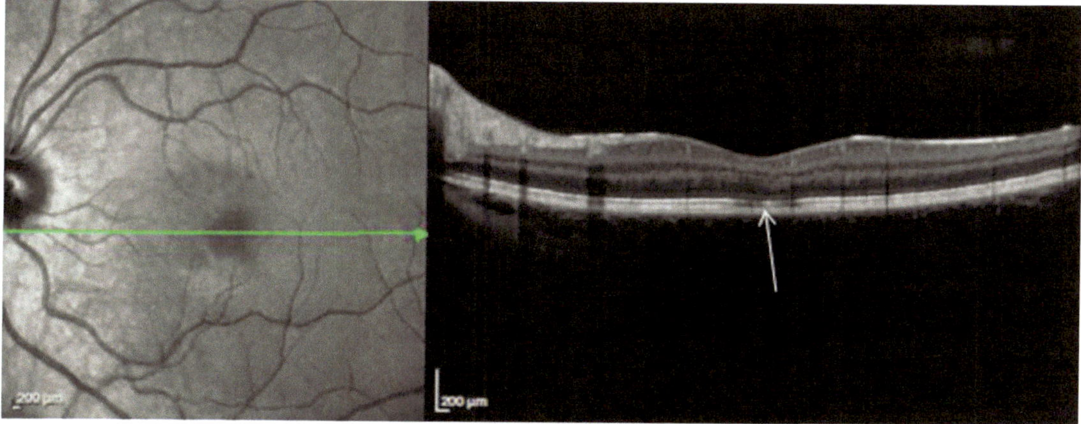

Fig. 25.14 Outer retinal acute macular neuroretinopathy. SD-OCT shows discontinuity of the EZ (*white arrow*) in the central macular area which corresponds to an area of decreased reflectivity on the infrared scout map

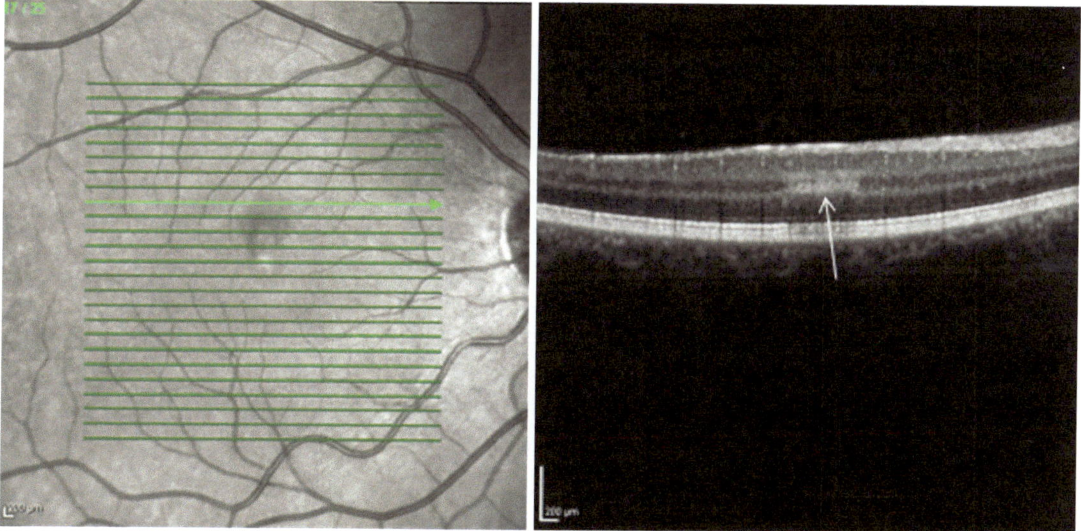

Fig. 25.15 Middle retina acute macular neuroretinopathy. SD-OCT shows hyper-reflectivity in the inner nuclear layer (*white arrow*) and corresponding to an area of decreased infrared reflectance on the scout map

vision, well-defined scotoma or enlarged blind spot without any visible fundus abnormality or features consistent with alternative diagnoses.

OCT in the acute phase shows diffuse loss of ellipsoid zone and interdigitation zone in the involved area as determined by ERG, visual field or autofluorescence (Li and Kishi 2007; Mrejen et al. 2014). Treatment with local or systemic immune suppression has been shown to promote at least partial reconstitution of these lamellae in areas with intact outer nuclear layers (Spaide et al. 2008).

In the chronic phase, patients develop a trizonal appearance with normal OCT outside the area of AZOOR, subretinal material in active areas and atrophy of photoreceptors, RPE and choroid in the chronic areas (Mrejen et al. 2014). Other studies with EDI-OCT report that choroidal thickness is unaffected but confirm the attenuation of the ellipsoid zone and reduced or absent outer nuclear layer (Fujiwara et al. 2010). Epiretinal membrane is common (Fujiwara et al. 2010).

25.3.9 Sarcoidosis

Sarcoidosis is a multisystem, idiopathic, non-caseating granulomatous disease. It may affect the anterior segment, retina, optic nerve or choroid. On OCT imaging, retinal and optic nerve head granulomas appear as inner retinal, hyper-reflective nodules protruding into the vitreous (Goldberg et al. 2015). The surrounding tissue is disturbed; there is reduced signal transmission to outer retinal structures, and there may be subretinal fluid (Goldberg et al. 2015). Lesions regress but may not ever completely dissolve (Goldberg et al. 2015). Choroidal granulomas may be identified on EDI-OCT as homogenous lesions that may be isoreflective or hyporeflective relative to the surrounding choroid (Invernizzi et al. 2015; Rostaqui et al. 2014). The overlying choriocapillaris is compressed (Modi et al. 2013). The lesions may be round or lobulated and only half will have well-defined margins (Invernizzi et al. 2015).

25.3.10 Vogt-Koyanagi-Harada (VKH) Syndrome and Sympathetic Ophthalmia

Given their clinical, ophthalmological, histopathological and imaging similarities, these two conditions shall be discussed together in the context of OCT appearance. Choroidal thickening, an undulating RPE and serous retinal detachments characterize the acute phase (Figs. 25.16

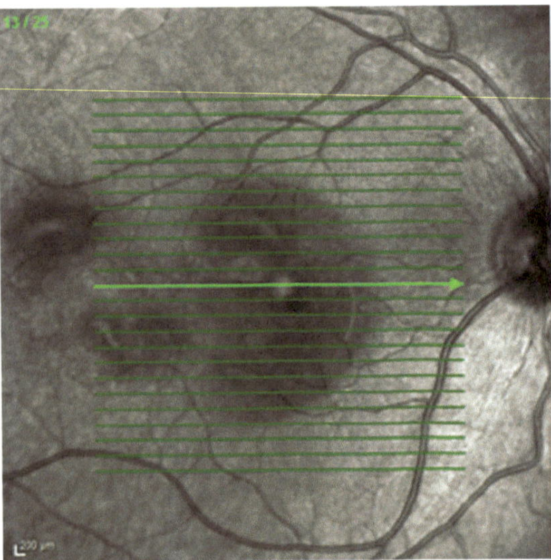

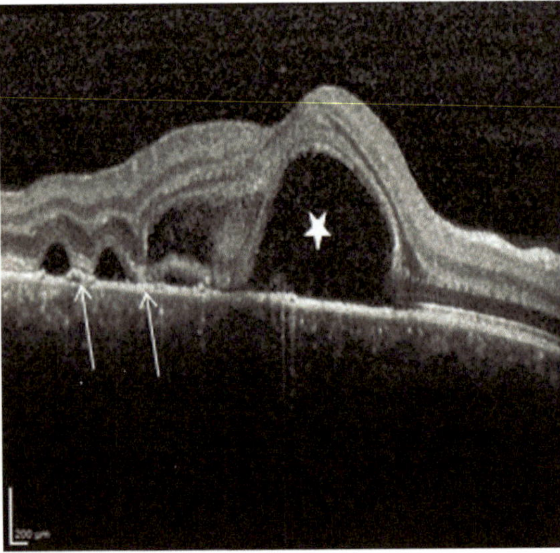

Fig. 25.16 Acute Vogt-Koyanagi-Harada (VKH) syndrome. SD-OCT shows serous detachment of the retina (*white star*) and loculated intra-retinal fluid divided by subretinal strands (*white arrows*)

and 25.17) (Fong et al. 2011; Ishihara et al. 2009). Wavy, hyper-reflective lines traversing and bridging the entirety of the subretinal fluid pockets can be seen (Tsjuikawa et al. 2005). These may represent fibrinous septa (de Smet and Rao 2005) and are responsible for the loculation of fluid compartments seen on fluorescein fundus angiography (FFA) (Yamaguchi et al. 2007). The EZ may be thickened and irregular (Gupta et al. 2009). Hyper-reflective dots, potentially representing small vessels of the choriocapillaris that are present in normal EDI-OCT, have been shown to be less numerous in the acute stage of disease (Fong et al. 2011). Single-layer RPE analysis demonstrates small elevations that correspond to areas of punctate hyperfluorescence on FFA, and troughs in the RPE correspond to hypofluorescent lines on FFA (Gupta et al. 2009). Within a week of steroid therapy, serous retinal detachment starts to resolve (Fig. 25.18), and by 1 month, 75 % of detachments are completely resolved (Ishihara et al. 2009). EZ integrity is reconstituted more gradually and may take 3 months (Ishihara et al. 2009). In the convalescent phase, there is marked, rapid reduction in the choroidal thickness to normal levels after initiation of steroid therapy within 3–14 days (Maruko et al. 2011). In chronic cases of VKH, the choroid is likely to be thinner than control eyes (da Silva et al. 2013). It may be possible to use EDI-OCT measurements of choroidal thickness to gauge treatment response or disease recurrence. Dalen-Fuchs nodules that are seen with both conditions have previously been characterized histologically into three types (Reynard et al. 1985). Type 1 consists of focal hyperplasia and aggregation of RPE cells. Type 2 consists of epithelioid cells and lymphocytes covered by intact dome of RPE. Type 3 consists of degeneration of RPE and release of disorganized Dalen-Fuchs nodule into the subretinal space. With SD-OCT, it is possible to distinguish between the types; however the clinical significance of the different types remains unclear (Figs. 25.19 and 25.20).

25.4 Infectious Posterior Uveitis

25.4.1 Bacterial Posterior Uveitis

25.4.1.1 Acute Syphilitic Posterior Placoid Chorioretinitis

In the acute phase of a macular placoid syphilitic lesion, the OCT demonstrates disruption or loss of the EZ and ELM (Brito et al. 2011) (Fig. 25.21). There may also be subretinal fluid (Joseph et al. 2007; Pichi et al. 2014). The choroid can appear infiltrated with hyper-reflective dots and reduction in the number and size of visible vascular structures (Brito et al. 2011; Pichi et al. 2014).

As the condition is treated, prominent nodular elevations of the RPE are seen (Pichi et al. 2014). After treatment is completed, the subretinal fluid resolves, and the normal foveal lamination is restored (Brito et al. 2011; Joseph et al. 2007; Pichi et al. 2014) (Fig. 25.22). The choroidal infiltration also resolves (Pichi et al. 2014). Rare

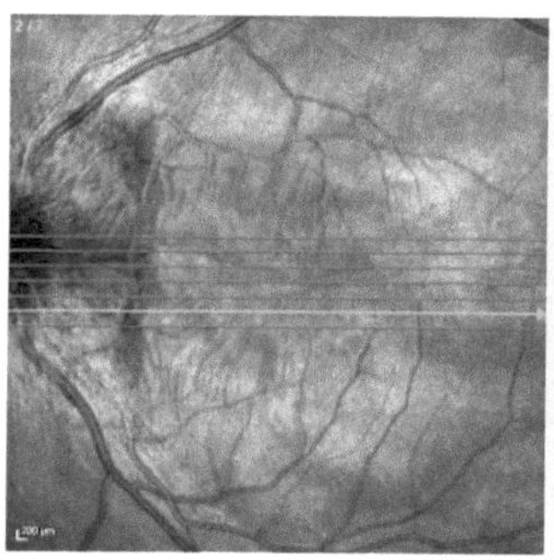

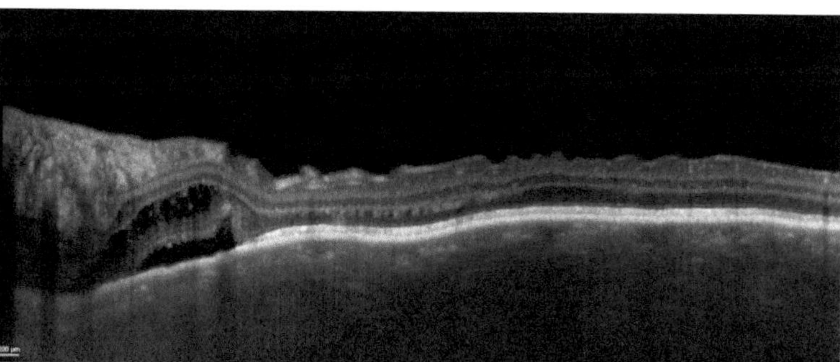

Fig. 25.17 Acute Vogt-Koyanagi-Harada syndrome. EDI-OCT shows a grossly thickened choroid in a patient with acute VKH

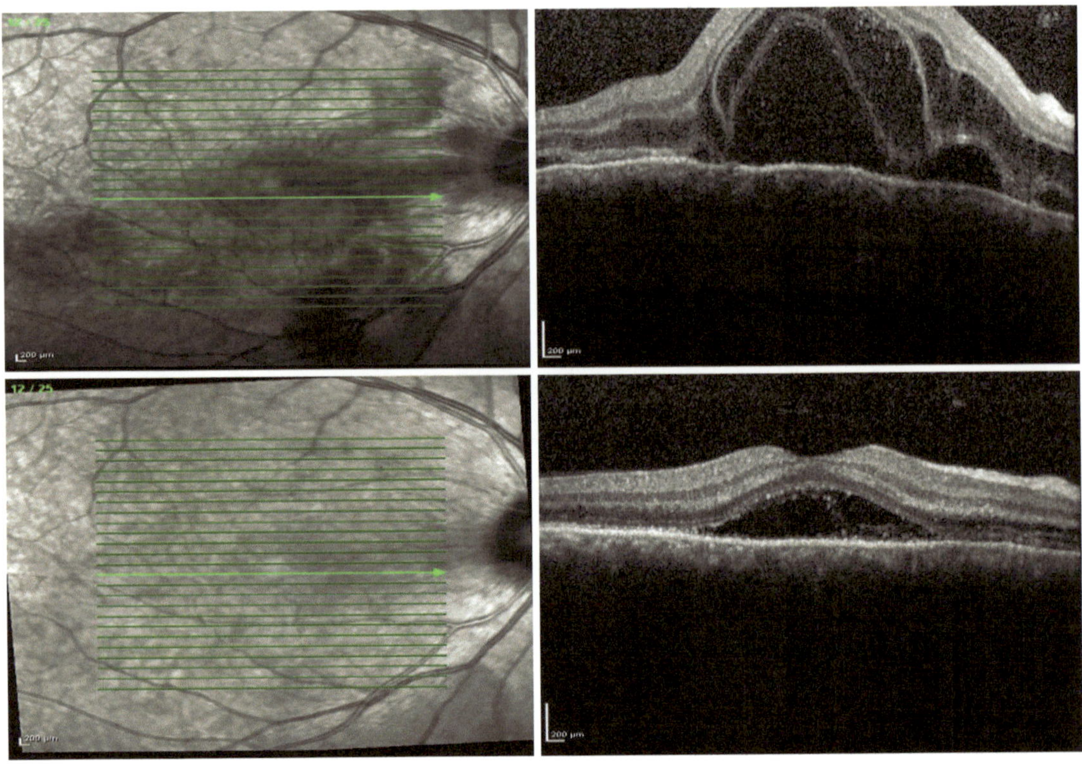

Fig. 25.18 Acute Vogt-Koyanagi-Harada (VKH) syndrome. Acute VKH at presentation and after 3 days of intravenous methylprednisolone. A dramatic reduction in the intra-retinal fluid and retinal thickening is seen

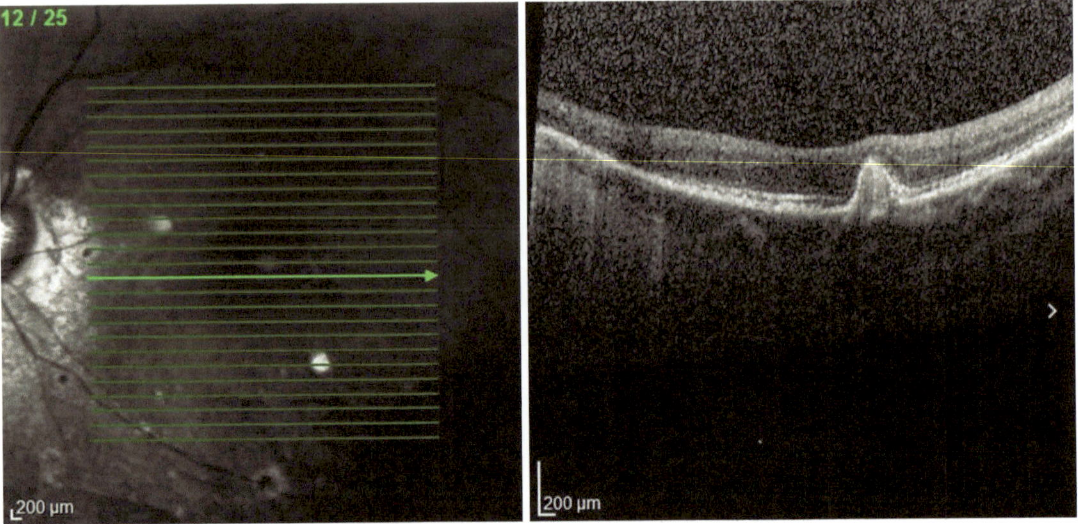

Fig. 25.19 Vogt-Koyanagi-Harada (VKH) syndrome. SD-OCT with corresponding red-free showing type 2 Dalen-Fuchs nodules. Here the dome-shaped elevation has displaced but not disrupted the overlying RPE

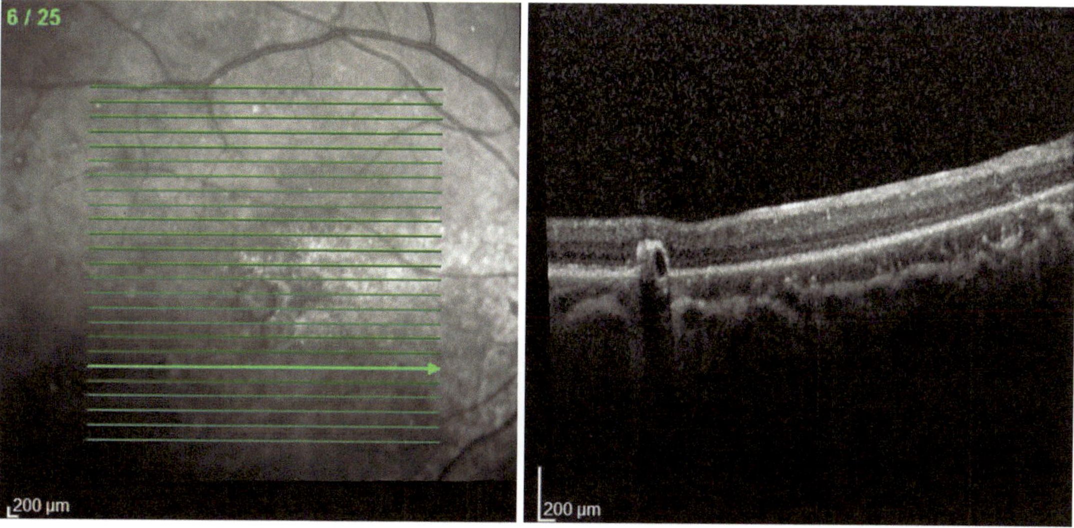

Fig. 25.20 Vogt-Koyanagi-Harada (VKH) syndrome. SD-OCT with corresponding red-free of the right eye showing type 3 Dalen-Fuchs nodule, a dome-shaped elevation that is associated with disruption of overlying retinal pigment epithelial layer

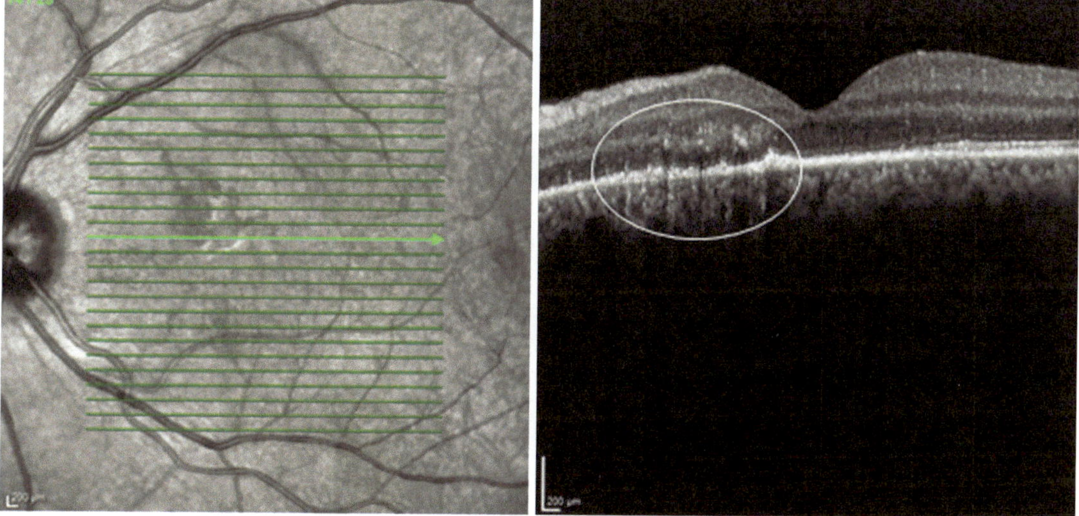

Fig. 25.21 Acute syphilitic posterior placoid chorioretinitis. SD-OCT shows loss of the outer retinal elements and an infiltrated appearance to the choroid (*white circle*)

cases may fail to recover normal foveal anatomy and are associated with a worse final acuity (Pichi et al. 2014).

25.4.1.2 Tuberculous Chorioretinitis

The principal difficulty with tuberculous (TB) uveitis is the confirmation of a case. As such, the literature contains many potential or probable cases rather than definite cases. The OCT imaging itself is therefore coupled with this diagnostic uncertainty, and there are no proven pathognomonic imaging features. The following paragraphs describe the various clinical appearances ascribed to TB uveitis and the corresponding imaging.

A. Focal TB chorioretinitis

A focal choroidal granuloma is seen as a localized elevation and thickening of the choroid with possible subretinal fluid (Goldberg and Jabs 2015; Saxena et al. 2013) (Fig. 25.23). Within the subretinal fluid area, there may be a point of adhesion between the neurosensory retina and RPE-Bruch's membrane with the overlying hyper-reflective retina (Salman et al. 2006) (Figs. 25.24 and 25.25).

B. Tuberculous serpiginous-like choroiditis (TB-SLC)

TB-SLC starts as unilateral, multifocal lesions that coalesce and involve the periphery (Vasconcelos-Santos et al. 2010) in comparison to the bilateral, disc centric lesions of classic serpiginous choroiditis (SC).

OCT imaging in TB-SLC is similar to classic SC. Active lesions show hyper-reflective and blurred outer retinal layers and RPE. There may be some elevation of the retina and RPE

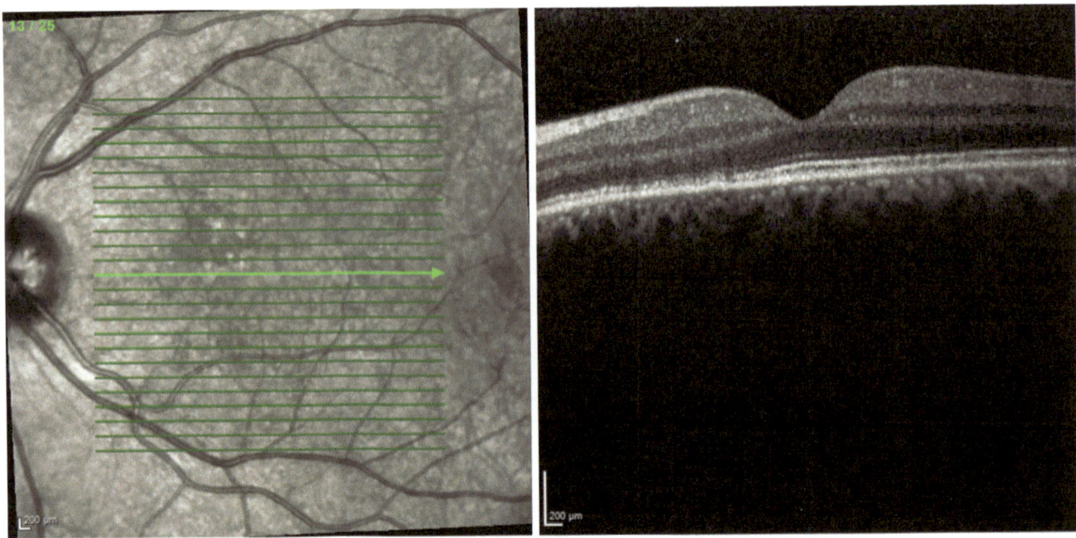

Fig. 25.22 Acute syphilitic posterior placoid chorioretinitis. SD-OCT 1 month after intravenous penicillin with almost complete reformation of the outer retinal lamellae

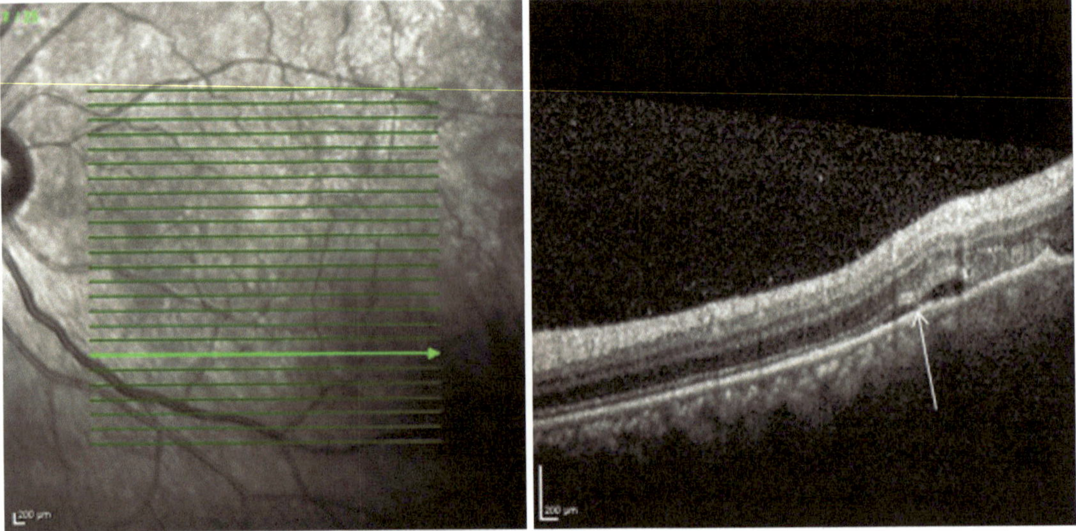

Fig. 25.23 Tuberculous chorioretinitis. SD-OCT showing a case of possible tuberculous choroidal granuloma. Evidence of subretinal fluid with an area of adhesion between the retina and RPE-Bruch's membrane (*white arrow*)

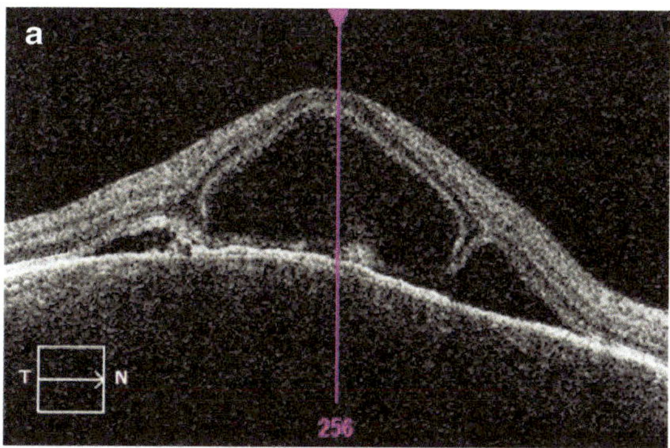

Fig. 25.24 Tubercular choroidal granuloma. (**a**) Pretreatment. SD-OCT showing elevated choroid with associated subretinal fluid and adhesion between the neurosensory retina and RPE-Bruch's membrane. (**b**) Post-antitubercular treatment. Significant reduction of both choroidal elevation and reduction in subretinal fluid with antitubercular treatment

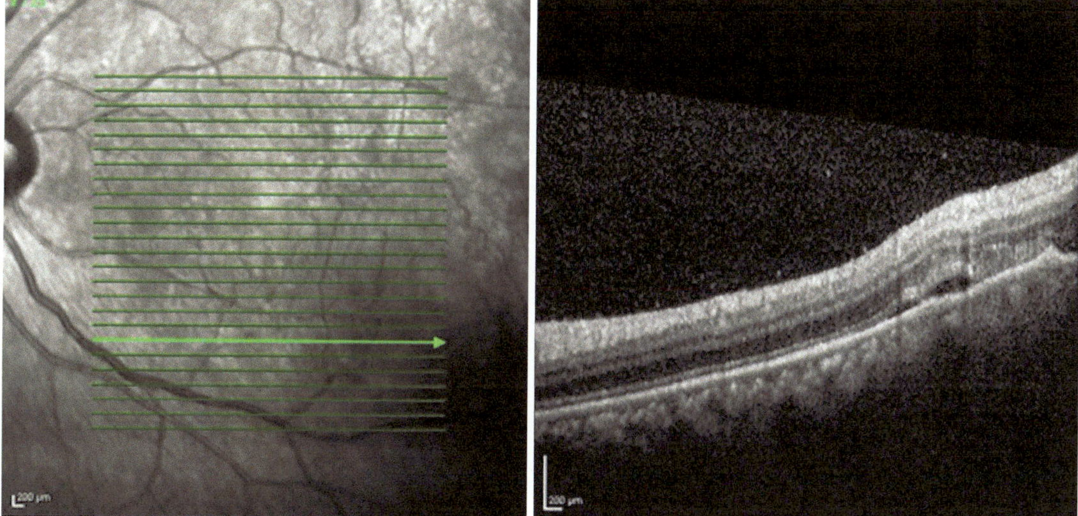

Fig. 25.25 Tuberculous choroidal granuloma. SD-OCT showing subretinal fluid with an area of adhesion between the retina and RPE-Bruch's membrane

by the underlying choroid (Rifkin et al.). As the lesions heal, the outer retina displays irregular lumpy elevations that progresses to atrophy of the outer retina, RPE and choroid (Bansal et al. 2011; Rifkin et al. 2015).

25.4.1.3 *Bartonella henselae* Neuroretinitis

Also called cat scratch disease (CSD), this condition is manifested clinically by optic nerve swelling with the appearance of a macular star of exudate. In the acute phase, OCT demonstrates outer plexiform cystic oedema emanating from the disc and macular serous detachment (Habot-Wilner et al. 2011; Stewart et al. 2005). As the fluid is reabsorbed in the convalescent phase, the lipid precipitates in the outer plexiform layer to form a macular star. The precipitates are seen as hyper-reflective elements in the outer plexiform layer (Habot-Wilner et al. 2011).

25.4.2 Viral Posterior Uveitis

25.4.2.1 Herpes Retinitis

Herpes simplex virus (HSV), herpes zoster virus and cytomegalovirus (CMV) are potential causes of infectious necrotizing retinitis. This may be manifested as various clinical syndromes including acute retinal necrosis (ARN) and progressive outer retinal necrosis (PORN). Most reports on OCT imaging relate to PORN and CMV retinitis because of difficulty obtaining quality OCT images of the peripheral retina and the presence of dense vitritis. Retinitis due to these herpes viruses all appears similar on OCT imaging in the acute phase. At presentation of an acute lesion with active white retinal necrosis, the OCT demonstrates outer retinal oedema and inner retinal hyper-reflectivity (Arichkia et al. 2016; Blair et al. 2007; Narayanan and Kuppermann 2006; Yeh et al. 2010) (Fig. 25.26). Over weeks to months with antiviral treatment, the retina undergoes cystic oedema and subsequent profound atrophy (Blair et al. 2007; Sun et al. 2012; Yeh et al. 2010). Due to the slower nature of CMV retinitis, the OCT images may display partial atrophy and inflammation simultaneously. Figure 25.27 shows a resolved CMV retinitis.

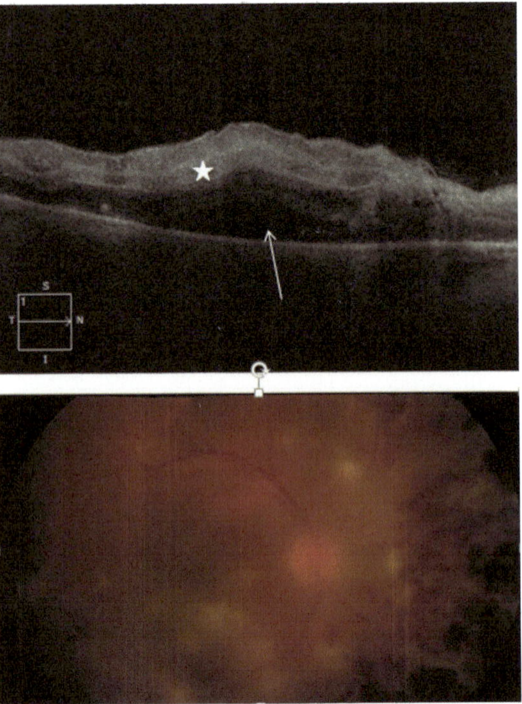

Fig. 25.26 Varicella zoster virus-related acute retinal necrosis (ARN). SD-OCT of the macula showing severe retinal thickening, inner retinal hyper-reflectivity (*white star*) and disruption of outer retinal layers with associated subretinal fluid (*white arrow*). Corresponding colour photo of the fundus showing vitreous haze, diffuse retinal oedema associated with scattered exudates and haemorrhages

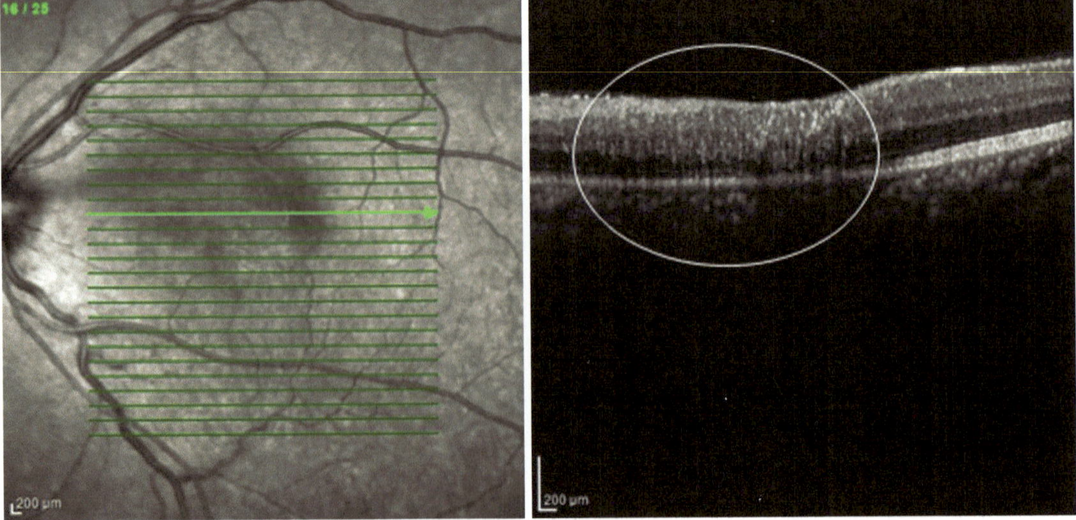

Fig. 25.27 Cytomegalovirus-related retinitis. SD-OCT shows full-thickness loss of the lamellar retinal structure, hyper-reflective inner retina and partial retinal thinning developing suggesting chronicity (*white circle*)

25.4.2.2 Coxsackie Virus Maculopathy

Also known as unilateral acute idiopathic maculopathy (UAIM), this condition has a strong association with coxsackievirus infection (Beck et al. 2004). Acute infection is seen as subfoveal neurosensory retinal detachment with hyper-reflective debris on the apical side of the RPE, possibly representing photoreceptor outer segments (Jung et al. 2012). During convalescence, the neurosensory detachment resolves, and the outer retinal layers appear disrupted (Jung et al. 2012).

In the resolved phase, there is almost complete restoration of foveal anatomy but with some residual disruption of the EZ (Srour et al. 2013). The RPE may appear slightly elevated and thickened (Srour et al. 2013).

25.4.2.3 Dengue Maculopathy

Dengue fever can cause ocular complications in up to 10 % of patients (Su et al. 2007). Acute macular findings in such cases can include diffuse retinal thickening, cystoid macular oedema or a foveolitis seen as thickening and high reflectivity of the outer retina (Teoh et al. 2010) (Fig. 25.28). Return to normal anatomy occurs over 1 month, but up to 60 % have persistent paracentral scotomas at 2 years (Teoh et al. 2010).

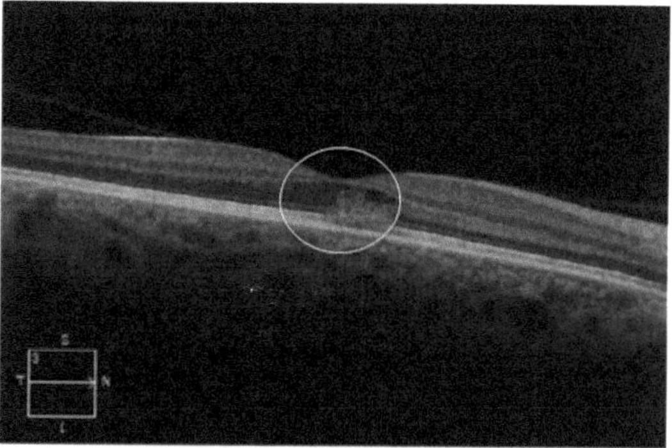

Fig. 25.28 Dengue maculopathy. SD-OCT shows 'foveolitis' and mild cystic oedema (*white circle*)

25.4.3 Fungal Posterior Uveitis

25.4.3.1 Candida Chorioretinitis

Ocular candidiasis may present with predominantly vitreal pathology with or without chorioretinal lesions. In cases with chorioretinal abscesses, early or small lesions show protrusion of material at the level of the RPE into the outer retina. More significant lesions may demonstrate a hyper-reflective, elevated lesion protruding into the vitreoretinal interface with significant shadowing of the underlying layers (Cho et al. 2007). Elevation of the adjacent RPE suggests a choroidal origin (Lavine and Mititelu 2015). In the resolved state, smaller lesions gradually regress with reformation of the external limiting membrane but with residual RPE irregularity (Cho et al. 2007). The more advanced lesions also regress with flattening of the vitreoretinal protrusion, and the affected retina is replaced by a full-thickness hyper-reflectivity indicative of scar formation (Lavine and Mititelu 2015).

25.4.4 Parasitic Posterior Uveitis

25.4.4.1 Toxoplasmic Retinochoroiditis

Acute toxoplasmosis infection by replicating tachyzoites may produce two clinical manifestations: classic toxoplasmic retinochoroiditis and punctate outer retinal toxoplasmosis (PORT).

A. Classic retinal toxoplasmosis

   Acute retinal infection will be represented on OCT as thickening, hyper-reflectivity and disruption of the entire neurosensory retina that gives a 'smudge'-like appearance (Fig. 25.29) (Goldenberg et al. 2013; Oréfice et al. 2006). The full-thickness involvement of the retina helps distinguish toxoplasmic retinal infection from a cotton wool spot that shows relative sparing of the outer retina (Kurup et al. 2014). Other findings include possible subretinal fluid (Diniz et al. 2011) and thickening of the posterior hyaloid with partial detachment over the lesion (Goldenberg et al. 2013). The underlying choroid is significantly thickened on enhanced depth imaging optical coherence tomography (EDI-OCT) scans, and this returns to normal during resolution (Goldenberg et al. 2013). In some eyes, hyper-reflective spherical deposits may be detected at the vitreoretinal interface.

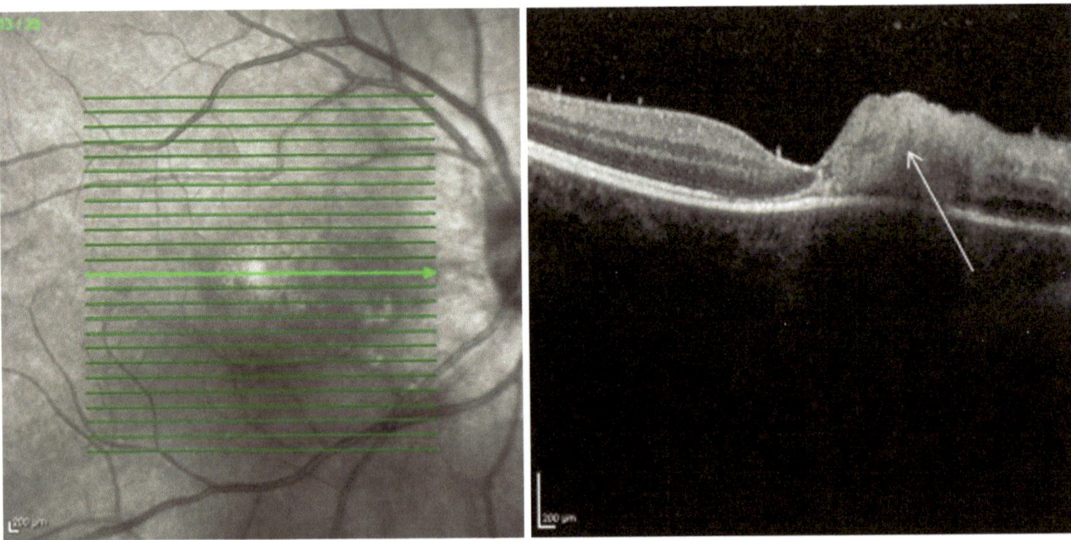

Fig. 25.29 Toxoplasmic retinochoroiditis. SD-OCT shows full-thickness involvement of neurosensory retina with a 'smudge-like' appearance in the acute phase (*white arrow*) and vitreal cells

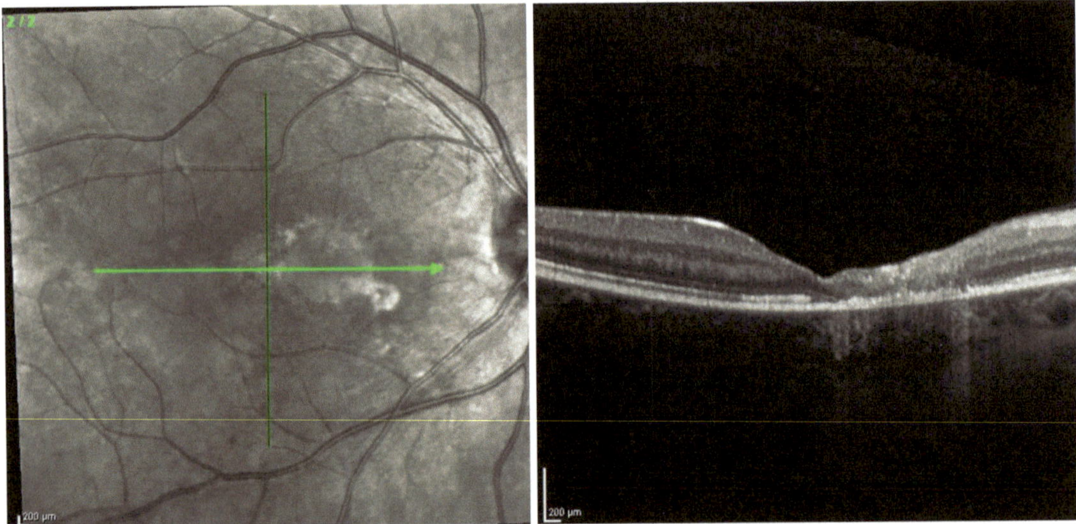

Fig. 25.30 Toxoplasmic retinochoroiditis. SD-OCT, 3 weeks after initial presentation and with treatment, shows full-thickness retinal disorganization and atrophy on the nasal side of the fovea

These may be remote from the infective focus and may occur along retinal vessels (Guagnini et al. 2007; Oréfice et al. 2013). As the lesion heals, these deposits may be incorporated into the inner retina and then dissolved (Goldenberg et al. 2013).

B. Punctate outer retinal toxoplasmosis (PORT)
Acute infection of the outer retina and RPE appears as hyper-reflectivity of the inner retina with shadowing of the outer retina and a focally detached posterior hyaloid face (Oréfice et al. 2007). There may also be subretinal fluid accumulation and fluid accumulation in the outer retina in a cystic-like appearance (Lujan 2014).

For both subtypes, as the lesion heals, there is further separation of the hyaloid, epiretinal membrane formation, retinal thinning and permanent loss and disorganization of the outer retinal elements (Fig. 25.30) (Diniz et al. 2011;

Oréfice et al. 2006). The residual scar may demonstrate various appearances including retinal atrophy and disorganization with thinning, an elevated retinal scar, deep (outer) retinal scar with excavation or a combination of these patterns (Goldenberg et al. 2013). Some patients may develop vitreomacular traction (Oréfice et al. 2006) or potential full-thickness macular hole (Panos et al. 2013).

25.4.4.2 Other Parasitic Infections

A. *Toxocara*

Acute *Toxocara* infection has been imaged as a mobile hyper-reflectivity on the inner retinal surface protruding into the vitreous (Sukuzi et al. 2005; Hashida et al. 2014). A significant granulomatous retinal reaction can occur and appears as hyper-reflectivity in the subretinal space or on the retinal surface (Shimzu et al. 2005). A tractional retinal fold emanating from the granuloma may be observed and on OCT appears as a diffusely hyper-reflective area of the elevated retina and surrounding subretinal fluid (Verallo et al. 2012; Shimzu et al. 2005).

B. Diffuse unilateral subacute neuroretinitis (DUSN)

This is a clinical presentation of unilateral retinal wipeout due to a retinal worm infection. OCT in late-phase disease demonstrates predominantly inner retinal thinning with loss of retinal nerve fibre layer (Garcia Filho et al. 2012). On OCT the worm may appear as a hyper-reflective outer retinal structure with surrounding disturbance of retinal lamellae (Garcia Filho et al. 2012). Another case has shown the worm residing on the retinal surface (Cunha et al. 2010).

25.5 Haemorrhagic Occlusive Retinal Vasculitis (HORV)

A recently described entity, haemorrhagic occlusive retinal vasculitis (HORV), occurs postoperatively and is associated with intraocular use of vancomycin (Witkin et al. 2015). Clinically, the condition may mimic viral retinitis, postoperative endophthalmitis or toxic anterior segment syndrome. The difference is the relative lack of pain and anterior segment inflammation in the presence of severe retinal changes. Prognostically, these patients have very poor visual outcome and often are complicated with neovascular glaucoma. Early OCT changes may show serous retinal detachment, disruption of the outer retinal layers and increased macular oedema with hyper-reflective inner retina (Witkin et al. 2015) (Fig. 25.31). Later OCT may show resolution of retinal oedema and hyper-reflectivity. Hyper-reflective lesions representing

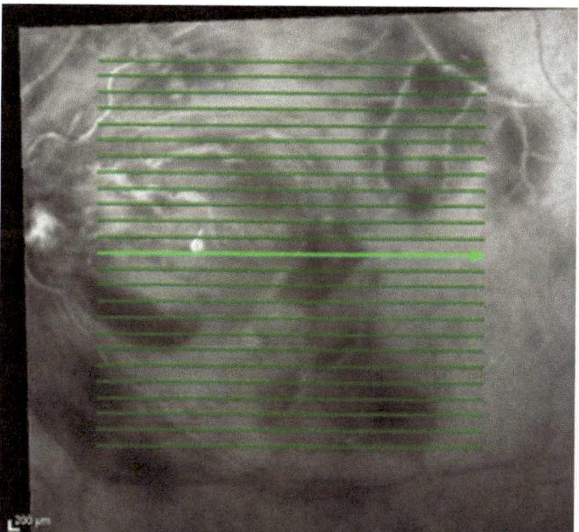

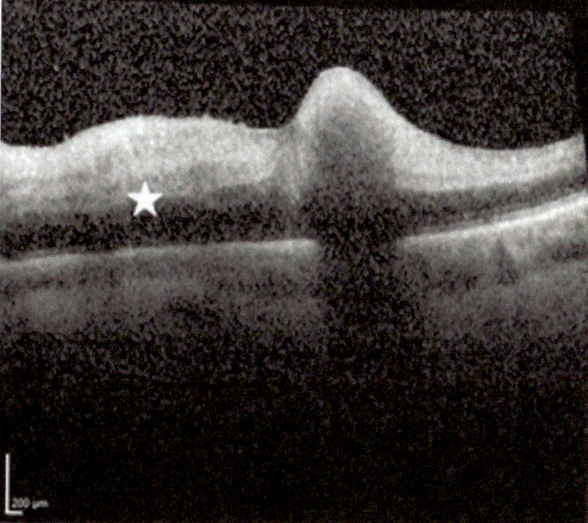

Fig. 25.31 Haemorrhagic occlusive retinal vasculitis (HORV). SD-OCT with corresponding red-free showing thickening of all retinal layers with hyper-reflectivity of the inner retinal layers (*white star*) suggesting retinal ischaemia

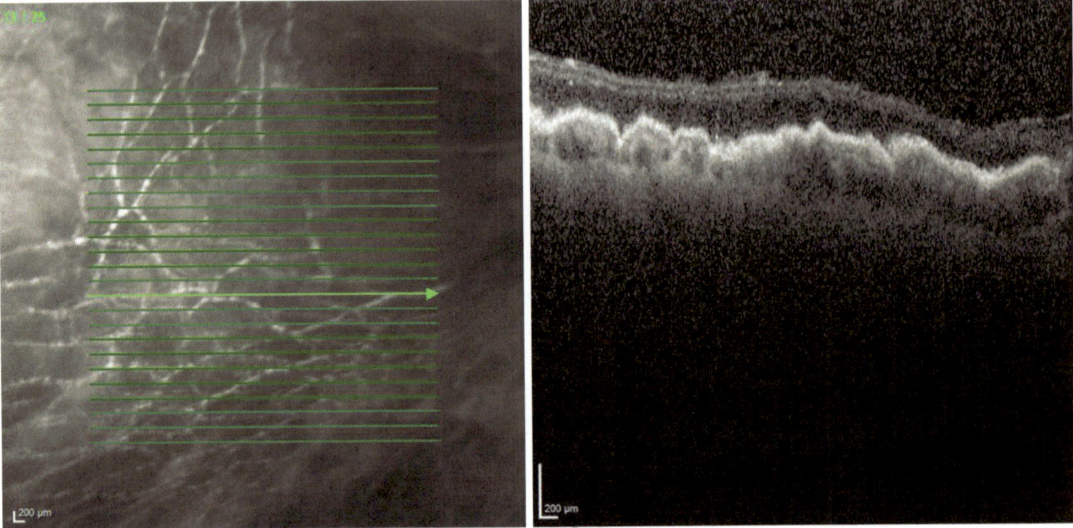

Fig. 25.32 Haemorrhagic occlusive retinal vasculitis. SD-OCT of the right eye 6 months following HORV shows severe retinal thinning of all layers with loss of outer retinal layers. Note hyper-reflective spot in the outer plexiform layer representing hard exudate

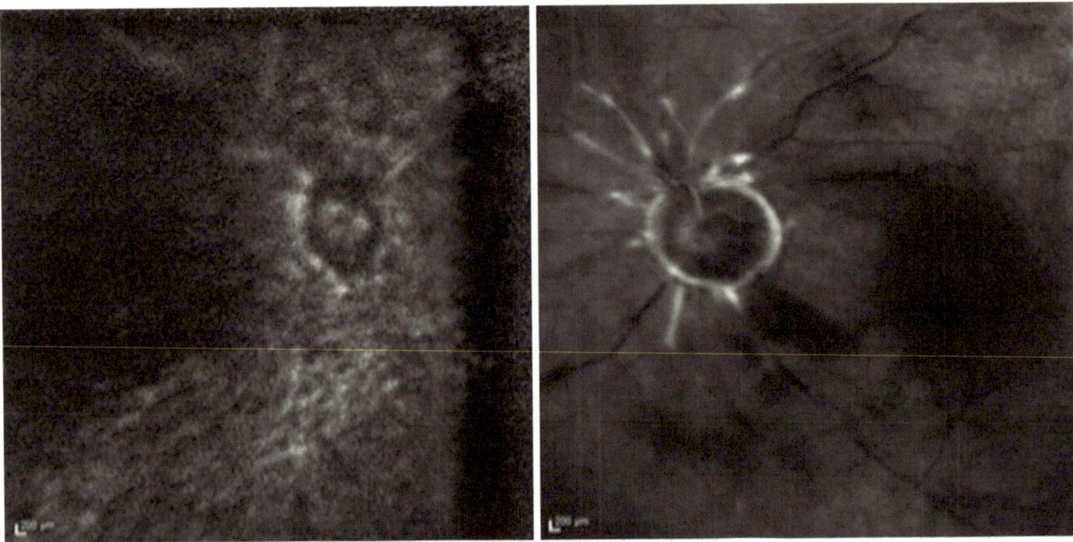

Fig. 25.33 Haemorrhagic occlusive retinal vasculitis. Corresponding FFA of both the left and right eye with HORV. The right showing complete non-perfusion of retinal circulation 6 months following HORV, whilst the left showing staining of retinal vessels with minimal perfusion beyond 1 disc diameter from the disc

hard exudates in the outer plexiform layer may persist (Witkin et al. 2015). Months after onset, OCT may show diffuse atrophy of all retinal layers and loss of outer retinal layers (Figs. 25.32 and 25.33).

25.6 Posterior Scleritis

Posterior scleritis is a specific form of scleral inflammation with very variable clinical presentation. Up to one third of patients with posterior

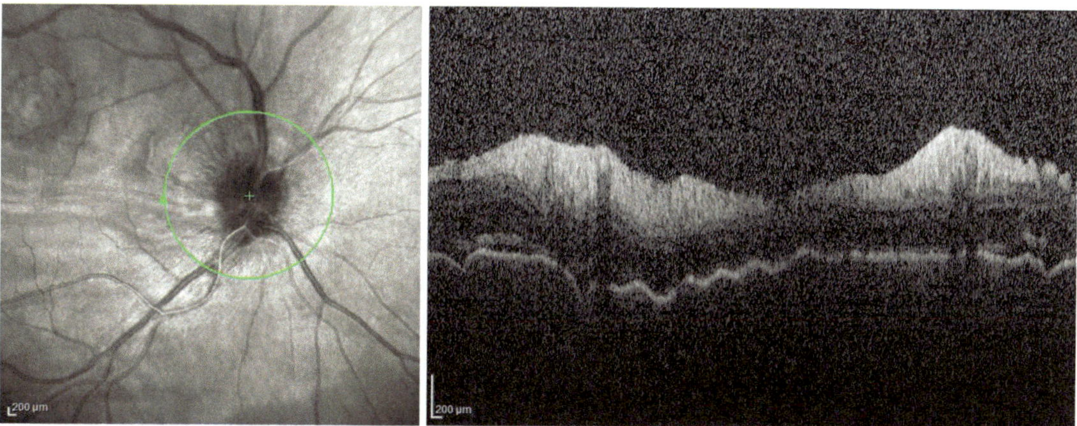

Fig. 25.34 Posterior scleritis. SD-OCT showing swollen optic disc associated with nodular posterior scleritis

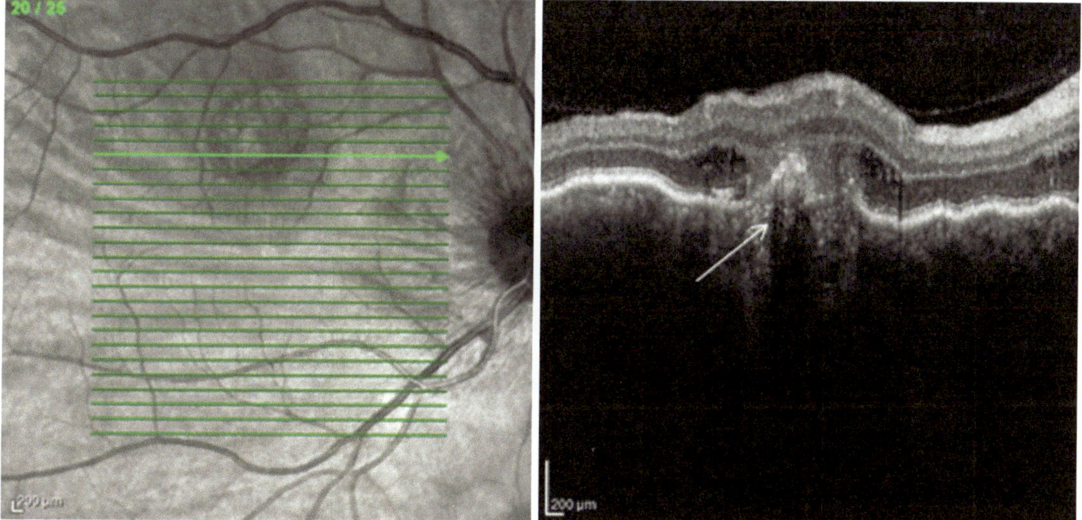

Fig. 25.35 Posterior scleritis. SD-OCT of the right optic nerve showing disc swelling associated with nodular posterior scleritis (*visible on red-free*). SD-OCT raster over the lesion showing focal choroidal elevation (*white arrow*) and intra-retinal fluid

scleritis have systemic association such as rheumatoid arthritis, granulomatosis with polyangiitis, relapsing polychondritis, etc. Clinical features of posterior scleritis are characterized most frequently by serous retinal detachment, swollen optic disc (Fig. 25.34), localized subretinal granuloma and uveitis. Nodular posterior scleritis presents as nodular subretinal mass which can be imaged on OCT (Fig. 25.35). This can be associated with retinal pigment epithelial changes, subretinal fluid, macular oedema and choroidal folds (Agrawal et al. 2016). OCT findings in scleritis are typically nonspecific, and other imaging modalities, e.g. ultrasound and CT, are used to show focal choroidal thickening. Studies reporting on OCT features in posterior scleritis are rare. OCT may show choroidal thickening with associated cystic subretinal spaces which typically resolves with treatment (Erdol et al. 2008).

25.7 Masquerade Syndromes

25.7.1 Intraocular Lymphoma

Primary CNS lymphoma is an important differential for panuveitis. Whilst confirmatory testing will require vitreous biopsy or lumbar puncture, various authors have described longitudinal OCT features that may point to a diagnosis of PCNSL (Liu et al. 2012). Early OCT may show hyper-reflective material within the outer retina that obscures EZ and ELM and increased irregularity in the RPE (Fig. 25.36). This is associated with disruption to the outer nuclear layer and outer plexiform layer (Liu et al. 2012). Later OCTs may show RPE elevation accompanied by heterogeneous, hyper-reflective sub-RPE deposits. Importantly, retinal and subretinal deposits may resolve with treatment-making OCT a useful modality to monitor treatment response (Forooghian et al. 2011) (Fig. 25.37).

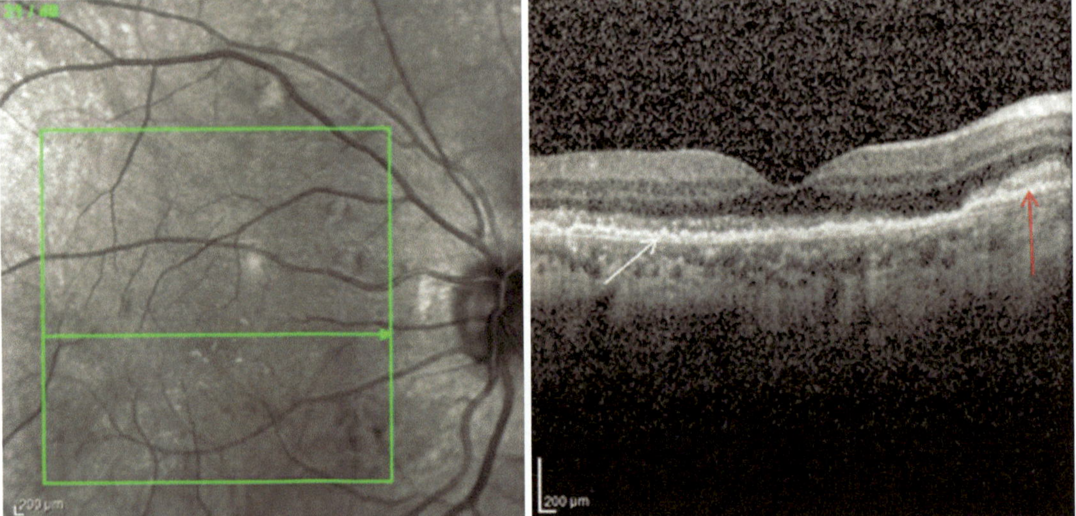

Fig. 25.36 Intraocular lymphoma. Pretreatment SD-OCT showing hyper-reflectivity above the RPE (*red arrow*) with loss of EZ and ELM. Note also the increase irregularity of RPE temporally (*white arrow*)

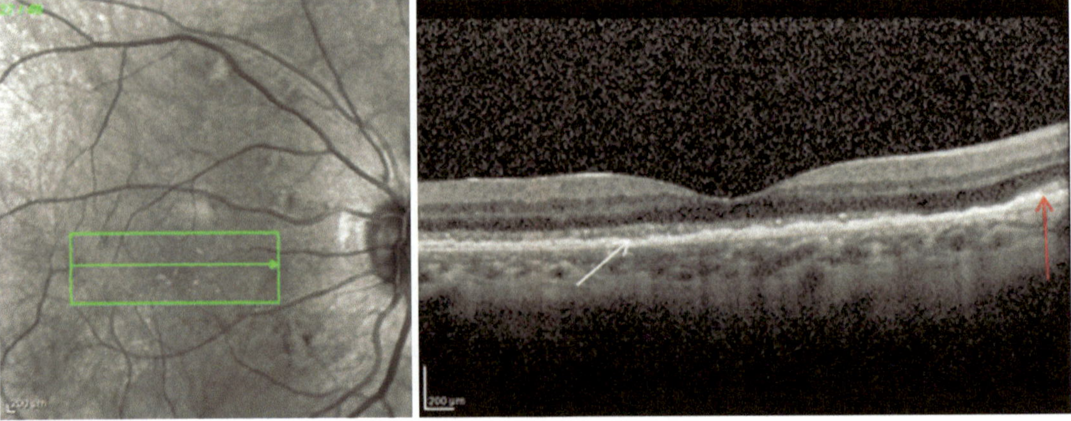

Fig. 25.37 Intraocular lymphoma. Posttreatment SD-OCT showing reduction in hyper-reflectivity deposit above RPE (*red arrow*) and significant reduction in RPE irregularity (*white arrow*)

References

Agrawal R, Lavric A, Restori M, Pavesio C, Sagoo MS (2016) NODULAR POSTERIOR SCLERITIS: clinico-sonographic characteristics and proposed diagnostic criteria. Retina 36(2):392–401

Amer R, Florescu T (2008) Optical coherence tomography in relentless placoid chorioretinitis. Clin Experiment Ophthalmol 36:388–390. doi:10.1111/j.1442-9071.2008.01773.x

Amin HI (2006) Optical coherence tomography findings in multiple evanescent white dot syndrome. Retina 26:483–484

Arantes TEF, Matos K, Garcia CR et al (2011) Fundus autofluorescence and spectral domain optical coherence tomography in recurrent serpiginous choroiditis: case report. Ocul Immunol Inflamm 19:39–41

Arichkia S, Uji A, Yoshimura N (2016) Retinal structural features of cytomegalovirus retinitis with acquired immunodeficiency syndrome: an adaptive optics imaging and optical coherence tomography study. Clin Experiment Ophthalmol 44(1):62–64. doi:10.1111/ceo.12577

Bansal R, Kulkarni P, Gupta A (2011) High-resolution spectral domain optical coherence tomography and fundus autofluorescence correlation in tubercular serpiginous like choroiditis. J Ophhtalmic Inflamm Infect 1:157–163

Beck AP, Jampol LM, Glaser DA et al (2004) Is coxsackie virus the cause of unilateral acute idiopathic maculopathy? Arch Ophthalmol 122:121–123

Birnbaum AD, Blair MP, Tessler HH et al (2010) Subretinal fluid in acute posterior multifocal placoid pigment epitheliopathy. Retina 30:810–814

Birnbaum AD, Fawzi AA, Rademaker A et al (2014) Correlation between clinical signs and optical coherence tomography with enhanced depth imaging findings in patients with birdshot chorioretinopathy. JAMA Ophthalmol 132:929–935

Blair MP, Goldstein DA, Shapiro MJ (2007) Optical coherence tomography of progressive outer retinal necrosis. Retina 27:1313–1314

Brito P, Penas S, Carneiro Â et al (2011) Spectral-domain optical coherence tomography features of acute syphilitic posterior placoid chorioretinitis: the role of autoimmune response in pathogenesis. Case Rep Ophthalmol 2:39–44

Channa R, Ibrahim M, Sepah Y et al (2012) Characterization of macular lesions in punctate inner choroidopathy with spectral domain optical coherence tomography. J Ophthalmic Inflamm Infect 2:113–120

Chen X, Rahimy E, Sergott RC et al (2015) Spectrum of retinal vascular diseases associated with paracentral acute middle maculopathy. Am J Ophthalmol 160:26–34

Cho M, Khanifar AA, Chan RV (2007) Spectral-domain optical coherence tomography of endogenous fungal endophthalmitis. Retina Cases Brief Rep 5:136–140

Cunha LP, Costa-Cunha LV, Souza EC et al (2010) Intraretinal worm documented by optical Coherence tomography in a patient with diffuse unilateral subacute neuroretinitis: case report. Arq Bras Oftalmol 73:462–463

da Silva FT, Sakata VM, Nakashima A et al (2013) Enhanced depth imaging optical coherence tomography in long-standing Vogt-Koyanagi-Harada disease. Br J Ophthalmol 91:70–74

de Bats F, Wolff B et al (2014) "En-Face" spectral-domain optical coherence tomography findings in multiple evanescent white dot syndrome. J Ophthalmol 2014:928028. doi:10.1155/2014/928028

de Smet MD, Rao NA (2005) Retinal cystoid spaces in acute Vogt-Koyanagi-Harada syndrome. Am J Ophthalmol 140:962

Diniz B, Regatieri C, Andrade R et al (2011) Evaluation of spectral domain and time domain optical coherence tomography findings in toxoplasmic retinochoroiditis. Clin Ophthalmol 5:645–650

Dolz-Marco R, Rodríguez-Ratón A, Hernández-Martínez P, Pascual-Camps I, Andreu-Fenoll M, Gallego-Pinazo R (2014) Macular retinal and choroidal thickness in unilateral relentless placoid chorioretinitis analyzed by swept-source optical coherence tomography. J Ophthalmic Inflamm Infect 4:24. doi:10.1186/s12348-014-0024-x

Erdol H, Kola M, Turk A (2008) Optical coherence tomography findings in a child with posterior scleritis. Eur J Ophthalmol 18:1007–1010

Fawzi AA, Pappuru RR, Sarraf D et al (2012) Acute macular neuroretinopathy: long-term insights revealed by multimodal imaging. Retina 32:1500–1513

Feigl B, Haas A (2000) Optical Coherence Tomography (OCT) in acute macular neuroretinopathy. Acta Ophthalmol Scand 78:714–716

Fong AH, Li KK, Wong D (2011) Choroidal evaluation using enhanced depth imaging spectral-domain optical coherence tomography in Vogt-Koyanagi-Harada disease. Retina 31:502–509

Forooghian F, Yeh S, Faia LJ, Nussenblatt RB (2009) Uveitic foveal atrophy: clinical features and associations. Arch Ophthalmol 127:179–186, doi:10.1001

Forooghian F, Merkur AB, White VA, Shen D, Chan CC (2011) High-definition optical coherence tomography features of primary vitreoretinal lymphoma. Ophthalmic Surg Lasers Imaging 42 Online:e97–e99. doi:10.3928/15428877-20110922-02

Fujiwara T, Imamura Y, Giovinazzo VJ et al (2010) Fundus autofluorescence and optical coherence tomographic findings in acute zonal occult outer retinopathy. Retina 30:1206–1216

Garcia Filho CA, Garcia CA, Arevalo JF (2012) Imaging in the diagnosis and management of diffuse unilateral subacute neuroretinitis. Int Ophthalmol Clin 52:283–289

Goldberg NR, Jabs DA (2015) Multimodal imaging of a tuberculous granuloma. Retina 35:1919–1920

Goldberg NR, Jabs DA, Busingye J (2015) Optical coherence tomography imaging of presumed sarcoid retinal and optic nerve nodules. Ocul Immunol Inflamm 24:1–4

Goldenberg D, Goldstein M, Loewenstein A et al (2013) Vitreal, retinal, and choroidal findings in active and scarred toxoplasmosis lesions: a prospective study by spectral-domain optical coherence tomography. Graefes Arch Clin Exp Ophthalmol 251:2037–2045

Guagnini AP, De Potter P, Levecq L et al (2007) Atypical spherical deposition on vitreoretinal interface associated with toxoplasmic chorioretinitis. Graefes Arch Clin Exp Ophthalmol 245:158–160

Gupta V, Gupta A, Gupta P et al (2009) Spectral-domain cirrus optical coherence tomography of choroidal striations seen in the acute stage of Vogt-Koyanagi-Harada disease. Am J Ophthalmol 147:148–153

Habot-Wilner Z, Zur D, Goldstein M et al (2011) Macular findings on optical coherence tomography in cat-scratch disease neuroretinitis. Eye (Lond) 25:1064–1068

Hashida N, Nakai K, Nishida K (2014) Diagnostic evaluation of ocular toxocariasis using high-penetration optical coherence tomography. Case Rep Ophthalmol 5:16–21

Hashimoto H, Kishi S (2015) Ultra-wide-field fundus autofluorescence in multiple evanescent white dot syndrome. Am J Ophthalmol 159:698–706

Hughes EG, Siow YC, Hunyor AP (2009) Acute macular neuroretinopathy: anatomic localization of the lesion with high-resolution OCT. Eye (Lond) 23: 2132–2134

Invernizzi A, Mapelli C, Viola F et al (2015) Choroidal granulomas visualized by enhanced depth imaging optical coherence tomography. Retina 35:525–531

Ishihara K, Hangai M, Kita M et al (2009) Acute Vogt-Koyanagi-Harada disease in enhanced spectral-domain optical coherence tomography. Ophthalmology 116:1799–1807

Joseph A, Rogers S, Browning A et al (2007) Syphilitic acute posterior placoid chorioretinitis in nonimmunocompromised patients. Eye (Lond) 21:1114–1119

Jung CS, Payne JF, Bergstrom CS (2012) Multimodality diagnostic imaging in acute idiopathic maculopathy. Arch Ophthalmol 130:50–56

Kanis MJ, van Norren D (2006) Integrity of foveal cones in multiple evanescent white dot syndrome assessed with OCT and foveal reflection analyser. Br J Ophthalmol 90:795–796

Keane PA, Allie M, Turner SJ et al (2013) Characterization of birdshot chorioretinopathy using extramacular enhanced depth optical coherence tomography. JAMA Ophthalmol 131:341–350

Kurup SP, Khan S, Gill MK (2014) Spectral domain optical coherence tomography in the evaluation and management of infectious retinitis. Retina 34:2233–2241

Lavine JA, Mititelu M (2015) Multimodal imaging of refractory Candida chorioretinitis progressing to endogenous endophthalmitis. J Ophthalmic Inflamm Infect 5:54

Lee GE, Lee BW, Rao NA et al (2011) Spectral domain optical coherence tomography and autofluorescence in a case of acute posterior multifocal placoid pigment epitheliopathy mimicking Vogt-Koyanagi-Harada disease: case report and review of the literature. Ocul Immunol Inflamm 19:42–47

Li D, Kishi S (2007) Loss of photoreceptor outer segment in acute zonal occult outer retinopathy. Arch Ophthalmol 125:1194–2000

Li D, Kishi S (2009) Restored photoreceptor outer segment damage in multiple evanescent white dot syndrome. Ophthalmology 116:763–770

Lim LL, Watzke RC, Lauer AK et al (2006) Ocular coherence tomography in acute posterior multifocal placoid pigment epitheliopathy. Clin Experiment Ophthalmol 34:810–812

Liu TY, Ibrahim M, Bittencourt M, Sepah YJ, Do DV, Nguyen QD (2012) Retinal optical coherence tomography manifestations of intraocular lymphoma. J Ophthalmic Inflamm Infect 2:215–218

Lujan BJ (2014) Spectral domain optical coherence tomography imaging of punctate outer retinal toxoplasmosis. Saudi J Ophthalmol 28:152–156

Markomichelakis NN, Halkiadakis I, Pantelia E et al (2004) Patterns of macular edema in patients with uveitis: qualitative and quantitative assessment using optical coherence tomography. Ophthalmology 111: 946–953

Maruko I, Iida T, Sugano Y et al (2011) Subfoveal choroidal thickness after treatment of Vogt-Koyanagi-Harada disease. Retina 31:510–517

Modi YS, Epstein A, Bhaleeya S et al (2013) Multimodal imaging of sarcoid choroidal granulomas. J Ophthalmic Inflamm Infect 3:58

Monnet D, Levinson RD, Holland GN (2007) Longitudinal cohort study of patients with birdshot chorioretinopathy. III. Macular imaging at baseline. Am J Ophthalmol 144:818–828

Monson BK, Greenberg PB, Greenberg E et al (2007) High-speed, ultra-high-resolution optical coherence tomography of acute macular neuroretinopathy. Br J Ophthalmol 91:119–120

Montero JA, Ruiz-Moreno JM, Fernandez-Munoz M (2011) Spectral domain optical coherence tomography findings in acute posterior multifocal placoid pigment epitheliopathy. Ocul Immunol Inflamm 19:48–50

Mrejen S, Khan S, Gallego-Pinazo R et al (2014) Acute zonal occult outer retinopathy: a classification based on multimodal imaging. JAMA Ophthalmol 132: 1089–1098

Narayanan R, Kuppermann BD (2006) Optical coherence tomography in progressive outer retinal necrosis. Ophthalmic Surg Lasers Imaging 37:506–507

Oréfice JL, Cost RA, Campos W et al (2006) Third-generation optical coherence tomography findings in punctate retinal toxoplasmosis. Am J Ophthalmol 142:503–505

Oréfice JL, Costa RA, Oréfice F et al (2007) Vitreoretinal morphology in active ocular toxoplasmosis: a prospective study by optical coherence tomography. Br J Ophthalmol 91:773–780

Oréfice JL, Cost RA, Scott IU et al (2013) Spectral optical coherence tomography findings in patients with ocular toxoplasmosis and active satellite lesions (MINAS Report 1). Acta Ophthalmol 91:e41–e47

Panos GD, Papageorgiou E, Kozeis N et al (2013) Macular hole formation after toxoplasmic retinochoroiditis. BMJ Case Rep bcr2013008915

Pichi F, Ciardella AP, Cunningham ET Jr et al (2014) Spectral domain optical coherence tomography findings in patients with acute syphilitic posterior placoid chorioretinopathy. Retina 34:373–384

Punjabi OS, Rich R, Davis JL et al (2008) Imaging serpiginous choroidopathy with spectral domain optical coherence tomography. Ophthalmic Surg Lasers Imaging 39:S95–S98

Rahimy E, Sarraf D, Dollin ML et al (2014) Paracentral acute middle maculopathy in nonischemic central retinal vein occlusion. Am J Ophthalmol 158:472–480

Reynard M, Riffenburgh RS, Minckler DS (1985) Morphological variation of Dalén-Fuchs nodules in sympathetic ophthalmia. Br J Ophthalmol 69: 197–201

Rifkin LM, Munk MR, Baddar D et al (2015) A new finding in tuberculous serpiginous-like choroidopathy. Ocul Immunol Inflamm 23:53–58

Rostaqui O, Querques G, Haymann P et al (2014) Visualization of sarcoid choroidal granuloma by enhanced depth imaging optical coherence tomography. Ocul Immunol Inflamm 22:239–241

Salman A, Parmar P, Rajamohan M et al (2006) Optical coherence tomography in choroidal tuberculosis. Am J Ophthalmol 142:170–172

Sarraf D, Rahimy E, Fawzi AA et al (2013) Paracentral acute middle maculopathy: a new variant of acute macular neuroretinopathy associated with retinal capillary ischemia. JAMA Ophthalmol 131:1275–1287

Saxena S, Singhal V, Ajduman L (2013) Three-dimensional spectral domain optical coherence tomography imaging of the retina in choroidal tuberculoma. BMJ Case Rep 2013. bcr2012008156

Scheufele TA, Witkin AJ, Schocket LS et al (2005) Photoreceptor atrophy in acute posterior multifocal placoid pigment epitheliopathy demonstrated by optical coherence tomography. Retina 25:1109–1112

Shimzu Y, Imai M, Fukasawa A et al (2005) Premacular membrane peeling without removal of subretinal granuloma in an eye with ocular toxocariasis. Acta Ophthalmol Scand 83:395–396

Souka AAR, Hillenkamp J, Gora F et al (2006) Correlation between optical coherence tomography and autofluorescence in acute posterior multifocal placoid pigment epitheliopathy. Graefes Arch Clin Exp Ophthalmol 244:1219–1223

Spaide RF, Koizumi H, Freund KB (2008) Photoreceptor outer segment abnormalities as a cause of blind spot enlargement in acute zonal occult outer retinopathy-complex diseases. Am J Ophthalmol 146:111–120

Spaide RF, Goldberg N, Freund KB (2013) Redefining multifocal choroiditis and panuveitis and punctate inner choroidopathy through multimodal imaging. Retina 33:1315–1324

Srour M, Querques G, Rostaqui O et al (2013) Early spectral-domain optical coherence tomography findings in unilateral acute idiopathic maculopathy. Retina 33:2182–2184

Staurenghi G, Sadda S, Chakravarthy U, Spaide RF (2014) International Nomenclature for Optical Coherence Tomography (IN•OCT) Panel. Proposed lexicon for anatomic landmarks in normal posterior segment spectral-domain optical coherence tomography: the IN•OCT consensus. Ophthalmology 121:1572–1578. doi:10.1016/j.ophtha.2014.02.023

Stewart MW, Brazis Paul W, Barrett KM et al (2005) Optical coherence tomography in a case of bilateral neuroretinitis. J Neuro Ophthalmol 25:131–133

Su DH, Bascl K, Chee SP et al (2007) Prevalence of dengue maculopathy in patients hospitalized for dengue fever. Ophthalmology 114:1743–1747

Sukuzi T, Joko T, Akao N et al (2005) Following the migration of a Toxocara lava in the retina by optical coherence tomography and fluorescein angiography. Jpn J Ophthalmol 49:159–161

Sun LL, Goodwin T, Park JJ (2012) Optical coherence tomography changes in macular CMV retinitis. Digit J Ophthalmol 18:1–4

Teoh SC, Chee CK, Laude A et al (2010) Optical coherence tomography patterns as predictors of visual outcome in dengue-related maculopathy. Retina 30:390–398

Tsjuikawa A, Yamashiro K, Yamamoto K et al (2005) Retinal cystoid spaces in acute Vogt-Koyanagi-Harada syndrome. Am J Ophthalmol 139:670–677

Vasconcelos-Santos DV, Rao PK, Davies JB et al (2010) Clinical features of tuberculous serpiginouslike choroiditis in contrast to classic serpiginous choroiditis. Arch Ophthalmol 128:853–8

van Velthoven MEJ, Onkosuwito JV, Verbraak FD et al (2006) Combined En-Face optical coherence tomography and confocal ophthalmoscopy findings in active multifocal and serpiginous chorioretinitis. Am J Ophthalmol 141:972–975

Vance SK, Khan S, Klancnik JM et al (2011a) Characteristic spectral-domain optical coherence tomography findings of multifocal choroiditis. Retina 31:717–723

Vance SK, Spaide RF, Freund KB (2011b) Outer retinal abnormalities in acute macular neuroretinopathy. Retina 31:441–445

Verallo O, Fragiotta S, Verboschi F et al (2012) Diagnostic aspects and retinal imaging in ocular toxocariasis: a case report from Italy. Case Rep Med 2012:984512, doi.org/10.1155/2012/984512

Wickremasighne S, Lim L (2010) Serous retinal detachment as a complication of acute posterior multifocal placoid pigment epitheliopathy. Retin Cases Brief Rep 4:129–131

Witkin AJ, Shah AR, Engstrom RE, Kron-Gray MM, Baumal CR, Johnson MW, Witkin DI, Leung J, Albini TA, Moshfeghi AA, Batlle IR, Sobrin L, Eliott D (2015) Postoperative hemorrhagic occlusive retinal vasculitis: expanding the clinical spectrum and possible association with vancomycin. Ophthalmology 122:1438–1451. doi:10.1016/j.ophtha.2015.03.016

Yamaguchi Y, Otani T, Kishi S (2007) Tomographic features of serous retinal detachment with multilobular dye pooling in acute Vogt-Koyanagi-Harada disease. Am J Ophthalmol 144:260–265

Yeh S, Wong WT, Weichel ED et al (2010) Fundus autofluorescence and OCT in the management of progressive outer retinal necrosis. Ophthalmic Surg Lasers Imaging 9:1–4

Yu S, Wang F, Pang CE et al (2014) Multimodal imaging findings in retinal deep capillary ischemia. Retina 4:636–646

Yu S, Pang CE, Gong Y et al (2015) The spectrum of superficial and deep capillary ischemia in retinal artery occlusion. Am J Ophthalmol 159:53–63

Ocular Tumors

26

Eduardo B. Rodrigues and Ana C. Garcia

Contents

26.1 Introduction

Advances in ophthalmic imaging improved diagnosis and management of ocular tumors. Optical coherence tomography (OCT) is a powerful imaging technique that provides cross-sectional imaging of the internal microstructures of biological tissues (Huang et al. 1991). Spectral domain OCT (SD-OCT) has replaced traditional time domain OCT providing high-resolution, high-sensitivity, and high-speed imaging (up to 40,000 scans per second). Such implementations enable noninvasive and noncontact visualization and measurement of the microstructures of the human eye. Recently, software upgrades and new imaging techniques have improved the ability to better evaluate intraocular tumors by allowing longer scan lengths, enhanced depth imaging (EDI), and three-dimensional reconstruction. In ocular oncology, OCT provides tools for diagnosis, treatment planning, and monitoring response.

26.2 Conjunctival and Corneal Tumors

Ocular surface lesions may be benign or carry significant morbidity. The correct diagnosis approach may demand clinical examination and adjunctive tests. The gold standard is obtaining a biopsy but it represents an invasive diagnostic technique. Anterior segment OCT can provide valuable information in the diagnosis of various tumors of the cornea and conjunctiva. Conjunctival nevi are one of the most common benign tumors of the ocular surface. On histopathology, a nevus typically consists of nests of nevus cells that are present in the junctional and subepithelial area of the conjunctiva. Conjunctival inclusion cysts are characteristic for nevi and may be observed clinically. Anterior segment OCT enables high-quality imaging of conjunctival nevi to reveal all margins, thickening of the conjunctiva, and the presence of the typical intrale-

E.B. Rodrigues, MD (✉) • A.C. Garcia, MD
Department of Ophthalmology, Federal University of São Paulo, São Paulo, Brazil
e-mail: rodriguesretina@gmail.com

C.H. Meyer et al. (eds.), *Spectral Domain Optical Coherence Tomography in Macular Diseases*,
DOI 10.1007/978-81-322-3610-8_26

sional cysts (Fig. 26.1). One of the main disadvantages of OCT is the optical shadowing of deeper structures caused by pigment in conjunctival nevi. Ultra-high-resolution spectral-domain reveals a highly reflective lesion, cysts within subepithelial tissue and an obscured posterior border due to the shadow caused by pigmentation (Shousha et al. 2013).

Clinically, ocular surface squamous neoplasia (OSSN) presents as elevated, papillary, gelatinous, or leukoplakic lesions. Diagnosis of these lesions can sometimes be challenging, and the use of noninvasive methods such as anterior segment OCT and ultrasound biomicroscopy has proven very useful (Thomas et al. 2014). A small pilot study involving the uterine cervix demonstrated the ability of OCT to distinguish abnormal epithelium from normal epithelium in the examination of cervical tissue (Gallwas et al. 2011). Kieval et al. (2012) investigated the use of an ultrahigh-resolution OCT as an adjuvant diagnostic tool in distinguishing ocular surface squamous neoplasia and pterygia (Fig. 26.2) (Kieval et al. 2012). Preoperative ultrahigh-resolution OCT images demonstrated similarities to the histopathologic specimens. Thomas et al. utilizing ultrahigh-resolution OCT demonstrated that OSSN presents a thickened layer of the epithelium, often with an abrupt transition from normal to neoplastic tissue. Differences in the measured epithelial thickness on ultrahigh-resolution OCT between squamous cell carcinoma and pterygia were statistically significant. Shousha et al. evaluated pterygia and through ultrahigh-resolution OCT imaging observed normal-thickness epithelium and a highly hyperreflective layer between the epithelium and Bowman's layer.

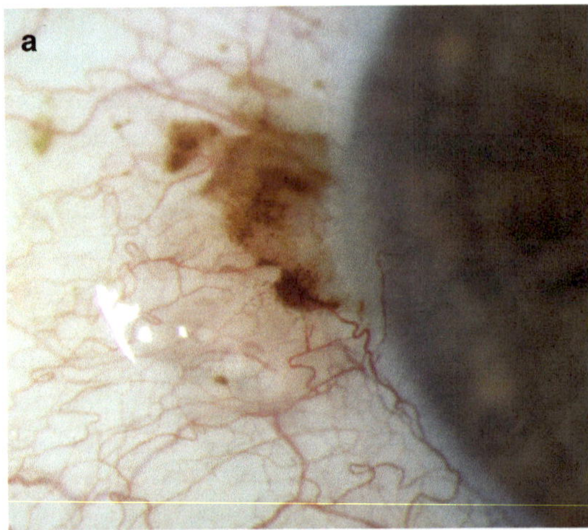

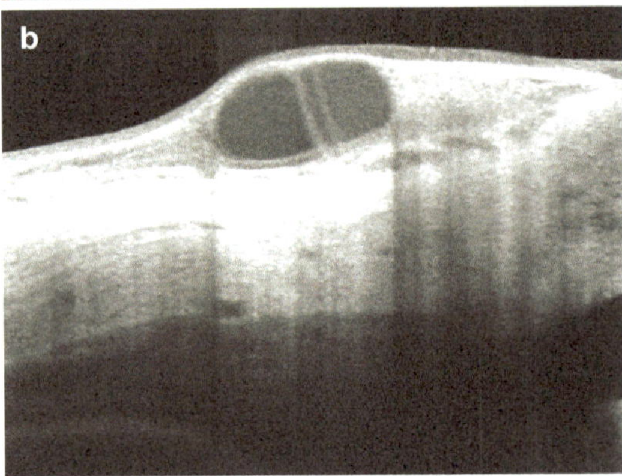

Fig. 26.1 (**a**) Conjunctival nevus with cyst. (**b**) Anterior segment OCT presents thickening of the conjunctiva and intralesional cyst

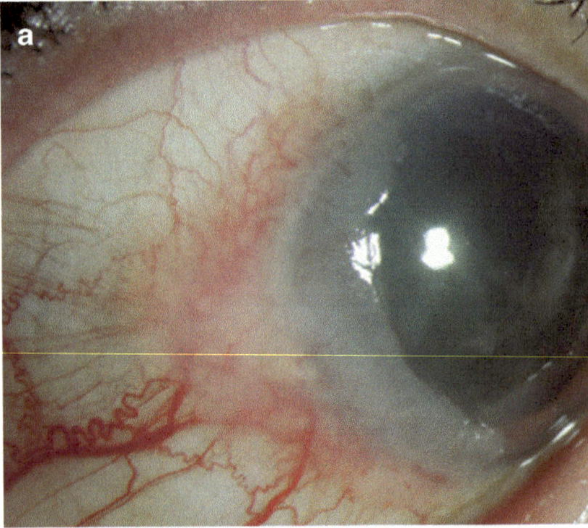

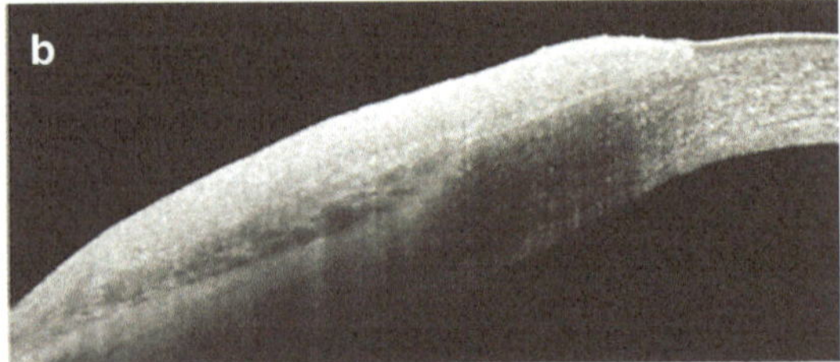

Fig. 26.2 (**a**) Ocular surface squamous neoplasia: clinical appearance. (**b**) Anterior segment OCT reveals thickened epithelium crossing the limbus from the conjunctiva to the cornea

Scleral lesions can be visualized partially by OCT (Shousha et al. 2013).

26.3 Anterior Uveal Tumors

Imaging technologies for anterior segment tumor evaluation provide useful information with regard to tumor size, shape, internal features, and extension. Anterior segment OCT has proven to be an important tool for diagnosis and analysis (Fig 26.3). Ultrasound biomicroscopy (UBM) represents another well-established method of imaging (Hood et al. 2011). Few clinical studies compared the usefulness of OCT and UBM in the evaluation of ciliary body and iris tumors. Siahmed et al. observed that UBM provided a precise measurement and regular surveillance capabilities compared with OCT (Razzaq et al. 2011). Pavlin et al. published a series of patients with iris and ciliary body tumors that were evaluated with both UBM and OCT and described that UBM had a superior ability to penetrate larger, highly pigmented tumors and those located in the ciliary body (Pavlin et al. 2009). Bianciotto and coworkers also reported UBM as a superior method for imaging of anterior segment tumors, such as ciliary body and iris melanoma, since it enabled visualization of all tumor margins and fewer problems with posterior shadowing and presented better resolution (Bianciotto et al. 2011).

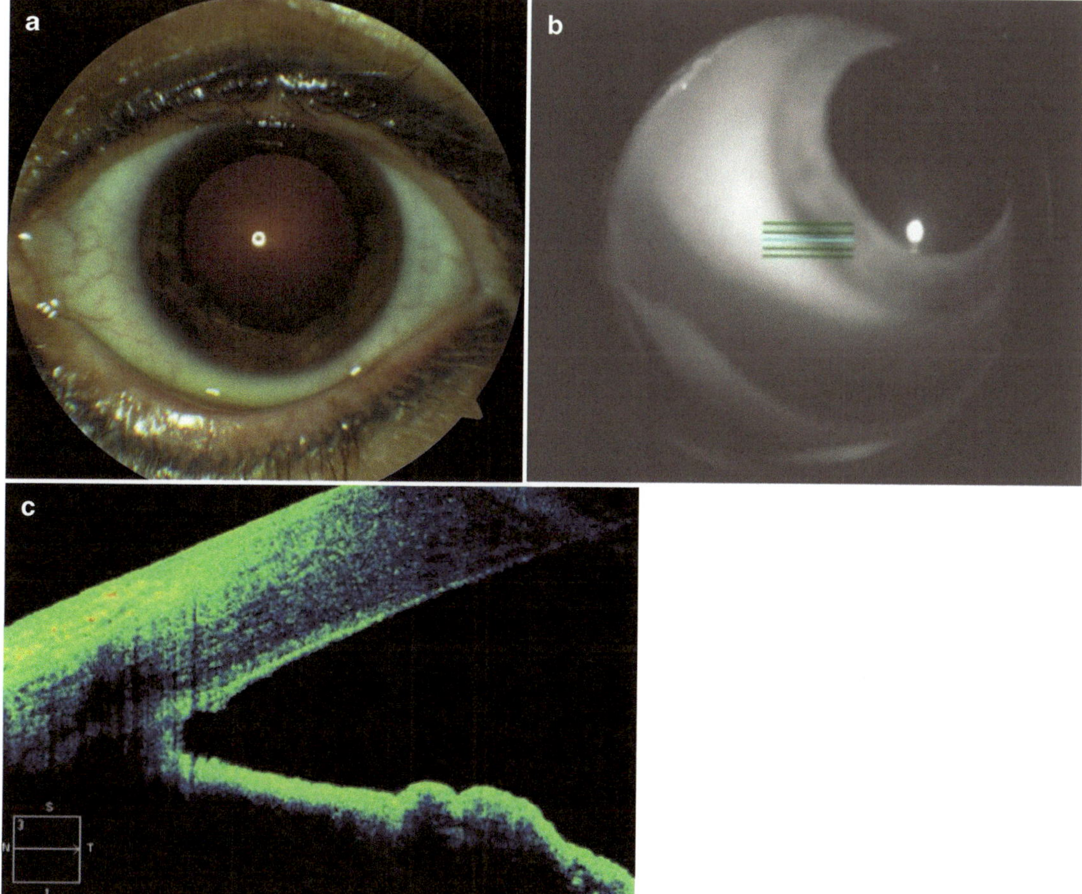

Fig. 26.3 (**a**) Pigmented iris melanocytoma. (**b, c**) Anterior segment OCT shows hyperreflectivity with shadowing and obscuration of the posterior margin

26.4 Intraocular Tumors

26.4.1 Retinal and Retinal Pigment Epithelial Tumors

26.4.1.1 Congenital Hypertrophy of the Retinal Pigment Epithelium

Congenital hypertrophy of the retinal pigment epithelium (CHRPE) presents as a pigmented lesion with benign behavior, rarely associated with visual symptoms. Usually it is unilateral but can occasionally be multifocal or grouped. Due to its peripheral location, OCT imaging is difficult but the typical appearance is of thickened RPE layer (Fig. 26.4). Shields and colleagues described overlying retinal thinning and photoreceptor loss in patients with CHRPE (Shields et al. 2006).

26.4.1.2 Combined Hamartoma of the Retina and Retinal Pigment Epithelium

Combined hamartoma of the retina and RPE presents as an elevated gray mass of the retina that blends with the surrounding retina and RPE without retinal detachment or vitreous inflammation. It is associated with preretinal fibrosis and traction on the adjacent retina. Spectral domain OCT reveals an elevated hyperreflective mass in the retina with mild attenuation of the retinal pigment epithelium and photoreceptor inner segment/outer segment junction and may be accompanied by a hyperreflective epiretinal membrane (Brue et al. 2013; Huot et al. 2009; Shields et al. 2005a). Schachat and associates from the Macula Society observed vascular tortuosity, vitreoretinal surface abnormalities, and pigmentation (Schachat et al. 1984).

26.4.1.3 Retinal Astrocytic Hamartoma

Retinal astrocytic hamartoma (astrocytoma) is a vascularized, benign, glial tumor of the retina that can be acquired or congenital. Acquired astrocytic hamartomas appear as yellow-white mass of the inner retina, lack calcification, and can be associated with macular edema, exudation, and retinal traction. Congenital astrocytic hamartomas acquire calcification and are associated with tuberous sclerosis. SD-OCT shows a thickened inner retina, some disorganization of the inner and outer retinal layers, and an intact RPE and choriocapillaris underlying the tumor (Fig. 26.5) (Kimoto et al. 2008). Calcified tumors have higher reflectivity.

26.4.1.4 Retinal Cavernous Hemangioma

Cavernous hemangioma is a benign retinal vascular tumor that presents as dark-red saccular

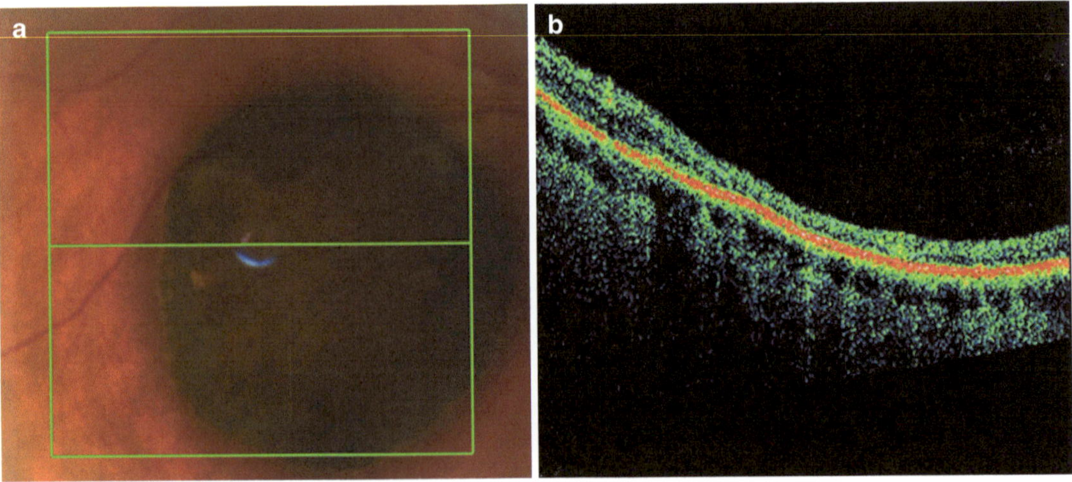

Fig. 26.4 (**a**) Fundus appearance of congenital hypertrophy of the retinal pigment epithelium (RPE). (**b**) OCT appearance of the thickened RPE layer

aneurysms. It can be associated with vitreous hemorrhage, preretinal fibrosis, or vascular occlusion. OCT shows a lobulated inner retina with optically clear spaces representing the saccular aneurysms. The underlying RPE is intact and subretinal fluid is typically absent (Fig. 26.6) (Andrade et al. 2005; Shields et al. 2005c).

26.4.1.5 Retinal Capillary Hemangioma

Retinal hemangioblastoma (capillary hemangioma) is an orange circumscribed vascular lesion with dilated feeding artery and draining vein that can affect any part of the ocular fundus. Small tumors appear as red dots or as retinal telangiectasia. They may occur sporadically or can be associated with Von Hippel-Lindau disease. The value of OCT evaluation of these lesions lies in identifying and monitoring retinal changes. OCT shows a hyperreflective lesion with little inner tumor detail, but is useful to detect associated macular edema, epiretinal membrane, and subretinal fluid (Shields et al. 2005c).

26.4.1.6 Retinal Vasoproliferative Tumor

Vasoproliferative tumors of the retina are usually unilateral, yellow-red colored, located in the inferotemporal periphery with minimally dilated

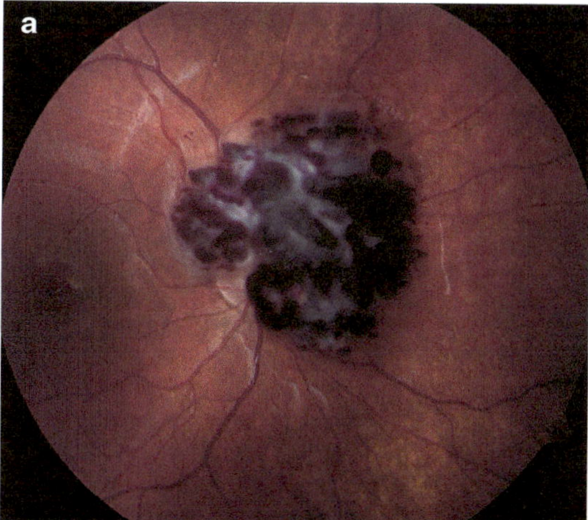

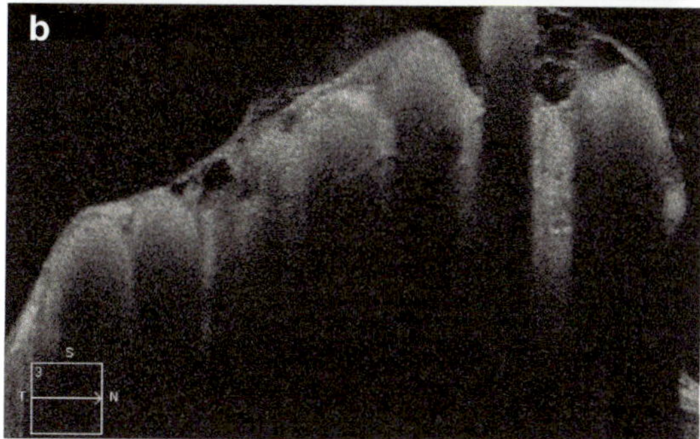

Fig 26.6 (**a**) Retina cavernous hemangioma. (**b**) Epiretinal membrane bridging over multiple cystic spaces within inner and outer retinal layers

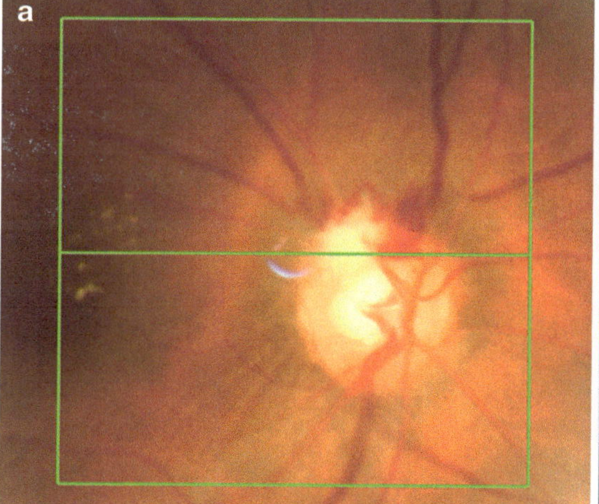

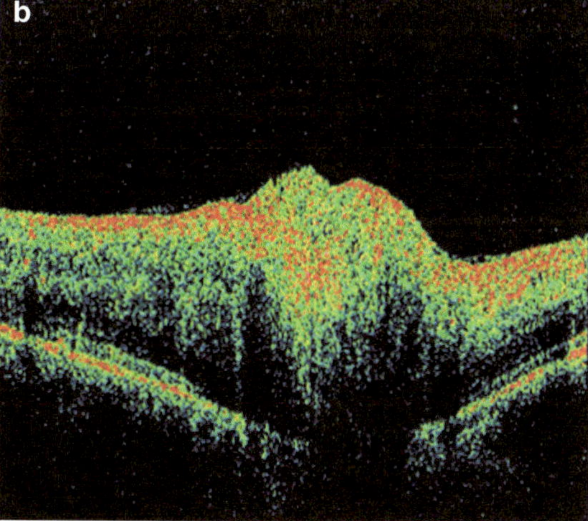

Fig. 26.5 (**a**) Retinal astrocytic hamartoma. (**b**) Thickened inner retina with disorganization of the inner and outer retinal layers

or nondilated feeding artery and draining vein in contrast to hemangioblastoma. Associated changes are exudative retinal detachment, macular edema, retinal fibrosis, hyper- and hypopigmentation of the RPE, and cellular infiltrates in the vitreous. Due to its peripheral location, many vasoproliferative tumors cannot be imaged requiring advanced changes in the OCT scan length. Posterior lesions demonstrate retinal inner layer disorganization and posterior shadowing. Vision loss is usually due to epiretinal membrane or exudative macular detachment, and OCT is useful to identify these changes and follow up during treatment. Following successful ablation of the vasoproliferative tumor, regression of the associated retinal exudative changes occurs.

26.4.2 Optic Disk Melanocytoma

Optic disk melanocytoma (ODM) is a benign deeply pigmented lesion that usually occurs in the optic nerve head. Histological studies have shown malignant transformation into melanoma in 1–2 % of cases, which causes progressive growth and severe visual loss. ODM sometimes causes complications such as central retinal vascular obstruction. OCT images show an elevated dome-shaped mass with dense posterior shadowing and a gradual slope at the tumor margin. Shields et al. examined optic disk melanocytomas using time domain OCT and found typical features of a gradually sloped nodular elevation with a hyperreflective anterior surface and dense posterior shadowing portraying an optically empty mass (Fig. 26.7) (Saxena et al. 2010; Shields et al. 2008).

26.4.3 Choroidal Tumors

26.4.3.1 Choroidal Nevus

Choroidal nevi are the most common intraocular tumors and usually do not cause visual symptoms. Nevi are pigmented round subretinal lesions, with smooth margins and frequently present with overlying drusen, measuring less than 5 mm in basal diameter and 1 mm in thickness. They are benign lesions but can undergo malignant transformation. Factors predictive of nevus transformation into melanoma are juxtapapillary location, orange pigment, thickness greater than 2 mm, the presence of subretinal fluid, and visual symptoms. OCT is able to detect retinal and anterior choroidal changes that include retinal thinning, retinal edema, subretinal fluid, RPE detachment, and drusen. The choroidal findings are limited to the anterior surface and include hyporeflectivity in most of the cases. OCT evaluation is more sensitive than clinical examination to detect retinal edema, subretinal fluid, retinal thinning, and RPE detachment.

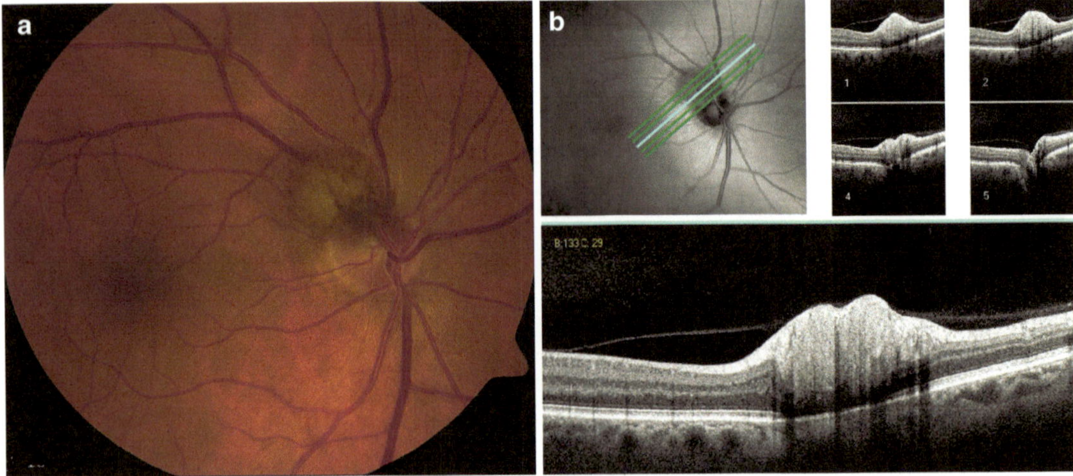

Fig. 26.7 (**a**) Optic disk melanocytoma. (**b**) The inner layers of the retina appear to be thickened with disorganization of outer layers. The RPE is intact with normal underlying choroid

Also, it helps to determine the status of photoreceptor and to characterize retinal edema (cystoid versus non-cystoid). Drusen, which are clinically visible, are evidenced by OCT as small dome-shaped elevations at the level of Bruch's membrane (Shields et al. 2005b).

26.4.3.2 Indeterminate Melanocytic Lesions

Indeterminate melanocytic lesions (IMLs) are pigmented choroidal lesions between 1 and 3 mm in thickness and present a diagnostic challenge. IML can correspond to a large nevus or a choroidal melanoma. OCT is able to detect some of the features predictive of growth such as thickness greater than 2 mm, presence of orange pigment and subretinal fluid, and absence of drusen. Singh and associates used spectral domain OCT to describe accumulation of subretinal deposits corresponding to orange pigment over a small IML that had not been observed with time domain OCT (Fig. 26.8) (Singh et al. 2010). Lesions less likely to grow present chronic retinal changes such as thinned retina with intraretinal cysts and RPE thickening. Hyperautofluorescence correlates to OCT findings of lipofuscin or subretinal fluid (Fig. 26.9) (Singh et al. 2010).

26.4.3.3 Choroidal Melanoma

Uveal melanoma is the most common primary intraocular malignant tumor, and 90 % develop in the choroid. They often present as a pigmented, elevated, choroidal mass. OCT imaging provides better evaluation of the retina and anterior surface of the tumor. The limitation of OCT for choroidal melanoma lies in the inability to image past the anterior choroidal surface. Subretinal fluid is an important characteristic

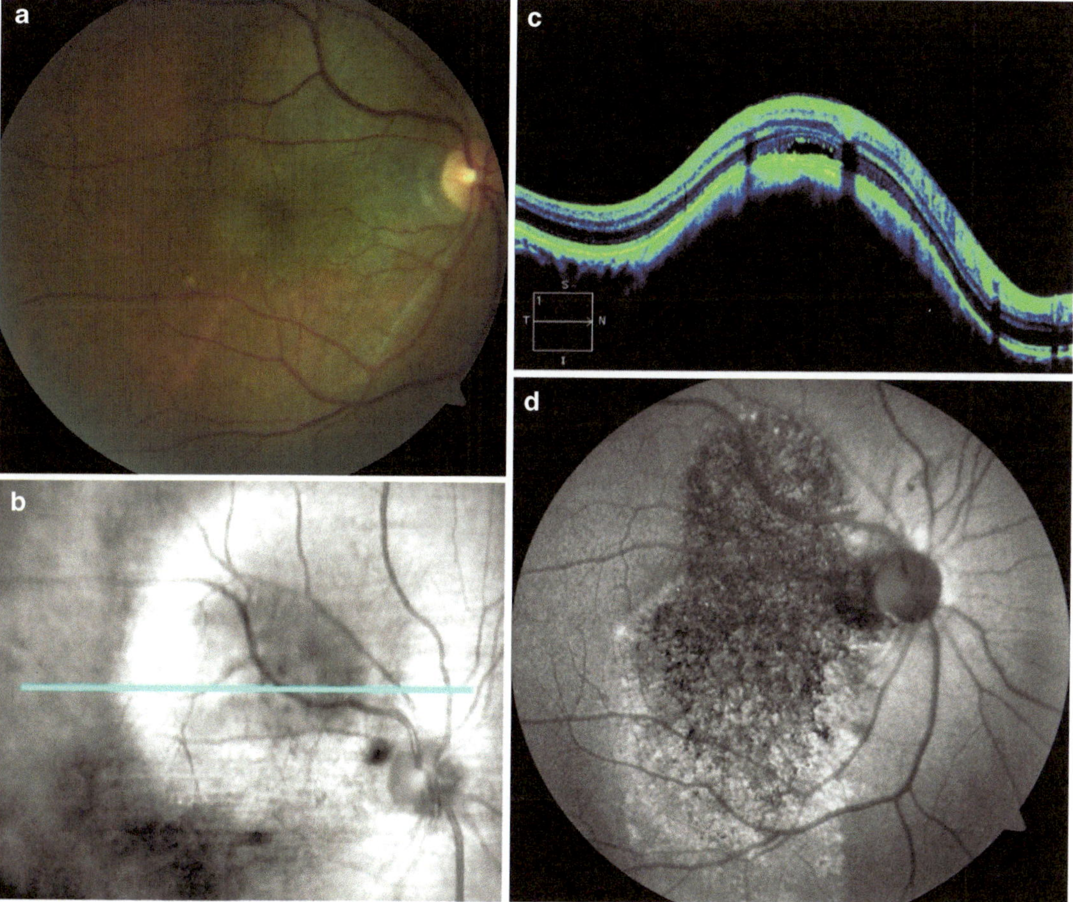

Fig. 26.8 (**a**) Indeterminate choroidal melanocytic lesion: fundus appearance. (**b**, **c**) Spectral domain OCT shows subretinal fluid and deposits. (**d**) Autofluorescence after transpupillary thermotherapy (TTT) treatment

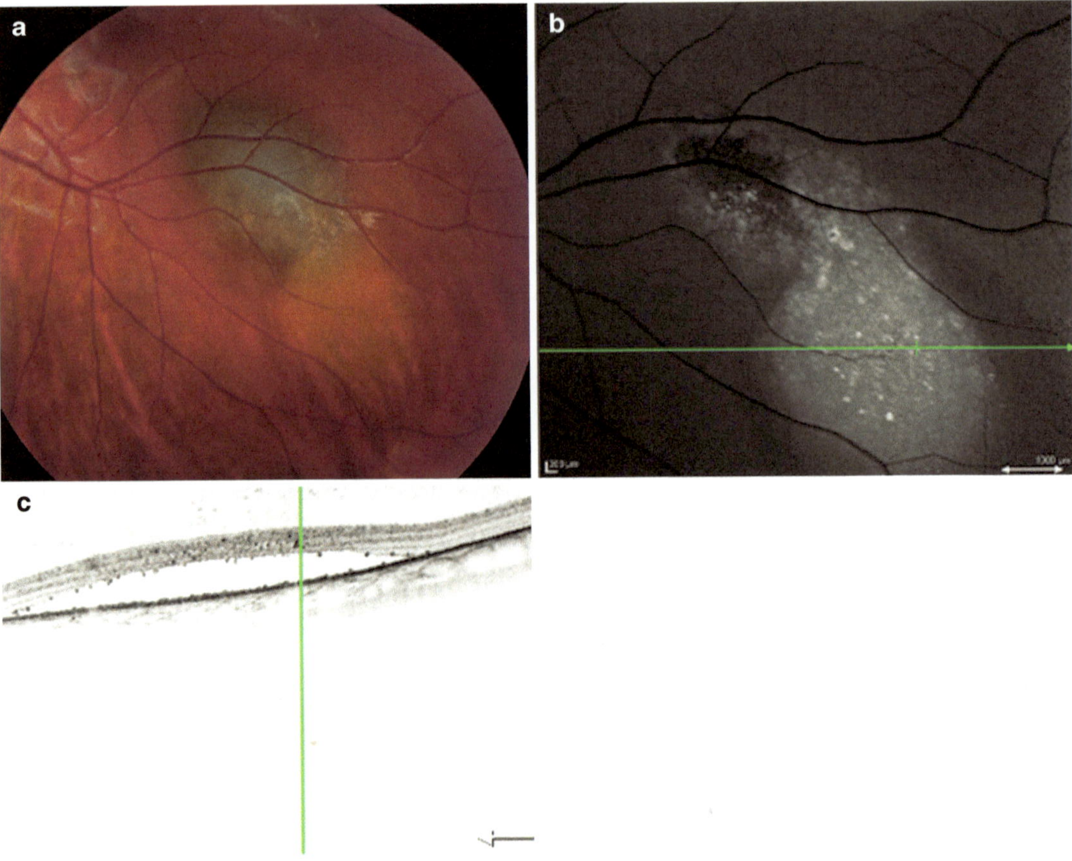

Fig. 26.9 (**a**) Indeterminate choroidal melanocytic lesion (small choroidal melanoma). Orange pigmentation (lipofuscin) on fundus photograph. (**b**) Hyperautofluorescent spots on fundus autofluorescence image. (**c**) Spectral domain OCT. Deposition of hyperreflective material near the retinal pigment epithelium and in the outer retina (Reproduced with permission from Singh et al. 2010)

related to underlying choroidal melanoma, may be detectable by OCT in almost all cases, and is a significant risk factor for metastasis (Muscat et al. 2004; Espinoza et al. (2004)). The clinical differentiation between small choroidal melanomas and choroidal nevi can be very challenging, and the use of OCT imaging can help elucidate the diagnosis. Shields et al. presented features that were more often found with small choroidal melanoma compared with choroidal nevus such as increased tumor thickness, subretinal fluid, subretinal lipofuscin deposition, and RPE atrophy (Shields et al. 2012). Sayanagi et al. used 3D spectral domain OCT and found a significantly higher prevalence of subretinal fluid (91 % versus 14 %), retinal edema (61 % versus 14 %), and subretinal deposits (61 % versus 11 %) in choroidal melanoma compared with nevi (Sayanagi et al. 2011). Spectral domain OCT was also capable of detecting early vitreous seeding as highly reflective spheroidal bodies in the vitreous. OCT has been used to monitor retinal changes related to complications of radiotherapy like macular edema, which can be present in 61 % of the cases, 24 months after treatment or retinal atrophy. Horgan et al. performed pre- and postplaque radiotherapy OCT and found that the mean time to the onset of radiation maculopathy was 12 months (Horgan et al. 2008).

26.4.3.4 Choroidal Osteoma

Choroidal osteoma is a benign osseous tumor reported in young females. The tumor is located in the juxtapapillary region or macula and presents an orange-yellow color when calcified and as a white tumor when decalcified. Complications of choroidal osteoma that cause

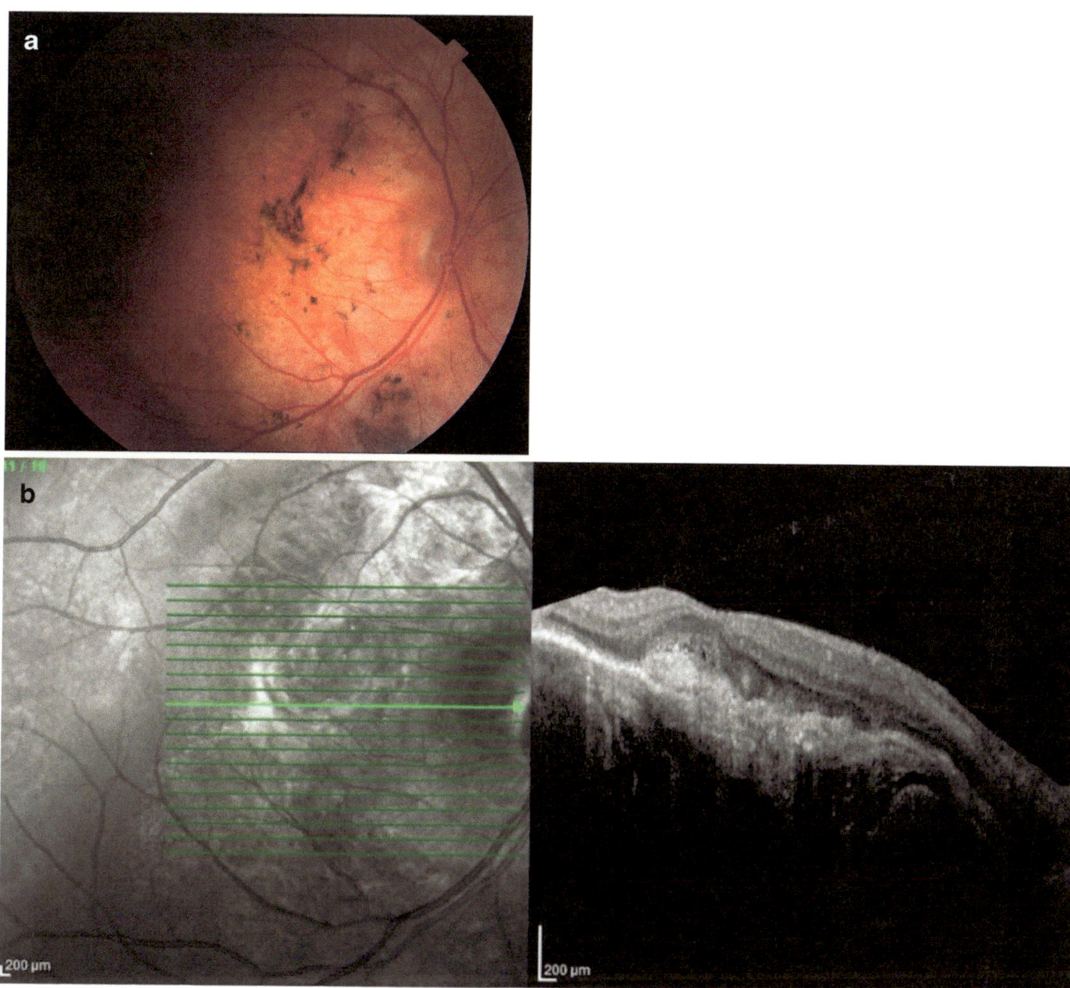

Fig. 26.10 (**a**) Choroidal osteoma. (**b**) OCT image reveals irregularity of external retinal layers, retinal pigment epithelium and choriocapillaris

vision loss are related to the tumor decalcification and include neovascular membranes and retinal changes (subretinal fluid or photoreceptor loss) both identifiable by OCT imaging. Shields and coworkers reported OCT features of choroidal osteoma that included heterogeneity that depended upon the amount of tumor calcification (Shields et al. 2007). The internal structure of choroidal osteoma is difficult to evaluate with OCT when hyperpigmentation is present. Another important characteristic that may limit OCT evaluation is calcification of the tumor. Calcified portions of the tumor reveal mostly intact inner (100 %) and outer (95 %) retinal layers, a distinct RPE (57 %), and mild transmission of light (95 %) (Fig. 26.10). In contrast, decalcified portions of the tumor reveal intact inner retinal layers (90 %), thinned outer retinal layers (100 %), an indistinct RPE (90 %), and marked light transmission into the tumor (70 %). The anterior tumor surface was hyperreflective in 48 % and isoreflective in 52 % if calcified, but was mostly hyperreflective (90 %) when decalcified (Shields et al. 2007).

26.4.3.5 Choroidal Metastasis

The choroid is a common site of metastasis due to its vascularization. Clinically, choroidal metastasis appears as a solitary, nonpigmented choroidal mass. On OCT examination, a dome-shaped elevation of the RPE and retina with adjacent subretinal fluid is observed. Retinal changes on OCT include retinal edema, intraretinal cysts, thickening, and detachment of the RPE. Arevalo and colleagues reviewed retinal changes associated with choroidal metastasis using time domain OCT and found highly reflective points within neurosensory detachment in 14.2 % of cases and concluded that these points "may correspond to retinal compromise by cancer cells or macrophages containing lipofuscin and melanin granules"(Arevalo et al. 2005). Demirci et al. presented enhanced depth imaging optical coherence tomography imaging features of 24 choroidal metastatic tumors such as thinning of the choriocapillaris over the metastatic tumor (100 %), plateau-shaped tumor elevation, low internal optical reflectivity, and partial choroidal shadowing deep to the tumor (Demirci et al. 2013). Spaide et al. demonstrated through enhanced depth imaging that choroidal metastasis revealed a low reflective band in the deeper choroid with enlargement of the suprachoroidal space (Spaide et al. 2008). OCT imaging is especially useful in small metastatic tumors, can be more sensitive than ultrasonography, and can monitor retinal changes after the treatment such as resolution of subretinal fluid and retinal atrophy.

26.4.3.6 Choroidal Hemangioma

Circumscribed choroidal hemangioma is a benign vascular tumor usually orange colored, round, and located in the posterior pole. These lesions are hyporeflective on OCT but usually exhibit overlying retinal edema, subretinal fluid, and RPE alterations secondary to tumor leakage (Shields et al. 2008). Ramasubramanian et al. described OCT findings in circumscribed choroidal hemangioma and found subretinal fluid (19 %), retinal edema (42 %), retinoschisis (12 %), macular edema (24 %), and localized photoreceptor loss (35 %) (Ramasubramanian et al. 2010). OCT shows preserved photoreceptors and normal retinal thickness if the leakage is acute and degenerated photoreceptors, retinoschisis, and intra-retinal edema if the leakage is chronic (Say et al. 2011). Spaide et al. described that circumscribed choroidal hemangioma presented low/medium reflectivity and a homogenous signal with large intrinsic spaces on enhanced depth imaging (Spaide et al. 2008).

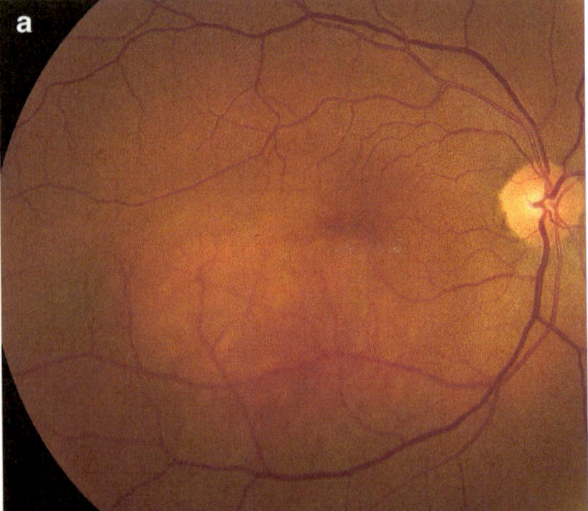

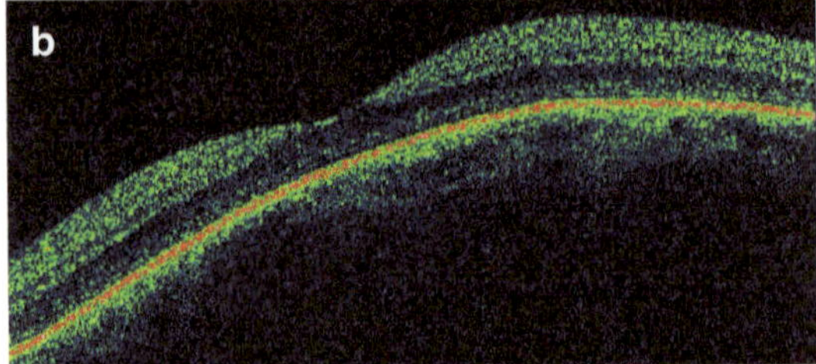

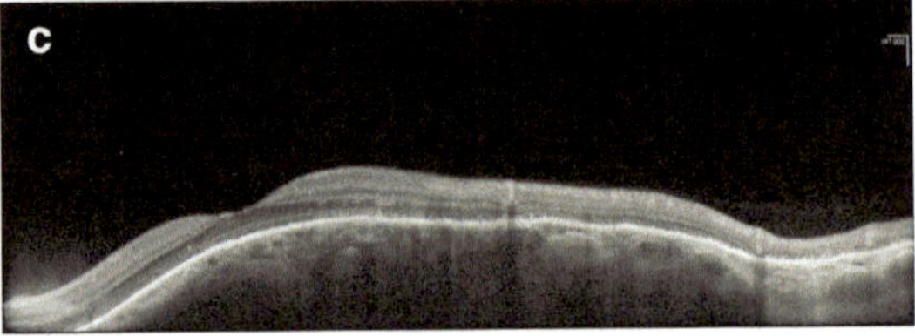

Fig. 26.11 (**a**) Circumscribed choroidal hemangioma. (**b**) Spectral domain OCT (Topcon1000). There is elevation of retina/choroid complex with nonspecific signals from the underlying choroid. (**c**) Spectral domain OCT – EDI technique (inverted). Note a low to medium reflective signal from the lesion. Small and large spaces (possibly vascular) are also identified within the tumor (Reproduced with permission from Torres et al. 2011)

OCT has been used to monitor response to treatment by photodynamic therapy, transpupillary thermotherapy, plaque radiation, or laser photocoagulation (Fig. 26.11).

Conclusions

OCT presents as pivotal in the practice of ophthalmology. Advances in imaging techniques enable faster and more precise diagnosis, treatment planning, and better follow-up. Through OCT, the ophthalmologist can identify tumor margin, surface, and alterations such as thickening of the overlying epithelium and recognition of secondary features like conjunctival cysts. In cases of posterior iris and ciliary body tumors, OCT tends to be inferior to UBM. The limitations of imaging in intraocular tumors are hyperpigmentation and calcification. Enhanced depth imaging (EDI) may enable better visualization of deep anterior segment tumors and choroidal tumors.

References

Andrade RE, Farah ME, Costa RA, Belfort R Jr (2005) Optical coherence tomography findings in macular cavernous haemangioma. Acta Ophthalmol Scand 83:267–269

Arevalo JF, Fernandez CF, Garcia RA (2005) Optical coherence tomography characteristics of choroidal metastasis. Ophthalmology 112:1612–1619

Bianciotto C, Shields CL, Guzman JM et al (2011) Assessment of anterior segment tumors with ultrasound biomicroscopy versus anterior segment optical coherence tomography in 200 cases. Ophthalmology 118:1297–1302

Brue C, Saitta A, Nicolai M et al (2013) Epiretinal membrane surgery for combined hamartoma of the retina and retinal pigment epithelium: role of multimodal analysis. Clin Ophthalmol 7:179–184

Demirci H, Cullen A, Sunstrom J (2014) Enhanced Depth Imaging Optical Coherence Tomography of Choroidal Metastasis. Retina 34(7):1354–1359

Espinoza G, Rosenblatt B, Harbour JW (2004) Optical coherence tomography in the evaluation of retinal changes associated with suspicious choroidal melanocytic tumors. Am J Ophthalmol 137:90–95

Gallwas JK, Turk L, Stepp H et al (2011) Optical coherence tomography for the diagnosis of cervical intraepithelial neoplasia. Lasers Surg Med 43:206–212

Hood CT, Schoenfield LR, Torres V, Singh AD (2011) Iris melanoma. Ophthalmology 118:221–222

Horgan N, Shields CL, Mashayekhi A et al (2008) Early macular morphological changes following plaque radiotherapy for uveal melanoma. Retina 28: 263–273

Huang D, Swanson EA, Lin CP et al (1991) Optical coherence tomography. Science 254:1178–1181

Huot CS, Desai KB, Shah VA (2009) Spectral domain optical coherence tomography of combined hamartoma of the retina and retinal pigment epithelium. Ophthalmic Surg Lasers Imaging 40:322–324

Kieval JZ, Karp CL, Abou Shousha M et al (2012) Ultrahigh resolution optical coherence tomography for differentiation of ocular surface squamous neoplasia and pterygia. Ophthalmology 119:481–486

Kimoto K, Kishi D, Kono H et al (2008) Diagnosis of an isolated retinal astrocytic hamartoma aided by optical coherence tomography. Acta Ophthalmol 86:921–922

Muscat S, Parks S, Kemp E, Keating D (2004) Secondary retinal changes associated with choroidal naevi and melanomas documented by optical coherence tomography. Br J Ophthalmol 88:120–124

Pavlin CJ, Vasquez LM, Lee R et al (2009) Anterior segment optical coherence tomography and ultrasound biomicroscopy in the imaging of anterior segment tumors. Am J Ophthalmol 147:214–219

Ramasubramanian A, Shields CL, Harmon SA, Shields JA (2010) Autofluorescence of choroidal hemangioma in 34 consecutive eyes. Retina 30:16–22

Razzaq L, Emmanouilidis-van SK, Luyten GP, Keizer RJ (2011) Anterior segment imaging for iris melanocytic tumors. Eur J Ophthalmol 21:608–614

Saxena S, Sharma B, Bhasker SK (2010) Three-dimensional spectral-domain optical coherence tomography of melanocytoma of the optic nerve head. J Ocul Biol Dis Infor 3:112–116

Say EAT, Shah SU, Ferenczy S, Shields C (2011) Optical coherence tomography of retinal and choroidal tumors. J Ophthalmol 2011:385058. doi:10.1155/2011/385058

Sayanagi K, Pelayes DE, Kaiser PK, Singh AD (2011) 3D Spectral domain optical coherence tomography findings in choroidal tumors. Eur J Ophthalmol 21:271–275

Schachat AP, Shields JA, Fine SL (1984) Combined hamartomas of the retina and retinal pigment epithelium. Ophthalmology 91:1609–1615

Shields CL, Shields JA (2008) Intraocular tumors: an atlas and textbook. Lippincott Williams & Wilkins, Philadelphia

Shields CL, Materin MA, Shields JA (2005a) Review of optical coherence tomography for intraocular tumors. Curr Opin Ophthalmol 16:141–154

Shields CL, Mashayekhi A, Materin MA et al (2005b) Optical coherence tomography of choroidal nevus in 120 patients. Retina 25:243–252

Shields CL, Mashayekhi A, Dai VV et al (2005c) Optical coherence tomographic findings of combined hamartoma of the retina and retinal pigment epithelium in 11 patients. Arch Ophthalmol 123:1746–1750

Shields CL, Materin MA, Walker C, Marr BP, Shields JA (2006) Photoreceptor loss overlying congenital hypertrophy of the retinal pigment epithelium by optical coherence tomography. Ophthalmology 113:661–665

Shields CL, Perez B, Materin MA et al (2007) Optical coherence tomography of choroidal osteoma in 22 cases: evidence for photoreceptor atrophy over the decalcified portion of the tumor. Ophthalmology 114:e53–e58

Shields CL, Perez B, Benavides R, Materin MA, Shields JA (2008) Optical coherence tomography of optic disk melanocytoma in 15 cases. Retina 28:441–446

Shields CL, Kaliki S, Rojanaporn D et al (2012) Enhanced depth imaging optical coherence tomography of small choroidal melanoma: comparison with choroidal nevus. Arch Ophthalmol 130:850–856

Shousha MA, Karp C et al (2013) Diagnosis of ocular surface lesions using ultra–high-resolution optical coherence tomography. Ophthalmology 120:883–891

Singh AD, Belfort RN, Sayanagi K, Kaiser PK (2010) Fourier domain optical coherence tomographic and auto-fluorescence findings in indeterminate choroidal melanocytic lesions. Br J Ophthalmol 94:474–478

Spaide RF, Koizumi H, Pozzoni MC (2008) Enhanced depth imaging spectral-domain optical coherence tomography. Am J Ophthalmol 146:496–500

Thomas BJ et al (2014) Ultra high-resolution anterior segment optical coherence tomography in the diagnosis and management of ocular surface squamous neoplasia. Ocul Surf 12:46–58

Torres VL, Brugnoni N, Kaiser PK, Singh AD (2011) Optical coherence tomography enhanced depth imaging of choroidal tumors. Am J Ophthalmol 151:586–593.e2

27 Retinal Trauma

Carsten H. Meyer, Fernando M. Penha, Michel E. Farah, and Peter Kroll

Contents

C.H. Meyer, MD, FEBO, FMH (✉)
Department of Ophthalmology, Pallas Klinik, Aarau, Switzerland
e-mail: meyer_eye@yahoo.com

F.M. Penha, MD, PhD
Bascom Palmer Eye Institute, University of Miami, Miami, FL, USA

M.E. Farah, MD
Department of Ophthalmology, Federal University of São Paulo, São Paulo, Brazil

P. Kroll, MD
Department of Ophthalmology, Philipps University, Marburg, Germany

27.1 Introduction

Non-penetrating or closed-globe injuries represent 50–80 % of traumatic eye injuries. Generally, the most affected population is the man under 30 years old. It may occur by several mechanisms thus damaging a variety of different retinal structures. The Ocular Trauma Classification Group defined a standardized classification for frequently used terms based on standard terminology and features of ocular injuries that have demonstrated prognostic significance. In a closed-globe injury, the eye wall does not have a full-thickness wound, and the mechanism of injury may be grouped into two main categories: the direct (anterior) type occurring at the site of the impact and an indirect (posterior) type at the contrecoup injury, which is more commonly found. Several groups investigated the mechanical impact of blunt ocular trauma and reported theories how defined anatomical structures can be damaged (Fig. 27.1). After a traumatic event, the vision can be unaffected or completely lost, depending on the location of the damaged anatomical structure, e.g., choroidal vessels, choriocapillaris, Bruch's membrane, retinal pigment epithelium (RPE), and neuroretina (Berg et al. 1989; Mennel et al. 2004; Williams et al. 1990).

The following chapter demonstrates a variety of closed-globe injuries on time and spectral

C.H. Meyer et al. (eds.), *Spectral Domain Optical Coherence Tomography in Macular Diseases*, DOI 10.1007/978-81-322-3610-8_27

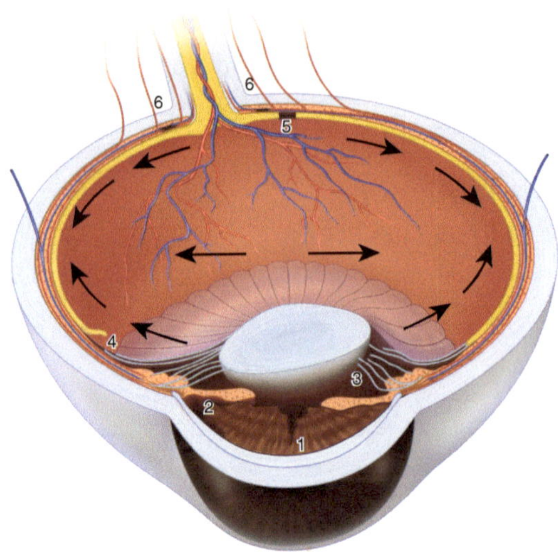

Fig. 27.1 Non-penetrating or closed-globe injuries may occur by several mechanisms thus damaging a variety of different retinal structures including the iris (*1*), trabecular mash work (*2*), lens fibers (*3*), retina (*4*), posterior pole (*5*), or optic nerve with the posterior ciliary vessels (*6*)

domain optical coherent tomography (OCT), fluorescein angiography (FA), autofluorescence (AF), and fundus photography.

27.2 Choroidal Folds

Choroidal folds were first described by Nettleship in 1884 and were initially considered as foldings of the entire retina (Nettleship 1884). They are visible striae at the posterior pole that radiate across the macula arranged in a parallel and horizontal fashion as dark and light lines. Later Norton investigated the typical fluorescein angiographic (FA) appearance and defined a clear distinction between choroidal and retinal folds (Norton 1969). The anatomical structure of choroidal folds can be explained by the typical fluorescein pattern traversing the folded choroidal vessels. Hyperfluorescent streaks occur in the early arteriovenous phase and persist throughout the late venous phase with no leakage. A stretching and atrophy of the RPE induce an increased filling of the choriocapillaris overlying this peak of the choroidal fold. Hypofluorescent streaks are on the bases of inclinated RPE in the valley of the fold, resulting to a compression of the pigment-containing base of the RPE cells and blockage of the underlying choroidal fluorescence. Histological studies confirmed a folding at the level of the RPE, Bruch's membrane, and choroid giving the retina above a "brain-like" configuration. Cross-sectional imaging by computer tomography (CT) or B-scan ultrasonography reveals an abnormal flattening of the posterior pole, a thickening of the sclera, and a consecutive axial shortening of the globe (Dailey et al. 1986). This characteristic picture is associated with a variety of orbital and ocular conditions including trauma, hypotony, orbital tumors, thyroid disease, papillitis, or uveal effusion syndrome.

Color fundus picture (Fig. 27.2a) and fluorescein traversing the folded choroidal vessels demonstrated hyperfluorescent streaks in the early and late phase with no signs of leakage, while adjacent hypofluorescent streaks remained dark throughout the entire angiography. In vivo measurements by OCT determined a significant folding of the hyperreflective RPE-choriocapillaris complex (Fig. 27.2b) in the papillomacular area. The thickness, reflectivity, and surface contour of the retina appeared within normal limits.

Differently patients with ocular hypotony may face severe impaired vision with metamorphopsia. On fundus examination there is a significant tortuous beading of the retinal and venous vessels (Fig. 27.3a). Fluorescein angiography (FA) demonstrates a fussy fluorescence in the early and late phase (Fig. 27.3b). OCT shows a mountain-like folding of the entire retina with moderate hyporeflective areas in the subretinal space corresponding with subretinal fluid (Fig. 27.3c). Between the RPE and the sclera, there are flat large areas corresponding with choroidal fluid.

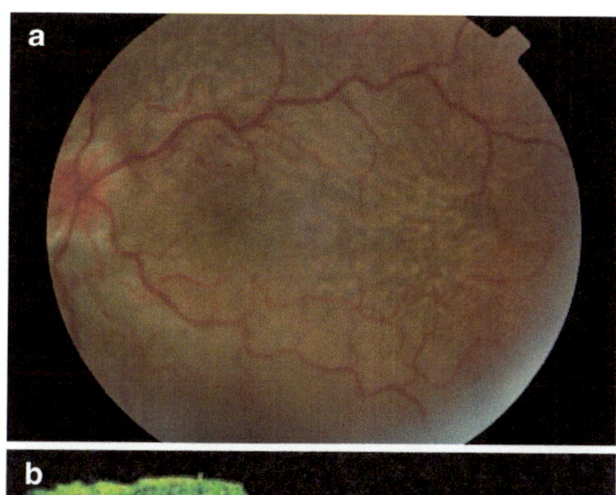

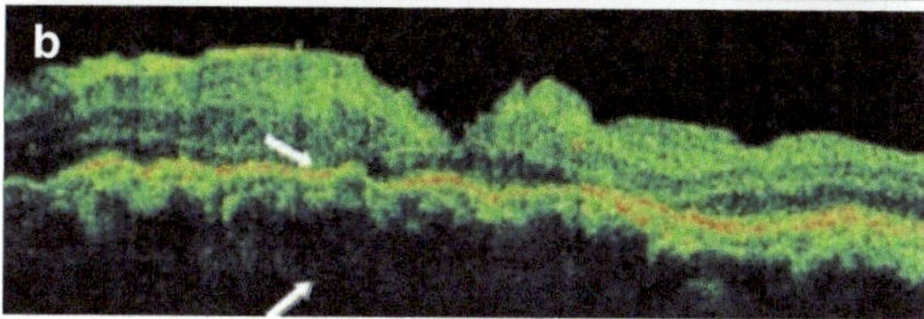

Fig. 27.2 Choroidal folds. (**a**) In the late venous phase of the fluorescein angiography, there are multiple parallel and horizontal lines of different fluorescence in the macular area. The hyperfluorescent streaks persist with no leakage and are caused by an increased filling of the choriocapillaris overlying the peak of the choroidal fold. The hypofluorescent streaks are in the valley of the fold, where the compressed RPE blocks the underlying choroidal fluorescence. (**b**) The vertical OCT scan of the choroidal folds in the papillomacular area. The inner surface of the retina is flattened by image analysis using Adobe Photoshop, so that the choroidal folds become more prominent. The neuroretina in the papillomacular bundle has a moderate reflectivity and normal thickness of approximately 225 μm. There is no intraretinal or subretinal fluid. The folded hyperreflective band, in red to white colors, corresponds to the RPE-choriocapillaris complex and is firmly attached to the underlying sclera, with no signs of pigment epithelium detachment (PED). Each fold has a height of approximately 45 μm. The dark and hyporeflective spots in the deep scleral layer under each fold (*white arrows*) may either correspond to compressed tissue or shadowing of the folded RPE-choriocapillaris complex

27.3 Commotio Retinae

Commotio retinae are defined as a transient gray-white opacification at the level of the deep sensory retina occurring after blunt ocular trauma, and it was first described by Berlin in 1873 (Berlin 1873). The whitening and elevation of the retina appear immediately after a trauma and can be limited to the central retina although it may even involve extensive areas of the peripheral retina progressing to retinal necrosis and chorioretinitis sclopetaria (Hesse et al. 1996).

Commotio retinae are grouped in two variations: a milder type (retinal concussion) with less dramatic gray-white changes and no visible pigment alterations, which later may progress to scarring. The more severe type (retinal contusion or chorioretinitis sclopetaria) can occur anterior at the point of impact (coup) or posterior at the remote impact site (contrecoup). A coup damage is therefore caused by local trauma directly at the site of impact, while a contusive contrecoup injury occurs at the opposite site of the blunt trauma creating damage at tissue interfaces. The consecutive whitening is more severe and a creamy discoloration of the RPE appears within 48 h after the injury. Fluorescein angiography typically demonstrates an alternated retinal vascular permeability, a bright leakage due to a partial breakdown of the outer blood-retina barrier at the level of the RPE. Visual acuity may be transiently or permanently reduced. The visual prognosis is good if the damaged location is outside the fovea. However, if the fovea is involved, vision loss may maintain permanently (Fig. 27.4) (Hesse et al. 1996; Sipperley et al. 1978).

The clinicopathologic features of retinal contusion or chorioretinitis sclopetaria include direct traumatic chorioretinal damage followed by marked fibrovascular proliferation with variable replacement of vascular and neuroretinal tissue (Fig. 27.4a). A visible retinal opacity at the site of the contrecoup injury is considered to be a severe injury. It may later progress to a "salt-and-pepper" appearance accompanied by a hypofluorescence on fluorescein angiography. The chorioretinal circulation disturbance corresponds with a delayed filling and narrowing of the choroidal veins and changes in choroidal vasculature causing obstruction and occlusion of the choriocapillaris (Fig. 27.4b, c). The breakdown of the outer blood-retina barrier in the RPE may increase permeability of the choriocapillaris.

Histopathologic studies demonstrated a partial loss of the nerve fiber and ganglion cell layers and loss of the photoreceptors with hypertrophy and hyperplasia of the RPE. Although the sclera

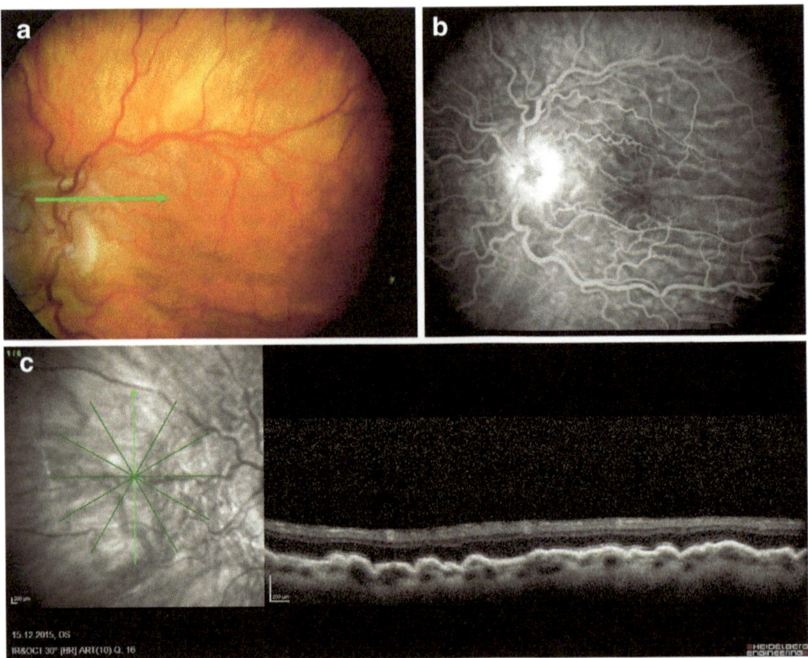

Fig. 27.3 (**a**) Fundus image of the right eye in patients with severe hypotony after blunt ocular trauma. Funduscopy demonstrates a chorioretinal folding of the entire retina (*green arrow*). (**b**) Fluorescein angiography demonstrates a moderate elevation of the retina with mild leakage. (**c**) On OCT there is a significant folding of the entire neuroretina (**X**) with some hyporeflective areas under the retina corresponding with subretinal fluid. Under the hyperreflective RPE-choriocapillaris complex, there is a broad hyperreflective area (*) presenting a second fluid compartment in the choroid adjacent to the sclera

and a long posterior ciliary nerve remained intact, a marked ingrowth of fibrovascular tissue may be extended from the choroid into the subretinal space where it was covered by retinal pigment epithelium. On OCT there is a marked thinning of the neuroretina in the affected area compared to the unaffected adjacent areas (Fig. 27.4d, f) (Dubovy et al. 1997; Pahor 2000).

There have been conflicting reports on histopathologic features of Berlin's edema or commotio retinae. Although Berlin originally hypothesized that the loss of the outer retinal transparency may relate to an extracellular edema, the origin and underlying pathogenesis remain controversial. Several postmortem studies on human and animal eyes confirmed a disruption of photoreceptor outer segments followed by phagocytosis of fragmented outer segments by the retinal pigment epithelium (RPE), while some authors reported a direct damage to the neurosensory retina as seen by swelling of Müller food processes and mitochondria in the nerve fiber layer. The gross anatomy revealed swollen inner segments with mitochondrial deposits of resembling calcium, indicating an increased permeability of the plasma membranes. The blunt ocular trauma may generate mechanical contrecoup distortion of the retina via vitreoretinal attachments. Mansour et al. hypothesized that hydraulic forces stretch the neuroretina at the level of the outer segments, while intact Müller cells hold the rest of the retina together (Mansour et al. 1992).

In vivo measurements by OCT revealed a traumatic lesion at the level of the photoreceptor-RPE complex, disclosing a detached sensory retina with fluid in the subretinal space. The reflectivity of the neuroretinal tissue was reduced and the architecture less compact. The neuroretina, held together by the Müller food processes, appears to be intact up to the photoreceptors. The uncommon hyperreflective inner retinal band possibly represents the photoreceptor inner segments, with less reflective outer segments underneath and in the subretinal space. Although the neuroretinal thickness was increased, the foveolar indentation remained still visible (Fig. 27.5b). Fundus biomicroscopy revealed a mild retinal

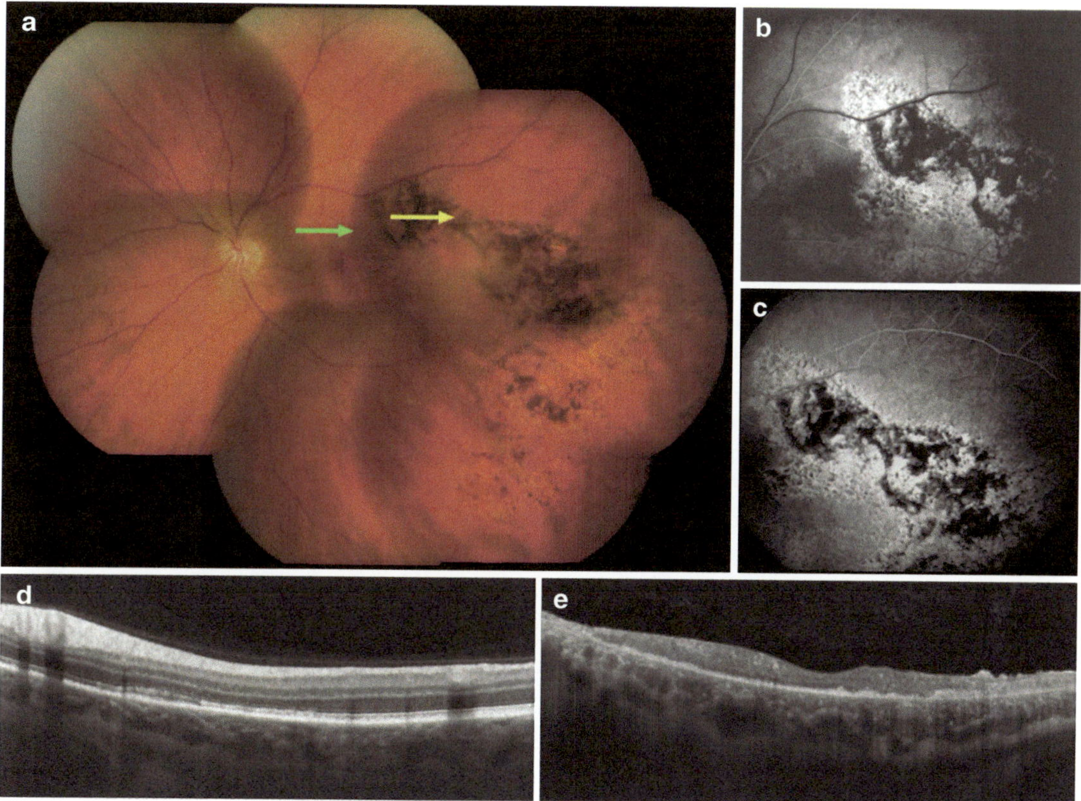

Fig. 27.4 Chorioretinitis sclopetaria. (**a**) Fundus image of the left posterior pole resulting from a localized destruction of both the retina and choroid (*yellow arrow*) with connective tissue proliferation adjacent to the impact site (*green arrow*). (**b, c**) Fluorescein angiography shows irregular filling of the choriocapillaris and partially obstructed by connective tissue plaques. (**d, e**) SD-OCT showing marked thinning of the entire neuroretina

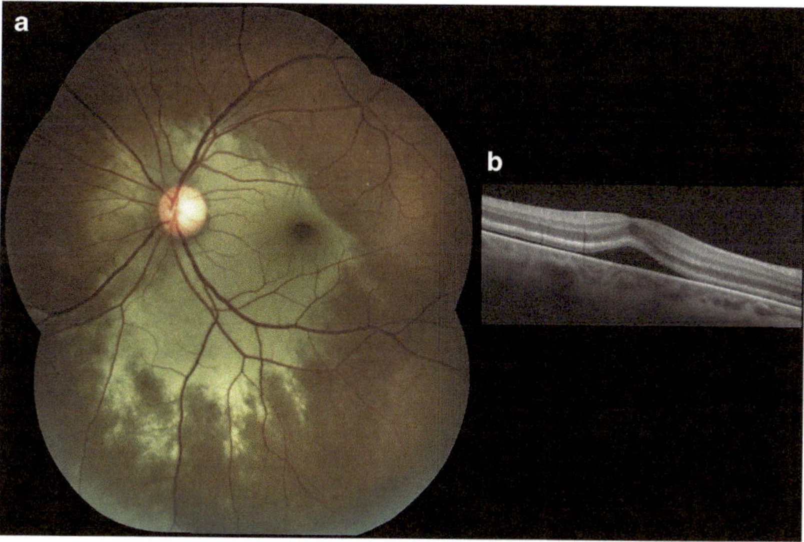

Fig. 27.5 (**a**) Fundus image of the left posterior pole showing dull foveal reflex and mild retinal elevation in the papillomacular region. (**b**) Horizontal OCT scan in the papillomacular area demonstrates a detachment of the entire neuroretina with hyporeflective space underneath, corresponding with subretinal fluid

elevation at the level of neurosensory retina and the RPE in the fovea with white concentric lines (Fig. 27.5b). The RPE phagocytoses damaged the outer segments and restore central vision within weeks. We determined a full anatomical and functional recovery of the macular lesion within 3 months. The patient's vision returned to 20/20 OU 5 months later (Meyer et al. 2003a).

Another complication that may occur after commotio retinae is the traumatic pigment epitheliopathy. It is possible to identify RPE atrophy with areas of discoloration and pigment clumping associated with patchy lesions, which represented post-traumatic pigment epitheliopathy. Fundus autofluorescence (FAF) examination demonstrated a well-defined reduced FAF patchy area with interposed granular increased autofluorescent areas in regions of the epitheliopathy (Fig. 27.6). OCT showed an area of increased reflectivity beneath the choriocapillaris/RPE complex and focal thinning of the retina. We also demonstrated the functional damage of traumatic pigment epitheliopathy using Humphrey's computerized visual field in one patient and compared these findings to autofluorescence imaging, which correlated to the area of decreased sensitivity of the visual field (Fig. 27.7). Therefore, alterations in autofluorescent pattern in these patients may be an indirect indication of the function of the retina and RPE and could be suggestive of poor prognosis in some cases of commotio retinae.

27.4 Choroidal Rupture

Choroidal rupture, first described by von Graefe in 1854, is a breach of Bruch's membrane, the choroid, and the RPE secondary to a blunt ocular trauma (Von Graefe 1854). They can be divided into two main categories: a direct (anterior) type occurring at the site of the impact is oriented parallel to the ora serrata. Indirect ruptures, which are more common, occur predominantly at the

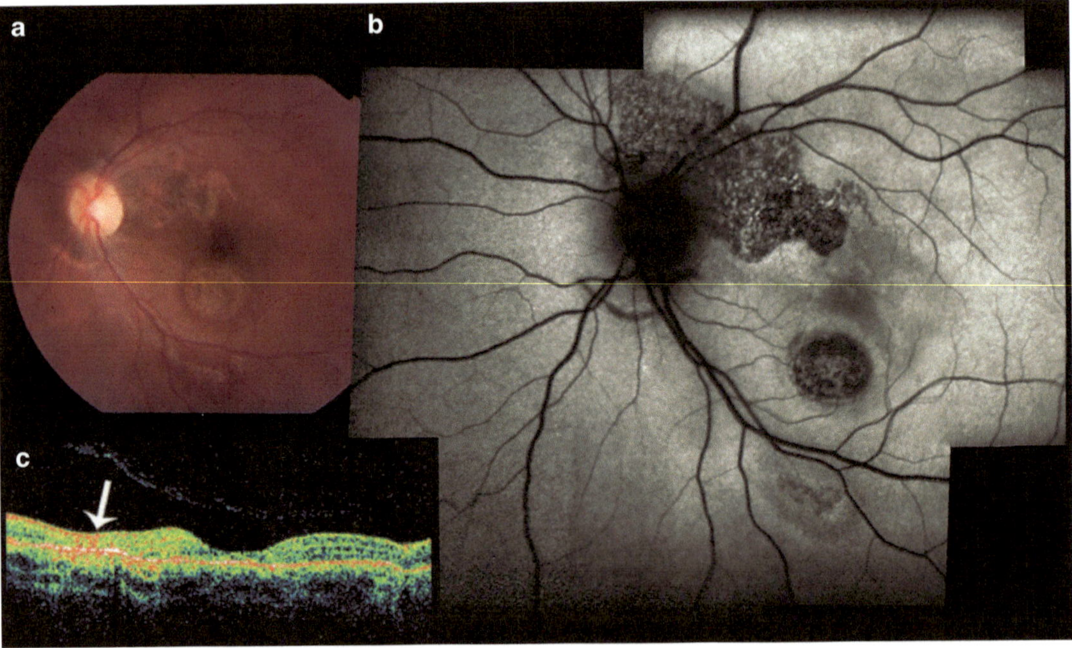

Fig. 27.6 (**a**) Color fundus picture showing peripapillary retinal pigment epithelium (RPE) atrophy with areas of discoloration and pigment clumping (Courtesy of Dr Daniel Lavinsky). (**b**) Fundus autofluorescence (FAF) demonstrates reduced FAF area in the same region of RPE atrophy with an increased granular autofluorescent pattern inside the lesion (Courtesy of Dr Daniel Lavinsky). (**c**) Optical coherence tomography (OCT) shows increased reflectivity of the choriocapillaris/RPE complex and local thinning of the retina (*white arrow*) (Courtesy of Dr Daniel Lavinsky)

posterior pole away from the site of impact. The rupture is here usually crescent shaped and concentrically aligned to the optic disk, with the convexity away from the optic disk. The majority (82 %) of ruptures run temporal to the optic disk may involve the macula.

Mechanical and vascular mechanisms are the two most frequently cited hypotheses explaining the damages in choroidal ruptures. During a closed-globe injury, the eyeball is first mechanically compressed and then rapidly hyperextended. The sclera's tensile strength resists this compression. The retina is elastic and stretches during such an injury. However, Bruch's membrane breaks because it does not have sufficient tensile strength or elasticity. The choriocapillaris is injured and bleeds into the sub-RPE and/or subretinal space. Such hemorrhage may hide the choroidal rupture initially. Over days, the blood clears and a whitish/yellowish, curvilinear, crescent-shaped subretinal streak is visible and concentric to the optic disk. Between 5 and 10 % of all blunt ocular trauma lead to indirect choroidal ruptures (Wagemann 1902).If there is a large amount of hemorrhage, surgery may be indicated with vitrectomy subretinal tissue plasminogen activator and gas displacement.

Over time, choroidal neovascularization (CNV) can develop. In most cases, the CNV involutes over time. Secretan et al. demonstrated that ruptures greater than 4000 μm in length and located within 1500 μm of the center of the fovea are more frequently associated with CNV (Secretan et al. 1998). In about 30 %, the CNV may recur, with a serous or hemorrhagic pigment epithelial detachment, anytime following the

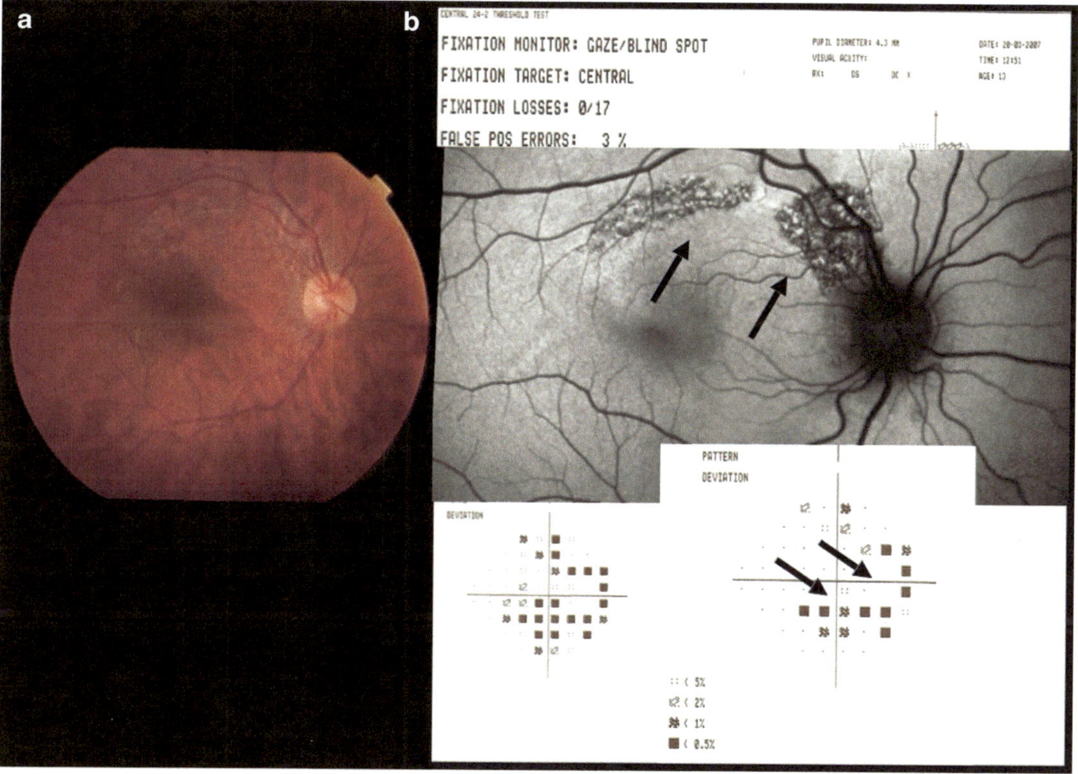

Fig. 27.7 (**a**) Ocular fundus photography of the right eye showing a mild pigmentary change at the temporal superior arcade (Courtesy of Dr Daniel Lavinsky). (**b**) Fundus autofluorescence (FAF) demonstrates two reduced autofluorescent areas with increased autofluorescent granular areas (*arrow*). Humphrey's 24-2 SITA-standard strategy perimetry demonstrates acceptable reliability scores and a significant decrease in the sensitivity of lower nasal fields, corresponding to the superior temporal pigment epitheliopathy evident on autofluorescence (*arrow*) (Courtesy of Dr Daniel Lavinsky)

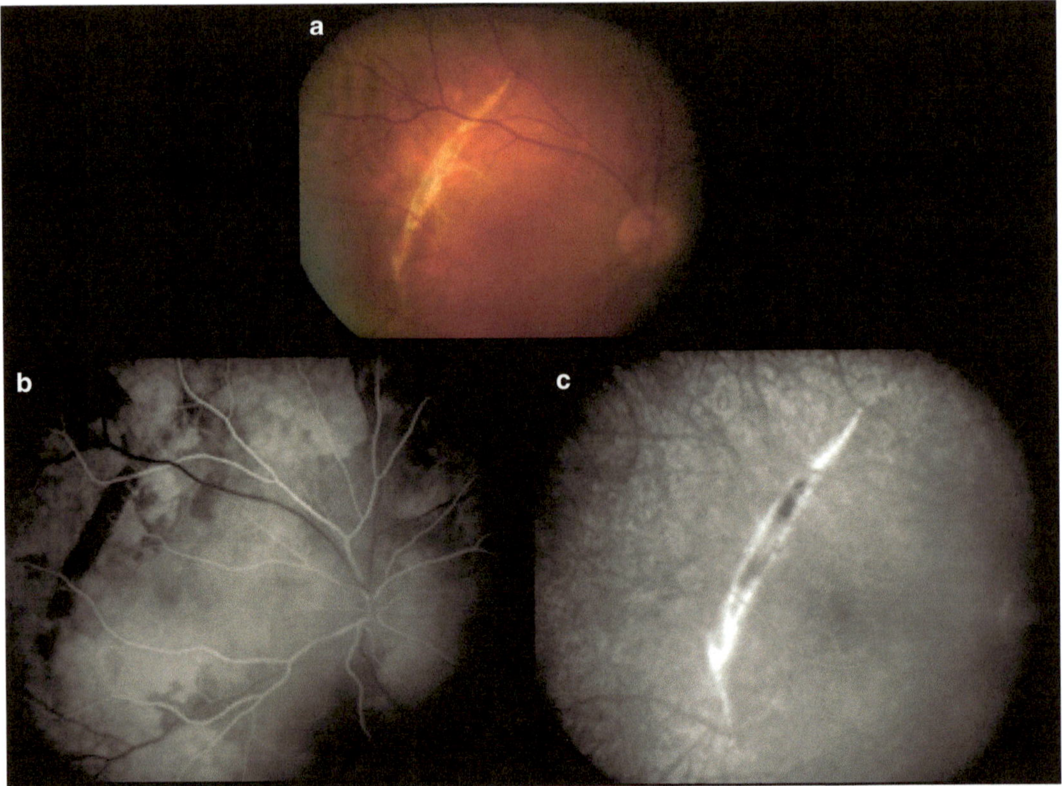

Fig. 27.8 Choroidal rupture. (**a**) Fundus image demonstrates a white crescent-like rupture of the choroid in the superior temporal quadrant. (**b**) Fluorescein angiography early phase showing an incomplete filling of the choroidal vasculature. In the area of the choroidal rupture, there is a dark hypofluorescence visible consistent with the rupture and loss of choroidal vessels. (**c**) Fluorescein angiography late phase showing sharp crescent-like hyperfluorescence due to leakage of choroidal vessels and a window defect at the choroidal rupture

formation of the choroidal rupture. If the rupture or CNV does not involve the foveal center, vision may not be affected. Late complications may also include migration of RPE cells, ERM (epiretinal membrane) formation, loss of photoreceptors, optic atrophy, and retinal detachment.

Fluorescein angiography demonstrates a crescent-shaped delay filling at the site of the choroidal rupture. Early on there is a hypoperfusion of the choroidal artery. Evidence of the choroidal rupture hyperfluorescent streak occurred in the late phase of the FA at the site of the choroidal rupture (Fig. 27.8a–c). In another case it is possible to observe besides the choroidal rupture and progressive hyperfluorescent lesion in the macular area corresponding to a secondary CNV (Fig. 27.9a–d). ICG may also disclose a hypofluorescent rim along the choroidal veins as signs of an increased permeability of the choriocapillaris. These feeder vessels seem to have a greater caliber and a higher tendency to proliferate and are therefore more resistant to photodynamic therapy (PDT) and selective feeder vessel treatment as demonstrated by us previously (Mennel et al. 2005). More recently some case reports have been published treating this secondary CNV with anti-VEGF therapy such as bevacizumab or ranibizumab (Janknecht 2011; Piermarocchi and BenettiE 2011).

SD-OCT highlights the cross-sectional features of choroidal ruptures. The first case demonstrated a mounted subretinal lesion corresponding with fibrovascular scar tissue and some fluid underneath and inside the retina showing an active CNV secondary to a choroidal rupture (Fig. 27.9e–f).

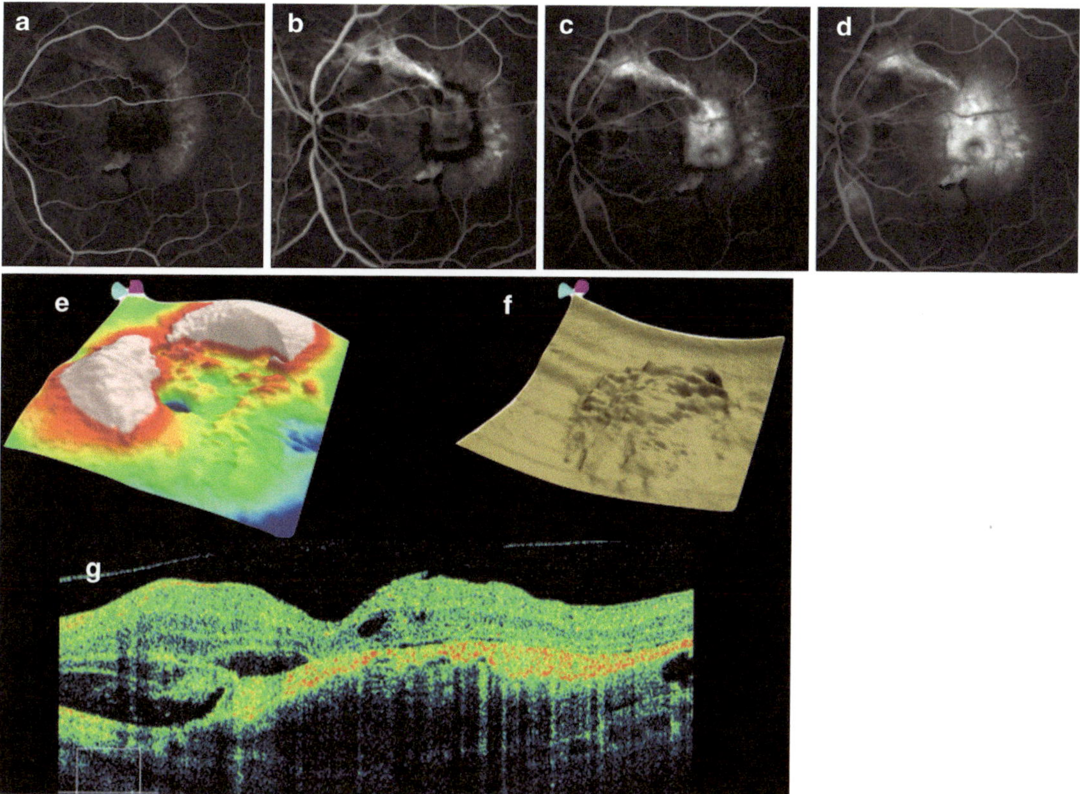

Fig. 27.9 Choroidal rupture. (**a**) Fluorescein angiography showing crescent-like hyperfluorescent lesion in the superior temporal region corresponding to the choroidal rupture. (**b–d**) Serial fluorescein angiography shows progressive hyperfluorescent lesion in the macular area corresponding to a secondary choroidal neovascularization (CNV). (**e**) The retinal thickness map shows some areas of increased retinal thickness corresponding to the fluid of the active CNV. (**f**) RPE map shows the irregularity of the RPE where the CNV membrane is placed. (**g**) The horizontal scan shows a fibrovascular RPE detachment, with the choroidal rupture subretinal and intraretinal fluid and posterior vitreous detachment (G)

In the second case, there was an irregular hyporeflective vertical failure corresponding to the choroidal rupture and a hyperreflective band radiating from the subretinal space through the entire neuroretina to the retinal surface, indicating a transretinal migration of fibrovascular cells (Fig. 27.10a, b).

27.5 Valsalva Retinopathy

The term "Valsalva retinopathy" was first used in 1972 by Duane to describe preretinal hemorrhages secondary to a sudden increase of intrathoracic pressure, in association after vomiting, coughing, heavy lifting, or straining stool, although in some instances no initiating event can be ruled out (Duane 1972). After the Valsalva maneuver, a sudden rise in the intraocular venous pressure causes retinal capillaries to spontaneously rupture; the consequence is the hemorrhage. A well-circumscribed, round, or dumbbell-shaped mound of preretinal blood is seen in or near the central macular area.

The most common site for this hemorrhage is the posterior pole, where the premacular bursa provides a preexisting anatomic space (Foos 1972). In addition the ILM (internal limiting membrane) has no firm attachments to the retina at the posterior pole, thus predisposing hemorrhagic detachments between both layers (Fig. 27.11a, b).

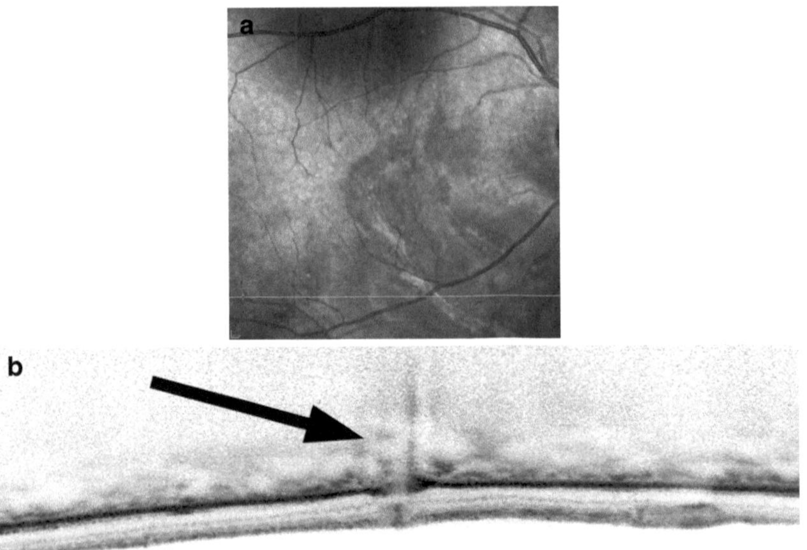

Fig. 27.10 (**a**) The red-free image shows a concentric whitish lesion in the inferior temporal area corresponding to the choroidal rupture. (**b**) The enhanced depth OCT imaging shows an irregular hyporeflective vertical lesion at the deep choroid corresponding the choroidal rupture (*arrow*). The retina has a normal thickness; however, there is a hyperreflective band extending from the outer retinal to throughout the entire retina to the retinal surface (Courtesy of Dr Daniel Lavinsky)

It is generally agreed that the sharply demarcated hemorrhage is located at the vitreoretinal interface either directly under the posterior hyaloid of the vitreous or under the internal limiting membrane (ILM) itself. The exact location of it cannot be determined biomicroscopically, although subhyaloid blood tends to shift by changing the head from an upright to flat position, and sublaminar retinal hemorrhage remains still (Choudhry and Rao 2014; Green et al. 1996) (Fig. 27.11c, d).

Patients commonly describe a sudden spontaneous loss of their vision. Part of the blood may decent in the preretinal bursa and turn yellow after several days. The prognosis is generally good, but resorption of the entrapped blood tends to be slow and may result in long-standing visual impairment. With a spontaneous rupture of the membrane, vision recovers rapidly. However, if the spontaneous resorption of preretinal blood is slow, laser puncturing or photodisruption of the posterior hyaloid face or the limiting membrane has been described by means of argon laser coagulation (Kroll and Busse 1986) or Nd:YAG laser (Ulbig et al. 1998) as an alternative to vitrectomy. The laser puncturing enables drainage through the focal opening of entrapped premacular blood into the vitreous cavity, where it is resorbed more quickly (Meyer et al. 2006).

Our group showed a patient that was submitted to focal membranotomy by argon laser and developed ERM with a superficial prominent sheen-like membrane. In these cases vitrectomy should be performed with ERM removal and ILM peeling with the use of vital dyes such as brilliant blue or indocyanine green for ILM and trypan blue for ERM (Meyer et al. 2004a; Schmidt et al. 2003). It has been shown that after performing a vitrectomy and histology in preretinal hemorrhages, it was possible to identify multiple layers of cells on the inside of the dome-shaped membrane (Garcia-Arumi et al. 1994).

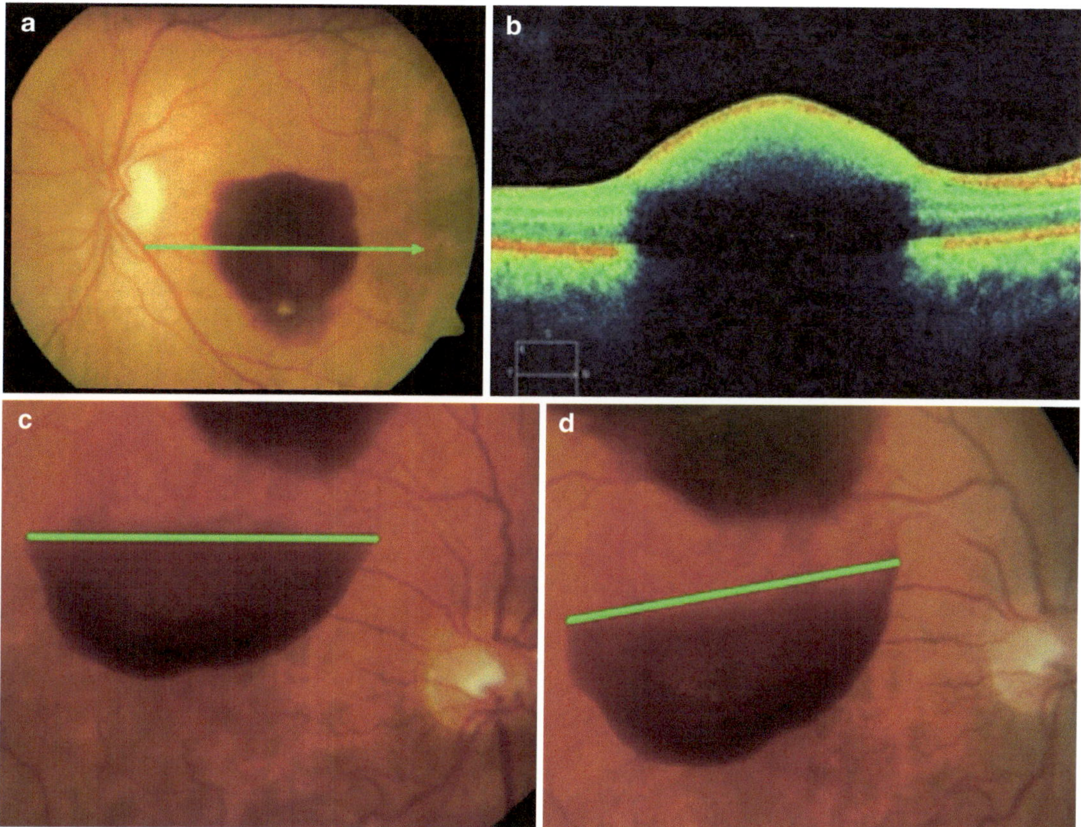

Fig. 27.11 Valsalva retinopathy. (**a**) Fundus image showing well-circumscribed, round, or dumbbell-shaped mound of preretinal blood in or near the central macular area. (**b**) The entrapped blood under the ILM presents on SD-OCT as hyperreflective band in the retina surface obscuring the underlying retinal structures. (**c**) Fundus image taken in an upright position. The preretinal hemorrhage has a horizontal direction. (**d**) Fundus image taken after the head was tilted to the right side. The preretinal blood has shifted to the right side in an oblique direction

27.6 Traumatic Optic Pit Maculopathy

Congenital pit of the optic nerve head is an excavation or regional depression of the optic nerve head resulting from an imperfect closure of the embryonic fissure. An unequal growth on both sides causes a delayed closure of the fissure at approximately 5 weeks of gestation. They were first described in 1882 as dark gray depressions in the optic nerve head, and they appear craterlike holes on the surface of the optic nerve head usually with a steep temporal wall, usually associated with posterior vitreous detachment and serous retinal detachment in the macular area (Kranenberg 1960).

The underlying mechanism optic pit maculopathy remains speculative, although many patients develop serous retinal detachments during life. As optic pits are congenital and the corresponding macular detachments develop later, certain unknown events may trigger macular detachments. It is known that most eyes with an optic pit maculopathy have a partial vitreous detachment (PVD) with firm attachments at the margin of the optic head (Sugar 1962). Therefore, one of the mechanisms that may trigger the serous detachment is the PVD associated or not with ocular trauma.

Many times, an optic pit is asymptomatic and is just an incidental finding on the examination of the eye by a physician. However, some patients may present with the symptoms of a posterior vitreous detachment or serous retinal detachment. This is because optic pits are associated with these disorders and are even speculated to be the actual cause of these disorders when they arise in patients with optic pits. The most common visual field defects include an enlarged blind spot and a scotoma. Visual acuity is typically not affected by the pit but may get worse if serous detachment of the macula occurs. Metamorphopsia may then result.

Funduscopy discloses a gray oval pit usually at the temporal margin of the disk (Fig. 27.12a). A shallow uniform opaque retinal detachment, about 4 disk diameters, extended from the edge of the optic nerve to the macula (Fig. 27.12a). OCT demonstrated an inner layer separation (ISL) with an outer layer detachment (OLD) of the retina (Fig. 27.12b). The non-reflective space between them corresponded to a large schisis-like cavity (Fig. 27.12b).

Lincoff et al. hypothesized a two-layered structure in optic pit maculopathy. The serous retinal elevations in optic pits primarily begin at the optic disk with a schisis-like separation of the inner retinal layers. The ILS appears clinically transparent, while the corresponding functional scotoma is mild and central vision may remain intact. When a hole in the outer layer develops, fluid may flow through into the subretinal space creating a secondary OLD (Lincoff and Kreissig 1998). Vigorous radial forces transmitted through abnormal vitreous attachment may have therefore exaggerate a schisis-like retinal detachment in our patients with a congenital optic pit (Meyer et al. 2003b; Meyer and Rodrigues 2004).

In general optic disk pits themselves do not need to be treated. However, patients with chronic serous retinal detachments with loss of visual acuity may be submitted to surgery. There are several case reports and case series treating those lesions with simple intravitreal gas injection or vitrectomy and fluid-gas exchange with functional and anatomical improvement with low

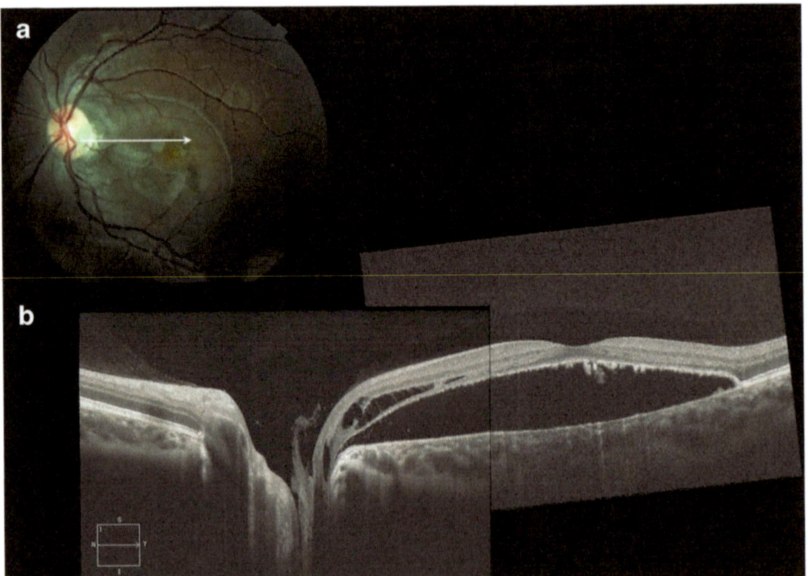

Fig. 27.12 Traumatic optic pit maculopathy. (**a**) Fundus picture shows an optic disk with a gray oval pit at the temporal side and a darker area in the papillomacular bundle (*arrow*). (**b**) The SD-OCT shows the pit inside the optic nerve head. In the papillomacular region, it is possible to observe an inner layer separation (ISL) in multiple layers. The outer layer detachment (OLD) of the neuroretina from the retinal pigment epithelium can be seen in a second hyperreflective band. The non-reflective space between the ILS and the OLD responds to a large schisis-like cavity. The RPE-choriocapillaris complex represents as a third hyperreflective band. The fluid under the OLD can leak through a hole in the outer layer into the subretinal space and the retinal schisis in multiple layers at the inner retina and subretinal fluid or a schisis in the outer retina (Courtesy of Dr Rodrigo Meirelles)

recurrence rates (Moreira Neto and Moreira Junior 2013; Akiyama et al. 2014).

27.7 Epiretinal Membrane

The proliferation of epiretinal membranes (ERMs) occurs spontaneously or as a complication of various diseases on the surface of the retina along the internal limiting membrane (ILM). Iwanoff first in 1865 considered ERM as the formation of endothelial cells (Iwanoff 1865). These cells mainly derive from retinal glial or RPE cell proliferating along the retinal surface and gain access to the ILM by unknown stimuli (Trese et al. 1983). The separation or peeling of ERM is a rare incidence. It may occur spontaneously without evidence of any intervention, by development of a PVD and Nd-YAG laser or after ocular trauma (Messner 1977).

Clinically ERMs are a semitransparent membrane that develops over the retina that may be asymptomatic or cause a contraction of the retinal tissue and consequent misalignment and damage to the retinal tissue (Fig. 27.13a). The final result is metamorphopsia, low visual acuity that may vary from almost normal to 20/400 or hand motion to the more severe and chronic cases. The diagnosis is clinical, but the use of SD-OCT is very important to the identification of the hyperreflective membrane on the retinal surface (Fig. 27.13b) and to the evaluation of the coexisting vitreoretinal traction that may be found in some cases (Fig. 27.14) (Bottós et al. 2012). Moreover the use of SD-OCT is also very important to evaluate the prognosis after surgery. It has been shown that edema of the inner retina correlates with poor prognosis and a disruption of the inner/outer segment layer (IS/OS) or the ellipsoid zone may also be associated with poor functional results after ERM removal (Fig. 27.15) (Kinoshita et al. 2012; Shiono et al. 2013).

The treatment for ERM is surgery; however, there are some reports of spontaneous ERM separation with visual acuity improvement (Meyer et al. 2004b). Usually vitrectomy is indicated when visual acuity is 20/40 or worse or if the patient has a remarkable metamorphopsia. Standard vitrectomy associated with ERM removal, with or without trypan blue staining, and today ILM peeling

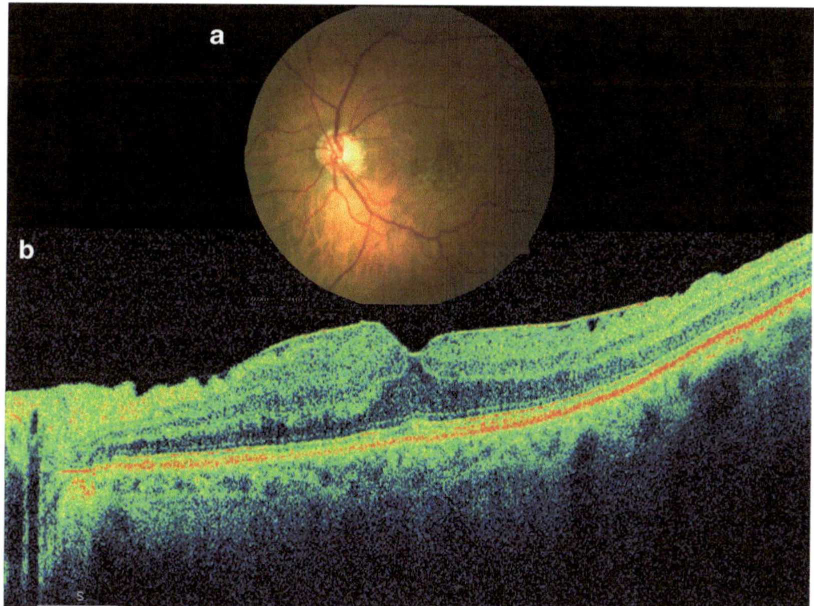

Fig. 27.13 Epiretinal membrane. (**a**) Fundus picture demonstrates loss of foveal reflex and the typical aspect of cellophane maculopathy. (**b**) Spectral domain OCT shows hyperreflective tissue over the retinal surface corresponding to the epiretinal membrane (ERM). There is an irregularity on the retinal surface and also some increase of the retinal thickness due to edema caused by the ERM

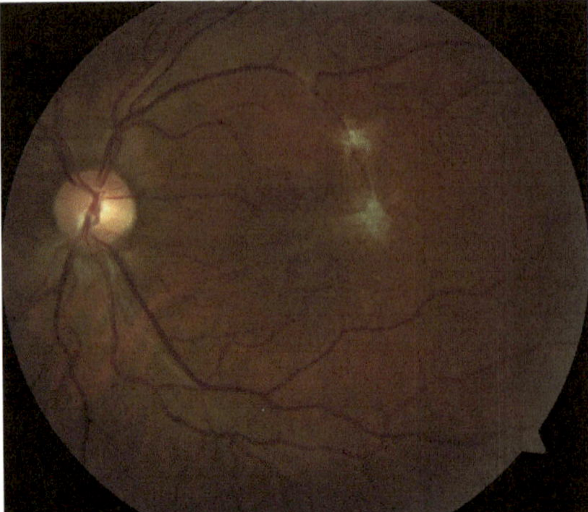

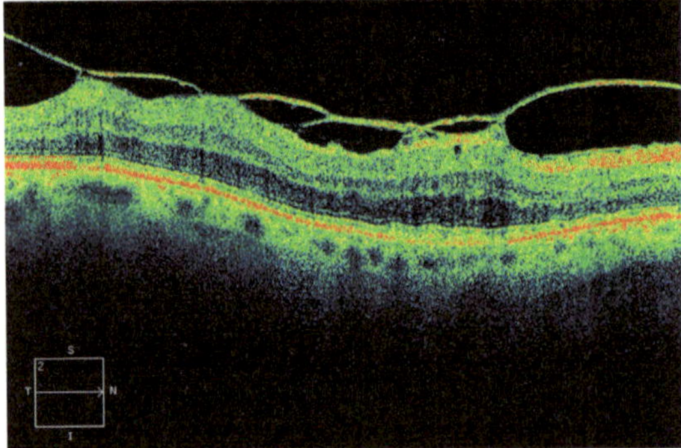

Fig. 27.14 Fundus picture and SD-OCT of a patient with vitreomacular traction and ERM. The first hyperreflective membrane is the vitreous traction and the second layer over the retinal surface is the ERM

with brilliant blue has also been performed to reduce the recurrence rate of ERM.

27.8 Traumatic Macular Hole

Macular hole (MH) can occur in either gender, at any age, with no racial predilection. The incidence in women is higher that may be attributed to the earlier onset of PVD due to premature vitreous liquefaction, probably associated with declining estrogen levels in the postmenopausal period. This profile is also seen in ERM, another condition considered to be a complication of PVD.

Vitreofoveal traction is believed to be important in the pathogenesis of idiopathic MH. Since Gass has described its early stages, the development of this pathology was attributed to tangential traction of the perifoveal vitreous cortex resulting in a foveal dehiscence that can progress from foveolar detachment to a mature full-thickness MH (Gass 1988, 1995). Some susceptible patients have abnormal and strong vitreomacular adherence, causing persistent foveal traction with perifoveal detachment, which is universally associated with the earliest MH stages. The continuous anterior traction of the slightly detached vitreous cortex appears to be a major contributing factor to MH formation. Both types of traction, anteroposterior and tangential, might be combined in some cases. Tangential traction may also be the result of glial cell proliferation onto the perifoveal internal limiting membrane and may explain the persistence and enlargement of MH, in some specific cases, even when the posterior hyaloid spontaneously detaches. The mechanisms of traumatic macular hole are slightly different from idiopathic MH. It has been postulated that it is formed by a necrotic cystoid degeneration of the foveal retinal tissue, associated with the subretinal hemorrhage and anterior vitreous traction.

Clinically the patients complain about loss of central vision, low visual acuity, and metamorphopsia. On the fundus exam, it is possible to identify a hole in the foveal area that could be confirmed on the slit lamp by the Watzke-Allen sign (Fig. 27.16a). With the fluorescein angiogram, it is possible to identify a hyperfluorescent lesion to the absence of the retinal tissue in the hole location. The spectral domain OCT may identify a true hole in the retina (Fig. 27.16b) and the presence of fluid in the edges, measure the size of the hole, and also evaluate the vitreoretinal interface to observe if the vitreous is still attached or the presence of ERM.

The main value of the SD-OCT is to help us understand the pathogenic theory (Fig. 27.17) and also clarify the possible therapeutic implications: a vitrectomy with the aim of resolving anteroposterior traction could be the main goal of a surgical procedure when the vitreous face is not totally separated from the edge of the MH. Otherwise, when no anteroposterior traction is shown by OCT or US, the surgeon would attempt to remove epiretinal tissue and internal limiting membrane to release the tangential traction. Moreover, the differentiation between VMT and PVD, by a

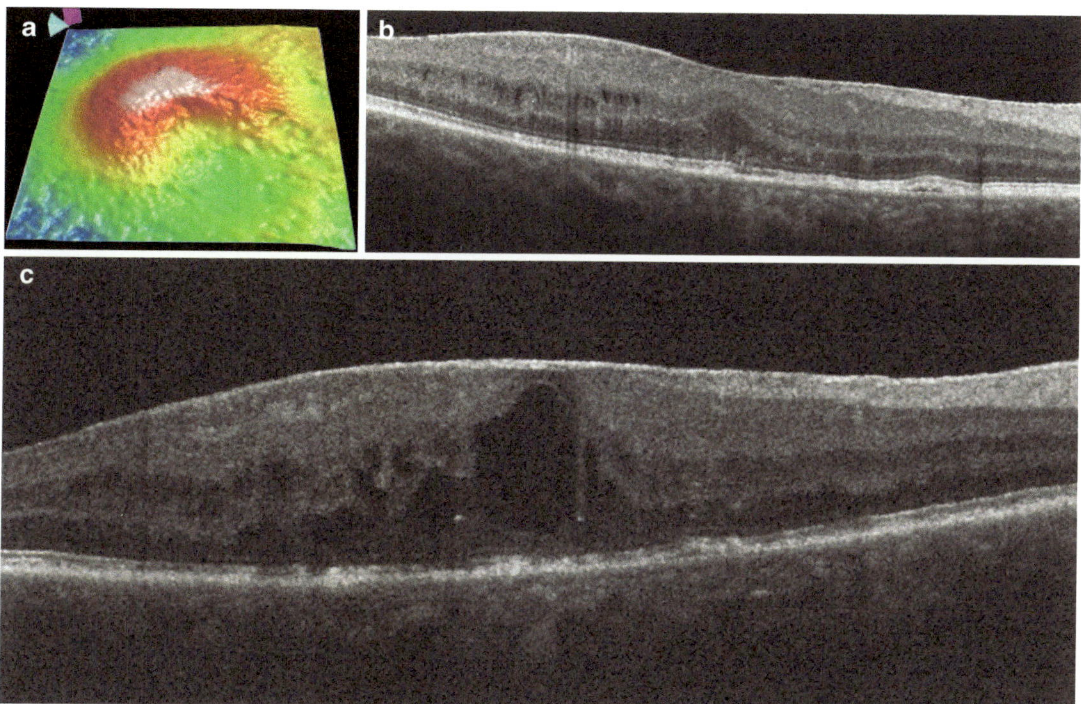

Fig. 27.15 In a patient with ERM at the initial presentation, the visual acuity was 20/50 with some increase in retinal thickness (**a**) and the SD-OCT scan shows a very adherent ERM with mild retinal edema (**b**). It was offered surgical treatment but the patient came back just 2 years later; now the visual acuity is 20/400 and the retinal anatomy is completely abnormal. Huge retinal cysts in the inner retina and disruption in the ellipsoid zone indicating a poor prognosis after surgery (**c**)

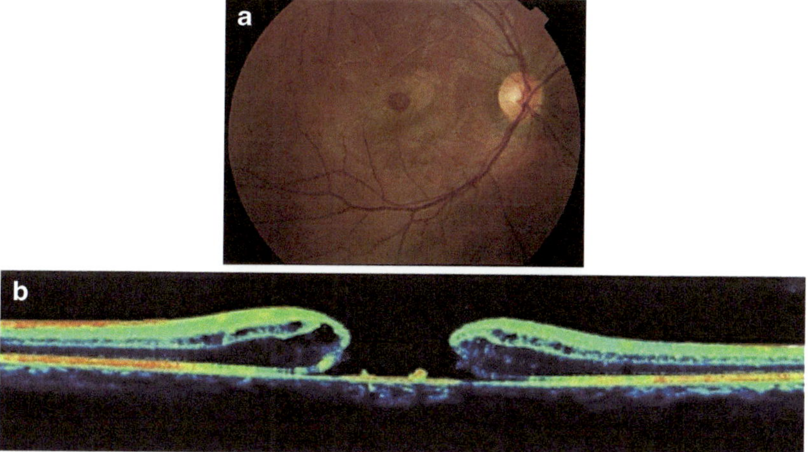

Fig. 27.16 Traumatic macular hole. (**a**) Fundus picture shows macular hole in the foveal area. (**b**) Spectral domain OCT showing complete disruption of all retinal layers revealing a macular hole. There are some cysts in the edges of the hole indicating a better prognosis after surgery

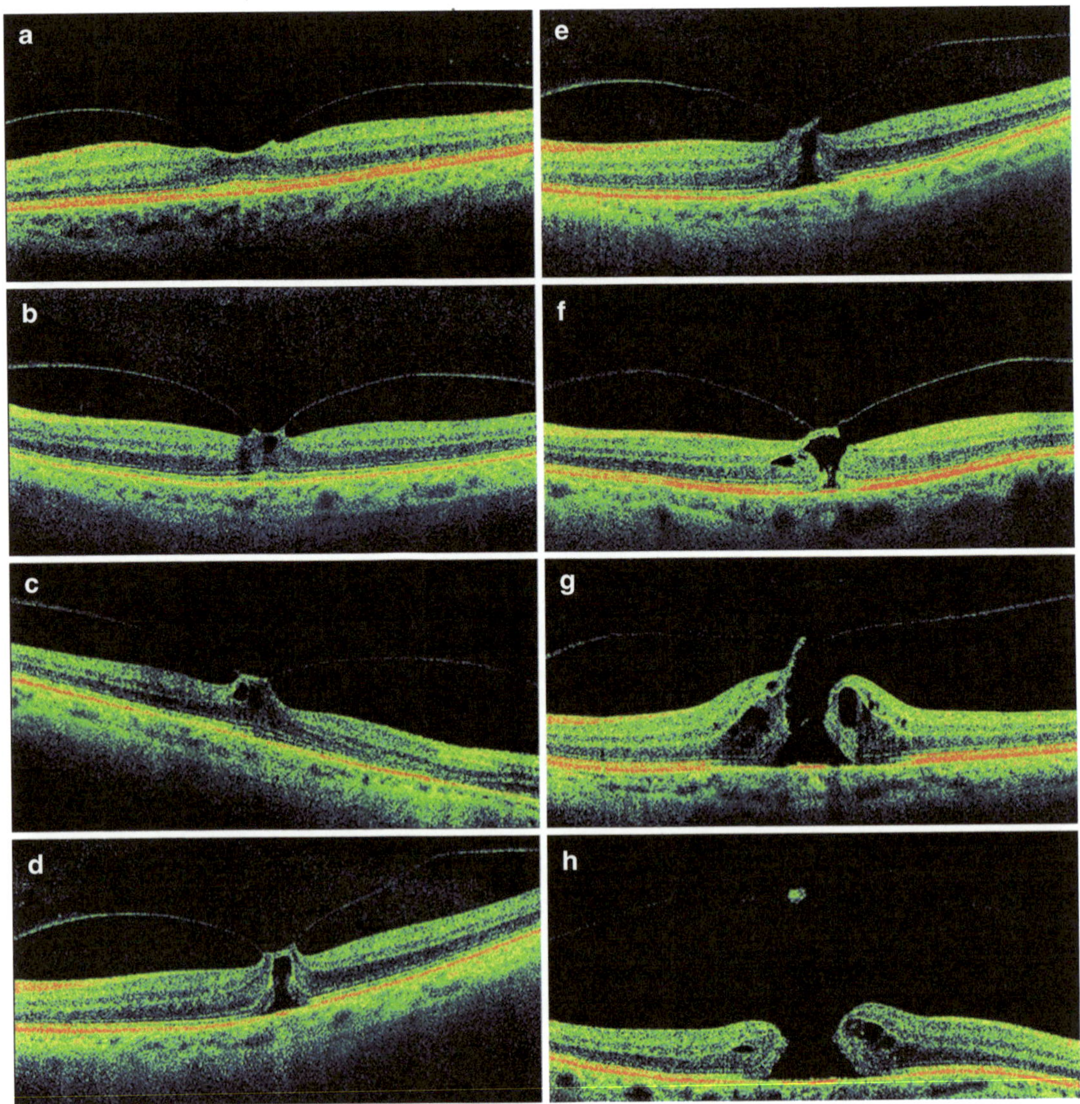

Fig. 27.17 Stages of macular hole. (**a**) SD-OCT shows that vitreous is still attached with almost no traction. (**b** and **c**) SD-OCT showing some anterior traction by the vitreous causing some changes in the retinal anatomy at the inner retina. (**d–h**) Showing evolution of the macular hole with progressive disruption of all retinal layers and enlargement of the hole and progressive release of the vitreous traction (Courtesy of Dr Juliana Bottós)

noninvasive technique, is inevitable and decisive for further surgical or pharmacological treatment.

Traumatic macular hole may close spontaneously but it also may require surgery (Yamashita et al. 2002). We describe a case of a 15-year-old boy that had a history of blunt ocular trauma due to a soccer ball. The initial visual acuity at his presentation 10 days after the trauma was 20/120 due to a traumatic macular hole. One month after the surgery, his visual acuity recovery was 20/60 with small amount of subretinal fluid that completely disappeared after 2 months, and his final visual acuity was 20/25 with a macular hole closure (Fig. 27.18).

27.9 Retinal Pigment Epithelium Tear

Retinal pigment epithelium tears occur most commonly in the posterior pole as a complication of age-related macular degeneration (AMD), and

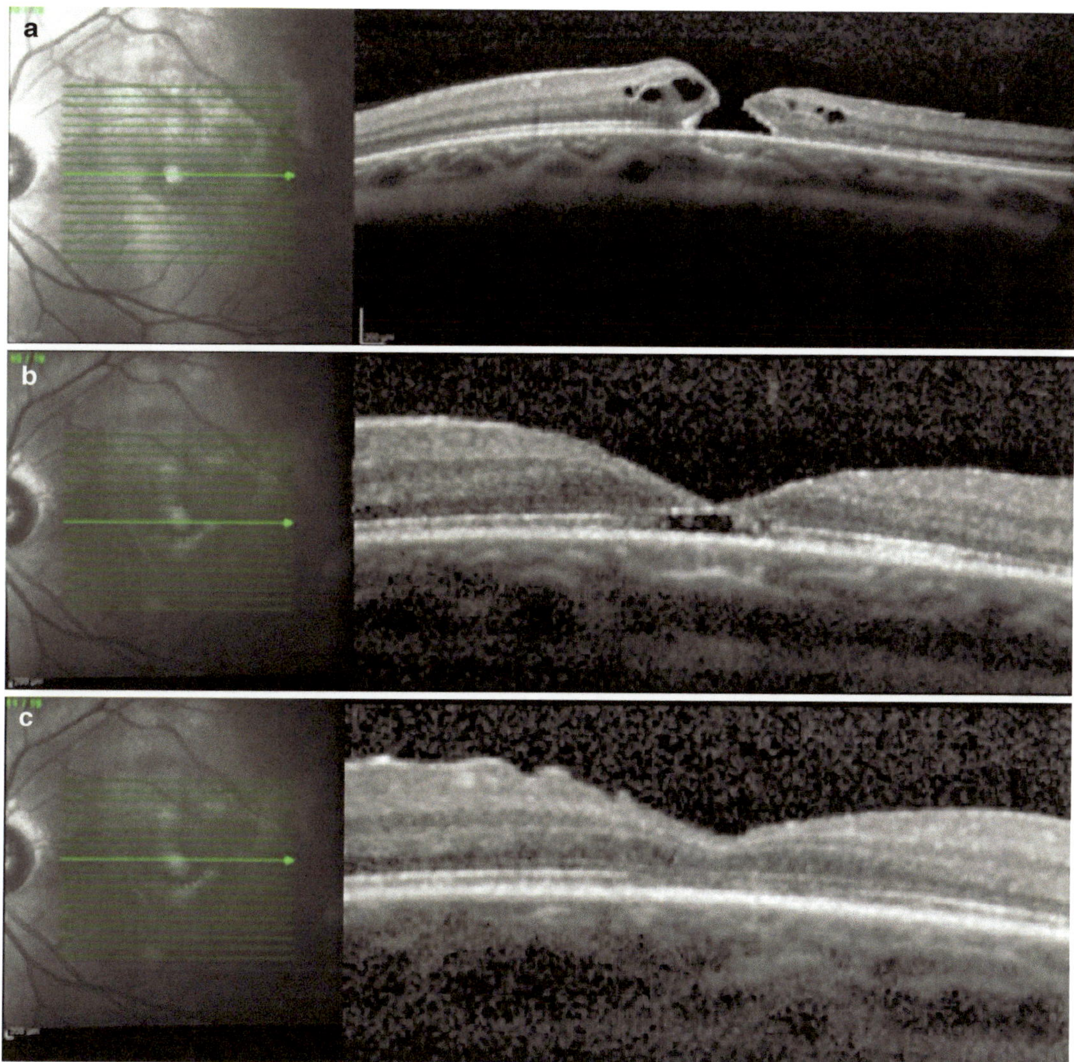

Fig. 27.18 Traumatic macular hole in a 15-year-old boy. (**a**) SD-OCT 10 days after the blunt ocular trauma shows full-thickness macular hole. (**b**) SD-OCT 1 month after the surgery shows small amount of subretinal fluid. (**c**) SD-OCT 2 months after the surgery shows complete disappearance of subretinal fluid and macular hole closure

it is generally associated with RPE detachments. RPE tears associated with blunt ocular trauma have been reported at the posterior pole and periphery (Doi et al. 2000; Levin et al. 1991). Levin et al. suggested that excessive force to the eye transmitting sufficient mechanical stress between the choroid and sclera and the RPE may induce RPE tears or choroidal ruptures (Levin et al. 1991).

We previously presented three patients with AMD and RPE tears in the presence of vitreomacular traction and postulated that shear and abnormal stresses from the vitreoretinal interface may trigger the development of RPE tears (Meyer and Toth 2001). Here we presented another case of a 68-year-old white man, who complained of low vision acuity. At presentation, his best-corrected VA was 20/23 OD and 20/400 OS. On biomicroscopy there was an area of subretinal elevation temporal to the fovea with hyperpigmentation superiorly consistent with folded RPE and CNV. Subretinal fluid extended superiorly and inferiorly to the lesion. The SD-OCT scan of the macula and the neurosensory retina was elevated as well as the RPE layer. It was possible to observe that the hyperreflective band correspondent to the

RPE was not continuous that was a failure corresponding to the tear. Adjacent to the reflective lesion was a well-demarcated area of low reflectivity in the subretinal space consistent with serous fluid. In the inner retina, it is possible to observe intraretinal cysts. The detached posterior hyaloid could be seen as a highly reflective band above the center of the fovea (Fig. 27.19).

27.10 Choroidal Excavation

Choroidal excavation or focal choroidal excavation (FCE) was first described in 2006, by Jampol et al., who reported a peculiar optical coherence tomography (OCT) finding in the macula, in which the choroid was excavated in an asymptomatic elderly woman (Jampol et al. 2006).

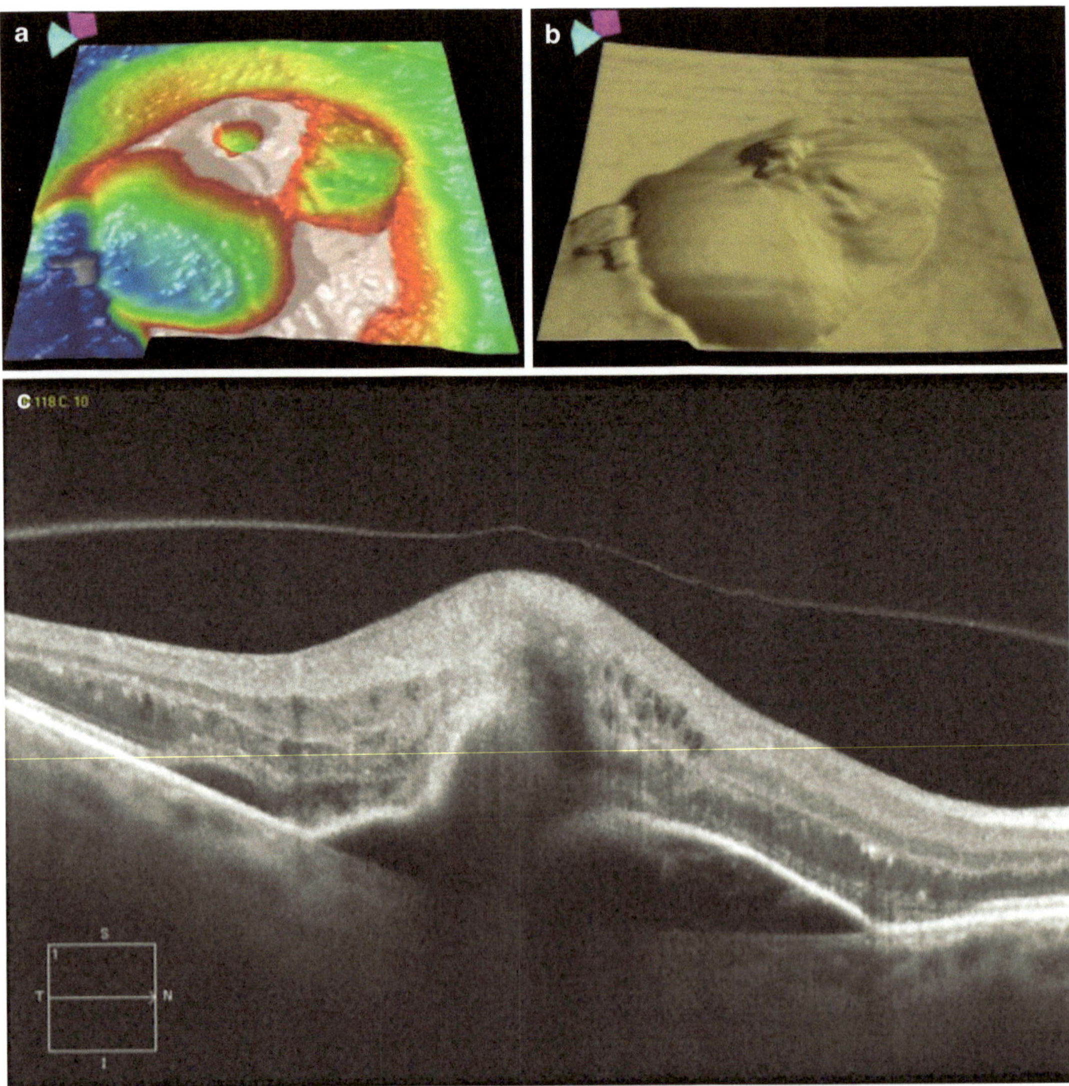

Fig. 27.19 Retinal pigment epithelium tear. (**a**) Spectral domain OCT shows subretinal fluid extending superiorly and inferiorly to the lesion that can be observed in the retinal thickness map. (**b**) The SD-OCT scan of the macula and the neurosensory retina is elevated as well as the RPE layer. (**c**) Shows noncontinuous hyperreflective RPE band corresponding to tear. Adjacent to the reflective lesion is a well-demarcated area of low reflectivity in the subretinal space consistent with serous fluid. In the inner retina, there are intraretinal cysts. The detached posterior hyaloid is seen as a highly reflective band above the center of the fovea

Later, Wakabayashi et al. identified three more patients with similar findings and called the lesions "unilateral choroidal excavation," because lesions were confined to only one eye (Wakabayashi et al. 2010). Margolis et al. found a bilateral case in their series of 12 patients and proposed the term "focal choroidal excavation" (FCE) (Margolis et al. 2011).

The cause of FCE is currently unknown. Occasional bilaterality and a relatively stable clinical course in the absence of any systemic or ocular conditions that may have disturbed the choroidal layer in the macula prompt investigators to suspect that FCE is a congenital abnormality. The clinical implications of FCE are largely unknown. Most patients appear to retain good visual acuity, but a few cases have been diagnosed with concurrent choroidal vascular disorders, including central serous chorioretinopathy (CSC), choroidal neovascularization (CNV), and polypoidal choroidal vasculopathy (PCV) (Lee et al. 2014).

We present a case of a 16-year-old woman complaining of a metamorphopsia and blurry vision for the last 4 months. She had a history of trauma 5 years ago. Her vision acuity was 20/40; in the fundus exam, it was possible to observe a grayish lesion temporal to the fovea with some pigmentary changes that correspond to a hyperfluorescent area on the fluorescein angiogram exam. The SD-OCT reveals a disruption of the outer retina and RPE with some fluid in the excavated area (Fig. 27.20). This is a case of a secondary CNV associated with FCE in a patient with ocular trauma in the past that was treated with anti-vascular endothelial growth factor intravitreal injections with good functional and anatomical recovery.

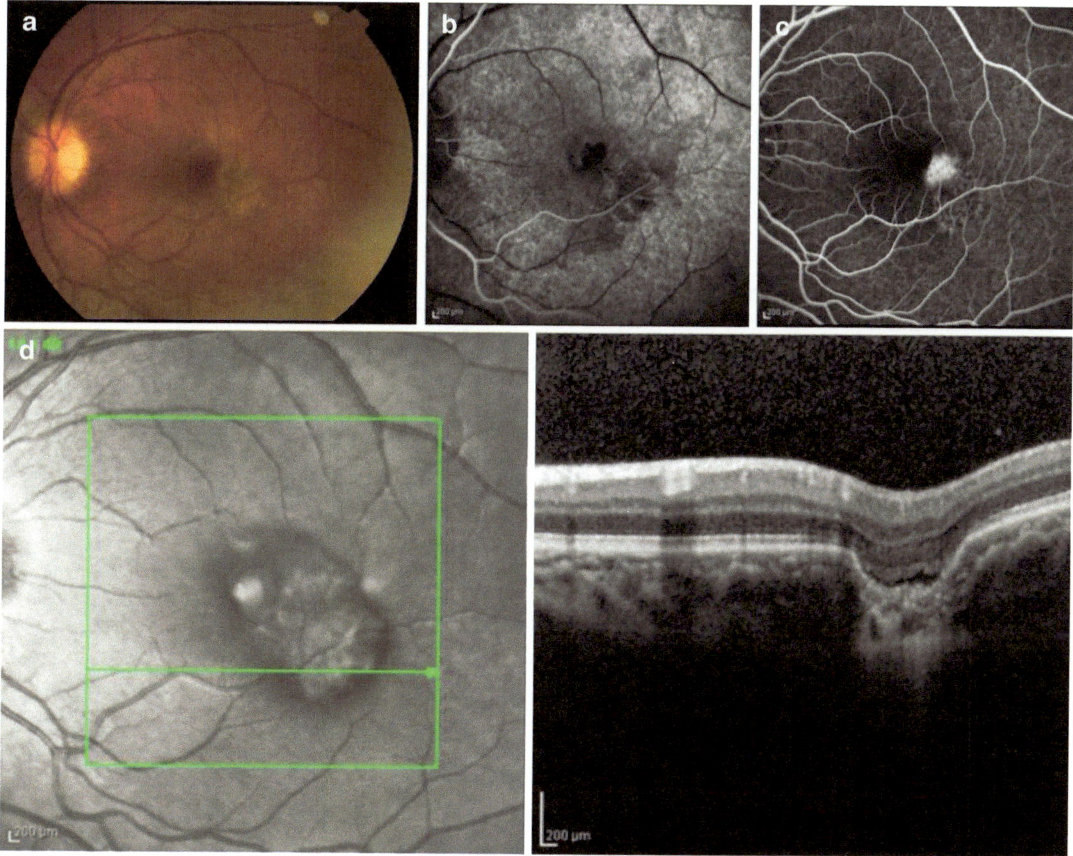

Fig. 27.20 Choroidal excavation. (**a**) The color fundus image shows a grayish lesion temporal to the fovea with some pigmentary changes. (**b**, **c**) The corresponding lesion is hyperfluorescent on fluorescein angiogram. (**d**) The SD-OCT reveals a disruption of the outer retina and RPE with some fluid in the excavated area

References

Akiyama H, Shimoda Y, Fukuchi M, Kashima T, Mayuzumi H, Shinohara Y, Kishi S (2014) Intravitreal gas injection without vitrectomy for macular detachment associated with an optic disc pit. Retina 34:222–227

Berg P, Kroll P, Krause K (1989) Pathogenic mechanism of contusio bulbi. Fortschr Ophthalmol 86:407–410

Berlin R (1873) Zur sogenannten commotio retinae. Klin Monatsbl Augenheilkd 1:42–78

Bottós JM, Elizalde J, Rodrigues EB, Maia M (2012) Current concepts in vitreomacular traction syndrome. Curr Opin Ophthalmol 23:195–201

Choudhry N, Rao RC (2014) Images in clinical medicine: valsalva retinopathy. N Engl J Med 370:1368

Dailey RA, Mills RP, Stimac GK, Shults WT, Kalina RE (1986) The natural history and CT appearance of acquired hyperopia with choroidal folds. Ophthalmology 93:1336–1342

Doi M, Osawa S, Sasoh M, Uji Y (2000) Retinal pigment epithelial tear and extensive exudative retinal detachment following blunt trauma. Graefes Arch Clin Exp Ophthalmol 238:621–624

Duane TD (1972) Valsalva retinopathy. Trans Am Ophthalmol Soc 70:298–311

Dubovy SR, Guyton DL, Green WR (1997) Clinicopathologic correlation of chorioretinitis sclopetaria. Retina 17:510–520

Fernández MG, Navarro JC, Castaño CG (2012) Long-term evolution of Valsalva retinopathy: a case series. Journal of medical case reports 6:1

Foos RY (1972) Vitreoretinal juncture, topographical variations. Invest Ophthalmol 11:801–809

Garcia-Arumi J, Corcostegui B, Tallada N, Salvador F (1994) Epiretinal membranes in tersons syndrome. A clinicopathologic study. Retina 14:351–355

Gass JD (1988) Idiopathic senile macular hole. Its early stages and pathogenesis. Arch Ophthalmol 106:629–639

Gass JD (1995) Reappraisal of biomicroscopic classification of stages of development of a macular hole. Am J Ophthalmol 119:752–759

Green MA, Lieberman G, Milroy CM, Parsons MA (1996) Ocular and cerebral trauma in non-accidental injury in infancy: underlying mechanisms and implications for paediatric practice. Br J Ophthalmol 80:282–287

Hesse L, Bodanowitz S, Kroll P (1996) Retinal necrosis after blunt ocular trauma. Klin Monatsbl Augenheilkd 209:150–152

Iwanoff A (1865) Beiträge zur normalen und pathologischen Anatomie des Auges. Archiv für Ophthalmologie 11:135–170

Jampol LM, Shankle J, Schroeder R et al (2006) Diagnostic and therapeutic challenges. Retina 26:1072–1076

Janknecht P (2011) Treatment of traumatic choroidal neovascularization with ranibizumab. Ophthalmology 108:57–59

Kinoshita T, Imaizumi H, Okushiba U, Miyamoto H, Ogino T, Mitamura Y (2012) Time course of changes in metamorphopsia, visual acuity, and OCT parameters after successful epiretinal membrane surgery. Invest Ophthalmol Vis Sci 53:3592–3597

Kranenberg EW (1960) Crater-like holes in the optic disc and central serous retinopathy. Arch Ophthalmol 64:912–924

Kroll P, Busse H (1986) Therapy of preretinal macular hemorrhages. Klin Monatsbl Augenheilkd 188: 610–612

Lee CS, Woo SJ, Kim YK et al (2014) Clinical and spectral-domain optical coherence tomography findings in patients with focal choroidal excavation. Ophthalmology 121:1029–1035

Levin LA, Seddon JM, Topping T (1991) Retinal pigment epithelial tears associated with trauma. Am J Ophthalmol 112:396–400

Lincoff H, Kreissig I (1998) Optic coherence tomography of pneumatic displacement of optic disk pit maculopathy. Br J Ophthalmol 83:367–372

Mansour AM, Green WR, Hogge C (1992) Histopathology of commotio retinae. Retina 12:24–28

Margolis R, Mukkamala SK, Jampol LM et al (2011) The expanded spectrum of focal choroidal excavation. Arch Ophthalmol 129:1320–1325

Mennel S, Meyer CH, Kroll P (2004) Dislocation of the lenses. N Engl J Med 351:1913–1914

Mennel S, Hausmann N, Meyer CH, Peter S (2005) Photodynamic therapy and indocyanine green guided feeder vessel photocoagulation of choroidal neovascularization secondary to choroidal rupture after blunt trauma. Graefes Arch Clin Exp Ophthalmol 243:68–71

Messner KH (1977) Spontaneous separation of preretinal macular fibrosis. Am J Ophthalmol 83:9–11

Meyer CH, Rodrigues EB (2004) Optic disc pit maculopathy after blunt ocular trauma. Eur J Ophthalmol 14:71–73

Meyer CH, Toth CA (2001) Retinal pigment epithelial tear with vitreomacular attachment: a novel pathogenic feature. Graefes Arch Clin Exp Ophthalmol 239:325–333

Meyer CH, Rodrigues EB, Mennel S (2003a) Acute commotio retinae determined by cross-sectional optical coherent tomography. Eur J Ophthalmol 13:816–818

Meyer CH, Rodrigues EB, Schmidt JC (2003b) Congenital optic nerve head pit associated with reduced retinal nerve fiber thickness at the papillomacular bundle. Br J Ophthalmol 87:1300–1301

Meyer CH, Rodrigues EB, Kroll P (2004a) Reduced concentration and incubation of intravitreal Indocyanine green can improve the functional outcome in macular hole surgery. Am J Ophthalmol 137:386

Meyer CH, Rodrigues EB, Mennel S, Schmidt JC, Kroll P (2004b) Spontaneous separation of epiretinal membrane in young subjects: personal observations and review of the literature. Graefes Arch Clin Exp Ophthalmol 242:977–985

Meyer CH, Mennel S, Rodrigues EB, Schmidt JC (2006) Persistent premacular cavity after membranotomy in

Valsalva retinopathy on optical coherence tomography. Retina 26:116–118

Moreira Neto CA, Moreira Junior CA (2013) Vitrectomy and gas-fluid exchange for the treatment of serous macular detachment due to optic disc pit: long-term evaluation. Arq Bras Oftalmol 76:159–162

Nettleship E (1884) Peculiar lines in the choroid in a case of post-papillitic atrophy. Trans Ophthalmol Soc UK 4:167

Norton EWD (1969) A characteristic fluorescein angiographic pattern in choroidal folds. Proc R Soc Med 62:119

Pahor D (2000) Changes in retinal light sensitivity following blunt ocular trauma. Eye 14:583–589

Piermarocchi S, BenettiE FG (2011) Intravitreal bevacizumab for posttraumatic choroidal neovascularization in a child. J AAPOS 15:314–316

Schmidt JC, Meyer CH, Rodrigues EB, Hörle S, Kroll P (2003) Staining of the internal limiting membrane in vitreoretinal surgery: a simplified technique. Retina 23:263–264

Secretan M, Sickenberg M, Zografos L, Piguet B (1998) Morphometric characteristics of traumatic choroidal ruptures associated with neovascularization. Retina 18:62–66

Shiono A, Kogo J, Klose G, Takeda H, Ueno H, Tokuda N, Inoue J, Matsuzawa A, Kayama N, Ueno S, Takagi H (2013) Photoreceptor outer segment length: a prognostic factor for Idiopathic epiretinal membrane surgery. Ophthalmology 120:788–794

Sipperley JO, Quigley HA, Gass DM (1978) Traumatic retinopathy in primates. The explanation of commotio retinae. Arch Ophthalmol 96:2267–2273

Sugar HS (1962) Congenital pits in the optic disc with acquired macular pathology. Am J Ophthalmol 53:307–311

Trese M, Chandler D, Machemer R (1983) Macular pucker. I Prognostic criteria. Graefes Arch Clin Exp Ophthalmol 221:12–15

Ulbig MW, Mangouritsas G, Rothbacher HH, Hamilton AM, McHugh JD (1998) Long-term results after drainage of premacular subhyaloid hemorrhage into the vitreous with a pulsed Nd:YAG laser. Arch Ophthalmol 116:1465–1469

Von Graefe A (1854) Zwei Fälle von Ruptur der Choroidea. Graefes Arch Clin Exp Ophthalmol 1:402

Wagemann A (1902) Zur pathologischen Anatomie der Aderhautruptur und Iridodialyse. Bericht Deutsche Ophthal Ges 30:278–282

Wakabayashi Y, Nishimura A, Higashide T et al (2010) Unilateral choroidal excavation in the macula detected by spectral-domain optical coherence tomography. Acta Ophthalmol 88:e87–e91

Williams DF, Mieler WF, Williams GA (1990) Posterior segment manifestations of ocular trauma. Retina 10(Suppl 1):S35–S44

Yamashita T, Uemara A, Uchino E, Doi N, Ohba N (2002) Spontaneous closure of traumatic macular hole. Am J Ophthalmol 133:230–235

28 Miscellaneous Disorders

Varun Gogia, Pooja Bansal,
and Pradeep Venkatesh

Contents

28.1 Macular Schisis

Splitting of the nerve fiber layer at the macular region is known as macular schisis. It is typically seen in X-linked juvenile retinoschisis and hence more common in males and is almost always bilateral (Eriksson et al. 2004). Characteristic features on fundus examination include radial plication of the internal limiting membrane and microcystoid-like spaces. This is hence often wrongly misdiagnosed as cystoid macular edema. Peripheral retinoschisis, pigmentary degeneration, and beaten metal appearance may be other associated findings (Apushkin et al. 2005).

On OCT (optical coherence tomography), cleavage of the retina in two planes, deep (outer retina) and superficial (Henle layer), is characteristic (Fig. 28.1). These two planes are connected by delicate vertical septa creating a pseudo-cystoid pattern (low reflectivity spaces). Lamellar macular defect due to dehiscence of cystoid spaces may be seen after several years.

28.2 Macular Infarction

Macular infarction may be a consequence of arterial occlusion, or occasionally it may arise as a complication of drug toxicity especially the aminoglycosides. On fundus examination there is a variable extent of foveal opacification along with retinal hemorrhages. HPE has shown lamellar lysosomal inclusion bodies in the retinal pigment epithelium and accumulation of an amorphous PAS-positive material in the subepithelial space. On OCT there is increased macular thickness with hyperreflectivity of the inner retinal layers, corresponding to the area of retinal pallor and edema. Neurosensory retina may be elevated

V. Gogia, MD • P. Bansal, MD
Senior Research Associates, R.P. Centre AIIMS, New Delhi, India

P. Venkatesh, MD (✉)
R.P. Centre AIIMS, New Delhi, India
e-mail: venkyprao@yahoo.com

C.H. Meyer et al. (eds.), *Spectral Domain Optical Coherence Tomography in Macular Diseases*,
DOI 10.1007/978-81-322-3610-8_28

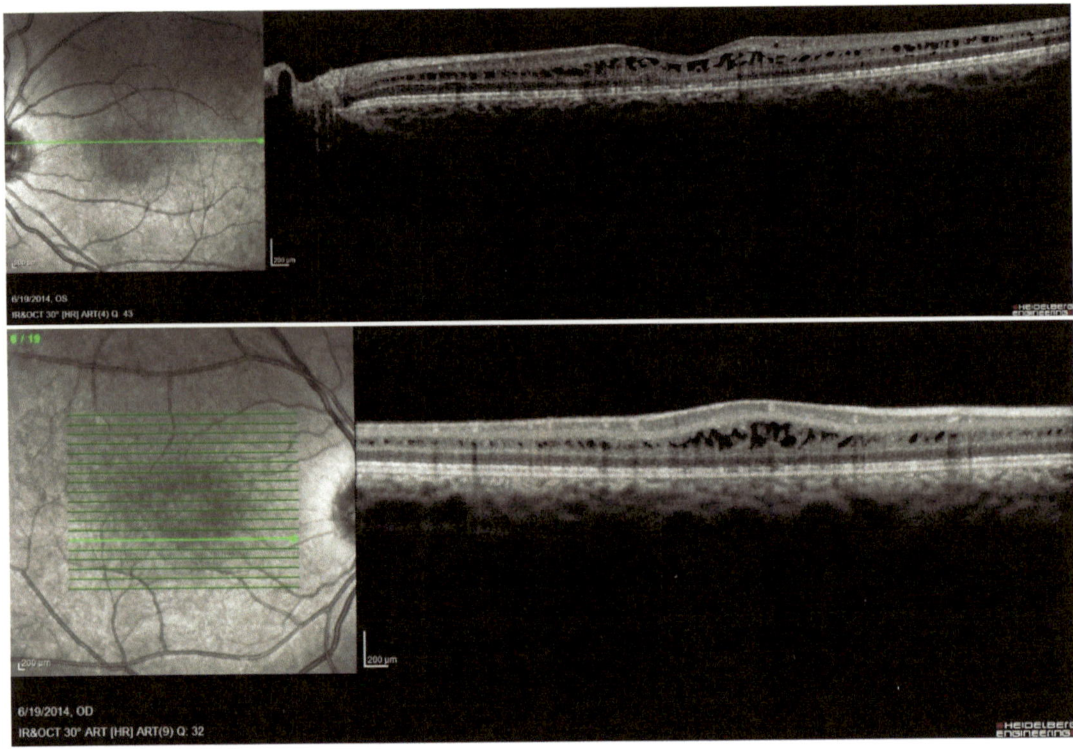

Fig. 28.1 Macular schisis. SD-OCT shows microcystoid-like spaces

with accumulation of hyperreflective material under the neurosensory retina (Fig. 28.2) (Venkatesh et al. 2005; Witkin et al. 2006). There is loss of normal alternate layers of hyperreflectivity that represent different layers of the retina. During follow-up OCT though a reduction in the macular edema is observed, the ischemic retina may still remain hyperreflective, and the alternate layers of hyperreflectivity that represent different layers of the retina are generally lost.

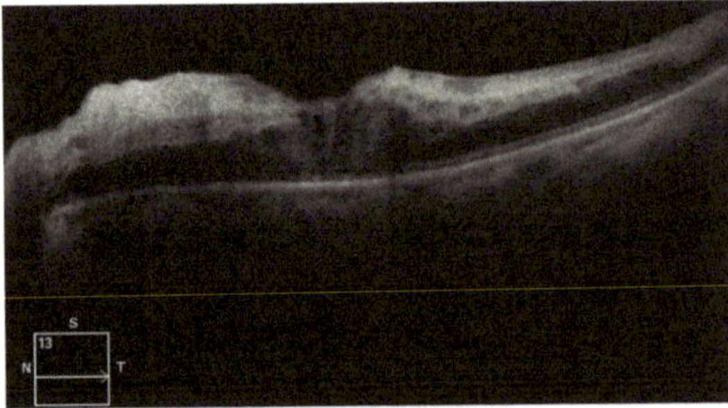

Fig. 28.2 Macular infarction. SD-OCT shows increased macular thickness with hyperreflectivity of the inner retinal layers. Neurosensory retina is elevated with accumulation of hyperreflective material underneath

28.3 Optic Nerve Head Drusen

Optic nerve head drusen (ONHD) are a common, benign, congenital anomaly of the optic nerve, which rarely lead to decreased visual acuity. Clinically, optic nerve head drusen may be visible on the disk surface or buried within the disk. These lesions often obscure the margins of the optic disk. Buried ONHD may simulate optic disk edema (ODE) and lead to diagnostic uncertainty. Various techniques to differentiate these two conditions include fundus examination, optic disk autofluorescence, fluorescein angiography, B-scan ultrasonography, and OCT. In recent years, there have been a number of reports evaluating OCT to distinguish between ODE and ONHD. The OCT appearance of optic disk drusen is characterized by an elevated optic nerve

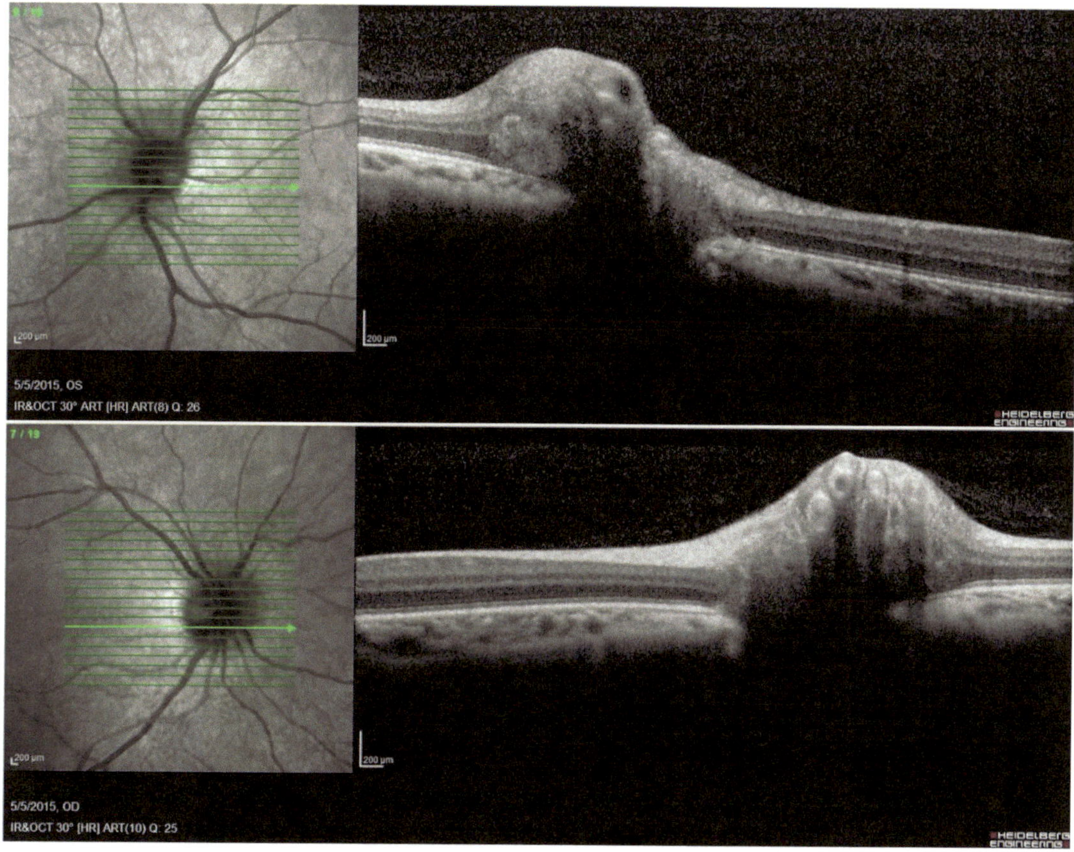

Fig. 28.3 Optic disk drusen. SD-OCT shows an elevated optic nerve head with an abrupt tapering of the hyporeflective space located between the sensory retina and the retinal pigment epithelium and choriocapillaris

head with a "lumpy-bumpy" internal optic nerve contour and an abrupt tapering of the hyporeflective space located between the sensory retina and the retinal pigment epithelium and choriocapillaris. Retinal nerve fiber layer thickness, especially in the nasal quadrant, has also been shown to be decreased in ONHD when compared with ODE (Davis and Jay 2003; Johnson et al. 2009; Karam and Hedges 2005) (Fig. 28.3).

28.4 Myelinated Nerve Fiber

Intraocular myelination of the retinal nerve fiber has been reported in 0.3–0.6 % of population by ophthalmoscopy and in 1 % by postmortem examination (Duke-Elder 1963). Normally myelination stops at the lamina cribrosa and does not extend intraocularly. Oligodendrocytes, which are responsible for myelination of the central nervous system, are not normally present in the human retina. However, histological sections confirm their presence in some areas of myelinated nerve fibers (Straatsma et al. 1981). The presence of myelinated nerve fiber has been associated with several ocular and systemic disorders. Extensive unilateral myelination of nerve fibers can be associated with anisometropic high myopia and dense amblyopia which is refractory to treatment by occlusion therapy (Ellis et al. 1987; Moradian and Karimi 2009). They may also be associated with occult microvascular abnormalities (Tabassian et al. 1995) and Gorlin syndrome (de Jong et al. 1985). Myelinated nerve fibers do not usually reduce visual acuity. However, it may produce relative scotomas depending upon their location and the number of fibers present. The scotomas are smaller than what the size of the myelinated fiber would suggest. The time domain and SD-OCT features of myelinated nerve fiber have been described by Salvatore et al. (Salvatore et al. 2011). Increased reflectivity and thickness of the retinal nerve fiber layer (RNFL) in the area of the myelinated fibers were reported. Furthermore this characteristic was accompanied by a posterior cone of shadowing. Three-dimensional OCT features of myelinated nerve fiber were described by Saxena and Jain. They observed an abrupt termination of the structures posterior to the hyperreflective RNFL due to the back shadowing produced by the thickened nerve fiber layer. The steeply elevated area of myelinated nerve fiber as observed on 3D-OCT acted as an optical barrier creating an area of non-reflectivity seen amidst the hyperreflective area as seen on the C-scan (Saxena and Jain 2011) (Fig. 28.4).

28.5 Solar Burn

Solar retinopathy is a retinal damage, particularly the macula that results from exposure to solar radiation. On fundus examination in the

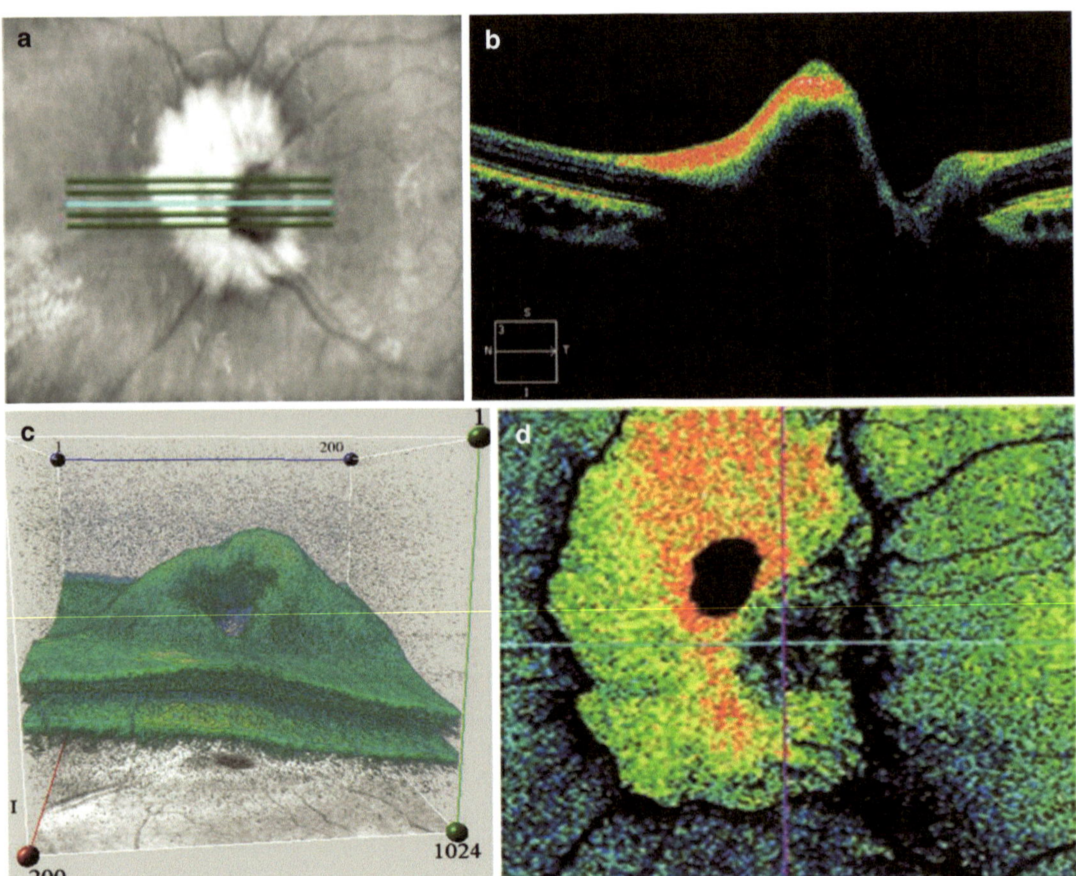

Fig. 28.4 Myelinated nerve fiber. (**a**) The five-line raster of the optic disk on OCT shows increased reflectivity of the retinal nerve fiber layer (RNFL). (**b**) The ellipsoid zone and the retinal pigment epithelium show an abrupt end at the beginning of the hyperreflective RNFL. (**c**) The 3D-OCT shows an elevation around the optic disk supranasally due to myelinated nerve fibers. (**d**) C-scan at the level of the retinal pigment epithelium shows areas of hyperreflectivity corresponding to the area of the myelinated fibers. The optic nerve head is seen as hyporeflective area. The retinal vessels and the most elevated part of the myelinated nerve fibers are seen as non-reflective areas (Figures reprinted with permission from A. Jain and S. Saxena)

initial period, there is a foveolar yellow spot. With the passage of time, this gets replaced by a very small sharply delimited red lesion or by a hypopigmented lesion with irregular margins. Solar burn is the smallest form of a macular hole. Visual acuity is relatively well maintained. Optical coherence tomography (OCT) is the most sensitive diagnostic imaging technique to detect the subtle macular changes in solar retinopathy which might get missed clinically and on fundus fluorescein angiography. It helps delineating the retinal injury site in vivo. Bechmann et al. for the first time described solar retinopathy as a hyperreflective area at the fovea with all retinal layers affected using time domain OCT (Bechmann et al. 2000).Acute changes seen on OCT predominantly include the RPE and outer photoreceptor segments, while chronic changes (more than 1 year from exposure) mainly affect the inner and outer photoreceptor segments. A tiny punched-out disruption of the pigment epithelial layer on OCT is pathognomonic of solar burn. Other OCT changes which have been observed include transient increase in foveal reflectivity and disruption of the inner and outer segments of the photoreceptor layers with or without underlying RPE defects. In many cases the changes are reversible, but solar retinopathy can lead to permanent visual impairment. Worse long-term vision is significantly related to the presence of photoreceptor layer damage on OCT (Chen et al. 2012; Codenotti et al. 2002; Garg et al. 2004; Hossein et al. 2011; Garg et al. 2004; Kaushik et al. 2004) (Fig. 28.5).

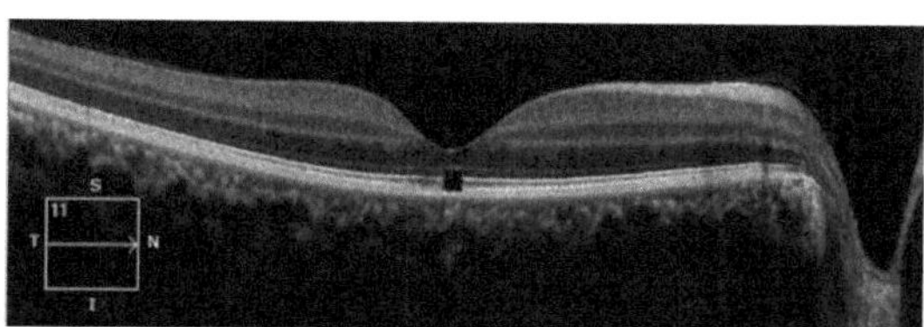

Fig. 28.5 Solar burn. SD-OCT shows punched-out disruption of the outer photoreceptor segment and retinal pigment epithelium

28.6 Electric Burn

Trauma to the ocular tissue following high-voltage electric current injury is a result of many factors that include disruption of the cell membrane, generation of heat, and vasoconstriction leading to tissue ischemia. Current traveling through the RPE is converted into thermal energy that is high enough to disrupt the retina. In initial acute response following electric shock injury, there is retinal opacification with increased retinal thickness. Subsequently this progresses to retinal atrophy. As the macula has a higher concentration of melanin, macular involvement is encountered more commonly following high-voltage electric current injury. Macular manifestations include macular edema, macular cyst, and full-thickness macular hole. Gass described that initial macular edema may be replaced later by a macular cyst or a macular hole. These macular changes are associated with loss of vision. Macular cysts may simulate a full-thickness macular hole clinically; OCT imaging is valuable in demonstrating the nature of such foveal lesions that resemble macular holes. The OCT shows thin residual inner retinal tissue and intact RPE suggestive of intraretinal macular cysts. Reports suggest that despite the appearance of various macular lesions and initial visual loss, the final visual recovery may be relatively good. Macular cysts may undergo spontaneous resolution and improvement in visual acuity. Thus OCT also helps in prognosticating these cases (Sony et al. 2005; Tandon et al. 2013).

28.7 Retained Intraocular Foreign Body

Standard imaging modalities available to detect RIOFB (retained intraocular foreign body) include orbital X-ray, ultrasound B-scan, computed tomography (CT) scan, and magnetic resonance imaging (MRI) especially in eyes with opaque media. OCT may serve as an important adjunctive imaging tool in the evaluation of injuries to the posterior segment associated with clear media. Metallic foreign body impacted near the macula and imaged by OCT appears as an area of hyperreflectivity with marked posterior shadowing. It can be useful in exact localization of depth of the foreign body on or within the retina or choroid, scanning the retina surrounding the RIOFB to assess consequent changes and postoperative assessment of the macula. OCT may also be used as a diagnostic tool for IOFBs that are not seen clinically or are too small for the detection limits of standard imaging techniques. Other subtle changes like posterior vitreous detachment status, detection of vitreomacular traction, epiretinal membranes, and quantification of increased macular thickness can also help in formulating a surgical plan and prognostication of treatment outcome. The main drawback of this technique, however, is the need for clear media, user dependency, limited assessment of highly reflective foreign bodies due to back shadowing and allowing scanning only in a limited area in the posterior pole near or within the retina (Pal et al. 2005; Rishi et al. 2009; Turkcuoglu and Turgut 2009).

References

Apushkin MA, Fishman GA, Janowicz MJ (2005) Correlation of optical coherence tomography findings with visual acuity and macular lesions in patients with X-linked retinoschisis. Ophthalmology 112:495–501

Bechmann M, Ehrt O, Thiel MJ et al (2000) Optical coherence tomography findings in early solar retinopathy. Br J Ophthalmol 84:547–548

Chen KC, Jung JJ, Aizman A (2012) High definition spectral domain optical coherence tomography findings in three patients with solar retinopathy and review of the literature. Open Ophthalmol J 6:29–35

Codenotti M, Patelli M, Brancato R (2002) OCT findings in patients with retinopathy after watching a solar eclipse. Ophthalmologica 216:463–466

Davis PL, Jay WM (2003) Optic nerve head drusen. Semin Ophthalmol 18:222–242

de Jong PT, Bistervels B, Cosgrove J, De Grip G, Leys A, Goffin M (1985) Medullated nerve fibers: a sign of multiple basal cell nevi (Gorlin's) syndrome. Arch Ophthalmol 103:1833–1836

Duke-Elder S (ed) (1963) Congenital deformities. In: System of ophthalmology. Mosby, St Louis

Ellis GS, Frey T, Gouterman RZ (1987) Myelinated nerve fibers, axial myopia, and refractory amblyopia: an organic disease. J Pediatr Ophthalmol Strabismus 24:111–119

Eriksson U, Larsson E, Holmstrom G (2004) Optical coherence tomography in the diagnosis of juvenile X-linked retinoschisis. Acta Ophthalmol Scand 82:218–223

Garg SJ, Martidis A, Nelson ML et al (2004) Optical coherence tomography of chronic solar retinopathy. Am J Ophthalmol 137:351–354

Hossein M, Bonyadi J, Soheilian R et al (2011) Spectral-domain optical coherence tomography features of mild and severe acute solar retinopathy. Ophthalmic Surg Lasers Imaging 42 Online:e84–86

Johnson LW, Diehl ML, Hamm CW et al (2009) Differentiating optic disc edema from optic nerve head drusen on optical coherence tomography. Arch Ophthalmol 127:45–49

Karam EZ, Hedges TR (2005) Optical coherence tomography of the retinal nerve fibre layer in mild papilloedema and pseudopapilloedema. Br J Ophthalmol 89:294–298

Kaushik S, Gupta V, Gupta A (2004) Optical coherence tomography findings in solar retinopathy. Ophthalmic Surg Lasers Imaging 35:52–55

Moradian S, Karimi S (2009) Unilateral myelinated retinal nerve fiber layer associated with axial myopia, amblyopia and strabismus. J Ophthalmic Vis Res 4:264–265

Pal N, Azad RV, Sony P et al (2005) Optical coherence tomography-assisted localization of retained intraocular foreign body. Eye (Lond) 19:717–719

Rishi P, Sharma T, Rishi E et al (2009) Optical coherence tomography for precise localization of in apparent retained foreign body in ocular coats. Retina Cases Brief Rep 3:275–278

Salvatore S, Iannetti L, Fragiotta S, Vingolo EM (2011) Optical coherence tomography and myelinated retinal nerve fibers: anatomical description and comparison between time-domain and spectral domain OCT. Minerva Oftalmol 53:31–38

Saxena S, Jain A (2011) Three-dimensional optical coherence tomography of the optic nerve head with myelinated nerve fibers. J Ocul Biol Dis Infor 4:145–148

Sony P, Venkatesh P, Tewari HK et al (2005) Bilateral macular cysts following electric burn. Clin Experiment Ophthalmol 33:78–80

Straatsma BR, Foos FY, Heckenlively JR et al (1981) Myelinated retinal nerve fibers. Am J Ophthalmol 91:25–38

Tabassian AR, Reddy CV, Folk JC (1995) Retinal vascular abnormalities associated with myelinated nerve fibers. Invest Ophthalmol Visc Sci 36:594

Tandon M, Agarwal A, Gupta V et al (2013) Peripapillary retinal thermal coagulation following electrical injury. Ind J Ophthalmol 61:240–242

Turkcuoglu P, Turgut B (2009) Optical coherence tomography in the detection of an intraocular foreign body. Acta Ophthalmologica 87:582–583

Venkatesh P, Sony P, Tewari HK, Garg SP (2005) Optical coherence tomography in Amikacin-induced macular infarction. Ind J Ophthalmol 53:269–270

Witkin AJ, Rogers AH, Ko TH et al (2006) Optical coherence tomography demonstration of macular infarction in sickle cell retinopathy. Arch Ophthalmol 124:746–747

Part V
Intraoperative Optical Coherence Tomography

Intraoperative Spectral Domain Optical Coherence Tomography: Technology, Applications, and Future Perspectives

29

Lyubomyr Lytvynchuk, Carl Glittenberg, and Susanne Binder

Contents

Electronic supplementary material The online version of this chapter (doi:10.1007/978-81-322-3610-8_29) contains supplementary material, which is available to authorized users.

L. Lytvynchuk, MD, PhD (✉) • C. Glittenberg, MD
S. Binder, MD
Department of Ophthalmology, Rudolf Foundation Clinic, Karl Landsteiner Institute for Retinal Research and Imaging, Vienna, Austria
e-mail: lubko_l@yahoo.co.uk

29.1 Overview

The implementation of spectral domain OCT diagnostic technique into the intraoperative process (iSD-OCT) has drastically improved our understanding of the behavior of ocular tissue during surgical intervention. Being fully integrated into the surgical microscope, iOCT systems allow the surgeon to perform iSD-OCT-guided eye surgery without any interruption of workflow. This chapter reveals the historical aspects of iSD-OCT development, specifics of its exploitation, technical characteristics, as well as its application for use in ophthalmic microsurgery. Multiple ongoing studies are going to determine the feasibility of iSD-OCT in everyday use for certain surgical procedures in the future.

29.2 Introduction

During the last two decades, optical coherence tomography (OCT) became an indispensable diagnostic method in ophthalmology, which dramatically revolutionized the field, allowing to diagnose and monitor eye diseases (Fercher et al.

C.H. Meyer et al. (eds.), *Spectral Domain Optical Coherence Tomography in Macular Diseases*, DOI 10.1007/978-81-322-3610-8_29

2003; Huang et al. 1991; Yaqoob et al. 2005). The evolution of OCT from time domain (TD-OCT) to spectral domain (SD-OCT) made this diagnostic technique more precise and accurate, which in turn provided us with so-called optical biopsy, a noninvasive and noncontact in vivo imaging of living tissue (Fercher et al. 2003; Fujimoto et al. 2000). Examination of ocular tissues during the surgery was always highly desirable for every practicing eye surgeon. The integration of OCT into the surgical process was a logical and irreversible step toward discovering the possibilities of this novel diagnostic approach. Therefore, an intraoperative OCT (iOCT) was developed that has made a tremendous impact on our perception of surgical procedures in situ.

The emergence of iOCT is linked to the concept of an image-guided intervention (IGI) method that facilitates high precision in clinical diagnosis (Huang et al. 2012; Yaqoob et al. 2006). Based on different computer systems, the IGI method aims to create image overlays during the surgical intervention in order to assist the surgeon to better visualize and manage living tissues. There are many well-known medical imaging techniques, such as computed tomography, magnetic resonance imaging, ultrasound, etc., which provide important information in the course of treatment. The OCT is one of the bio-imaging techniques that deliver the image visualization with high sensitivity and high resolution.

Being a well-accepted diagnostic imaging modality in different medical specialties, OCT started to be used not only before and after treatment but also during surgical interventions and invasive diagnostic examinations (Ehlers et al. 2014b, d, f; Feldchtein et al. 1998; Li et al. 2000a, b; Rollins et al. 1999; Sergeev et al. 1997; Sivak et al. 2000; Zivelonghi et al. 2014). The feasibility of performing clinical OCT imaging has been demonstrated in a number of studies which show a broad range of current and future clinical applications. Among the medical fields where iOCT is already used are ophthalmology, neurosurgery, otorhinolaryngology, cardiology, breast cancer surgery, dentistry, gastroenterology, and respiratory tract diseases (Ehlers et al. 2014a, b, c, g; Feldchtein et al. 1998; Hanna et al. 2005; Kraft et al. 2008; Li et al. 2000a, b; Rollins et al. 1999; Sergeev et al. 1997; Sivak et al. 2000; Terashima et al. 2012; Zivelonghi et al. 2014). For example, the intraoperative SD-OCT (iSD-OCT) implementation into neurosurgical procedures has improved the diagnostic value of this technology in the detection of residual tumor tissue within the wall of a resection cavity, as it is able to distinguish between diffuse growth pattern and a low inherent contrast of a tumor and adjacent normal brain tissue (Boppart et al. 1998; Giesea et al. 2006). In breast cancer surgery, iOCT became an alternative imaging technique to X-ray mammography (Nguyen et al. 2010). The big advantage is that iOCT may replace the microscopic postoperative tissue assessment to a real-time intraoperative assessment of the tumor margin containing a larger amount of samples. In the field of dental oncology, OCT was found to be useful as it facilitates noninvasive imaging of near-surface abnormalities in complex tissue (Aggarwal et al. 2013). In cardiology, iOCT can provide detailed information about dissection, tissue prolapse, thrombi condition, and stent position during percutaneous coronary intervention (PCI), etc. (Regar et al 2011, Zivelonghi et al. 2014).

However, ophthalmology remains one of the first medical fields in which intraoperative OCT became a rapidly developing diagnostic tool, facilitating the examination of almost all ocular tissues (Ehlers et al. 2014d, e, f).

29.3 History

The idea of mobile OCT systems arose from the necessity to create the conditions in which OCT examination would be possible in uncooperative pediatric patients or those with limited mobility (musculoskeletal disorders, unconsciousness) and limited access (hospital floor patients, those in isolation). Therefore, a noncontact intraoperative imaging system is needed to become available for patients that are in a supine position.

The first intraoperative OCT scans were performed with standard OCT systems that were mounted to a modified holder and draped with

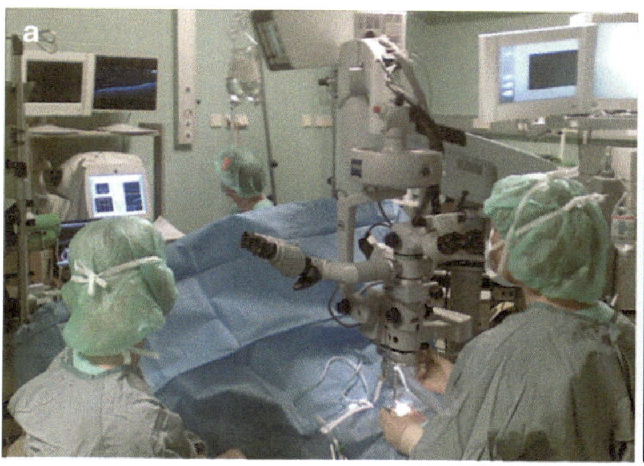

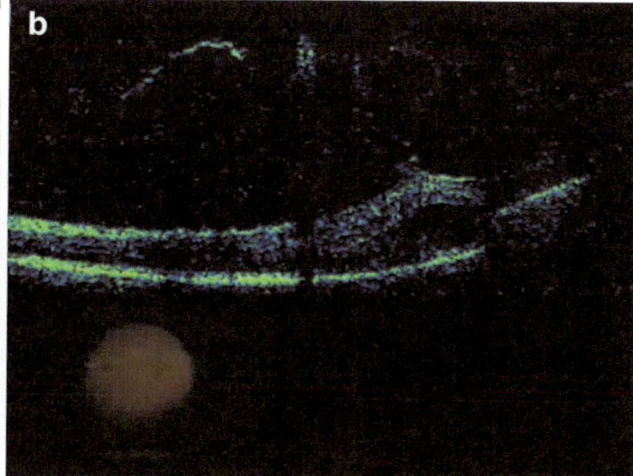

Fig. 29.1 (**a**) The prototype of the first surgical microscope-integrated iSD-OCT system based on Cirrus HD-OCT™ source and running the 4.5.1.11 Cirrus HD-OCT™ acquisition software adapted to the optical pathway of a Zeiss OPMI VISU 200™ SM (Carl Zeiss Meditec, Oberkochen, Germany). (**b**) iSD-OCT scan of an epiretinal membrane with a vitreomacular traction

sterile tissues during surgery (Dayani et al. 2009; Fujimoto et al. 2000). Endoscopic OCT probes have also been developed for diagnostic purposes. These small-gage probes became possible due to their single-mode fiber (SMF) of light delivery in OCT systems, which is important for small-gage surgery (Bouma and Tearney 1999).

Cynthia Toth is considered to be the pioneer of iOCT and world expert in retinal imaging with optical coherence tomography (Dayani et al. 2009; Scott et al. 2009; Tao et al. 2010). At Duke University, Toth and her group were the first who reported findings about a handheld spectral domain OCT system for research purposes using the Bioptigen Spectral Domain Ophthalmic Imaging System (SDOIS) (Bioptigen Inc., Research Triangle Park, NC, USA).[1] The examination of an area of interest was performed during a pause in surgery with a noncontact handheld OCT device, covered in a sterile drape, while the microscope was moved away from the surgical field (Tao et al. 2010). Toth was also the first who reported about the use of a handheld iOCT for infant examination and the use of swept source OCT (SS-OCT) imaging during macular surgery (Chavala et al. 2009; Hahn et al. 2011; Maldonado and Toth 2013; Maldonado et al. 2010; Toth et al. 2015).

At the Cleveland Clinic, Sunil Srivastava and Justis Ehlers were the first to report about the use of a microscope-mounted OCT system (Ehlers et al. 2011a, b; Srivastava 2010; Srivastava et al. 2011). The enhanced imaging was improved by implementation of higher stability and better control of the device. They also initiated the prospective intraoperative and perioperative OCT (PIONEER) study, which is aimed at discovering the possible applications for use of intraoperative OCT imaging (Ehlers et al. 2014a, 2015; Mehta 2011).

In 2008, our group, led by Susanne Binder, started to use the prototype of the first surgical microscope integrated iOCT system, using a spectral domain-based Cirrus HD-OCT™ (Carl Zeiss Meditec, Oberkochen, Germany) (Fig. 29.1). In our experience, the iOCT facilitated OCT imaging during surgery without interruption of the surgical procedure (Binder et al. 2010, 2011; Matz et al. 2012). Targeting and imaging of desired areas were controlled via an external monitor. There was therefore no direct OCT control using the foot pedal. Later in 2014, Binder and her group were the first to start the clinical use of a commercially available spectral domain iOCT system that was fully integrated into the microscope (Rescan 700, Carl Zeiss

[1] Bioptigen Spectral Domain Ophthalmic Imaging System (SDOIS) (Bioptigen, Morrisville, NC, USA).

Meditec, Oberkochen, Germany).[2] The integration of the iOCT image in the ocular of the microscope and foot pedal control enables performing iOCT scanning without interruption of the surgical procedure. This is the main advantage compared to the previous prototype. Since then, various OCT systems, which are described below, were adapted for intraoperative use.

29.4 Equipment

29.4.1 Intraoperative Optical Coherence Tomography Probes

A wide range of OCT systems provide imaging of eye structures that are perpendicular to the scanning beam, including the cornea, iris, lens, macula, optic nerve, retinal nerve fibers, and choroid. Straight beam delivery, however, lacks the ability to image peripheral structures. Additionally, the OCT signal becomes degraded and distorted in eyes with dense media, such as mature cataracts or vitreous opacities, which result in low-quality images (Fercher et al. 2003). The ability of forward-imaging intraocular OCT probes to provide real-time cross-sectional scanning of inner ocular structures gives this method a unique value during eye microsurgery. The main advantage of the iOCT probe is that it can scan almost any part of the anterior and posterior eye segments depending on the placement through the bypassing mechanism with a direct view of structures that are unreachable using external OCT systems (Li et al. 2000a, b; OKT 1300-E BioMedTech; Sun et al. 2014).

According to the direction of the optical scanning mechanism, the OCT probes can be divided into two main types: side-imaging probes and forward-imaging probes (Sun et al. 2014). The three main probe parameters are field of view, scanning range, and scanning rate. OCT side-scanning probes with different sizes have been designed to examine tissues within tubular structures. Those OCT probes are being successfully utilized in imaging of the esophagus, coronary arteries, etc., with a lateral resolution up to 10 μm. The first side imaging, 27-gage needle probe OCT, was designed by Li et al. in 2000 for interstitial imaging of different organs (Li et al. 2000a, b). A forward-imaging OCT probe, with relatively large diameter, has also been used to image bladders (Feldchtein et al. 1998). Usually, two-dimensional (2D) data imaging is provided by forward-imaging probes. By using 2D imaging with a combination of probe rotation or linear movement, three dimensional (3D) images can be obtained. A forward-imaging probe would be most desirable to examine the inner structures of a hollow organ such as the eye, in order to evaluate the retina.

The capability of OCT probes for real-time cross-sectional extraocular and intraocular imaging is considered to be effective for intraoperative diagnosis and surgery. The diameter of the probe is also an important issue, as it has to fit through a standard surgical entry port, preferably 23- or 25-gage. An important issue that is specific to the probe is that the tip must be positioned within close proximity to delicate tissues, such as the retina (Binder et al. 2011). A wide range of iOCT probes has been developed to visualize posterior pole and peripheral inner eye structures (Li et al. 2000a, b; OKT 1300-E BioMedTech;Stolyarenko et al. 2011; Sun et al. 2014). The average scanning range is 1–2 mm with an axial resolution of 4–6 μm and a lateral resolution of 25–35 μm. The distance between imaged structures and the probe tip has to be 1.6–4 mm, and the acquisition quality is dependent on the surgeon's ability to hold the probe steadily.

In 2007, at the Posterior Eye Segment Diagnostics and Surgery Center in Moscow, Russia, G. Stolyarenko and his group started to use the OKT 1300-E (BioMedTech, Russia) – a universal OCT system that can be used with both anterior and posterior segment probes (23- and 25-gage) (Fig. 29.2). The OKT 1300-E has scan depth of 1.8–2 mm, a depth resolution of 10 μm in air, with an acquisition rate 20,000 A-scans/s (Table 29.1) (OKT 1300-E BioMedTech; Stolyarenko et al. 2011). The main application

[2] Rescan 700 (Carl Zeiss Meditech, Oberkochen, Germany).

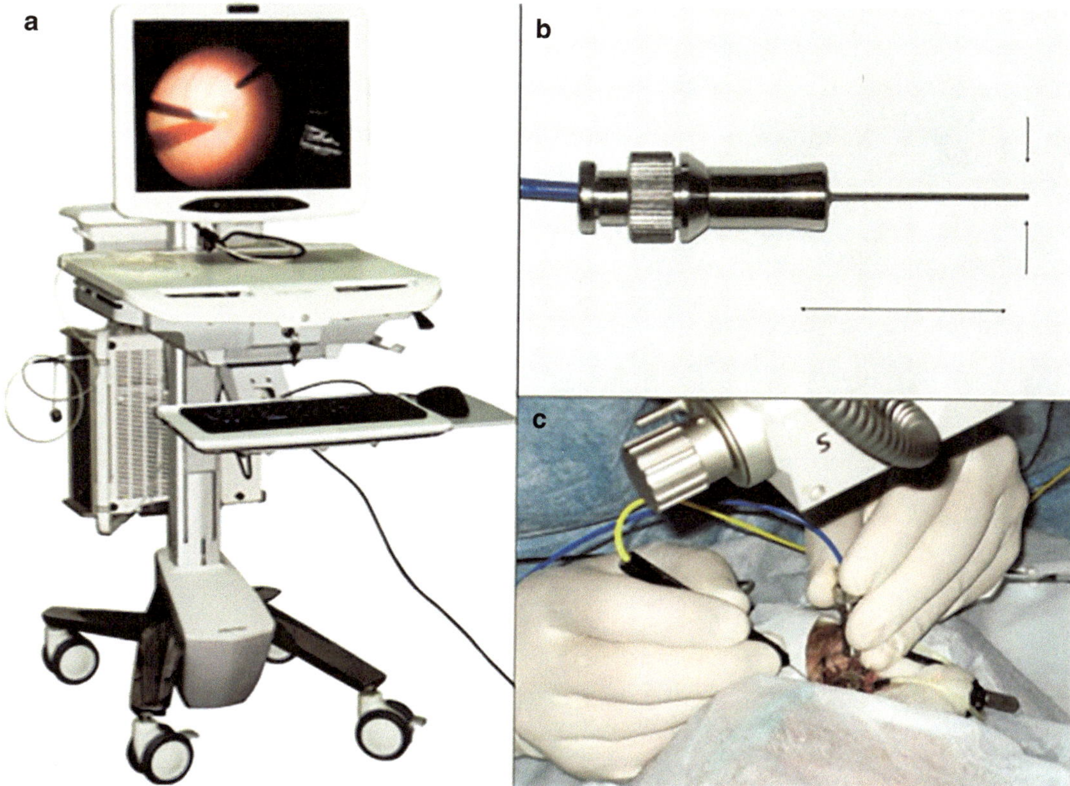

Fig. 29.2 iOCT system OKT 1300-E (BioMedTech, Russia) (**a**) with a 23-gage posterior segment endoprobe (**b**). Acquisition of the iOCT with endoprobe during pars plana vitrectomy (**c**) (Photos printed with the permission of Prof. G. Stolyarenko)

for anterior segment use was the differentiation of malignancies of the conjunctiva, localization of the site of biopsy, visualization of the cornea, iris, and anterior chamber, as well as intraoperative control during tumor resection. During posterior segment surgery, it was used intraoperatively to detect epiretinal membranes, assess vitreomacular traction, and control surgical maneuvers and outcome (Fig. 29.3).

In 2013, K. Joos and J. Shen reported the use of the smallest self-contained 25-gage handheld forward-imaging B-scan OCT probe for ophthalmic examination (Joos and Shen 2013). This new iOCT probe was adapted to an SD-OCT system Bioptigen Inc.[1]which delivered 700 μW of power, central wavelength of 870 nm, with 2,000 A-scans per B-scan. Optimal working distance was 3–4 mm from the probe tip to the targeted tissue. The intraocular OCT probe was meant to permit evaluation of structures beyond the central posterior pole of the eye, such as the peripheral retina and ciliary body. The possibility of iOCT probes to scan the peripheral structures of the eye is a very promising capability for the understanding of certain eye diseases. However, the narrow field of the OCT image and interruption of the surgical workflow in order to perform the scanning limit its use.

29.4.2 Handheld Optical Coherence Tomography Systems

29.4.2.1 Bioptigen Envisu SDOIS

Their Bioptigen Envisu Spectral Domain Ophthalmic Imaging System (SDOIS) was developed to capture, process, display, and save depth-resolved images of ocular tissue microstructures based on a spectral domain OCT source Bioptigen Inc.[1] (BioptigenEnvisu 2015)

Table 29.1 Technical characteristics of the OCT systems that are used during ophthalmic surgery

Characteristics	OKT 1300-E (BioMedTech, Russia)	Bioptigen SDOIS (Bioptigen, Morrisville, NC, USA)	iVue scanner (Optovue, Fremont, CA, USA)	iOCT® (Optomedical Technologies GmbH, Lübeck, Germany)	Rescan 700 (Zeiss, Oberkochen, Germany)
OCT source	Spectral domain	Spectral domain	Spectral domain	Spectral domain	Spectral domain
OCT image	20,000 A-scan/s	32,000 A-scans/s	28,000 A-scan/s	10,000 A-scans/s	27.000 A-scans/s
Frame rate	20 frames/s		256–1024 A-scan/frame	10 frames/s	
Depth resolution	10 μm in air	3.3 μm in air (2.4 μm in tissue)	5.0 μm in tissue	10 μm in air	5.5 μm in tissue
Traverse resolution	15 μm (retina)		15 μm (retina)		
Scan range depth	1.8–2 mm	3.4 mm (2.5 mm in tissue)	2–2.3 mm (retina)	4.2 mm	2.0 mm
Scan beam wavelength	1310 nm	830 ± 30 nm	840 ± 10 nm	800 nm	840 nm
Exposure power at pupil		700 μW (1500 μW max)	750 μW		
Lateral scan width	1.6–2.4 mm		13 × 9 mm external image	5–30 mm dependent on microscope zoom	3–16 mm (scan rotation 360°)
Recording options	Videos, snapshots, and 3D images	Videos, snapshots	Videos, snapshots, 3D en face analysis upgrade	Videos, snapshots, and 3D images	Videos, snapshots
Working distance	4 mm		22 mm/15 mm		
Motorized focus range		+10D to −12D	−15D to ± 12D		

Bioptigen SDOIS is a noncontact, portable, handheld SD-OCT system. The SD-OCT engine is connected via a 1.3-m flexible cable to the imaging handpiece that is used by the operator. The OCT unit is mounted on a trolley cart to increase the mobility in the operating room, as well as a screen, keyboard, and printer. A reference arm position adjuster with digital readout is also included into the OCT system. The handheld probe has a focus adjustment system and a diopter scale bar with a range of +10 to −12 D. The custom software (Bioptigen, Durham, NC, USA) enables imaging, analyzing, and archiving of the acquired data. The technical characteristics of Bioptigen SDOIS are a wavelength of 830 ± 30 nm, an axial resolution of 3.3 μm (2.4 μm in tissue), a scan depth of 3.4 mm (2.5 mm in tissue), and an acquisition rate of 32,000 A-scans/s (Table 29.1).

In 2009, C. Toth and her group reported the use of an FDA-approved portable, noncontact, handheld SD-OCT unit by Bioptigen Inc.[1] (Bouma and Tearney 1999; Scott et al. 2009). The OCT system consisted of an imaging handpiece connected to an SD-OCT engine and mounted on a trolley cart. To adjust the reference arm position, a calibrated knob was used. The focus correction adjustment of the handheld probe ranged from +10 to −12 D. J. Ehlers and his group at the Cole Eye Institute reported the use of two different prototype microscope-mounted systems. In the first one,

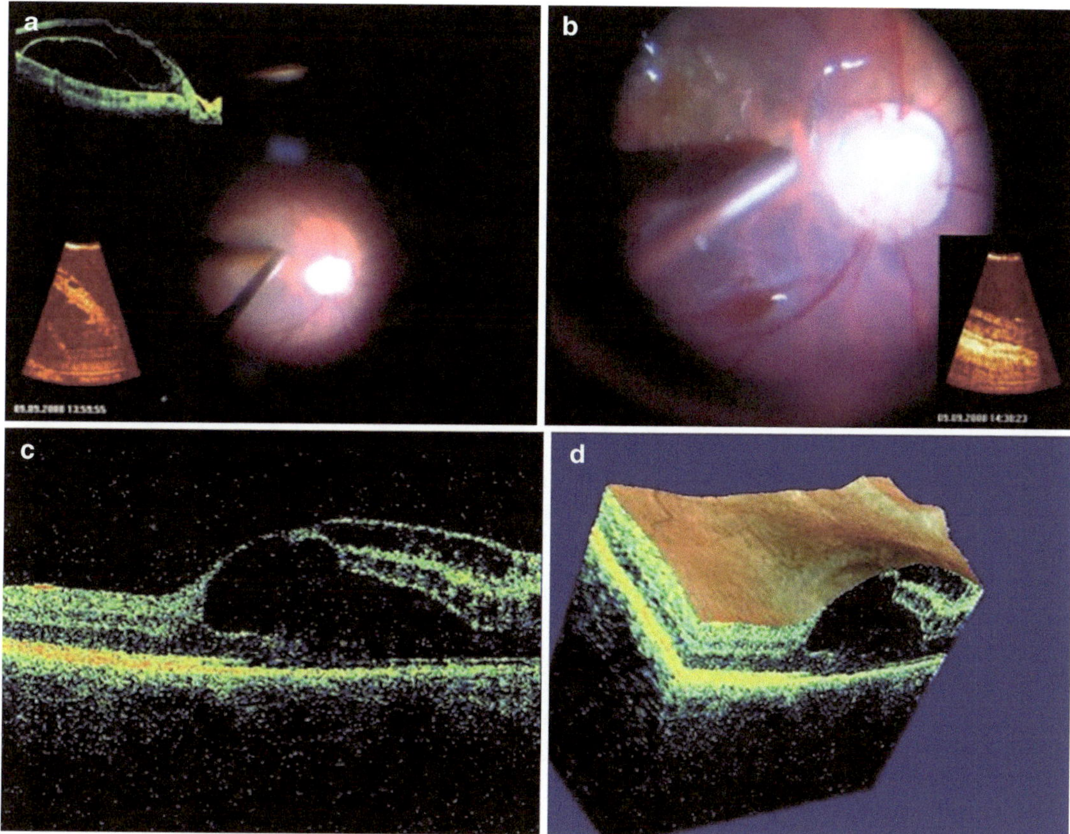

Fig. 29.3 iOCT imaging of the retina (**a**, **b**) with a 23-gage probe (OKT 1300-E (BioMedTech, Russia) in comparison to the preoperative OCT (*color scale*, **a**). A 2D (**c**) and a 3D (**d**) visualization of the retina with the OKT 1300-E endoprobe (Photos printed with the permission of Prof. G. Stolyarenko)

the handheld system was fixed below the lens of the microscope. The surgeon was therefore able to use an undraped microscope. In the second system, a modified plate was used to position the OCT probe to the side of the scope, and the entire system had to be draped (Ehlers et al. 2011a, b; Srivastava 2010; Srivastava et al. 2011).

29.4.2.2 iVue® SD-OCT

The iVue® SD-OCT (Optovue, Fremont, CA, USA) is a commercially available, portable, compact OCT system with the capability to perform a quantitative analysis of the obtained data (Optovue, iVue. SD-OCT 2015). The iVue includes a spectral domain source and provides a complete posterior and anterior segment scanning with an axial depth resolution of 5 μm, a traverse resolution for retina of 15 μm, and an OCT A-scan acquisition rate of 28,000 A-scans/s (Table 29.1). The depth of the OCT scan is 2–2.3 mm. Minimum pupil diameter required is 2.5 mm. The working distance is 22/15 mm. The motorized focus can be adjusted in a range from −15D to ± 12D (Optovue). The software enables the creation of retina, glaucoma, and cornea scans and reports live video and en face images. The iVue® SD-OCT software can be upgraded with ganglion cell complex analysis which provides the ability to identify ganglion cell loss. The 3D en face analysis upgrade provides virtual dissection of the retina and the optic disk with 67 million data points within a 512 × 128 dense cube and high-density 3D volume for visualization and analysis of the eye tissue structures. The iVue can be mounted to the iStand, a rolling floor stand option which enables scanning of the patients in different positions, including the supine position and moving the OCT system around.

The use of handheld OCT systems leads to a number of difficulties. For example, it is difficult to reach a proper stabilization of the units in order to obtain good images. The use of handheld systems can adversely affect the sterility of the surgical field with the risk of potential complications. The surgeon has to interrupt the surgery, remove the microscope, and adjust the OCT system, making the procedure time-consuming. Even with the custom microscope mount, the microscope has to be removed from the surgical field. In addition, with handheld OCT systems, it is impossible to image surgical maneuvers themselves. The quantitative data analysis also has to be improved.

29.4.3 Microscope-Integrated Intraoperative Optical Coherence Tomography Systems

29.4.3.1 Microscope-Integrated OCT (Mi-OCT)

A custom microscope-integrated OCT (Mi-OCT) system was developed by the team led by Toth and Izatt at Duke Eye Center, by implementing the OCT scanner into the surgical microscope (Hahn et al. 2013a, b). For OCT imaging, a commercially available SD-OCT engine Bioptigen Inc.[1] (Table 29.1) with a near-infrared light source, 700 μW of power, and a 5.2 μm axial resolution in air was integrated into the surgical microscope Leica M844 (Leica Microsystems, Switzerland) using a Leica digital imaging color module (DI C800). The Mi-OCT system enables simultaneous, wide-field noncontact, real-time, cross-sectional iOCT imaging of retinal structures including intraocular surgical manipulations without impairing the surgeon's view through the surgical microscope. Recently, the Mi-OCT was upgraded with a swept source OCT (SS-OCT) engine and customized with tracking hardware and software to target the OCT beam to the area of interest. The SS-OCT makes it possible to obtain many individual scans in the same time needed to obtain only a single scan using SD-OCT. With the new software, 3-dimensional real-time visualization of the retina is possible.

29.4.3.2 iOCT® OPMedT

Universal iOCT® camera by OPMedT (Optomedical Technologies GmbH, Lübeck, Germany) can be mounted to the standard camera port on a surgical microscope (HS Hi-R Neo 900A NIR, Haag-Streit Surgical GmbH) (iOCT®) (iOCT. Haag-Streit 2015). An additional M.DIS touch screen is available. The system has an SD-OCT source, 800 nm wavelength, 10,000 A-scans/s, and 10 μm axial resolution in air. As the iOCT engine itself is not directly integrated into the microscope stand, future upgrades and multiple screens are possible (Table 29.1). The iOCT images are injected into both oculars where they are superimposed over the microscopic view. The system ensures the same focus for iOCT and microscope. The zoom in the microscope can also magnify the iOCT image. The scan window depth is 4.2 mm. The second microscope-mounted display is installed close to the oculars. The microscope and iOCT adjustment is enabled via foot control for which the settings can be customized and saved. It can be used in both anterior and posterior segment surgeries, as well as in ENT and neurosurgery (Fig. 29.4). But up to the date, the use of OPMedT OCT system is widely described in the field of keratoplasty (iOCT®). The software enables the standard recording and editing of the surgery films and snapshots. Also, the generation of 3-dimensional images out of 30 consecutive images is possible.

29.4.3.3 Rescan 700

The Carl Zeiss Meditec Rescan 700 is the first commercially available CE approved iOCT system which is fully integrated into the foot stand of the operating microscope OPMI LUMERA 700 Carl Zeiss Meditec.[2] (Fig. 29.5a) (Rescan 700 Carl Zeiss Meditech 2015, Ehlers et al. 2014b). The system has a spectral domain OCT engine with a wavelength of 840 nm and a scanning speed of 27,000 A-scans per second and is incorporated into the head of the microscope without causing any loss of function. The main scan parameters are the following: A-scan depth (2.0 mm in tissue), axial resolution (5.5 μm in tissue), scan length adjustable from 3 to 16 mm,

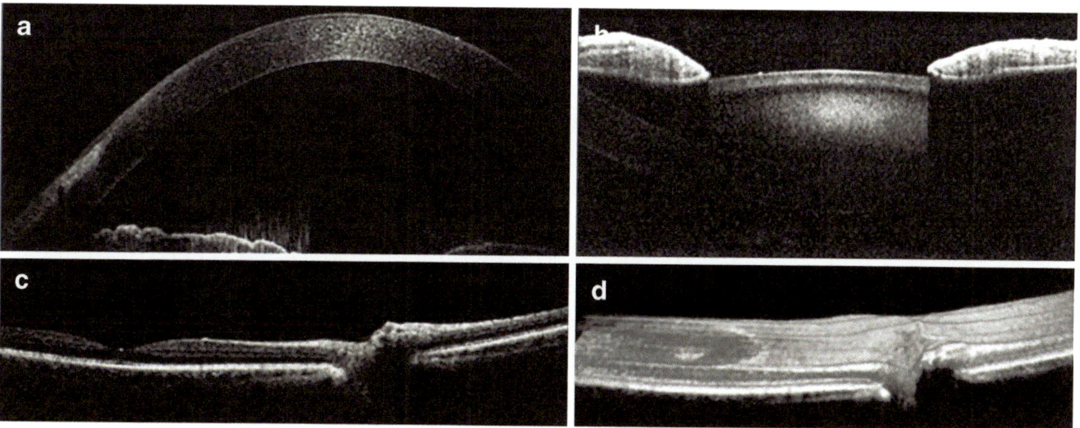

Fig. 29.4 iOCT imaging of a healthy cornea (**a**) lens, (**b**) retina, (**c**) and 3D visualization of the retina (**d**) with iOCT® camera by OPMedT (Optomedical Technologies GmbH, Lübeck, Germany) (Photos printed with the permission of Prof. C. Cursiefen and Prof. J. Szaflik)

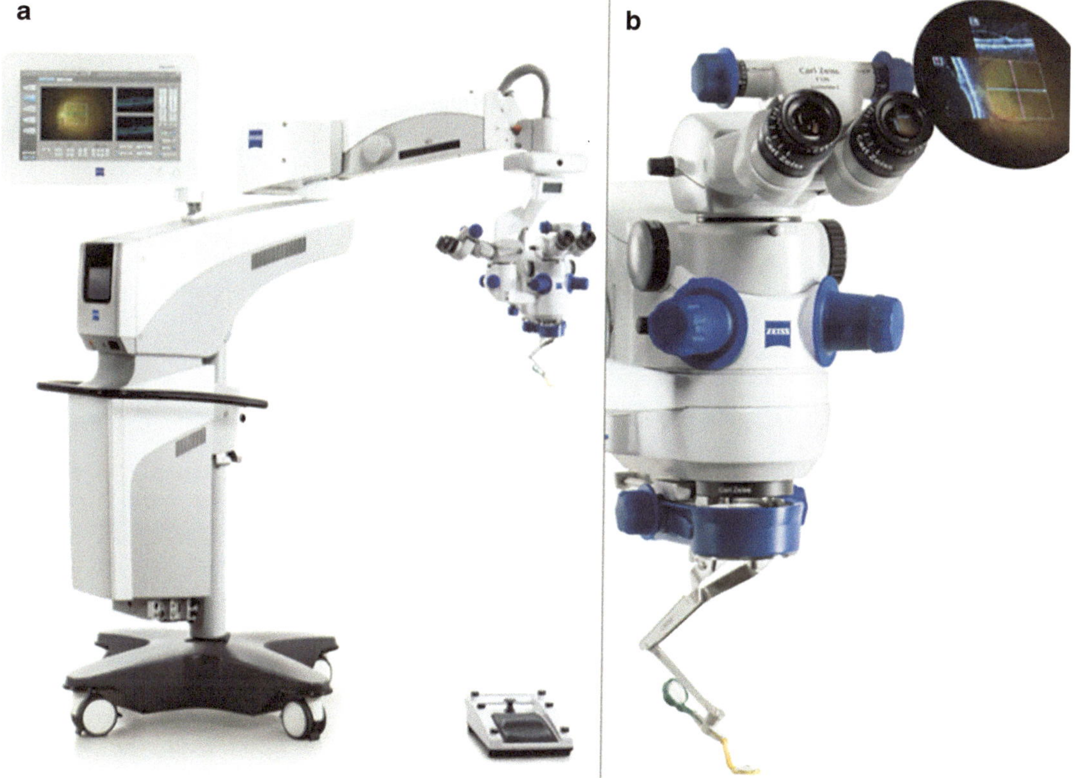

Fig. 29.5 iSD-OCT system Rescan 700 fully integrated into the foot stand of OPMI LUMERA 700² (Rescan 700 (Carl Zeiss Meditec, Oberkochen, Germany)). (**a**) Head-up display built into the ocular of OPMI LUMERA 700² (Rescan 700 (Carl Zeiss Meditec, Oberkochen, Germany)) (**b**)

and scan rotation adjustable 360° (Table 29.1). Scan modes for live film acquisition and snapshot capture are available (1-line, 5-line, cross hair). The Callisto eye system includes a touch screen and a 500 GB hard drive. The Callisto eye software adapts the iOCT acquisition to the different optics used with the Resight viewing system (60 D, 128 D lenses are included) and contact lenses for macular surgery. Due to the live iOCT images being directly injected into one of the surgeon's oculars, the surgeon does not need to change the direction of his gaze during surgery in order to see the iOCT images (Fig. 29.5b). The surgeon can easily control the key options of the Rescan 700 OCT system from the microscope's foot pedal, quickly turning it on and off, triggering OCT videos, and capturing SD-OCT images without looking up or interrupting the surgery.

29.5 Intraoperative Optical Coherence Tomography Imaging

While performing iOCT, the surgeon needs to be aware of the two main scanning modes: filming and snapshots. Both modes allow the surgeon to observe, analyze, and process the data in real time and after the surgery.

29.5.1 Acquisition

Anterior segment iOCT visualization usually can be achieved directly by handheld iOCT systems or through the objective lens of the ophthalmic surgical microscope into which the iOCT is integrated (Fig. 29.6a). By using the macular surgery contact lens, a wider and better visualization of the anterior segment can be achieved (Fig. 29.6b). The two most important prerequisites to obtain high-quality posterior segment iOCT are clear optical media and normal intraocular pressure (IOP). To obtain an iOCT image using a probe, it has to be placed close to the desired ocular structure at a distance of 1.6–4 mm. In handheld and microscope-integrated OCT systems, posterior segment iOCT scanning is possible without any additional optics but with an inferior quality and magnification. The wide angle, noncontact viewing systems, such as Resight 700 (Carl Zeiss Meditec, Germany), EIBOS II (Haag-Streit Surgical GmbH, Germany), and Oculus BIOM 3 (OCULUS Optikgeräte GmbH, Germany) with

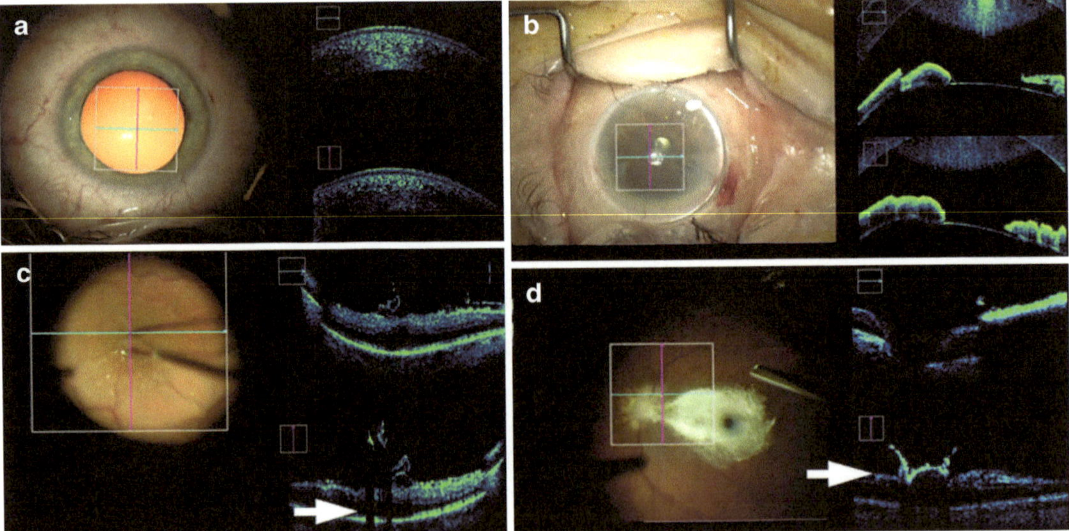

Fig. 29.6 iSD-OCT imaging of healthy cornea through the objective lens of the ophthalmic surgical microscope (**a**). Anterior segment iOCT visualization with the use of a contact macular lens (**b**). iOCT scanning of the ERM through a contact lens for macular surgery (**c**). Shadowing from the end-gripping forceps (**c**, *arrow*). Visualization of the vitreoretinal adhesion enhanced by triamcinolone acetonide (**d**, *arrow*). iOCT images made with iSD-OCT system Rescan 700[2] (Rescan 700 (Carl Zeiss Meditec, Oberkochen, Germany))

wide-field ophthalmic lens, can be used together with iOCT units. Any contact lens for macular surgery could also facilitate iOCT capturing with a higher magnification (Fig. 29.6c). The type of optics used has to be taken into consideration and adjusted in the iOCT systems settings if possible.

For imaging posterior retina, the best quality of iSD-OCT scans can be obtained in patients with clear cornea, pseudophakia, and no posterior capsule or vitreous opacities. The intraoperative swelling of the lens or cornea can influence on the quality of iOCT scans. Therefore, caution has to be maintained while manipulating close to them. Additionally, the surgery duration has to be optimal. It was shown that enhancement of the visualization of semitransparent tissues and tissue planes with triamcinolone acetonide or indocyanine green (ICG) may provide further improvement in surgeon feedback (Fig. 29.6d), Video 29.1 (3) (Ehlers et al. 2010, 2014c).

Any type of anesthesia is suitable for iOCT scanning. In the case of local drop anesthesia, the patient can be asked to fixate or follow the illuminated target point produced by iOCT machine if the preoperative vision is sufficient. The best conditions for iOCT imaging are complete akinesia and straight alignment of the eye. In addition, the centering of the iOCT image can be adjusted by centering the eye with the forceps or a fixation ring. Acquisition of the iOCT images usually is controlled via foot pedal or with help of an assistant. After activating the iOCT, a real-time video of OCT imaging starts running. Snapshot mode allows the acquisition of separate scans of a selected area. All data can be recorded and post-processed with supplementary software.

Besides the ocular tissues that can be visualized with iOCT, any anterior or posterior segment instrument that is introduced into the eye can produce hyperreflectivity and shadowing in the iOCT image (Fig. 29.6c) (Hahn et al. 2013a, b). The ability to image the instruments while using them within the eye is a unique feature that can help to control the safe distance to the ocular tissues and prevent any undesirable contact that may result in iatrogenic trauma. Tracking the instruments with iOCT during the entire surgery would be challenging as the surgeon rarely stays steady with the hands while performing a lot of tiny maneuvers.

The visualization of ophthalmic surgical maneuvers could also be improved with the use of iOCT enhanced with special additional lenses and mechanical enhancements. Tao and his group have demonstrated the use of an integrated electrically tunable lens that allows rapid focal plane focusing and iOCT imaging of ocular tissues of anterior and posterior segments in enucleated porcine eye (Tao et al. 2014). The real-time surgical maneuvers were visualized by acquiring spatially compounded volumetric data sets which allowed segmentation of the surface of a diamond-dusted scraper and retina on individual cross-sectional images (Hahn et al. 2013a, b). The study data provide integrative visualization of the membrane scraper position relative to the retina surface.

29.5.2 Calibration

The lack of calibration in iOCT systems limits the analysis of acquired data. The problem of iOCT system calibration is due to the constantly changing optical media during the surgery. The system would have to be recalibrated every time a different lens is used during surgery as well as at every change in magnification of the microscope. Nevertheless, some graphic software does offer substantial measurements of the tissues that can be used to show the difference, time dynamics in length, width, height, or volume. Due to the calibration issue, these measurements are only relative and not absolute.

Toth used a handheld SD-OCT unit by Bioptigen Inc.[1] to image the retina of infants. The iSD-OCT system was complemented with a calibrated knob to adjust the reference arm position with a digital readout. A manufacturer-supplied calibration factor was used to convert the readout units to optical distance in millimeters (Maldonado et al. 2010).

29.5.3 Post-processing

iOCT data post-processing is a very important step that usually is time-consuming but also reveals additional information about the intra-surgical tissue behavior. The main aim of post-processing of iOCT data is a deeper analysis obtained by the use of special software and algorithms (Hahn 2014; Koprowski and Wróbel 2011). Since the iOCT images have a low signal to noise ratio and movement artifacts, the post-processing also serves to improve data presentation. Each microscope-integrated iOCT system is supplemented with hardware and software with a built-in camera system to facilitate the generation of images for information, documentation, teaching, and presentation purposes.

29.5.4 Three-Dimensional Visualization and Animation

With the goal of enhancing the clarity of subtle structures inside the iOCT data, two different post-processing and 3D visualization systems can be used. Both of them employ ray-traced shading, which enhances small structures by throwing a shadow from the virtual light source or light sources onto the data behind or below the illuminated structure, making the structure stand out from its surroundings and thereby increasing the contrast of the visualization. The first system is voxel-based and has relatively low preprocessing time and can if necessary use unprocessed raw data directly from the iOCT. The raw iOCT data sets are exported, z-aligned, and noise-reduced in post-processing. The resulting data is imported into Cinema 4D™ and rendered using a custom-made plug-in which renders the data as voxels with ray-traced shading and a single customizable light source direction. The second system is based on triangle mesh representation of the data. This requires full nonplanar segmentation of the data, and a large amount of preprocessing is therefore necessary. Segmented meshes are created in Cinema 4D™ using a fluid dynamics particle generator/mesher and rendered using a CUDA GPU (Fig. 29.7, Video 29.2).

29.6 Application of Intraoperative Optical Coherence Tomography

29.6.1 Anterior Segment Application

The iOCT scanning of the cornea and anterior segment structures is the most used examination. The images are the highest quality images the iOCT system can offer, because these structures are the first ocular tissues that scatter the light beam. The iris blocks the OCT scan penetration, limiting the examination of the ciliary body and the lens. The iOCT can be used for all anterior segment surgery. While being used for different types of keratoplasties (DMEK, DSAEK, DALK, PKP), it can assist the surgeon to orient the donor's graft by assessing its position (Fig. 29.8). It can also aid in the search for residual fluid, viscoelastic, or air in between the host and donor corneal tissues, as well as improving the sutures. In cases with opaque cornea, the use of an iOCT probe can help to discover and recognize the structures behind the cornea and to find the most convenient entry side. The iOCT provides the surgeon with precise and accurate imaging of the entire anterior chamber including detailed information about apposition of the graft (De Benito-Llopis et al. 2014; Juthani et al. 2014; Miyakoshi et al. 2014; Steven et al. 2013, 2014; Xu et al. 2014).

In Descemet's membrane endothelial keratoplasty (DMEK), the technique can help recognize the donor graft edge curling that leads to incorrect graft positioning and damage of the endothelial cell layer (Fig. 29.8a). The iOCT-guided unfolding and correct positioning of the donor graft facilitate shortening of the surgical procedure (Steven et al. 2013). The iOCT is also useful for DMEK to determine whether the posterior lamella is attached in all regions of the cornea. Performing Descemet's stripping automated endothelial keratoplasty (DSAEK), it is essential to control the complete attachment of the graft to the host cornea at the end of the surgery (Fig. 29.8b). The utility of iOCT in DSAEK allows detecting the residual fluid between the host cornea and the graft after the graft was

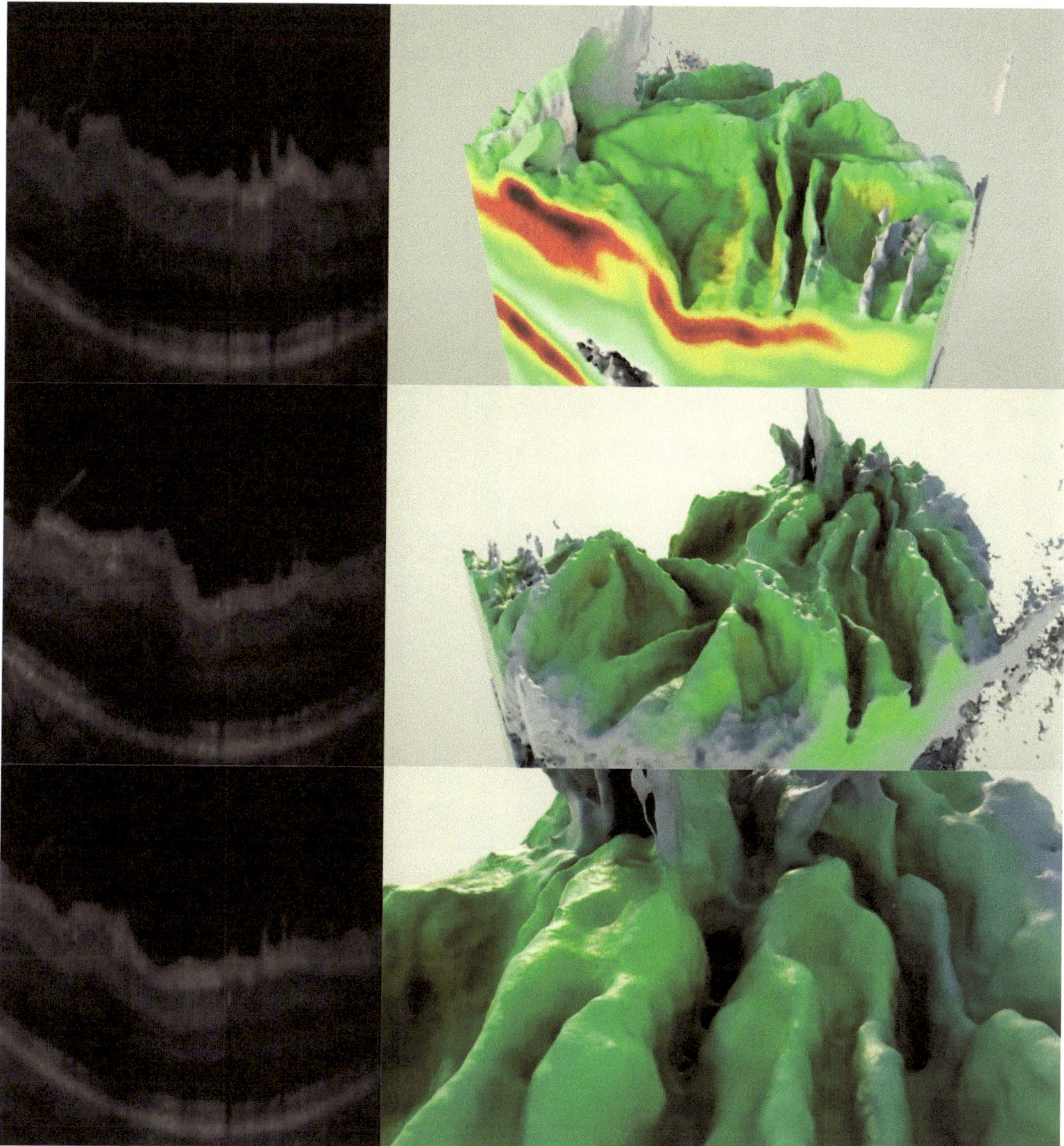

Fig. 29.7 Triangle-meshed CUDA-based 3D iOCT visualization of an ERM after peeling. A residual membrane "sail" is still visible. The raw iOCT data is on the left. The reconstructions are on the right

attached by air injection, which can be treated with fluid drainage through corneal incisions. (Juthani et al. 2014; Miyakoshi et al. 2014; Xu et al. 2014).

Deep anterior lamellar keratoplasty (DALK) is another application for iOCT, where all the preparation steps can be visualized and therefore controlled (Fig. 29.8c) (De Benito-Llopis et al. 2014; Steven et al. 2014). The use of iOCT during DALK was demonstrated by De Benito-Llopis L and his group (De Benito-Llopis et al. 2014). For intraoperative imaging, they used an iVue 100-2 (Optovue, Fremont, CA, USA). With the help of iOCT, it was possible to assess and control manual dissection, to detect the position of the needle before air injection, and to evaluate the location of the Descemet's membrane.

Additionally, iOCT can visualize intrastromal retention of fluid or viscoelastic that is usually not detectable by the operating microscope. Implementation of iOCT-assisted DALK facilitates the high-resolution imaging of the cornea and is useful to control every step of the procedure.

iOCT scanning is useful to assess the stability and improve the suturing of the donor graft after penetrating keratoplasty (PKP) (Fig. 29.9a, Video 29.3 (1)).

In cataract surgery, iOCT can be used to control the positioning of the intraocular lens (IOL) (Fig. 29.9b). One of the most common

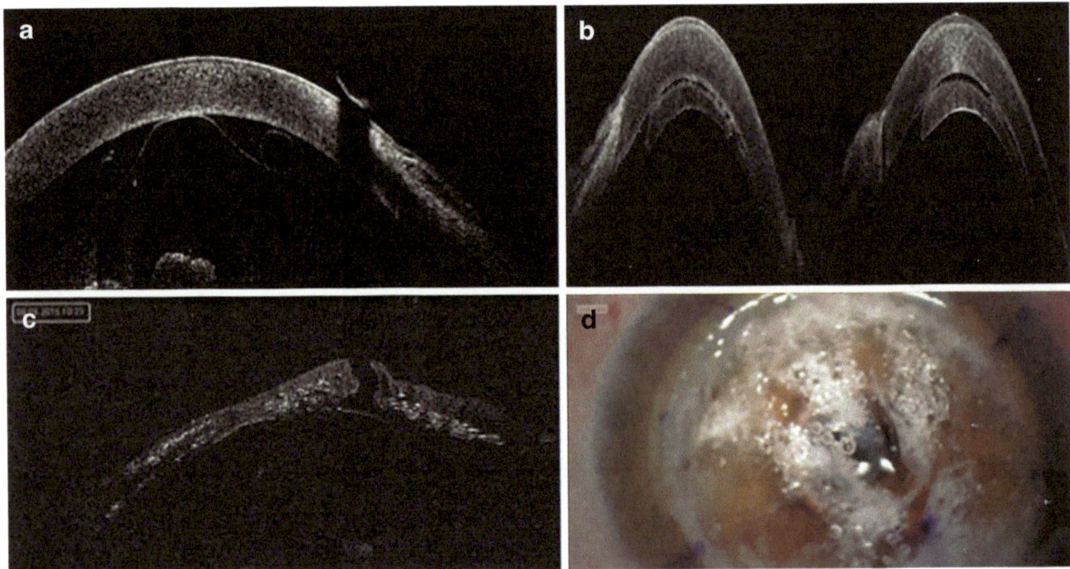

Fig. 29.8 iOCT imaging of DMEK, (**a**) DSAEK, (**b**) and DALK (**c**) by iOCT® camera by OPMedT. Color photo of the cornea (**d**) during DALK, same as on (c) (Optomedical Technologies GmbH, Lübeck, Germany) (Photos were used with the permission of Prof. C. Cursiefen) (Photos printed with the permission of Prof. C. Cursiefen and Dr. F. Price Jr.)

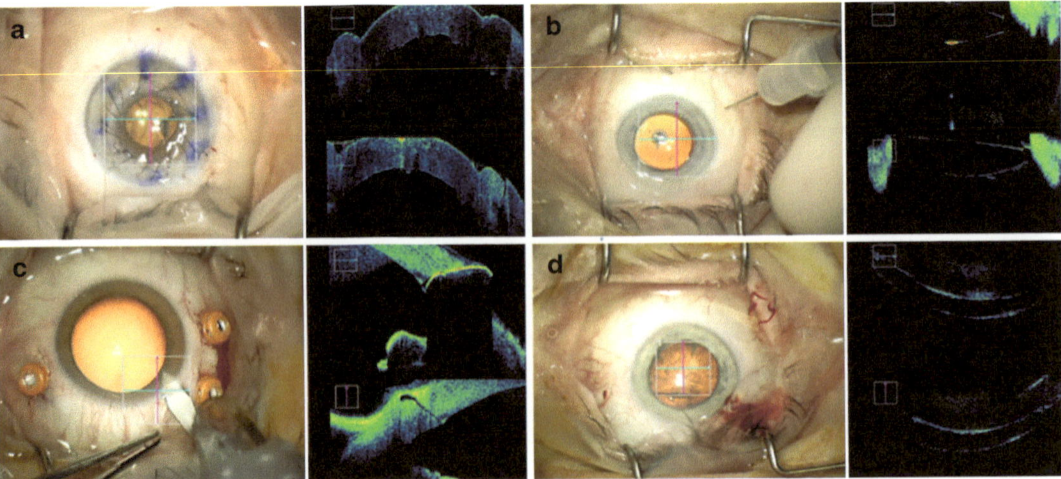

Fig. 29.9 iSD-OCT imaging of the corneal graft after penetrating keratoplasty, (**a**) intraocular lens position, (**b**) incision shape, (**c**) and completeness of the hydrodissection during phacoemulsification (**d**) with iSD-OCT system Rescan 700[2] (Rescan 700 (Carl Zeiss Meditec, Oberkochen, Germany))

applications of iOCT in refractive surgery is the qualitative assessment of the height of the vault during phakic IOL implantation for myopia or hyperopia correction. With the help of iOCT anterior chamber scanning, the surgeon is able to determine whether over vaulting or no vaulting of the phakic lens is present in order to prevent postoperative anterior chamber angle narrowing or contact with the crystalline lens. Studies on this topic are currently running.

Intraoperative measurements of the anterior lens capsule position after implanting a capsular tension ring (CTR) using iOCT can optimize the prediction of the postoperative refractive outcome. Hirnschall and his group showed that the predictive power of the intraoperative OCT-assisted measurements can be calculated better in comparison to IOL power calculations using only standard formulas (Holladay I, Hoffer Q, SRK/T, Haigis) (Hirnschall et al. 2013, 2015).

In standard phacoemulsification, iOCT can be utilized to control the shape of the incisions, completeness of the hydrodissection, depth of the groove, asses the movements of the lens fragments, and control the position of the IOL in the end of the surgery (Fig. 29.9b–d, Video 29.3 (2,3)).

An evaluation of iOCT's role in glaucoma surgery during phacotrabeculectomy, Ahmed glaucoma valve implantation, gonio-synechiolysis, and bleb needling was performed by Kumar and his group (Kumar et al. 2015). Intraoperative imaging facilitated the visualization and control of the scleral flap dissection, the triplanar entry wound, the deep sclera block removal, and the bleb at the end of the surgery. It was also possible to assess, in real time, the extent of peripheral anterior synechiae and the repositioning of the iris after the synechiae release in gonio-synechiolysis. The iOCT assisted the evaluation of the scleral flap adhesion, episcleral fibrosis, and restoration of the bleb after bleb needling. Therefore, the use of iOCT can help to visualize nearly blind glaucoma surgery without a gonioscopy lens, resulting in better control of the surgical maneuvers and efficacy of the procedures. Nevertheless, there are certain limitations in this approach due to specific technical specifications that have been offered by current iSD-OCT systems, such as straight scanning or defined wave length. It makes it difficult to visualize the anterior chamber angle or trabecular meshwork, which is essential for glaucoma surgery.

The use of iSD-OCT imaging in anterior segment surgery can improve the visualization of ocular structures during all surgical steps delivering a broad range of new information about tissue behavior and positioning of the implants.

29.6.2 Posterior Segment Applications

Implementation of iOCT has changed the understanding of certain retinal diseases. It can be used during almost every vitreoretinal surgical intervention with some essential benefit to the efficacy of the procedure and patient safety. With its use, the surgeon can judge the completeness of epiretinal membrane (ERM) peeling, the reestablished contact of a detached retina, the intraoperative management of a macular hole, etc (Ehlers et al. 2013; Lee and Srivastava 2011). Intraoperative SD-OCT imaging can provide the surgeon with the retinal imaging through different vitreous substitutes such as balanced salt solution (BSS), perfluorocarbon liquids (PFCLs), air, gas, or silicone oil of different densities.

The iSD-OCT systems are very useful and efficient for scanning the retina in infants or patients who for any reason are in a supine position. Toth has been able to image infant's retina with the portable handheld SD-OCT workstation by Bioptigen Inc.[1] in an incubator with a noncontact probe held over the eye (Cabrera et al. 2012, 2013; Chavala et al. 2009; Lee et al. 2011; Maldonado and Toth 2013; Maldonado et al. 2010, 2011; Moreno et al. 2013). For SD-OCT acquisition, the examiner had to open and hold the eyelids using fingertips but was also used under constant moisturizing of the cornea (Maldonado et al. 2010). The duration of the imaging session was restricted to 15 min, and the vital indices (heart rate, respiratory rate, and oxygen saturation) were monitored every minute to ensure the infant's safety. In the study, the authors have shown the dynamics of the axial length (AL) in children. Their data revealed that in the neonatal period, the AL increases rapidly growing 0.16 mm per week during the first 2 years (1 mm/year), from 2 to 5 years (0.4 mm/year), from 5 to 15 years (0.1 mm/year), and after age 15 without no significant further growth. The advantage of SD-OCT handpiece was the possibility to use it within the incubator; therefore, infants were not moved for imaging nor was it necessary to remove the continuous positive airway pressure (CPAP) mask.

The feasibility of the first microscope-integrated iSD-OCT system was reported by S. Binder and her group (Fig. 29.1) (Binder et al. 2010, 2011; Matz et al. 2012). During vitreoretinal surgery, additional information was acquired concerning the completeness of epiretinal membrane (ERM) removal, the condition of the macular area after membrane peeling, the presence of residual subretinal or sub-silicone fluid in retinal detachment (RD) cases, and the presence of macular edema in age-related macular degeneration (AMD) patients after cataract surgery was performed. With the help of real-time intra-surgical SD-OCT imaging, it became possible to influence certain surgical steps, decrease the amount of iatrogenic trauma to the tissues, and accomplish the surgery with additional treatment, such as intravitreal injection of anti-VEGF. The iSD-OCT system that was integrated into surgical microscope prevailed over handheld prototypes as it can be used without jeopardizing the sterility. The interruption of the surgery was not needed, and the OCT scanning stability was improved.

Falkner-Radler and our group reported the use of real-time iSD-OCT-assisted vitrectomy for macular surgery (Falkner-Radler et al. 2015). This prospective single-center interventional study showed that in 40 % of ERM and/or internal limiting membrane (ILM) peeling cases, it was possible to remove membranes without using any retinal dyes. During pars plana vitrectomy (PPV) on eyes with vitreomacular traction syndrome (VMTS), iSD-OCT revealed the cases with high risk of macular hole (MH) formation after ERM removal; hence, additional intraocular tamponade was considered. It was also shown on iSD-OCT scans that during membrane peeling, the strength of the tractional force induces subretinal hyporeflectance without immediate changes to the external limiting membrane or ellipsoid zone (Fig. 29.10a, Video 29.1 (1)). The difficulties were met when scanning flat ERM, so additional staining was needed. All these iSD-OCT findings can support the surgeon with real-time information about the behavior of retinal layers during membrane peeling, which can partially explain the postoperative outcomes.

Secondary membranes after peeling of an initial ERM can be detected using iOCT scanning. The internal limiting membrane itself is rarely visible in iSD-OCT but can usually be seen after peeling was initiated. Intraoperative SD-OCT imaging is useful in identifying tissue changes after the surgical manipulations that cannot be detected using the microscope. In VMTS, there is a risk of MH creation during vitrectomy and ERM peeling. With the use of iSD-OCT, it became possible to visualize in real time and prevent the increase of anteroposterior traction on the retinal areas with the strong ERM adhesion. The relief of macular traction surrounding the area of vitreoretinal adhesion is visible with iSD-OCT imaging. In 2013, G. Stolyarenko and his group reported the technique of 3D en face iOCT-guided isolation of ERM or ILM around the previously detected vulnerable zones with increased vitreoretinal adhesion (Stolyarenko et al. 2011). With the use of an iOCT probe, the incomplete peeling of the membranes was performed, and spots of ERM with the strongest adhesion were left over. The epiretinal remnants disappeared gradually over time. The iOCT probe utilization provided a more controlled ERM removal, avoiding the unnecessary intraoperative traction on the retina.

The utility of iOCT during PPV for VMTS was studied on 12 patients by Ehlers and his group (Ehlers et al. 2014e). They observed micro architectural changes after surgical release of the vitreomacular traction that appeared as increased subretinal hyporeflectivity in the outer retina. In 42 % of cases, iOCT findings influenced the decision-making in surgical procedures with additional ILM peeling and gas tamponade to treat occult new formed full-thickness macular hole

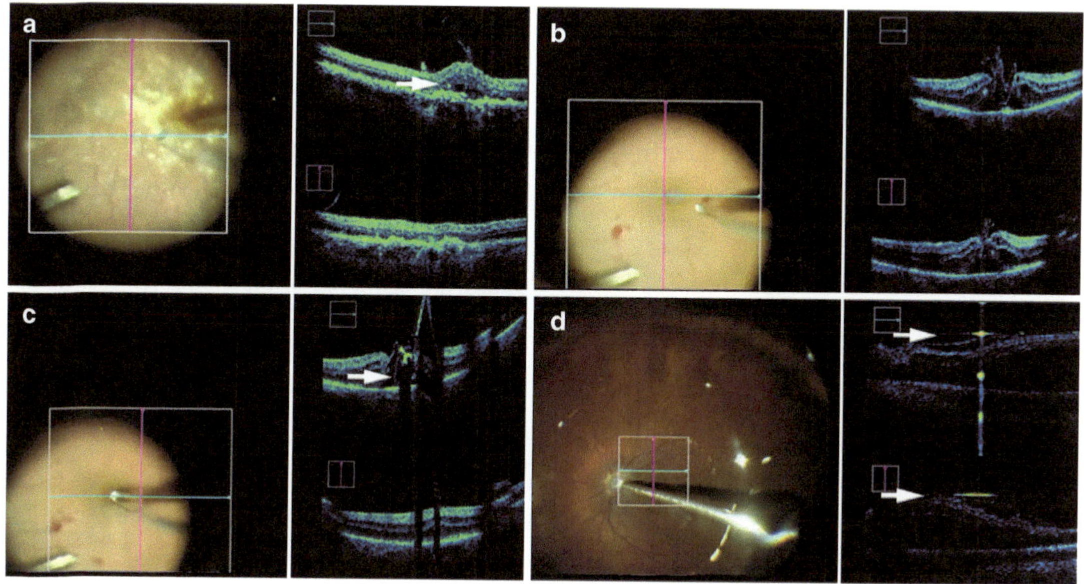

Fig. 29.10 Zone of subretinal hyporeflectance (**a**, *arrow*). Management of large macular hole with inverted ILM flap technique (**b**). Imaging of the tip of end-gripping forceps in order to keep a safe distance between the instrument and retina (**c**, *arrow*). Residual fluid meniscus after fluid-air exchange (**d**, *arrow*). iOCT images made with iSD-OCT system Rescan 700[2] (Rescan 700 (Carl Zeiss Meditec, Oberkochen, Germany))

and residual membranes. In macular hole surgery, iOCT findings revealed the influence of ILM peeling on intraoperative MH size and on the microstructure of retinal layers. It was shown that macular geometry was changed after the peeling associated with tractional forces. In spite of the decrease of the area of the top of the MH which is usually seen after the ILM removal, the base area and MH volume have a tendency to increase with the appearance of visible hyporeflective zones (Ehlers et al. 2014a, g; Hayashi et al. 2011; Wykoff et al. 2010). Additionally, it was noticed that there is some correlation between the extension of alteration and the functional and anatomical outcomes. During the surgery on large MH, with inverted ILM flap technique, the iSD-OCT can facilitate better control while inverting the ILM remnants into the macular hole (Fig. 29.10b). Also with real-time OCT imaging, a safe distance between the tip of the instruments and the retina can be maintained (Fig. 29.10c, Video 29.1 (2)).

The use of iSD-OCT can reveal new information about rare and difficult diseases, such as an optic pit and a morning glory disk anomaly (Video 29.1 (3)). Ehlers and his group analyzed iOCT-assisted PPV for optic pit-associated retinal schisis. The data demonstrated a potential communication between the vitreous cavity and the intraretinal fluid which can partially explain the pathogenesis of the disease (Ehlers et al. 2011a).

The iOCT utilization demonstrated the ability of this technique to identify the residual subretinal fluid meniscus under any type of endotamponade (BSS, PFCL, air, gas, silicone oil) (Fig. 29.10d). In the case of air or air-gas mixture, the quality of scans decreases due to additional OCT light scattering.

The presence of mature cataract or opaque vitreous makes it impossible to visualize the central retina before the surgery. Therefore, the iOCT scanning can influence the decision-making while bringing the new indications for further surgical steps, like ERM removal, macular hole surgery, or intravitreal injection of medication (Puliafito 2010).

Anterior segment iOCT mode may also be used after the PPV to assess the self-sealing of the beveled sclerotomy. This can prevent postoperative hypotony and reduce the risk of endophthalmitis. With the assistance of iOCT, it becomes possible to reveal the presence of macular edema and confirm the need for ILM peeling and evaluate the macula after retinal reattachment or macular surgery. However, further studies will show in which area the use of iOCT reaches clinical significance.

29.7 Future Perspectives

The implementation of iSD-OCT into everyday practice is being established (Ehlers et al. 2011, 2014f). There are many questions that can be addressed about intra-surgical use of this novel technique, but the main question would be how the intraoperative OCT visualization can influence the postoperative anatomical and functional outcomes. The future use of longer wavelengths such as 1310 and oblique scanning can improve the visualization of anterior chamber angle and trabecular meshwork providing greater control over the surgical maneuvers during glaucoma surgery (Heindl et al. 2014). The utilization of iOCT systems can reduce the use of potentially toxic dyes to avoid retinal damage. With the routine use of iSD-OCT, the surgeon will be able to assure the accuracy of the membrane peeling. The detection of the safest place to initiate the ERM flap during ERM removal already became a very useful approach that reduces the risk of retinal injury. During the vitrectomy on eyes with severe proliferative diabetic retinopathy, the iSD-OCT can provide the surgeon with real-time information flow about the condition of the retina, the choroid, and the risk of iatrogenic hole creation. Also, the residual traction that is not clearly distinguishable with just the microscopic view can be detected and treated without the delay. The iOCT systems are of great interest in the field of ocular oncology, as the technique can provide the useful information about the positing of the radioactive plaques in choroidal melanoma treatment. There is also a potential use of iOCT in following and controlling almost every step of anterior and posterior segment surgery with educational purposes starting from wound architecture during cataract surgery up till detection of the residual ERM.

With the implementation of 3D iOCT imaging, it will be possible to control surgical manipulations in real time, avoiding unnecessary iatrogenic trauma. The development of a real-time tracking iOCT mode will be of great importance, as it will facilitate the computer guided following of the tip of the instruments, thus preventing unnecessary contact with the living tissues. The iOCT will surely have a great potential further, when it will be combined with remote-automated robotic pars plana vitrectomy based on da Vinci® surgical system and IRISS (Bourla et al. 2008; Rahimy et al. 2013). With the use of adaptive optics, it is possible to scan the retinal layers with OCT (AO-OCT) up to the level of a single cell, as it increases the imaging capability of OCT through increased lateral resolution and enhanced sensitivity (Miller et al. 2011; Mujat et al. 2009). The implementation of AO-OCT into ophthalmic surgery will provide the surgeon with ultrahigh-resolution 3D imaging ($3 \times 3 \times 3$ μm^3), and this technology continues to be developed.

The field of iOCT technology is rapidly developing, especially after the implementation of swept source engines and adaptive optics. Additionally, the clinical interest in the new diagnostic tool is growing fast. The novel iOCT approach reveals many intra-surgical findings that increase our knowledge of certain eye diseases. The most important task would be to integrate the information obtained by the iOCT systems with postoperative findings in order to influence the postoperative anatomical and functional results. The future implementation of iOCT will serve as a tool to improve our surgery. The development of iOCT approach is unlimited as far as development of its technology, but the cost will limit the use in everyday practice.

References

Aggarwal A, Panat S, Agarwal N, Sowmya G, Alok A, Kishore M (2013) Optical coherence tomography: an emerging perspective. J Dent Sci Oral Rehabil p. 4–7

Binder S, Falkner-Radler C, Hauger C, Matz H, Glittenberg C (2010) Clinical applications of intra-surgical SD-optical coherence tomography. Poster

presented at Association for Research in Vision and Ophthalmology, Fort Lauderdale, 2–6 May 2010
Binder S, Falkner-Radler C, Hauger C, Matz H, Glittenberg C (2011) Feasibility of intrasurgical spectral-domain optical coherence tomography. Retina 31:1332–1336
BioptigenEnvisu. http://www.bioptigen.com/products/b-envisutm-s4410-for-contact-len-metrology. Accessed 09 July 2015
Böhringer HJ, Boller D, Leppert J, Knopp U, Lankenau E, Reusche E, Hüttmann G, Giese A (2006) Time-domain and spectral-domain optical coherence tomography in the analysis of brain tumor tissue. Lasers Surg Med 38(6):588–597
Boppart S, Brezinski M, Pitris C, Fujimoto J (1998) Optical coherence tomography for neurosurgical imaging of human intracortical melanoma. Neurosurgery 43:834–841
Bouma B, Tearney G (1999) Power-efficient nonreciprocal interferometer and linear scanning fiber-optic catheter for optical coherence tomography. Opt Lett 24:531–533
Bourla D, Hubschman J, Culjat M, Tsirbas A, Gupta A, Schwartz S (2008) Feasibility study of intraocular robotic surgery with the da Vinci surgical system. Retina 28:154–158
Cabrera M, Maldonado R, Toth C, O'Connell R, Chen B, Chiu S, Farsiu S, Wallace D, Stinnett S, Panayotti G, Swamy G, Freedman S (2012) Subfoveal fluid in healthy full-term newborns observed by handheld spectral-domain optical coherence tomography. Am J Ophthalmol 153:167–175
Cabrera M, O'Connell R, Toth C, Maldonado R, Tran-Viet D, Alling-ham M, Chiu S, Farsiu S, MaradiagaPanayotti G, Swamy G, Freed-man S (2013) Macular findings in healthy full-term Hispanic newborns observed by hand-held spectral-domain optical coherence tomography. Ophthalmic Surg Lasers Imaging Retina 44:448–454
Chavala S, Farsiu S, Maldonado R, Wallace D, Freedman S, Toth C (2009) In-sights into advanced retinopathy of prematurity using handheld spectral domain optical coherence tomography imaging. Ophthalmology 116:2448–2456
Dayani P, Maldonado R, Farsiu S, Toth C (2009) Intraoperative use of handheld spectral domain optical coherence tomography imaging in macular surgery. Retina 29:1457–1468
De Benito-Llopis L, Mehta J, Angunawela R, Ang M, Tan D (2014) Intraoperative anterior segment optical coherence tomography: a novel assessment tool during deep anterior lamellar keratoplasty. Am J Ophthalmol 157:334–341
Ehlers J (2011) Intraoperative OCT and vitreoretinal surgery. Retina Today, Sept, 50-23. http://retinatoday.com/2011/09/intraoperative-oct-and-vitreoretinal-surgery. Accessed 09 July 2015
Ehlers J, Gupta P, Farsiu S, Maldonado R, Kim T, Toth C, Mruthyunjaya P (2010) Evaluation of contrast agents for enhanced visualization in optical coherence tomography. Invest Ophthalmol Vis Sci 51:6614–6619
Ehlers J, Kernstine K, Farsiu S, Sarin N, Maldonado R, Toth C (2011a) Analysis of pars plana vitrectomy for optic pit-related maculopathy with intraoperative optical coherence tomography: a possible connection with the vitreous cavity. Arch Ophthalmol 129:1483–1486
Ehlers J, Tao Y, Farsiu S, Maldonado R, Izatt J, Toth C (2011b) Integration of a spectral domain optical coherence tomography system into a surgical microscope for intraoperative imaging. Invest Ophthalmol Vis Sci 6:3153–3159
Ehlers J, Ohr M, Kaiser P, Srivastava S (2013) Novel microarchitectural dynamics in rhegmatogenous retinal detachments identified with intraoperative optical coherence tomography. Retina 33:1428–1434
Ehlers J, Itoh Y, Xu L, Kaiser P, Singh R, Srivastava S (2014a) Factors associated with persistent subfoveal fluid and complete macular hole closure in the PIONEER study. Invest Ophthalmol Vis Sci 56:1141–1146
Ehlers J, Kaiser P, Srivastava S (2014b) Intraoperative optical coherence tomography using the RESCAN 700: preliminary results from the DISCOVER study. Br J Ophthalmol 98:1329–1332
Ehlers J, McNutt S, Dar S, Tao Y, Srivastava S (2014c) Visualisation of contrast-enhanced intraoperative optical coherence tomography with indocyanine green. Br J Ophthalmol 98:1588–1591
Ehlers J, Srivastava S, Feiler D, Noonan A, Rollins A, Tao Y (2014d) Integrative advances for OCT-guided ophthalmic surgery and intraoperative OCT: microscope integration, surgical instrumentation, and heads-up display surgeon feedback. PLoS One 9:e105224
Ehlers J, Tam T, Kaiser P, Martin D, Smith G, Srivastava S (2014e) Utility of intraoperative optical coherence tomography during vitrectomy surgery for vitreomacular traction syndrome. Retina 3:1341–1346
Ehlers J, Tao Y, Srivastava S (2014f) The value of intraoperative optical coherence tomography imaging in vitreoretinal surgery. Curr Opin Ophthalmol 25:221–227
Ehlers J, Xu D, Kaiser P, Singh R, Srivastava S (2014g) Intrasurgical dynamics of macular hole surgery: an assessment of surgery-induced ultrastructural alterations with intraoperative optical coherence tomography. Retina 34:213–221
Ehlers J, Petkovsek D, Yuan A, Singh R, Srivastava S (2015) Intrasurgical assessment of subretinal tPA injection for submacular hemorrhage in the PIONEER study utilizing intraoperative OCT. Ophthalmic Surg Lasers Imaging Retina 46:327–332
Falkner-Radler C, Glittenberg C, Gabriel M, Binder S (2015) Intrasurgical microscope-integrated spectral domain optical coherence tomography-assisted membrane peeling. Retina 35(10):2100–2106
Feldchtein F, Gelikonov G, Gelikonov V, Kuranov R, Sergeev A, Gladkova N, Shakhov A, Shakhova N, Snopova L, Terent'eva A, Zagainova E, Chumakov Y, Kuznetzova I (1998) Endoscopic applications of optical coherence tomography. Opt Express 3:257–270
Fercher A, Drexler W, Hitzenberger C, Lasser T (2003) Optical coherence tomography principles and applications. Rep Prog Phys 66:239–303

Fujimoto J, Pitris C, Boppart S, Brezinski M (2000) Optical coherence tomography: an emerging technology for biomedical imaging and optical biopsy. Neoplasia 2:9–25

Hahn P (2014) Microscope-integrated OCT provides 3-D images in real-time. Ophthalmology Times. http://ophthalmologytimes.modernmedicine.com/ophthalmologytimes/news/micros cope-integrated-oct-provides-3-d-images-real-time?page=full. Accessed 09 July 2015

Hahn P, Migacz J, O'Connell R, Maldonado R, Izatt J, Toth C (2011) The use of optical coherence tomography in intraoperative ophthalmic imaging. Ophthalmic Surg Lasers Imaging 42:S85–S94

Hahn P, Migacz J, O'Donnell R, Day S, Lee A, Lin P, Vann R, Kuo A, Fekrat S, Mruthyunjaya P, Postel E, Izatt JA, Toth C (2013a) Preclinical evaluation and intraoperative human retinal imaging with a high-resolution microscope integrated spectral domain optical coherence tomography device. Retina 33:1328–1337

Hahn P, Migacz J, O'Connell R, Izatt J, Toth C (2013b) Unprocessed real-time imaging of vitreoretinal surgical maneuvers using a microscope-integrated spectral-domain optical coherence tomography system. Graefes Arch Clin Exp Ophthalmol 251:213–220

Hanna N, Saltzman D, Mukai D, Chen Z, Sasse S, Milliken J, Guo S, Jung W, Colt H, Brenner M (2005) Two-dimensional and 3-dimensional optical coherence tomographic imaging of the airway, lung, and pleura. J Thorac Cardiovasc Surg 129:615–622

Hayashi A, Yagou T, Nakamura T, Fujita K, Oka M, Fuchizawa C (2011) Intraoperative changes in idiopathic macular holes by spectral-domain optical coherence tomography. Case Rep Ophthalmol 2:149–154

Heindl L, Siebelmann S, Dietlein T, Hüttmann G, Lankenau E, Cursiefen C, Steven P (2015) Future prospects: assessment of intraoperative optical coherence tomography in ab interno glaucoma surgery. Curr Eye Res 40(12):1288–1291

Hirnschall N, Amir-Asgari S, Maedel S, Findl O (2013) Predicting the postoperative intraocular lens position using continuous intraoperative optical coherence tomography measurements. Invest Ophthalmol Vis Sci 54:5196–5203

Hirnschall N, Norrby S, Weber M, Maedel S, Amir-Asgari S, Findl O (2015) Using continuous intraoperative optical coherence tomography measurements of the aphakic eye for intraocular lens power calculation. Br J Ophthalmol 99:7–10

Huang D, Swanson EA, Lin CP, Schuman JS, Stinson WG, Chang W, Hee MR, Flotte T, Gregory K, Puliafito CA (1991) Optical coherence tomography. Science 22:1178–1181

Huang Z, Liu X, Song C, Kang J (2012) Motion-compensated hand-held common-path Fourier-domain optical coherence tomography probe for image-guided intervention. Biomed Opt Express 3:3105–3118

iOCT® Haag-Streit. http://www.haag-streitsurgical.com/products/ophthalmology/ioct.html. Accessed 09 July 2015

Joos K, Shen J (2013) Miniature real-time intraoperative forward-imaging optical coherence tomography probe. Biomed Opt Express 4:1342–1350

Juthani V, Goshe J, Srivastava S, Ehlers J (2014) Association between transient interface fluid on intraoperative OCT and textural interface opacity after DSAEK surgery in the PIONEER study. Cornea 33:887–892

Koprowski R, Wróbel Z (2011) Image processing in optical coherence tomography using Matlab. University of Silesia, Katowice

Kraft M, Glanz H, von Gerlach S, Wisweh H, Lubatschowski H, Arens C (2008) Clinical value of optical coherence tomography in laryngology. Head Neck 30:1628–1635

Kumar R, Jariwala M, SA V, Venugopal J, Puttaiah N, Balu R, Rao A, Shetty R (2015) A pilot study on feasibility and effectiveness of intraoperative spectral-domain optical coherence tomography in glaucoma procedures. Transl Vis Sci Technol 4:2

Lee A, Maldonado R, Sarin N, O'Connell R, Wallace D, Freedman S, Cotten M, Toth C (2011) Macular features from spectral-domain optical coherence tomography as an adjunct to indirect ophthalmoscopy in retinopathy of prematurity. Retina 31:1470–1482

Lee L, Srivastava S (2011) Intraoperative spectral-domain optical coherence tomography during complex retinal detachment repair. Ophthalmic Surg Lasers Imaging 42 Online:e71–e74

Li X, Boppart S, Van Dam J, Mashimo H, Mutinga M, Drexler W, Klein M, Pitris C, Krinsky M, Brezinski M, Fujimoto J (2000a) Optical coherence tomography: advanced technology for the endoscopic imaging of Barrett's esophagus. Endoscopy 32:921–930

Li X, Chudoba C, Ko T, Pitris C, Fujimoto J (2000b) Imaging needle for optical coherence tomography. Opt Lett 25:1520–1522

Maldonado R, Toth C (2013) Optical coherence tomography in retinopathy of prematurity: looking beyond the vessels. Clin Perinatol 40:271–296

Maldonado R, Izatt J, Sarin N, Wallace D, Freedman S, Cotten C, Toth C (2010) Optimizing hand-held spectral domain optical coherence tomography imaging for neonates, infants, and children. Invest Ophthalmol Vis Sci 51:2678–2685

Maldonado R, O'Connell R, Sarin N, Freedman S, Wallace D, Cotten C, Winter K, Stinnett S, Chiu S, Izatt J, Farsiu S, Toth C (2011) Dynamics of human foveal development after premature birth. Ophthalmology 118:2315–2325

Matz H, Binder S, Glittenberg C, Scharioth G, Findl O, Hirnschall N, Hauger C (2012) Intraoperative applications of OCT in ophthalmic surgery. Biomed Tech (Berl) 57:297

Mehta N (2011) Intraoperative spectral-domain OCT in posterior segment surgery. Retina Today, Sept, 54–56. http://retinatoday.com/2011/09/intraoperative-spectral-domain-oct-in-posterior-segment-surgery. Accessed 09 July 2015

Miller D, Kocaoglu OP, Wang Q, Lee S (2011) Adaptive optics and the eye (super resolution OCT). Eye (Lond) 25:321–330

Miyakoshi A, Ozaki H, Otsuka M, Hayashi A (2014) Efficacy of intraoperative anterior segment optical coherence tomography during descemet's stripping automated endothelial keratoplasty. ISRN Ophthalmol 2014:562062

Moreno T, O'Connell R, Chiu S, Farsiu S, Cabrera M, Maldonado R, TranViet D, Freedman S, Wallace D, Toth C (2013) Choroid development and feasibility of choroidal imaging in the preterm and term infants utilizing SD-OCT. Invest Ophthalmol Vis Sci 54:4140–4147

Mujat M, Ferguson R, Iftimia N, Hammer D (2009) Compact adaptive optics line scanning ophthalmoscope. Opt Express 17:10242–10258

Nguyen F, Zysk A, Chaney E, Adie S, Kotynek J, Oliphant U, Bellafiore F, Rowland K, Johnson P, Boppart S (2010) Optical coherence tomography: the intraoperative assessment of lymph nodes in breast cancer. IEEE Eng Med Biol Mag 29:63–70

OKT 1300-E BioMedTech. http://www.biomedtech.biz/products.html. Accessed 09 July 2015

Optovue, iVue® SD-OCT. http://optovue.com/products/ivue/. Accessed 09 July 2015

Puliafito C (2010) Optical coherence tomography: a new tool for intraoperative decision making. Ophthalmic Surg Lasers Imaging 41:6

Rahimy E, Wilson J, Tsao T, Schwartz S, Hubschman J (2013) Robotassisted intraocular surgery: development of the IRISS and feasibility studies in an animal model. Eye (Lond) 27:972–978

Regar E1, Ligthart J, Bruining N, van Soest G (2011) The diagnostic value of intracoronary optical coherence tomography. Herz 36(5):417–429

Rescan™ 700 Carl Zeiss Meditech. http://www.zeiss.com/meditec/en_de/products---solutions/ophthalmology-optometry/glaucoma/therapy/surgical-microscopes/opmi-lumera-700.html#technical-data. Accessed 09 July 2015

Rollins A, Ung-Arunyawee R, Chak A, Wong C, Kobayashi K, Sivak M, Izat J (1999) Real-time in vivo imaging of human gastrointestinal ultrastructure by use of endoscopic optical coherence tomography with a novel efficient interferometer design. Opt Lett 24:1358–1360

Scott A, Farsiu S, Enyedi L, Wallace D, Toth C (2009) Imaging the infant retina with a hand-held spectral-domain optical coherence tomography device. Am J Ophthalmol 147:364–373

Sergeev A, Gelikonov V, Gelikonov G, Feldchtein F, Kuranov R, Gladkova N, Shakhova N, Snopova L, Shakov A, Kuznetzova I, Denisenko A, Pochinko V, Chumakov Y, Streltzova O (1997) In vivo endoscopic OCT imaging of precancer and cancer states of human mucosa. Opt Express 1:432–440

Sivak M, Kobayashi K, Izatt JA, Rollins A, Ung-Runyawee R, Chak A, Wong R, Isenberg G, Willis J (2000) High-resolution endoscopic imaging of the GI tract using optical coherence tomography. Gastrointest Endosc 51:474–479

Srivastava S (2010) Intraoperative diagnostic techniques. Paper presented at the American Academy of Ophthalmology Retina Subspecialty Day, Chicago, 15–16 Oct 2010

Srivastava S, Ray R, Hubbard B et al (2011) Intraoperative optical coherence tomography. Paper presented at the American Society of Retina Specialists Annual Meeting, Boston, 20–24 Aug 2011

Steven P, Le Blanc C, Velten K, Lankenau E, Krug M, Oelckers S, Heindl L, Gehlsen U, Hüttmann G, Cursiefen C (2013) Optimizing descemet membrane endothelial keratoplasty using intraoperative optical coherence tomography. JAMA Ophthalmol 131:1135–1142

Steven P, Le Blanc C, Lankenau E, Krug M, Oelckers S, Heindl LM, Gehlsen U, Huettmann G, Cursiefen C (2014) Optimising deep anterior lamellar keratoplasty (DALK) using intraoperative online optical coherence tomography (iOCT). Br J Ophthalmol 98:900–904

Stolyarenko G, Doroschenko D, Mazurina N, Unes H, Ledeneva M (2011) Surgical isolation of epimacular structures based on OCT en-face. Retina Mapping Annual meeting 2011 of American academy of Ophthalmology, Orlando, 22–25 Oct 2011

Sun CW, Lee SY, Lin KF (2014) Review: optical scanning probe for optical coherence tomography. J Med Biol Eng 34:95–100

Tao Y, Ehlers J, Toth C, Izatt J (2010) Intraoperative spectral domain optical coherence tomography for vitreoretinal surgery. Opt Lett 35:3315–3317

Tao Y, Srivastava S, Ehlers J (2014) Microscope-integrated intraoperative OCT with electrically tunable focus and heads-up display for imaging of ophthalmic surgical maneuvers. Biomed Opt Express 5:1877–1878

Terashima M, Kaneda H, Suzuki T (2012) The role of optical coherence tomography in coronary intervention. Korean J Intern Med 27:1–12

Toth C, Carrasco-Zevallos O, Keller B, Shen L, Viehland C, Nam D, Hahn P, Kuo A, Izatt J (2015) Surgically integrated swept source optical coherence tomography (SSOCT) to guide vitreoretinal (VR) surgery. Invest Ophthalmol Vis Sci 56:3512

Wykoff C, Berrocal A, Schefler A, Uhlhorn S, Ruggeri M, Hess D (2010) Intraoperative OCT of a full-thickness macular hole before and after internal limiting membrane peeling. Ophthalmic Surg Lasers Imaging 41:7–11

Xu D, Dupps W, Srivastava S, Ehlers J (2014) Automated volumetric analysis of interface fluid in descemet stripping automated endothelial keratoplasty using intraoperative optical coherence tomography. Invest Ophthalmol Vis Sci 55:5610–5615

Yaqoob Z, Wu J, Yang C (2005) Spectral domain optical coherence tomography: a better OCT imaging strategy. Biotechniques 39:S6–S13

Yaqoob T, Wu J, McDowell E, Heng X, Yang C (2006) Methods and application areas of endoscopic optical coherence tomography. J Biomed Opt 11:063001

Zivelonghi C, Ghione M, Kilickesmez K, Loureiro RE, Foin N, Lind-say A, de Silva R, Ribichini F, Vassanelli C, Di Mario C (2014) Intra-coronary optical coherence tomography: a review of clinical applications. J Cardiovasc Med (Hager-stown) 15:543–553